The BMT Data Book

Including Cellular Therapy

Third edition

The BMT Data Book

Including Cellular Therapy

Third edition

Edited by:

Reinhold Munker, MD
Associate Professor of Medicine, Department of Medicine, Division of Hematology – Oncology, Louisiana State University, Shreveport, LA, USA

Gerhard C. Hildebrandt, MD
Associate Professor of Medicine, University of Utah School of Medicine, Division of Hematology and Hematologic Malignancies, Huntsman Cancer Institute, Salt Lake City, UT, USA

Hillard M. Lazarus, MD, FACP
Professor of Medicine, Case Western Reserve University, The George and Edith Richman Professor and Distinguished Scientist in Cancer Research, University Hospitals Case Medical Center, Cleveland, OH, USA

Kerry Atkinson, MD, FRCP, FRACP
Professor of Medicine, Division of Hematology – Oncology, University of Queensland, South Brisbane, Australia; Head, Stem Cell Biology, Regenerative Medicine, and Novel Therapeutic Anti-Cancer Agents Group, Mater Medical Research Institute, Queensland, Australia

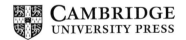

CAMBRIDGE
UNIVERSITY PRESS

University Printing House, Cambridge CB2 8BS, United Kingdom

Published in the United States of America by
Cambridge University Press, New York

Cambridge University Press is part of the University of Cambridge.

It furthers the Universitys mission by disseminating knowledge
in the pursuit of education, learning and research at the
highest international levels of excellence

www.cambridge.org
Information on this title: www.cambridge.org/9781107617551

Second edition © Cambridge University Press 2009
Third edition © Cambridge University Press 2013

Second Edition first published 2009
Third Edition first published 2013
Reprinted 2013

Printed in the United Kingdom by Bell and Bain Ltd.

A catalogue record for this publication is available from the British Library

Library of Congress Cataloging-in-Publication Data

The BMT data book : including cellular therapy / edited by
Reinhold Munker ... [et al.]. – 3rd ed.
      p. ; cm.
   Includes bibliographical references and index.
   ISBN 978-1-107-61755-1 (Paperback)
   I. Munker, Reinhold.
   [DNLM: 1. Bone Marrow Transplantation.   2. Decision Making.
3. Hematopoietic Stem Cell Transplantation.   4. Treatment Outcome.
WH 380]
   617.4′40592–dc23

                                                              2012029267

ISBN 978-1-107-61755-1 Paperback

Contents

Contributors

Klemens Angstwurm, MD
Associate Professor of Neurology,
University of Regensburg, Bezirksklinikum,
Regensburg, Germany

Kerry Atkinson, MD, FRCP, FRACP
Professor of Medicine, University of
Queensland, South Brisbane, Australia

Nicholas Barber, MD
Oncology Fellow, University of Nebraska
Medical Center, Omaha, NE, USA

Jaap J. Boelens, MD
Associate Professor of Pediatrics,
University Medical Center, Utrecht,
the Netherlands

Saurabh Chhabra, MD
Assistant Professor of Medicine, University
of South Carolina, Charleston, SC, USA

Richard W. Childs, MD
Senior Investigator, Hematology Branch,
National Heart, Lung, and Blood Institute,
National Institutes of Health, Bethesda,
MD, USA

Jill M. Comeau, PharmD, BCOP
Assistant Professor of Hematology/
Oncology, University of Louisiana at
Monroe, College of Pharmacy,
Monroe, LA; Gratis Assistant Professor
of Medicine, Louisiana State University,
Shreveport, LA, USA

Daniel R. Couriel, MD
Director, Adult Blood and Marrow
Transplant Program, University of
Michigan, Ann Arbor, MI, USA

Tina Dietrich-Ntoukas, MD
Associate Professor of Ophthalmology,
University of Regensburg, Regensburg,
Germany

Nicholas R. DiPaola, PhD
Ohio State University Medical Center,
Columbus, OH, USA

Ulrich Duffner, MD
Director, Blood and Bone Marrow
Transplant Program, Michigan State
University, Grand Rapids, MI, USA

Carolina Escobar, MD
Assistant Professor of Medicine, Baylor
University Blood and Marrow Transplant
Program, Dallas, TX, USA

Alison G. Freifeld, MD
Professor of Medicine, University of
Nebraska Medical Center, Omaha,
NE, USA

Gerhard C. Hildebrandt, MD
Associate Professor of Medicine, University
of Utah School of Medicine, and Huntsman
Cancer Institute, Salt Lake City, UT, USA

Hans-Jochem Kolb, MD
Professor of Medicine and Senior
Consultant, Klinikum Rechts der Isar,
Munich, Germany

Nebu V. Koshy, MD
Assistant Professor of Medicine, Louisiana
State University, Shreveport, LA, USA

Ginna G. Laport, MD
Associate Professor, Stanford University,
Blood and Marrow Transplantation,
Stanford, CA, USA

Mary J. Laughlin, MD
Professor of Medicine, University of
Virginia, Section Head for Stem Cell
Transplantation, Charlottesville, VA, USA

Hillard M. Lazarus, MD, FACP
Professor of Medicine, The George
and Edith Richman Professor and
Distinguished Scientist in Cancer Research,
University Hospitals Case Medical Center,
Case Western Reserve University,
Cleveland, OH, USA

Anna Locasciulli, MD
Professor of Pediatrics, Ospedale
S. Camillo-Forlanini, Rome, Italy

Reinhold Munker, MD
Associate Professor of Medicine, Louisiana
State University, Shreveport, LA, USA

Binu Nair, MD
Assistant Professor of Medicine, Louisiana
State University, Shreveport, LA, USA

Pavan Reddy, MD
Associate Professor of Medicine, University
of Michigan, Ann Arbor, MI, USA

Muhammad A. Saif, MD
Clinical Fellow, University of Manchester,
Manchester, UK

Vishwas Sakhalkar, MD
Director, Pediatric Hematology/Oncology,
Medical Center of Central Georgia, Macon,
GA, USA

Shalini Shenoy, MD
Associate Professor of Pediatrics,
Washington University, St. Louis,
MO, USA

Michael Stadler, MD, PhD
Attending Physician, Hannover
Medical School, Department of
Hematology, Hemostasis, Oncology
and Stem Cell Transplantation,
Hannover, Germany

Amanda Sun, MD, PhD
Chief of Hematology/Oncology,
Group Health Physicians, Tacoma,
WA, USA

Daniel Wolff, MD
Professor of Medicine,
University of Regensburg,
Regensburg, Germany

Robert F. Wynn, MD
Director of Blood and Marrow
Transplant, University of Manchester,
Manchester, UK

Foreword

It is over 50 years since the basic concepts underpinning bone marrow transplantation were revealed in radiation protection experiments in mice. It seems curious now that in the 1950s the idea that marrow cells could grow and reconstitute hematopoiesis in an irradiated recipient was so revolutionary that it took a series of critical experiments to prove the "cellular theory" and disprove the "humoral theory" of radiation protection. Equally remarkable is the fact that within a few years (and at a time when our knowledge of lymphocytes was sketchy) the unique allotransplant-associated phenomena of graft-versus-host disease, graft rejection, and graft-versus-leukemia effects were teased out, paving the way for human transplant studies in the 1960s.

Fast forward to today, bone marrow transplantation has become stem cell transplantation (SCT), incorporating the use of umbilical cord and peripheral blood as stem cell sources. The complexity of the field has increased exponentially as transplant biology is defined increasingly at the molecular level. SCT or HCT (hematopoietic cell transplantation) is continually being extended to new malignant and nonmalignant diseases and is increasingly used because more unrelated donors and cord blood donations are available, and mismatched transplants can be performed more safely. Currently, over 25 000 SCTs are performed annually in over 70 countries. As confidence to deliver transplants with low mortality has grown, SCTs are being applied increasingly to older patients. Luckily, expertise in the clinical transplant community has kept pace with this expansion. There has been an overall increase in transplant "know how" and many procedures and approaches are standardized worldwide. To maintain our standards of care at the cutting edge, clinicians need a reference volume for the many algorithms of treatment we now handle in treating our patients. The editors of *The BMT Data Book*, Drs Munker, Hildebrandt, Lazarus, and Atkinson, have striven to produce a book that fulfills the stem cell transplanter's need for a practical guide and data source. Particularly, attention has been given to the practical issues of who should have a transplant and what type of transplant approach should be chosen.

However, no medical discipline can afford to stand still and textbooks must also move with advances or perish. SCT is no exception–in fact, there is a sense that the pace of development, both in new concepts and new clinical practice, has quickened in the last decade. In particular, improvements in transplant and nontransplant approaches, which are never in step with each other, have altered the indications for transplant. There has been ever-increasing use and success of umbilical cord blood transplantation and the emergence of safer regimens for haploidentical transplants. Progress has also been made in cell therapy with the use of mesenchymal stromal cells and regulatory T-cells to treat graft-versus-host disease and antigen-specific T-cell lines to treat viral infections. The third edition of this volume, therefore, is both timely and necessary. The editors have excelled in updating the indications for transplantation and incorporating the newest developments into this completely updated book.

So let us welcome this new edition of *The BMT Data Book Including Cellular Therapy*. It will continue to serve the stem cell transplantation community well and will play its part in the constant honing of our clinical practice so as to deliver the best and most advanced care to our patients.

John Barrett
Bethesda, MD

Preface

The last 15 years have seen a major change, expansion, and improvement in the discipline of clinical bone marrow and blood stem cell transplantation. Unifying bone marrow and peripheral blood stem cell transplants, the term hematopoietic cell transplantation has been proposed. New data have become available to support the decision for or against transplantation. The future has started already. Basic science has made progress: new genes and microRNAs have been characterized as risk factors in the outcomes of hematologic malignancies. The involvement of natural killer cells in the graft-versus-tumor reactions has been recognized. New cell populations like dendritic cells and mesenchymal stem cells have been characterized. Clinical science has made progress. New indications for transplants have been developed and evaluated. Examples are renal cell cancer, autoimmune disorders, and amyloidosis. New stem cell sources (e.g., from cord blood) were implemented. Owing to sophisticated typing methods, unrelated transplants have become safer. Because of increased donor numbers, matched unrelated transplants can now be offered to more than 70% of patients who do not have a family match. Old indications (breast cancer) have become obsolete or are being reevaluated (chronic myelogenous leukemia) because of advances in the nontransplant arena. In the first edition of this book, transplant for multiple myeloma was put into context against "conventional" treatments. Now, autologous transplant has become the standard of care for multiple myeloma, which has to compete and will join forces with antiangiogenic agents or proteasome inhibitors. New treatment protocols for older patients or those who have significant comorbidities were introduced (reduced-intensity conditioning).

Overall, in the United States more than 17 000, in Europe more than 30 000, and in Australia 1200 hematopoietic stem cell transplants are being performed each year. In addition to Europe and North America, South America, Mexico, China, and India have all started active transplant programs. The registry data evaluating the outcomes of autologous and allogeneic transplants now are based on thousands of patients instead of hundreds of patients. Therefore, in many instances, the promise of cure is being replaced or is supported by realistic long-term survival data.

Reacting to these many new developments, we decided to publish a third edition of *The BMT Data Book*. The basic structure is conserved. In the first section, the global trends in hematopoietic cell transplantation, the biology of stem cells, and the science underlying transplantation are discussed. Next, the indications for transplant in different diseases (malignant and non-malignant) are given. Pediatric aspects are noted when indicated. In a new chapter, pediatric neurologic and metabolic disorders treated with transplant are discussed. We review in detail the established and novel cellular therapies. Coauthors specialized in different areas have made contributions. All chapters are concise. The nontransplant options are mentioned briefly. Registry data are given when available. As in the first two editions, major articles from respected journals were chosen for each topic and with the permission of the authors, some figures were reproduced. These articles not only support our recommendations but also illustrate current controversies. In the other two major sections, the practical aspects and the complications of allogeneic and autologous transplantation are discussed. The "BMT pharmacopoeia" is updated with many new drugs, whereas standard-dose protocols (available in other textbooks) were removed. Finally, current transplant protocols and certain aspects of laboratory medicine are included. As in the second edition, *The BMT Data Book* has a guide to the internet and printed databases. This book is a work in progress. Owing to the enormous amount of literature and information available, it cannot be 100% complete or free from errors. However, we hope, by providing recent and solid data, to help the physicians and patients to make informed decisions and choose the best individual treatment.

Reinhold Munker
Gerhard C. Hildebrandt
Hillard M. Lazarus
Kerry Atkinson

Preface to the first edition

The use of hemopoietic stem cell transplantation to support high-dose chemotherapy or chemoradiotherapy is rapidly developing and fast changing. During the 1980s and 1990s, many marrow transplantation physicians had to start treating diseases they may not have treated for many years. Examples would be the use of autologous transplantation for breast, testicular, and ovarian cancer. Likewise, medical oncologists had to start becoming familiar with marrow and blood stem cell transplantation medicine.

In addition, effective new nontransplant treatments were introduced and made therapeutic decision making for an individual patient even more difficult. Examples included α-interferon for chronic myeloid leukemia and fludarabine for chronic lymphatic leukemia and low-grade non-Hodgkin lymphoma.

All this change occurred against a background of shrinking hospital budgets and an increasing concern for cost constraint.

These elements spurred the production of this book. Many long but useful hours were spent arguing such issues for individual patients in the weekly meeting of the marrow transplant program at St. Vincent's Hospital. It became clear that "change" was becoming the norm and marrow transplant physicians, like everyone else, had to adapt quickly. It thus seemed important to provide data-driven outcome analyses to help therapeutic decision making for individual patients.

Kerry Atkinson

Disclaimer: As in the first two editions, the authors have attempted to provide the most accurate data and guidance possible. We recognize, however, that there may be unforeseen errors in drug dosage and modification recommendations. We always encourage treating physicians and their staff to consult the original source documents when developing specific treatment plans.

Acknowledgments

Nicholas Dunton, Joanna Chamberlin, Caroline Mowatt, and Christopher Miller (Cambridge University Press) helped realize the third edition of *The BMT Data Book*. Talicia Tarver and John Cyras reviewed selected chapters. More than 60 authors (and their respective publishers) gave permission to use figures or graphs and provided valuable suggestions. We would especially like to thank our patients and their families for their motivation, courage, and trust.

Chapter 1

Hematopoietic cell transplantation: past, present, and future

Reinhold Munker

The transplantation of hematopoietic stem cells (derived from the bone marrow of healthy donors) in the 1970s was considered a highly experimental procedure and was offered only to patients with late-stage leukemia. Later, it was recognized that only a small fraction of the transplanted cells were true stem cells and that the cure effected by allogeneic transplant was mediated by an immune reaction (graft-versus-leukemia reaction). In the last 20 or 30 years, hematopoietic cell transplantation (HCT) became a routine procedure both in the United States and worldwide. It is estimated that currently 60 000 or more patients globally undergo HCT every year. Overall, both allogeneic and autologous transplants have found their indications in the everyday practice of hematology/oncology. As can been seen in the following figures, allogeneic and autologous transplants have enjoyed a huge increase both in the United States and worldwide. In this book, the terms HCT, HSCT (hematopoietic stem cell transplantation), and HPCT (hematopoietic progenitor cell transplantation) will be used interchangeably.

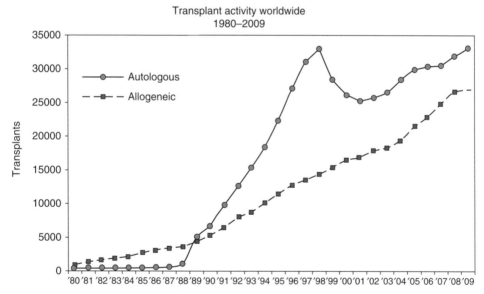

The BMT Data Book, Third Edition, ed. Reinhold Munker et al. Published by Cambridge University Press. © Cambridge University Press 2013.

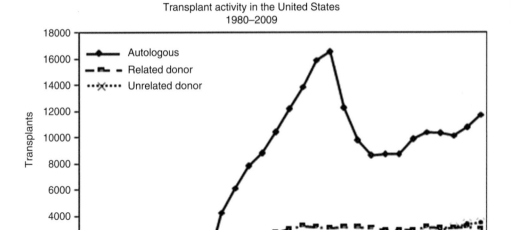

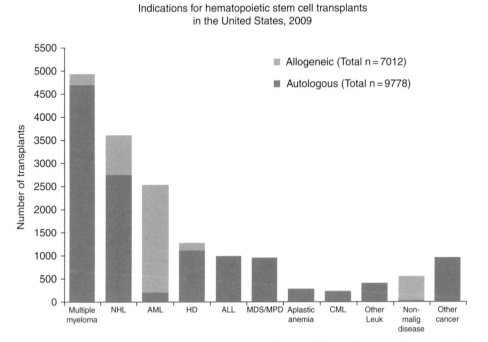

Reproduced with permission from the Center for International Blood and Marrow Transplant Research (CIBMTR) and kindly provided by Tanya Pedersen.

Although the reporting of autologous transplants is voluntary, all accredited transplant centers in the United States submit data to the CIBMTR. Since 2007, when a Stem Cell Transplant Outcomes Database was created, the reporting of allogeneic transplants is mandatory in the United States. In previous years, unrelated transplants facilitated by the National Marrow Donor Program (NMDP) were reported through the NMDP. It was estimated by the CIBMTR that currently more than half of autologous transplants in the United States are reported to a registry.

Overall, allogeneic and autologous transplants in a global perspective have a comparable frequency. The huge increase of autologous transplants in the early and mid-1990s was a result of transplants for breast cancer and multiple myeloma (in the World Health Organization [WHO] classification designated as plasma cell myeloma). The later decrease was caused by the reduced frequency of transplants for breast cancer. More recently, the autologous transplants increased again due to increased salvage transplants for lymphoma (including transplants for older patients). For multiple myeloma, autologous transplant is still the standard of care for most patients, although in older patients its role is challenged now by the introduction of new drugs. Another issue in multiple myeloma is timing of autologous transplantation.

HCT in its autologous form is performed in virtually all cases as a transplantation of mobilized peripheral stem cells. The majority of allogeneic transplantation procedures are performed with peripherally harvested cells, although some indications (severe aplastic anemia, possibly chronic myelogenous leukemia [CML]) still rely upon bone marrow as the graft source.

As seen in the previous figures, allogeneic transplantation has enjoyed a steady growth over the last two decades. During this time, the transplants for CML have decreased significantly due to the introduction of tyrosine kinase inhibitor (TKIs). Other indications like acute leukemias have increased. This correlates with the introduction of reduced-intensity conditioning (RIC) transplants for older patients or patients with comorbidities. At least in the United States, matched-unrelated transplants are about equal with matched-related transplants (or slightly more). This correlates with better outcomes for both types of transplants due to improved typing techniques resulting in better matches and better supportive treatment. In children who need a transplant, a significant number receive stem or progenitor cells from a matched or partially matched cord blood unit.

The European Group for Blood and Marrow Transplantation (EBMT) database reported more than 31 000 HCTs for 2009. Among the 28 000 first transplants, 41% were allogeneic and 51% were autologous. As in the North American database, matched unrelated transplants are now more frequent than matched sibling transplants (51% versus 43%). Large differences still exist between the high- and middle-income countries as far as the transplant frequency is concerned. As can be seen in the following figure, the transplant frequency in Western and Middle Europe varies between 50 and more than 400 cases per year among 10 million inhabitants.

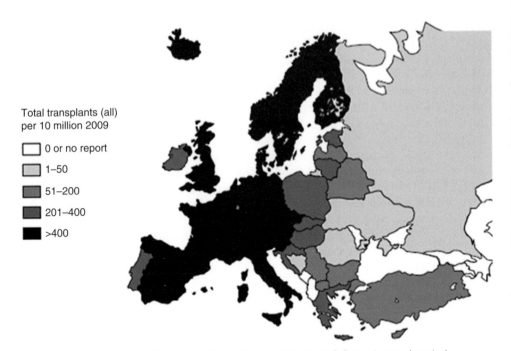

Total transplants (all)
per 10 million 2009

☐ 0 or no report

▨ 1–50

▨ 51–200

▨ 201–400

■ >400

Relative transplant frequency in Europe in 2009 (combining autologous and allogeneic transplantation). (Reproduced with permission from Baldomero et al., 2011.)

Autologous transplants following high-dose chemotherapy are generally considered safe. In most centers and for most indications, the transplant-related mortality (TRM) in 2012 is between 1% and 5% at day 100.

As far as complications of allogeneic transplants are concerned, a clear improvement occurred over the last 10–15 years. When a large transplant center in the United States compared the mortality at day 200 (excluding relapses) between the time periods 1993–1997 and 2003–2007, the mortality decreased by 60%. The overall mortality at seven years also decreased by 41%–52%. Generally, allogeneic transplant is now safer despite older and more high-risk patients being treated. The improvement is due to a lower risk of hyperacute acute graft-versus-host disease, fewer severe infections, and fewer liver, kidney, and pulmonary complications.

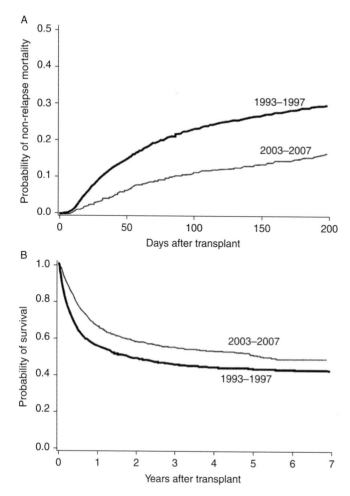

The probability of death not preceded by relapse at day 200 (A) and the probability of overall survival (OS) at seven years (B) in the two time periods are shown. (Reproduced with permission from Gooley et al., 2011.)

Allogeneic transplantation also has become an option for patients older than 60 years. In a multicenter study using conditioning with low-dose total body irradiation (TBI) ± fludarabine, a five-year risk of non-relapse mortality (NRM) of 27% (95% CI, 22%–32%), of relapse of 41% (95% CI, 36%–46%) and an OS of 35% (95% CI, 30%–40%) were reported (Sorror et al., 2011).

What is next? A survey initiated by the American Society of Blood and Marrow Transplantation shows that a growth in transplant activities of 5%–10% per year can be expected over the next decade (Schriber et al., 2010). This growth will result in a need for training of specialists and new facilities, especially in the developing world. It can be expected that more specific cellular therapies will be developed, and ultimately, the promises of gene therapy will be realized.

Details on the indications in 2012, complications and methods of stem cell and bone marrow transplantation, as well as new cellular therapies will be given in the subsequent chapters in this book.

References and further reading

Baldomero H, Gratwohl M, Gratwohl A, et al. 2011. The EBMT activity survey 2009: trends over the past 5 years. *Bone Marrow Transplant* **46**: 485–501.

Gooley TA, Chien JW, Pergam SA, et al. 2011. Reduced mortality after allogeneic hematopoietic-cell transplantation. *N Engl J Med* **363**: 2091–2101.

Gyurkozka B, Rezvani A, & Storb RF. 2010. Allogeneic stem cell transplantation: the state of the art. *Expert Rev Hematol* **3**: 285–299.

Körbling M & Freireich EJ. 2011. Twenty-five years of peripheral blood stem cell transplantation. *Blood* **117**: 6411–6416.

Moreau P, Avet-Loiseau H, Harousseau JL, et al. 2011. Current trends in autologous stem-cell transplantation for myeloma in the era of novel therapies. *J Clin Oncol* **29**: 1898–1906.

Pasquini MC & Wang Z. 2011. Current use and outcome of hematopoietic stem cell transplantation: CIBMTR summary slides. Available at: http://www.cibmtr.org.

Schriber JR, Anasetti C, Heslop HE, et al. 2010. Preparing for growth: current capacity and challenges in hematopoietic stem cell transplantation programs. *Biol Blood Marrow Transplant* **16**: 595–597.

Sorror ML, Sandmaier BM, Storer BE, et al. 2011. Long-term outcomes among older patients following non-myeloablative conditioning and allogeneic hematopoietic cell transplantation for advanced hematologic malignancies. *JAMA* **306**: 1874–1883.

Basic science

Reinhold Munker and Kerry Atkinson

The human hemopoietic system

Understanding of the human hemopoietic and immune systems has advanced markedly during the past 30 years. The key components of the human hemopoietic system are the hemopoietic growth factors, the hemopoietic stem cell, and the marrow microenvironment. Transcription factors direct hematopoietic differentiation. Each of these components is detailed further in the following sections.

Hemopoietic growth factors

- Colony-stimulating factors (CSFs)
  Granulocyte colony-stimulating factor (G-CSF)
  Granulocyte–macrophage colony-stimulating factor (GM-CSF)
  Macrophage colony-stimulating factor (M-CSF)
  Interleukin (IL)-3
  Erythropoietin
  Thrombopoietin
  IL-5

The BMT Data Book, Third Edition, ed. Reinhold Munker et al. Published by Cambridge University Press. © Cambridge University Press 2013.

- Stem cell factors
  Kit ligand (stem cell factor)
  Flt ligand
- Synergistic factors
  IL-1
  IL-6
  IL-7
  IL-9
  IL-10
  IL-11
  IL-12
  Leukemia inhibitory factor (LIF)
- Inhibitors/bidirectional regulators
  Tumor necrosis factor-alpha (TNF-α)
  Transforming growth factor-beta (TGF-β)
  Macrophage inflammatory protein-1β (MIP-1β)
  Interferon gamma (IFN-γ)

Registered hematopoietic growth factors

Native molecule	Form	Generic name	Brand name	Dosage	Manufacturer
G-CSF	Non-glycosylated	Filgrastim	Neupogen®	5 µg/kg/d	Amgen
Peg-G-CSF	Non-glycosylated	Pegfilgrastim	Neulasta®	6 mg/14 d	Amgen
G-CSF	Glycosylated	Lenograstim	Granocyte®	5 µg/kg/d	Chugai/Sanofi-Aventis, and others
GM-CSF	Non-glycosylated	Molgramostim	Leukomax®	250 µg/m²/d	Novartis, Schering-Plough, and others
GM-CSF	Glycosylated	Sargramostim	Leukine®	250 µg/m²/d	Genzyme
EPO		Epoetin α	Procrit®	50–150 U/kg 3 times weekly	Amgen/Ortho
EPO		Epoetin β	NeoRecormon®	60–150 U/kg (1–3 times weekly)	Roche
Darbepoietin-α		Darbepoietin	Aranesp®	25–500 µg/kg/week or 50 µg/kg/d	Amgen
IL-11		Oprelvekin	Neumega®	5–30 µg/kg/d	Pfizer
Stem cell factor		Ancestim	Stemgen®	20 µg/kg/d*	Amgen
Romiplostim (thrombomimetic)			Nplate®	1–5 µg/kg/wk sq	
Eltrombopag (thrombomimetic)			Promacta®	50–75 mg po/d	Glaxo-Smith-Kline

* Dosage for stem cell mobilization; not licensed in the United States.

The hemopoietic stem cell

- 1 in 2000 bone marrow cells
- 2000-fold increase in ability to confer radioprotection
- The murine phenotype is Sca-1$^+$ Thy 1^{lo} Lin$^-$. Sca-1$^+$ Thy 1^{lo} LinMac$^-$ 1^{-1} CD4$^-$ is the phenotype of stem cells with long-term repopulating ability. These have extensive self-renewal capacity and represent 80% of stem cells. Only 4%, however, are in the S/G$_2$/M phases of the cell cycle at any one time (0.005% of bone marrow cells)
- Sca 1$^+$ Thy 1^{lo} Lin-Mac 1^{lo} CD4$^-$ and Sca-1$^+$ Thy 1^{lo} Lin$^-$Mac 1^{lo} CD4$^+$ are the phenotypes of stem cells with short-term repopulating ability, representing 20% of stem cells in the marrow
- The human phenotype is CD34$^+$ Thy 1^{lo} Lin$^-$Rho$^{123\ lo}$ (rhodamine^{123} is a mitochondrial dye, the uptake of which correlates with self-renewal capacity)
- Phenotype variations: CD34$^+$, HLA-DR$^{+/-}$, CD38$^{+/-}$, Thy 1$^{+/-}$, Lin$^-$, c-kit$^+$, Rho$^{123\ dull}$; CD34$^+$/HLA-DR$^+$ do not produce long-term culture initiating cells (LTCIC); CD34$^+$/HLA-DR–do produce LTCIC

The phenotypic markers of human hematopoietic progenitor and stem cells were recently reviewed by Beksac and Preffer (2012).

- Human multipotential stem cell characteristics:
  Multilineage differentiation
  Self-renewal capacity
  Ability to reconstitute myeloablated patient
- Lineage negativity includes absence of the following:

Lineage	Cell surface antigens
T-cell	CD7, 2, 3, 4, 8
B-cell	CD19, 20
NK cell	CD56, 57
Myeloid	CD33, 15
Erythroid	Glycophorin

Hematopoietic stem cell differentiation is regulated by transcription factors.

Hematopoietic stem cell differentiation

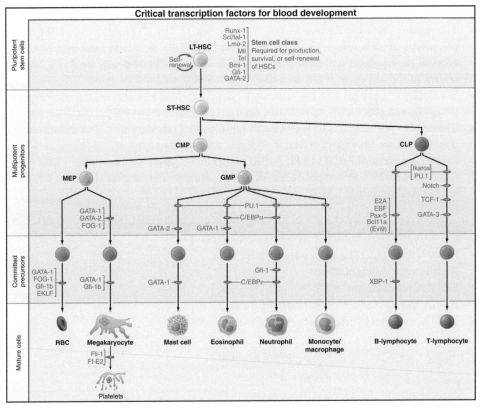

The stages at which hematopoietic development is blocked in the absence of a certain transcription factor (as determined by conventional gene knockouts) are indicated by solid bars. Often these factors have been associated with oncogenesis. Factors depicted in a light font have not yet been found translocated or mutated in human or rodent hematologic malignancies. CLP, common lymphoid progenitor; CMP, common myeloid progenitor; GMP, granulocyte/ macrophage progenitor; LT-HSC, long-term hematopoietic stem cell; MEP, megakaryocyte/ erythroid progenitor; RBC, red blood cell; ST-HSC, short-term hematopoietic stem cell. (Reproduced with permission from Orkin and Zon, 2008.)

The human bone marrow microenvironment

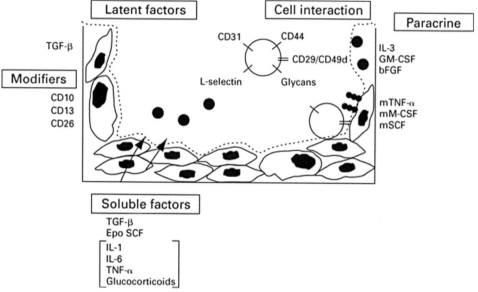

A schematic diagram of features of the human marrow environment. The major types of progenitor–stromal interactions thought to be important are boxed. Examples of each are listed beside the heading. The diagram illustrates stromal cells (arbitrarily drawn) and extracellular matrix. *Latent factors*: TGF-β, transforming growth factor β. *Modifiers*: CD10, CD13, CD26 represent the cluster of differentiation (CD) nomenclature for cell surface proteases and tuftsin endocarboxypeptidase. *Soluble factors*: Epo, erythropoietin; SCF, stem cell factor (c-kit ligand, mast cell growth factor); IL, interleukin; TNF-α, tumor necrosis factor-α. The factors in brackets are in serum at increased concentrations during infections and other systemic stresses. *Cell interaction*: CD, cluster of differentiation nomenclature for adhesion molecules; CD49d and CD29 are the α and β chains of α4β1-integrin, respectively; L-selectin, leukocyte-expressed member of the selectin family; glycans, saccharide structures that can act as ligands for molecules with lectin activity (e.g., selectins). *Paracrine*: bFGF, basic fibroblast growth factor; m-TNF-α, transmembrane form of TNF-α; mM-CSF, transmembrane isoform of M-CSF; m-SCF, transmembrane SCF; GM-CSF, granulocyte-macrophage colony-stimulating factor. (Reproduced with permission from Atkinson et al., 2003.)

Stem cell homing

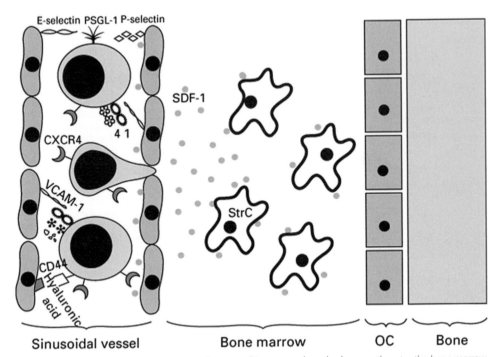

Human hematopoietic stem cells (HSCs) are administered intravenously and subsequently enter the bone marrow sinusoidal vessels. Cell adhesion molecules on the surface of HSCs bind to a variety of ligands on sinusoidal endothelial cells (ECs), allowing rolling and firm adhesion to occur. The HSCs then transmigrate the sinusoidal endothelial cells, following a stromal derived factor (SDF)-1 gradient, into the bone marrow where they establish residence within the endosteal niche, adjacent to osteoblastic cells (OCs). PSGL-1: P-selectin glycoprotein ligand-1; StrC: stromal cell; VCAM-1: vascular cell adhesion molecule-1. (Reproduced with permission from Chute, 2006.)

The cell cycle

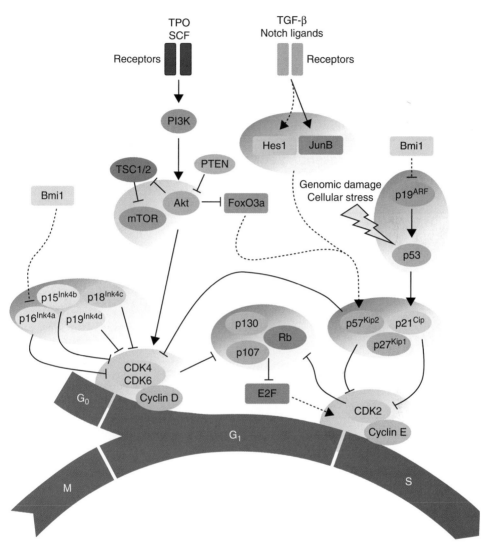

The HSC cell cycle entry is regulated by a complex network of cell-intrinsic and cell-extrinsic factors. The entry of quiescent HSCs from G0 into the G1 phase of the cell cycle is governed primarily via competing activating and inhibitory mechanisms that regulate the activity of cyclin–Cdk complexes. The PI3K/Akt/mTOR pathway, which is activated in response to numerous extrinsic signals, is considered a central activator of HSC cell cycle activity, primarily via activation of the cyclin D–Cdk4/6 complex. This pathway is heavily regulated, primarily by PTEN and TSC1/2. Moreover, the Ink4 CKI family inhibits cyclin D–Cdk4/6 activity and the CIP/KIP family. CKIs are also capable of inhibiting Cdk4 activity. Progression from the G1 to the S phase of the cell cycle is regulated by Cyclin E–Cdk2. This complex is regulated via the CIP/KIP family of Cdk inhibitors, as well as by the Rb family. Expression of CIP/KIP family members is in turn regulated by transcription factors such as Hes1, JunB, and FoxO3a, which are activated by extrinsic growth-repressive signals. Furthermore, HSC cell cycle activity is subject to regulation via p53, either in response to cellular damage or p19ARF activity. Solid arrows indicate direct activation/inhibition events; dashed arrows indicate transcriptional regulation events. (Reproduced with permission from Pietras et al., 2011.)

The human immune system

In the last 20 or 30 years, it was realized that the immune system plays an important role in eradicating minimal residual malignant disease (MRD) after marrow-ablative chemo-/radiotherapy and allogeneic or autologous stem cell transplantation (auto-SCT). For that reason, an understanding of the components of the immune system is important for the clinical transplant hematologist. A key event is the presentation of antigen to T-cells by antigen-presenting cells (APCs) using molecules of the MHC.

Antigen presentation by the major histocompatibility complex (MHC)

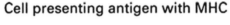

Cell presenting antigen with MHC

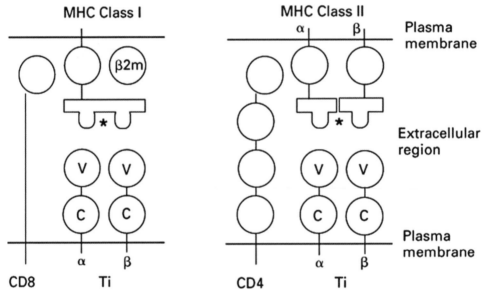

Antigen presentation by the MHC; intercellular interaction between T-cells and antigen presented by the MHC. The left part of the figure indicates antigen presentation by MHC Class I, and the right indicates antigen presentation by MHC Class II. The position of the peptide antigen is indicated by an asterisk. Each large circle represents an immunoglobulin-like domain of approximately 100 amino acids. The α and β chains of Class II are shown. β2m indicates β_2 microglobulin. The V (variable) and C (constant) regions of the Ti chains are shown.

T-cell–B-cell collaboration

T-cells also collaborate with B-cells to help them produce antigen-specific antibody.

Collaboration between B-cells and T-cells

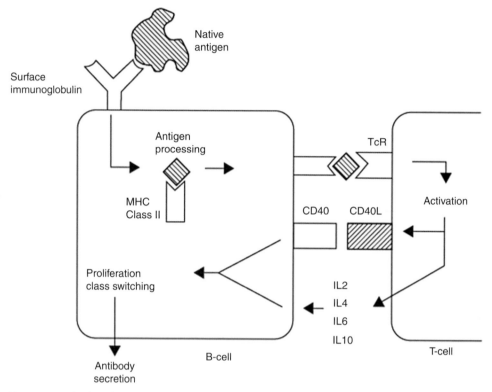

Native antigen binds surface immunoglobulin and is internalized and processed by B-cells. Antigen binds to Class II MHC and is presented to T-cells that become activated after the T-cell antigen receptor complex (TCR) recognizes the antigen. T-cells help B-cells by secreting several cytokines, including those shown, and by expressing the CD40 ligand (CD40L), which stimulates B-cells by binding to the surface marker CD40. The B-cell responses of proliferation, class switching, and antibody secretion are shown.

Cluster of differentiation markers and currently recognized leukocyte surface antigens

Another key component of the immune system is the array of molecules on the surface of leukocytes, known as cluster of differentiation (CD) antigens. The currently recognized human leukocyte differentiation antigens (see Zola et al., 2007 and updated by a conference in Barcelona in 2010) can be accessed online at www.hcdm.org.

Adhesion molecules

Adhesion molecules are important in promoting interactions between leukocytes and for attachment of leukocytes to endothelium.

Adhesion molecules

Group	Molecular characteristics	Example (function)	Ligand	Function
Integrins	Transmembrane α and β chains	LFA-1 (intercellular adhesion), CR3, CR4 (opsonization), VLA-1–6 (binding lymphocytes to extracellular matrix)	ICAM-1,-2 C3b Various	Firm attachment
Selectins (leccams)	Terminal lectin-like domain, thought to bind sugar residues	E-selectin (ELAM-1) L-selectin (Mel-14) P-selectin (GMP-140, CD62)	Sialyl Lewis-X Sulfated glycoprotein	Rolling (superficial attachment)
Intercellular adhesion molecules	Members of immunoglobulin gene superfamily	ICAM-1, ICAM-2, VCAM	LFA-1 LFA-2 VLA-4	Extravasation
Addressins	Single chain	Endothelial receptors for lymphocyte homing		

Cytokines and their function

In addition to T-cells, natural killer (NK) cells, and cell surface molecules, cytokines represent a third major component of the immune system that the marrow transplant physician should understand and be able to exploit therapeutically.

Cytokine production by the TH1 and TH2 subsets of helper T-cells (data established in murine systems)

T_H1	T_H2
IL-2	IL-3
IL-3	IL-4
GM-CSF	IL-5
IFN-γ	IL-6
	IL-10
	GM-CSF

Chemokines

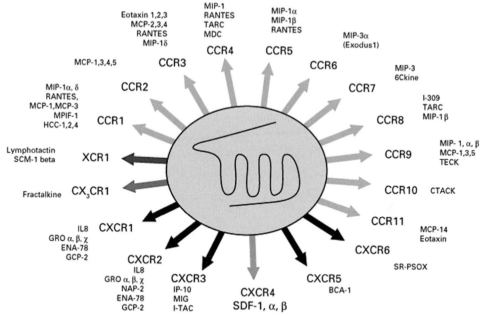

Schematic overview of chemokine receptors and their ligands. About 50 chemokines have been identified to date. Chemokines are chemotactic and are characterized by structural similarities, redundancy, and functional duality. Chemokines are produced by a great number of hematopoietic and non-hematopoietic cells such as leukocytes, platelets, endothelial cells, stromal cells (fibroblasts, osteoblasts), and keratinocytes. Chemokines are classified into four different subgroups characterized by their chemokine domains defined by the presence of two cysteines in highly conserved positions. The two largest chemokine subfamilies are the "CXC" and "CC" groups, depending on the presence or absence of any amino acid called "X." Two exceptions, lymphotactin and fractalkine, are characterized by a "C" and "CX3C" structure, respectively. (Reproduced with permission from Lataillade et al., 2004.)

Natural killer (NK) cells

NK cells are mononuclear cells that are the effectors of innate immunity. Natural killer cells function to eliminate virally infected cells, eliminate some tumor cells, secrete cytokines and chemokines, and perform contact-dependent co-stimulation. The phenotype of NK cells is $CD3^-$ and $CD56^+$. Among NK cells, the $CD56^{dim}$ subpopulation, which expresses high levels of CD16 and perforin, has the most avid killing activity. In recent years, it was discovered that NK cells have an array of activating and inhibitory receptors on their cell surface. The activating receptors, if triggered, lead to cytolysis of the target cells, while the inhibitory receptors, when binding with their appropriate ligands, prevent this from happening. In the following figure, the principle of NK cell activation and inhibition is shown schematically. The "missing self" hypothesis indicates that activated NK cells eliminate cells that do not or no longer express human leukocyte antigens (HLAs) (which is a characteristic of some tumor cells and virally infected cells). Indeed, the killer immuno-globulin (Ig) receptors (KIR) on NK cells interact with HLAs on target cells. Currently, at least 14 genes of KIR are known to be expressed in human NK cells. In the figure depicting human KIR family receptors and their ligands (page 19), the human KIR and their ligands are represented graphically. Recently, it was recognized that NK cells play a role in the graft-versus-leukemia effect (especially important in haploidentical or mismatched transplantation with maximum immunosuppression [Ruggeri et al., 2007]). For details see figure on donor recipient NK identity and mismatch (page 20).

NK cell inhibition and activation

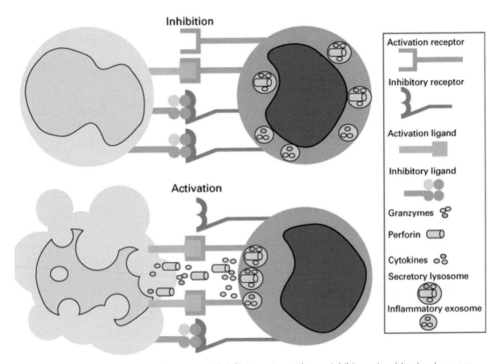

When an NK cell (right) interacts with a target cell (left), it receives either an inhibitory signal (top) or becomes activated (bottom). In inhibition, both activating as well as inhibitory receptors can be ligated, but the inhibitory receptor interaction dominates. In the inhibitory interaction, the balance favors the ligation of the inhibitory receptors and the secretory lysosomes containing perforin and granzymes, and the exosomes containing cytokines remain evenly distributed within the cytoplasm. In the NK cell-activating interaction, a preponderance of activating receptors dominates over inhibitory receptor signaling. This results in a reorganization of the cell surface molecules and cytoskeleton, leading to the polarization of the secretory bodies to the contact site. Once polarized, the granules can be exocytosed to exert their cytotoxic effect. (Reproduced with permission from Orange and Ballas, 2006.)

Human KIR family and their ligands

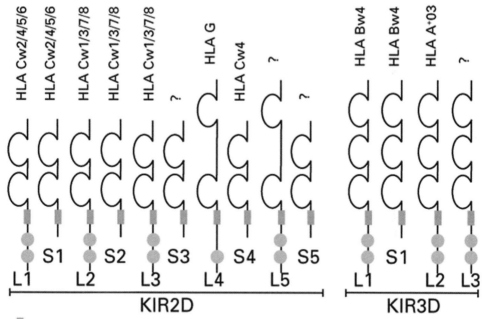

■ Transmembrane domain
● ITIM

Each of the 14 human KIRs is represented graphically. The KIR2D group having two Ig-like domains (represented by the "C" shaped loops) is shown on the left, and the KIR3D group having three Ig-like domains is shown on the right. Beneath each KIR is a letter designating whether it possesses a long (L) tail or a short (S) tail, and a number (1–5) designating to which cytoplasmic tail group it belongs. The long-tailed KIRs can be distinguished from the short-tailed KIRs in the diagram on the basis of length beneath the transmembrane domain. The immunoreceptor tyrosine-based inhibition motifs (ITIMs) contained within the cytoplasmic tails of the KIRs are noted with an octagon. Important ligand specificities for the given KIRs are shown above each KIR ("?" denotes an uncertain specificity). In general, the specificity for HLA-C alleles is conferred by the amino acids present at positions 77 and 80. Those HLA-C molecules with Asn 77/Lys 80 (HLA Cw2/4/5/6/) bind to KIR2D1, whereas those with Ser 77/Asn 80 (HLA Cw1/3/7/8) bind to KIR2D2 and KIR2D3. (Reproduced with permission from Orange and Ballas, 2006.)

Donor recipient NK cell identity and mismatch

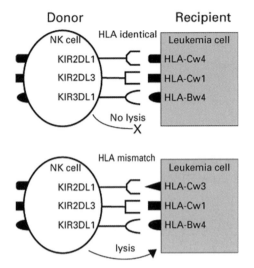

Role of the KIR system in regulating the graft-versus-leukemia effect in hematopoietic stem cell transplantation. In this example, hematopoietic stem cells from an individual having the "A" KIR haplotype (which includes KIR2DL1, KIR2DL3, and KIR3DL1) have been transferred into an HLA-identical (top) or HLA-mismatched (bottom) tumor-bearing recipient. The resulting donor-derived NK cells are depicted, and all receptors are shown on a single NK cell to represent the NK cell repertoire. In the example provided for HLA identity, all of the donor KIRs recognize a cognate MHC ligand present in the recipient. The resulting inhibitory signals block any graft-versus-tumor effect that would be mediated via NK cell cytotoxicity. In contrast, in the example of HLA mismatch, there is no ligand present for KIR2DL1 in the recipient. Thus, the KIR2DL1-expressing NK cells will not receive an inhibitory signal and can kill the tumor cell. (Reproduced with permission from Orange and Ballas, 2006.)

Dendritic cells

Dendritic cells are derived from bone marrow CD34$^+$ stem cells and are capable of initiating a primary MHC-restricted immune response. Dendritic cells belong to the class of antigen-presenting cells. Several cytokines promote the generation of dendritic cells (among them GM-CSF, TNF-α, IL-4, and FLT-3). Dendritic cells appear promising for the immunotherapy of cancer as they can increase the immune response to tumor antigens. For details about the clinical use of dendritic cells, see page 221.

The mesenchymal stem cells

Mesenchymal stem cells (MSCs) are also referred to as mesenchymal multipotent progenitor cells (MMPCs).

Human MSC characteristics:

- Plastic adherent, large (>20 μm) fibroblast-like cells
- Easily expanded in vitro
- Ability to differentiate into cell types of mesodermal origin in vitro including chondrocytes, adipocytes, and osteocytes
- Immunoinhibitory

The human MSC phenotype is CD73$^+$, CD90$^+$, and CD105$^+$, and lack of CD45$^-$.

- Stro-1 has also been used as a marker in combination with VCAM-1
- Murine phenotype is Sca-1$^+$, CD90+, Lin$^-$

MSC phenotypic markers are not unique and thus differentiation ability is generally used in combination with phenotype.

MSCs have been isolated from bone marrow, placenta, adipose tissue, liver, and umbilical cord blood (UCB).

Frequency of differentiation is $1:10^5$ to 10^6 from human bone marrow. MSCs can be greatly expanded with in vitro culture.

- MSCs can be grown in simple media, such as DMEM (low glucose) with FCS
- Fibroblast growth factor (FGF-2) and platelet-derived growth factor (PDGF) have been reported to substitute for FCS
- MSCs do not have unlimited self-renewal capacity (unlike hematopoietic stem cells [HSCs])

MSCs preferentially home to sites of inflammation when injected intravenously.

- Freshly isolated murine bone marrow-derived MSCs, but not culture-expanded MSCs have been reported to home to bone marrow when re-infused intravenously

MSCs possess immune suppressive properties.

- Mechanism is thought to be via T-cell inhibition
- IDO (indoleamine 2, 3-dioxygenase), IL-10, TGFβ, and HLA-G have all been implicated in the mechanism
- In large outbred animals, MSCs have been successfully transplanted across MHC barriers without the need for immune suppression
- MSCs that are HLA-matched, HLA-haploidentical, or HLA-unmatched (mismatched) have successfully been used in clinical trials for treatment of drug-refractory graft-versus-host disease (GVHD)

MSCs are actively studied in trials as being cellular therapeutic for a range of conditions including

- Myocardial infarct
- Stroke
- GVHD (see page 317)
- Osteogenesis imperfecta
- Cartilage repair

Purification strategies for isolating MSCs from human and mouse bone/bone marrow

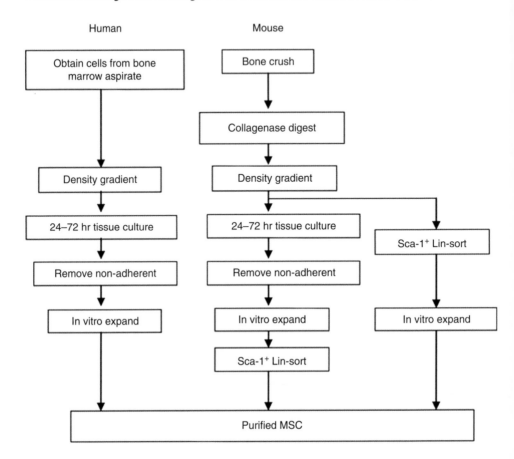

Factors required for in vitro differentiation of MSCs

A

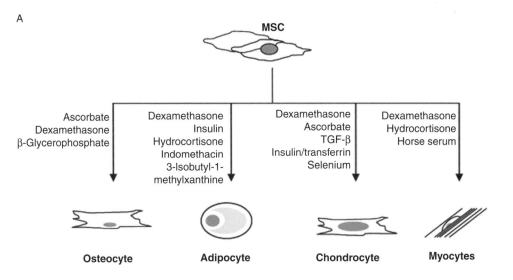

B

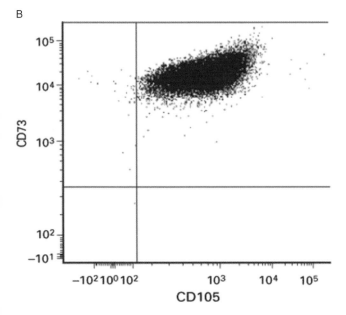

Expression of CD73 and CD105 on MSCs from human bone marrow (cells were lineage negative)
Further details about the clinical use and properties of MSCs are given on pages 222–223.

References and further reading

Atkinson K, ed. 2003. *Clinical Bone Marrow and Blood Stem Cell Transplantation: A Reference Textbook*. Cambridge: Cambridge University Press.

Beksac M & Preffer F. 2012. Is it time to revisit our current hematopoietic progenitor cell quantification methods in the clinic? *Bone Marrow Transplant* [Epub ahead of print].

Chute JP. 2006. Stem cell homing. *Curr Opin Hematol* **13**: 399–406.

Laine SK, Hentunen T, & Laitala-Leinonen T. 2012. Do microRNAs regulate bone marrow stem cell niche physiology? *Gene* **497**: 1–9.

Laiosa CV, Stadtfeld M, & Graf T. 2006. Determinants of lymphoid myeloid lineage differentiation. *Annu Rev Med* **24**: 705–738.

Lataillade JJ, Domenech J, & Le Bousse-Kerdilès MC. 2004. Stromal cell derived factor-1 (SDF-1)\CXCR4 couple plays multiple roles on haematopoietic progenitors at the border between the old cytokine and new chemokine worlds: survival, cell cycling and trafficking. *Eur Cytokine Netw* **15**: 177–188.

Orange JS & Ballas ZK. 2006. Natural killer cells in human health and disease. *Clin Immunol* **118**: 1–10.

Orkin SH & Zon LI. 2008. Hematopoiesis: an evolving paradigm for stem cell biology. *Cell* **132**: 631–644.

Pietras EM, Warr MR, & Passagué E. 2011. Cell cycle regulation in hematopoietic stem cells. *J Cell Biol* **195**: 709–720.

Ruggeri L, Mancusi A, Burchielli E, et al. 2007. Natural killer cell alloreactivity in allogeneic hematopoietic transplantation. *Curr Op Oncol* **19**: 142–147.

Zola H, Swart B, Banham A, et al. 2007. CD Molecules 2006 – human cell differentiation molecules. *J Immunol Methods* **319**: 1–5.

Chapter

3

Therapeutic decision making in BMT/SCT for acute myeloid leukemia

Reinhold Munker, Gerhard C. Hildebrandt, and Kerry Atkinson

Classification of acute myeloid leukemia (AML)

The French–American–British (FAB) classification of AML

FAB-type	Morphological features	POX	ANAE	Frequency (%)
M0	Undifferentiated lymphoid markers negative, reactive with some myeloid markers (CD33, CD13), ultrastructural peroxidase	0	0	<5
M1	Myeloid, no maturation, poorly differentiated blasts with rare azurophilic granules	+/−	0	15–20

The BMT Data Book, Third Edition, ed. Reinhold Munker et al. Published by Cambridge University Press. © Cambridge University Press 2013.

(cont.)

FAB-type	Morphological features	POX	ANAE	Frequency (%)
M2	Myeloid with maturation myeloblasts, promyelocytes, occasionally eosinophils and basophils, often Auer rods	++	0	25–30
M3	Promyelocytic, two variants: hypergranular (90%) and atypical microgranular (10%)	+++	0	10
M4	Myelomonocytic leukemic myeloblasts and monoblasts, variant: M4Eo with abnormal eosinophils	++	++	15
M5	Monoblastic leukemic monoblasts (two variants: M5a, M5b)	0	+++	2–9
M6	Erythroleukemia: >50% abnormal erythropoietic cells, >30% myeloblasts among all nonerythroid cells	0	0	< 5
M7	Megakaryoblastic usually associated with myelofibrosis, platelet markers present	0	0	2–10

POX, peroxidase; ANAE, α-naphthyl acetate esterase.

Common cytogenetic abnormalities in AML and their prognostic impact

Cytogenetic (molecular) marker	Association with FAB-type	Prognostic impact
t(8;21) Runx1-Runx1T1	AML M2	Good*
Inv(16)/ t(16;16) CBFB-MYH11	AML M4Eo	Good*
t(15;17)	AML M3	Good
Normal karyotype, del of Y chr.	Various	Intermediate
del(7q), del(9q), t(9;11), del (11q), isolated +8, +11, +13, +21, del (20q)	Various	Probably intermediate
Complex karyotype	Various	Poor
11q23 or t(11;19)	AML M4, M5	Poor
Inv(3)	AML M1, M4	Poor
Del5/5q- or 7/7q- or del7	Various	Poor
t (6;9) (p23; q34) DEK-NUP214	AML M2	Poor
Monosomal karyotypes (two or more distinct autosomies or one monosomy with other structural abnormalities)	Various	Very poor

* t(8;21), Inv16, t(16;16) plus c-kit mutation: intermediate risk.

Molecular abnormalities and their prognostic impact

NPM1 mutation with normal cytogenetics and in the absence of FLT3: good

Biallelic CEBPA mutation: good

Monoallelic CEBPA mutation:

- plus NPM1 mutation: additional beneficial effect
- plus NPM1 wildtype: no additional effect
- plus FLT3: no additional effect

FLT3 ITD mutation with normal cytogenetics: poor

IDH1, IDH2, TET2: poor (not yet considered for routine treatment decision making)

World Health Organization classification of AML (2008)

AML and related neoplasms
AML with recurrent genetic abnormalities
AML with t(8;21)(q22;q22); *RUNX1-RUNX1T1*
AML with inv(16)(p13.1q22) or t(16;16)(p13.1;q22); *CBFB-MYH11*
Acute promyelocytic leukemia (APL) with t(15;17)(q22;q12); *PML-RARA*
AML with t(9;11)(p22;q23); *MLLT3-MLL*
AML with t(6;9)(p23;q34); *DEK-NUP214*
AML with inv(3)(q21q26.2) or t(3;3)(q21;q26.2); *RPN1-EVI1*
AML (megakaryoblastic) with t(1;22)(p13;q13); *RBM15-MKL1* *Provisional entity: AML with mutated NPM1* *Provisional entity: AML with mutated CEBPA*
Acute myeloid leukemia with myelodysplasia-related changes
Therapy-related myeloid neoplasms
AML, not otherwise specified
AML with minimal differentiation
AML without maturation
AML with maturation
Acute myelomonocytic leukemia
Acute monoblastic/monocytic leukemia
Acute erythroid leukemia
Pure erythroid leukemia
Erythroleukemia, erythroid/myeloid
Acute megakaryoblastic leukemia
Acute basophilic leukemia
Acute panmyelosis with myelofibrosis

(cont.)

Myeloid sarcoma
Myeloid proliferations related to Down syndrome
Transient abnormal myelopoiesis
Myeloid leukemia associated with Down syndrome
Blastic plasmacytoid dendritic cell neoplasm
Acute leukemias of ambiguous lineage
Acute undifferentiated leukemia
Mixed phenotype acute leukemia with t(9;22)(q34;q11.2); *BCR-ABL1*
Mixed phenotype acute leukemia with t(v;11q23); *MLL* rearranged
Mixed phenotype acute leukemia, B-myeloid, NOS (not otherwise specified)
Mixed phenotype acute leukemia, T-myeloid, NOS

Cytochemical and immunohistochemical stains used for the classification of acute leukemia

Myeloperoxidase (MPO), an enzyme found in the primary (azurophilic) granules of cells of the granulocytic and monocytic series, is vital for distinguishing between lymphoid leukemia and myeloid leukemia. The granules are stained a dark blue to dark brown color when free oxygen liberated by the peroxidase reacts to change a benzidine dye from its clear state to a colored state.

Nonspecific esterase (NSE), prominent in monocytes and their precursors, employs α-naphthyl butyrate or α-naphthyl acetate, following pretreatment with sodium fluoride, as substrate for enzymatic cleavage of the naphthyl group, which is then reacted with a diazo dye. Although staining is prominent in the monocytic series, there can be weak staining in some acute lymphoblastic leukemia (ALL) cases and in some cases of AML-M3.

The periodic acid–Schiff (PAS) reaction depends on the liberation of carbohydrate radicals, which are oxidized to aldehydes and then reacted with Schiff reagent. Positivity in hemopoietic cells usually denotes glycogen, which is prominent in malignant erythroid precursors (blush and block positive). Granules can also be seen in some lymphoid and some myeloid leukemias.

Sudan black B (SBB) stains the phospholipids of monocytes and granulocytes but is not as specific as MPO in distinguishing lymphoid leukemia from myeloid leukemia (1.6% of ALL cases have 5% or greater SBB positivity).

Naphthol AS-D chloroacetate esterase (NASD), found in granulocytic precursors, cleaves the naphthyl group, which combines with a diazonium salt to give an azo dye. This enzyme can be absent in very early granulocytic differentiation and is therefore not as sensitive as MPO.

Terminal deoxynucleotidyltransferase (Tdt), detected by immunofluorescence or immunoperoxidase techniques, is a nuclear enzyme that allows for template-independent addition of deoxynucleotides on to DNA chains. Although not specific for non-B-cell ALL (10% of AML patients have more than 10% Tdt-positive cells), it is considered a valuable marker for immature lymphoid neoplasms (i.e., lymphoblastic lymphoma (LBL) and ALL).

Cytochemical, cytogenetic, and immune phenotype features of AML

The molecular, cytogenetic, morphologic, and surface marker features have significant prognostic implications for outcomes with both conventional chemotherapy and bone marrow or stem cell transplantation.

Other variants

In addition to the recognized FAB subtypes of AML (or acute non-lymphocytic leukemia), the following variants can occur.

Acute undifferentiated leukemia

- Blasts are not typical for AML or ALL
- Cytochemical stains are negative by light microscopy
- Electron microscopic findings are negative for MPO and platelet peroxidase
- Surface phenotype is negative for CD13, CD14, CD33, CD19, CD22, CD2, CD3, CD10, CD37, and glycophorin A; it may be positive for HLA-DR, CD34, CD7, and Tdt, because these are not considered solely lineage specific

Acute mixed lineage leukemia (acute leukemias of ambiguous lineage)

- Demonstrates unequivocal characteristics for more than one lineage (myeloid and lymphoid) on the same blasts and/or
- Separately on two or more populations of blasts
- Example: MPO positivity, plus two or more lymphoid lineage-associated immune phenotype markers. (For further details about acute leukemias of ambiguous lineage see Béné et al., 2012.)

Prognostic factors

Prognostic factors for outcome with conventional therapy

Favorable	Unfavorable
De novo AML	AML secondary to myelodysplasia (sAML) AML related to prior treatment (tAML)
Favorable cytogenetics	Unfavorable cytogenetics
For intermediate group: no genetic evidence of FLT3 ITD mutation, positive for NPM1 mutation in normal cytogenetic karyotype, positive for biallelic CEBPA mutation, no other unfavorable features	For intermediate group: showing abnormality in FLT3 gene (ITD FLT3 mutation), high BAALC expression
Panmyeloid phenotype (CD13, CD33, CD117, CD65, MPO)	CD7, CD11b, CD34?
Younger age (<45 years)	Age >60 years or <2 years
No CNS leukemia	CNS leukemia
WBC count at diagnosis $<20 \times 10^9$/L	WBC count at diagnosis $>100 \times 10^9$/L

CNS, central nervous system; WBC, white blood cell.

Risk categories are updated according to Estey (2012), Oran and Weisdorf (2011), and Paun and Lazarus (2012).

The assessment of risk and who benefits most from allogeneic (related versus unrelated) transplant is slightly discrepant between Europe and the United States (Hübel et al., 2011).

Results with conventional (nontransplant) therapy in adults
Summary

Age	CR1 achieved (%)	DFS (%)
<45 years	75–80	35
45–60 years	70–75	25
>60 years	30–60	5–10

CR1, first complete remission; DFS, disease-free survival.
Note: Results vary widely according to cytogenetic and other risk factors.

Outcome of induction and post-remission therapy in younger adults with AML with normal karyotype: a cancer and leukemia group B study

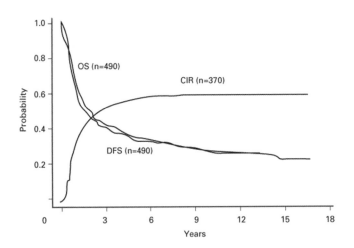

A total of 490 patients with AML and a normal karyotype received induction chemotherapy with cytarabine and daunorubicin (DA) or escalated doses of daunorubicin and etoposide ± a multidrug-resistance modulator. Four different types of post-remission chemotherapy were given. The figure shows the outcome of all patients included in the analysis. CIR, cumulative incidence of relapse. (Reproduced with permission from Farag et al., 2005.)

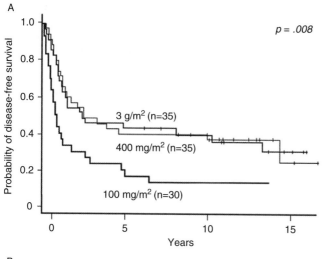

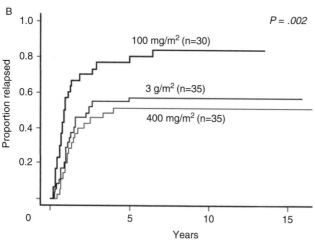

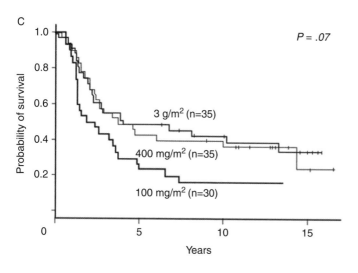

The three figures show that in the same study the outcome differed by the dose intensity of post-remission cytarabine. (A) disease-free survival; (B) cumulative incidence of relapse; and (C) overall survival. The best post-remission strategy was to give either four cycles of intermediate-dose or high-dose cytarabine or one cycle of high-dose cytarabine–etoposide followed by auto-SCT. In this study, allogeneic transplant was offered only at relapse. (Reproduced with permission from Farag et al., 2005.)

Results with allogeneic and autologous transplant
Matched unrelated donor versus HLA-identical sibling HCT in adults with AML

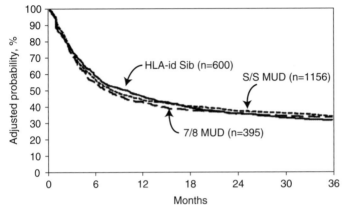

In this study from the CIBMTR, 2223 patients with AML who underwent allogeneic transplant between 2002 and 2006 were investigated for outcome. As can be seen in the graph, the survival free from leukemia was not different in the three transplant categories, HLA-identical siblings, 8/8 matched unrelated donors (MUD), and 7/8 MUD. (Reproduced with permission from Saber et al., 2012.)

Matched unrelated transplants with RIC for AML patients in complete remission (CR): comparison of blood versus bone marrow (Data from the Acute Leukemia Working Party of the EBMT)

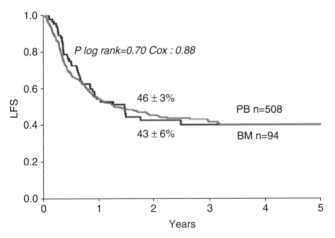

In somewhat older patients or patients with comorbidities, RIC is considered as standard of care by many centers. In the graph, the leukemia-free survival (LFS) of 508 patients transplanted with peripheral blood (PB) stem cells was compared with 94 patients who received bone marrow (BM) stem cells and found to be comparable. In the PB group, grade >II GVHD was significantly higher; in the BM group, the relapse incidence was significantly higher. (Reproduced with permission from Nagler et al., 2012.)

Allogeneic transplantation for therapy-related myelodysplastic syndrome (MDS) and AML

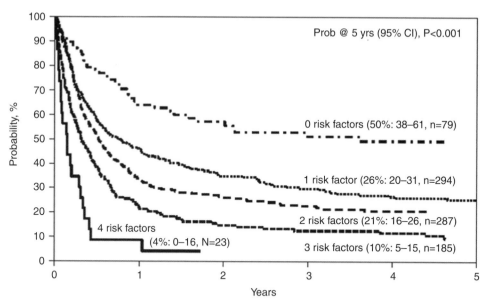

The outcome of treatment-related AML (t-AML) and treatment-related MDS (t-MDS) is generally poor. Litzow et al. (2010) analyzed 868 patients reported to the CIBMTR; 545 patients had t-AML and 323 had t-MDS. Most patients (77%) underwent a myeloablative transplant. The OS in this multicenter cohort was 22% at five years, the LFS 21% at five years. The authors defined four risk factors for a poor outcome (age >35 years, high-risk cytogenetics, t-AML not in remission or t-MDS at an advanced stage, donor other than an HLA-identical sibling or a partially or well-matched unrelated donor). The OS in the presence of zero, one, two, or three risk factors is shown in the graph. (Reproduced with permission.) The authors recommend that patients with zero to two risk factors should be considered for allogeneic transplantation.

Auto-transplantation versus HLA-matched unrelated donor (URD) transplantation for AML: a retrospective analysis from the CIBMTR

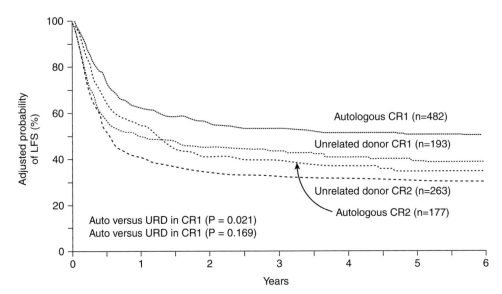

In this international registry study, 668 autotransplants performed in first or second complete remission (CR1/CR2) were compared with 476 unrelated matched transplants. In multivariate analyses, TRM was significantly higher and relapse lower with unrelated donor (URD) transplantation. Adjusted three-year survival probabilities were 57% (53%–61%) with autotransplants and 44% (37%–51%) with URD (P=0.002) transplants in CR1 and 46% (39%–53%) and 33% (28%–38%) (P=0.006) in CR2, respectively. Adjusted three-year LFS probabilities were 53% (48%–57%) with autotransplants and 43% (36%–50%) with URD (P=0.021) transplants in CR1 and 39% (32%–46%) and 33% (27%–38%) (P=0.169) in CR2, respectively. Both autologous and URD transplantation produced prolonged LFS. High TRM offsets the superior antileukemia effect of URD transplantation. This retrospective, observational database study showed that autotransplantation, in general, offered higher three-year survival for AML patients in CR1 and CR2. Cytogenetics, however, were known in only two-thirds of patients and treatment bias cannot be eliminated. The OS (LFS) is compared for autologous (auto) versus unrelated donor (URD) transplants separating patients in first remission (CR1) from patients in second remission (CR2). (Reproduced with permission from Lazarus et al., 2005.)

Role of autologous transplantation for AML: comparison with chemoconsolidation

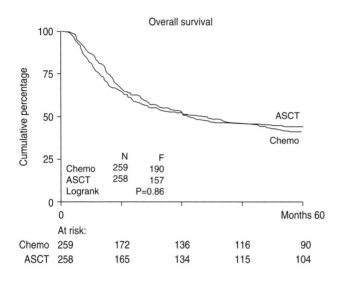

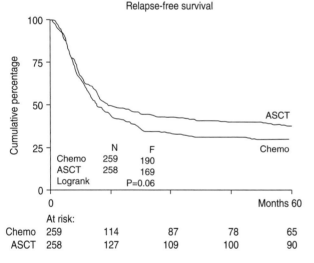

In this study from Europe, patients with AML in CR1 and not eligible for allogeneic SCT were randomized to intensive chemoconsolidation and autologous SCT. Two hundred and fifty-nine patients received intensive chemoconsolidation with etoposide and mitoxantrone, whereas 258 patients received an auto-SCT following conditioning with busulfan and cyclophosphamide. This study showed that relapse-free survival was improved after five years in the transplant arm; however, the OS was similar in both arms due to salvage transplants. Overall, the study establishes or confirms the value of autologous transplant as a treatment for patients who are unable or unwilling to undergo allogeneic transplantation. ASCT, autologous stem cell transplantation; Chemo, chemoconsolidation. (Reproduced with permission from Vellenga et al., 2011.)

CIBMTR database: results for AML

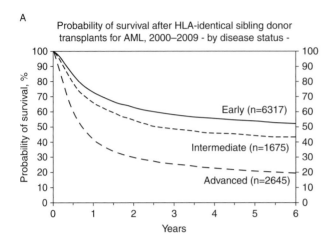

A

Probability of survival after HLA-identical sibling donor transplants for AML, 2000–2009 - by disease status -

Early (n=6317)

Intermediate (n=1675)

Advanced (n=2645)

The CIBMTR has data for 20 934 patients receiving an HLA-matched sibling (n=10 637) or URD (n=10 297) transplant for AML between 2000 and 2009. Their disease status at the time of transplant and the donor type are major predictors of posttransplant survival. The three-year probabilities of survival after HLA-matched sibling transplant in this cohort were 58%±1%, 48%±1%, and 25%±1% for patients with early, intermediate, and advanced disease, respectively. The probabilities of survival after a URD transplant were 46%±1%, 44%±1%, and 20%±1% for patients with early, intermediate, and advanced disease, respectively. Early disease is defined as CR1, intermediate as CR2 or later, advanced as induction failure or active disease.

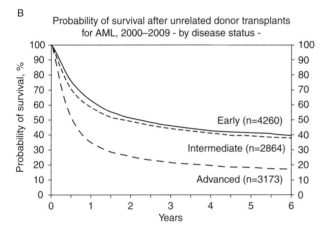

B

Probability of survival after unrelated donor transplants for AML, 2000–2009 - by disease status -

Early (n=4260)

Intermediate (n=2864)

Advanced (n=3173)

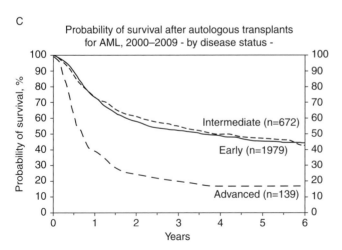

C

Probability of survival after autologous transplants for AML, 2000–2009 - by disease status -

Intermediate (n=672)

Early (n=1979)

Advanced (n=139)

The CIBMTR has data for 2 790 autologous transplants performed for patients with AML between 2000 and 2009. Autologous transplants are rarely performed in patients with active AML. The three-year probabilities of survival for patients with early, intermediate, and advanced AML were 52%±1%, 55%±2%, and 20%±4%, respectively. (Data kindly provided by Tanya Pedersen and Zhiwei Wang [CIBMTR website accessed 2/25/2012]).

Indications for transplant

HLA-identical family member transplant

	Indication	DFS(%)
1.	AML in CR1 (in presence of risk factors)	50–70
2.	AML in first relapse or second or subsequent remission	15–35
3.	Primary refractory AML	10–30

Note: for patients >55 years old or with significant comorbidities, a transplant with RIC in the context of a clinical trial should be considered. Results are age- and risk factor dependent.

DFS, as above, but subtract 10%
(Nine of ten HLA-identical family member transplants)

Autologous blood/marrow SCT

	Indication	DFS(%)
1.	AML in CR1	40–50
2.	AML in untreated first relapse or CR2	20–30
3.	APL in CR2	50–80

Autologous HSCT is currently considered as the recommended alternative consolidation strategy mainly for good risk patients with AML (DFS 50%–80%) and in APL CR2, if PML/RAR-α PCR (promyelocytic leukemia/retinoic acid alpha receptor; polymerase chain reaction) negative.

HLA-identical URD transplant

	Indication	DFS(%)
1.	AML in CR1, with poor prognostic features	40–50
2.	AML beyond CR1	15–30

Transplantation in patients of over sixty years of age with AML

The outcome of AML in the older patient is historically very poor. Conventional chemotherapy achieved a five-year OS rate in older AML patients with good-, intermediate-, and poor-risk cytogenetics of 19%, 7%, and 0%, respectively. These results may be improved in older patients who are in good performance status and who undergo an allogeneic transplant.

Comorbidities are important for the outcome of patients with AML undergoing an allogeneic transplant

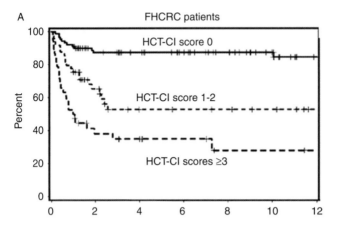

In these graphs, the Kaplan–Meier curves for OS are shown in two groups of patients (Fred Hutchinson Cancer Research Center [FHCRC] and MD Anderson Cancer Center [MDACC]). The survival is stratified by HCT-CI (comorbidity index) scores of 0, 1, 2, and ≥3 among patients transplanted. (For details about the HCT-CI see page 237.) (Reproduced with permission from Sorror et al., 2007).

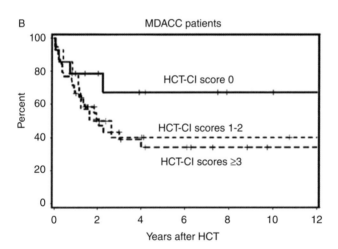

Transplantation for children with AML

The treatment of acute leukemias in children has made significant progress over the last 25 years. Likewise, the risk of allogeneic transplantation (matched related or well-matched unrelated) is generally lower than in adults. Like in adult patients with AML, the risk stratification has become more sophisticated. The indications and strategies for pediatric patients with AML were recently reviewed (Carpenter et al., 2012; Shenoy & Smith, 2008). Children with low-risk disease or standard-risk disease who are negative for minimal residual disease would not get an allogeneic transplant even if a matched family donor is available. The other patients in first remission would be offered an allogeneic transplant in first remission if a sufficiently matched donor is available. As for adults, all patients with relapsed AML would be investigated or considered for allogeneic transplant.

Pretransplant workup

1. Evaluation of PB and BM:

morphology, cytochemistry, immune phenotype, cytogenetics, and molecular testing.

2. See the general pretransplant workup (page 239).

Monitoring posttransplant

1. Bone marrow aspirate, with cytogenetic evaluation (chimerism and molecular evaluation, as appropriate) at 1, 3, 6, 12, and 24 months.

Treatment algorithm for AML

Induction

Standard anthracycline + cytarabine (3 + 7) or similar (if no contraindications).

Exception: APL–treat with ATRA + chemotherapy + arsenic trioxide consolidation + maintenance.

Consolidation in remission

Favorable cytogenetics: high-dose cytarabine or a similar agent for two to four cycles; alternatively, autologous HSCT.

Exception: APL–follow APL protocols.

Intermediate cytogenetics: allogeneic transplant as soon as possible (especially if molecular risk factors are present) or patient's choice–high-dose cytarabine consolidation or similar agent for two to four cycles–if HLA-matched family donor is available.

High-dose cytarabine consolidation or similar agent for two to four cycles if no HLA-matched sibling donor is available; alternatively, auto-HSCT if patient is not eligible for allogeneic HSCT.

Unfavorable cytogenetics: allogeneic transplant as soon as possible if matched related or unrelated donor is available.

High-dose cytarabine consolidation or similar agent for two to four cycles ± autologous transplant if no HLA-matched donor is available.

Comment: in patients who are 55–75 years old, consider non-myeloablative allogeneic transplantation if in remission. In patients with poor performance status, consider palliative options.

Relapsed or refractory AML

If remission of >6 to 12 months, consider original protocol.

In other cases, consider salvage protocol.

Consider allogeneic related or unrelated SCT.

If matched related or unrelated donor is unavailable, consider CBT or haploidentical SCT.

Comment: for relapsed APL, consider arsenic trioxide containing regimen; if patient comes into second remission and stem cells can be harvested and are negative for PML/RAR-α on PCR, consider auto-SCT. In support of this strategy, a small series of patients with relapsed APL had a 100% DFS when transplanted with PCR-negative PB stem cells (Kanimura et al., 2011). If a patient is not negative for PML/RAR-α, consider allogeneic transplantation.

References and further reading

Béné MC & Porwit A. 2012. Acute leukemias of ambiguous lineage. *Sem Diagnost Pathol* **29**: 12–18.

Carpenter PA, Meshinchi S, & Davies SM. 2012. Transplantation for AML in children. *Biol Blood Marrow Transplant* **18**: S33–S39.

Estey EH. 2012. Acute myeloid leukemia: 2012 update on diagnosis, risk stratification and management. *Am J Hematol* **87**: 90–99.

Farag SS, Ruppert AS, Mrózek K, et al. 2005. Outcome of induction and postremission therapy in young adults with acute myeloid leukemia with normal karyotype: a cancer and leukemia group B study. *J Clin Oncol* **23**: 482–493.

Hübel K, Weingart O, Neumann F, et al. 2011. Allogeneic stem cell transplant in adult patients with acute myelogenous leukemia: a systematic analysis of international guidelines and recommendations. *Leuk Lymphoma* **52**: 444–457.

Kamimura T, Miyamoto T, Nagafuji K, et al. 2011. Role of autotransplantation in the treatment of acute promyelocytic leukemia patients in remission: Fukuoka BMT Group observations and literature review. *Bone Marrow Transplant* **46**: 820–826.

Lazarus HM, Pérez WS, Klein JP, et al. 2005. Autotransplantation versus HLA-matched unrelated donor transplantation for acute myeloid leukaemia: a retrospective analysis from the Center for International Blood and Marrow Transplant Research. *Br J Haematol* **132**: 755–769.

Litzow MR, Tarima S, Pérez WS, et al. 2010. Allogeneic transplantation for therapy-related myelodysplastic syndrome and acute myeloid leukemia. *Blood* **115**: 1850–1857.

Nagler A, Labopin M, Shimoni A, et al. 2012. Mobilized peripheral blood stem cells compared with bone marrow as the stem cell source for unrelated donor allogeneic transplantation with reduced-intensity conditioning in patients with acute myeloid leukemia in complete remission: an analysis from the Acute Leukemia Working Party of the European Group for Blood and Marrow Transplantation. *Biol Blood Marrow Transplant* **89**: 206–213.

Oran B & Weisdorf DJ. 2011. Allogeneic stem cell transplantation in first complete remission. *Curr Opin Hematol* **18**: 395–400.

Paun O & Lazarus HM. 2012. Allogeneic hematopoietic cell transplantation for acute myeloid leukemia in first complete remission: have the indications changed? *Curr Opin Hematol* **19**: 95–101.

Saber W, Opie S, Rizzo JD, et al. 2012. Outcomes after matched unrelated donor versus identical sibling hematopoietic cell transplantation in adults with acute myelogenous leukemia. *Blood* **119**: 3908–3916.

Shenoy S & Smith FO. 2008. Hematopoietic stem cell transplantation for childhood malignancies of myeloid origin. *Bone Marrow Transplant* **41**: 141–148.

Song KW & Lipton J. 2005. Is it appropriate to offer allogeneic hematopoietic stem cell transplantation to patients with primary refractory acute myeloid leukemia? *Bone Marrow Transplant* **36**: 183–191.

Sorror ML, Giralt S, Sandmaier BM, et al. 2007. Hematopoietic cell transplantation specific comorbidity index as an outcome predictor for patients with acute myeloid leukemia in first remission: combined FHCRC and MDACC experiences. *Blood* **110**: 4606–4613.

Vellenga E, van Putten W, Ossenkoppele GJ, et al. 2011 Autologous peripheral blood stem cell transplantation for acute myeloid leukemia. *Blood* **118**: 6037–6042.

Therapeutic decision making in BMT/SCT for acute lymphoblastic leukemia

Reinhold Munker, Vishwas Sakhalkar, Hillard M. Lazarus, and Kerry Atkinson

Classification of acute lymphoblastic leukemia (ALL)

FAB classification

- ALL-L1: MPO-negative, with small cells predominating. Cells have a high nuclear–cytoplasmic (N/C) ratio (scant amount of cytoplasm), regular nuclear borders, and inconspicuous nucleoli. Tdt is usually positive
- ALL-L2: MPO-negative heterogeneous population, often with larger blasts. The cells have a low N/C ratio (moderate amount of cytoplasm), with irregular nuclear borders and prominent nucleoli. Tdt is usually positive
- ALL-L3, Burkitt type: MPO-negative, homogeneous population of large blasts. The cells have a moderate amount of deeply basophilic cytoplasm and prominent cytoplasmic vacuolation. The nuclei are regular, with one or more prominent nucleoli. The blasts are Tdt-negative and may be associated with t(2;8), t(8;14), or t(8;22) chromosomal abnormalities

---

The BMT Data Book, Third Edition, ed. Reinhold Munker et al. Published by Cambridge University Press. © Cambridge University Press 2013.

Immune phenotype classification

ALL is also classified on the basis of the cell surface immune phenotype:

- T-ALL
- B-ALL, also designated as mature ALL
- Pre-B-ALL
- Pre-pre-B-ALL (or pro-B-ALL)

Note: "Null ALL" (CD10-, non-B, non-T, with expression of early B-cell antigens, e.g., CD19) predominantly represents pre-pre-B-ALL. The term "null ALL" is no longer in use.

Many conventional chemotherapy protocols for ALL currently stratify treatment according to risk status. This status, in turn, is determined by the immune phenotype and cytogenetic abnormality present.

Immune phenotype of ALL

Type	HLA-DR	Tdt	CD10	CD19	CyIg	SIg	CD7	cyCD3	Frequency (%) Adults	Children
Pre-pre-B-ALL	+	+	0/+	+*	0	0	0	0	55–65	75
Pre-B-ALL	+	+	+	+*	+	0	0	0	10	15
T-ALL	0	+	0/+	0	0	0	+#	+	20–25	10

CD, cluster of differentiation; CyIg, cytoplasmic immunoglobulin; SIg, surface immunoglobulin; cyCD3, cytoplasmic CD3; * as accessory markers for B lineage CD79a and/or CD22 are useful; # accessory markers for T lineage are CD1a, CD2, and (surface) CD3.

Prognostic factors

As for AML, therapeutic decision making must include consideration of prognostic factors.

Prognostic factors for outcome with conventional therapy in adults

Better prognosis	Worse prognosis
Younger age (especially 2–10 years)	Infants, older age
Hyperdiploidy	Hypodiploidy
t(12;21)	t(9;22), t(4;11), t(1;19), del (11q23), BAALC+, MLL/AF4 rearranged, complex karyotypes, possibly CD20 positivity
No coexpression of myeloid or stem cell marker	Coexpression of CD13, CD20, CD33, and/or CD34
WBC at diagnosis <30 × 10⁹/L	WBC at diagnosis >30 × 10⁹/L or >100 × 10⁹/L in T-ALL
Time to induce CR1 <4 weeks	Time to induce CR1 >4 weeks
No CNS leukemia	CNS leukemia
No MRD	Persistence of MRD

MRD, minimal residual disease.

Results with conventional therapy in adults

Risk factor	CR1 (%)	DFS (%)
Age <60 years	80	40
Age >60 years	50	10–25
t(9;22) or bcr/abl +*	80	20–50

* With treatments incorporating TKIs.

Clinical relevance of MRD in adult ALL

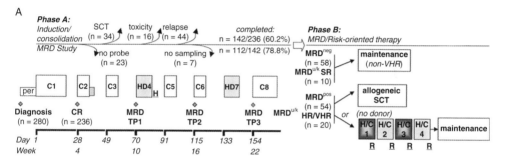

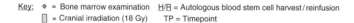

Key: ◆ = Bone marrow examination   H/R = Autologous blood stem cell harvest / reinfusion
☐ = Cranial irradiation (18 Gy)   TP = Timepoint

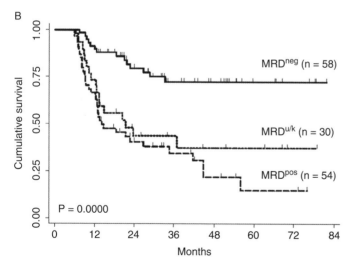

In this study from Italy, 280 patients with adult ALL (median age, 38 years) were investigated for MRD. The treatment sequence is outlined in (A). Patients with t(9;22) or t(4;11) were referred early for allogeneic transplant. MRD was investigated by real-time quantitative PCR at 10, 16, and 22 weeks with one or several sensitive probes. Among the 142 patients eligible for MRD at the end of consolidation, 54 were positive, 58 were negative, and 30 were not evaluable. As shown in (B), the DFS of MRD-positive and MRD-negative patients was clearly different. (Reproduced with permission from Bassan et al., 2009.)

Adolescents with acute lymphoblastic leukemia: outcome on U.K. national pediatric (ALL97) and adult (UKALLXII/ E2993) trials

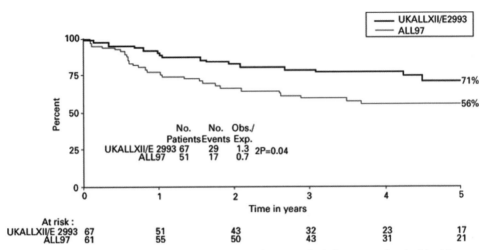

Overall survival of patients with ALL aged 15–17 years entered into a pediatric (upper curve) and adult trial (lower curve). This study shows that adolescents have a better outcome on the more aggressive pediatric protocols. (Reproduced with permission from Ramanujachar et al., 2007.)

Outcome of 609 adults after relapse of ALL: an MRC UKALL12/ECOG 2993 study

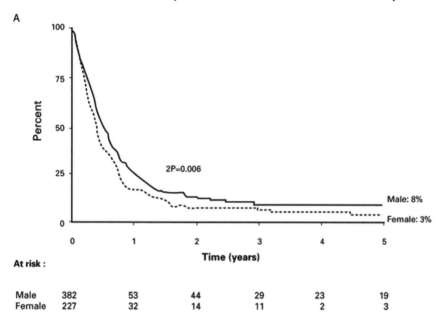

A

At risk :

Male	382	53	44	29	23	19
Female	227	32	14	11	2	3

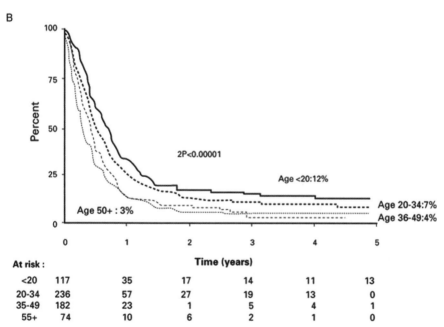

B

At risk :

<20	117	35	17	14	11	13
20-34	236	57	27	19	13	0
35-49	182	23	1	5	4	1
55+	74	10	6	2	1	0

Probabilities of survival from first relapse: an analysis of prognostic factors. A: gender; B: age at diagnosis. (Reproduced with permission from Fielding et al., 2007.)

It is clear from these curves and the following publication that the outcome of relapsed ALL is poor even for young adults; therefore, every attempt should be made to induce a lasting remission.

Probability of survival according to therapy given in relapse (patients who died within 100 days of relapse and who had undergone prior transplantation in first remission were excluded from this analysis)

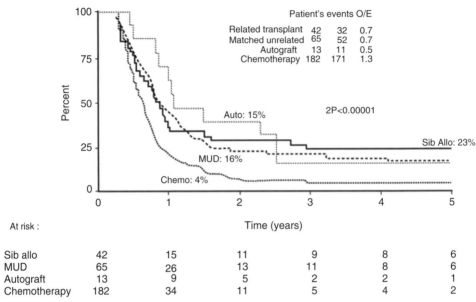

In this large study from two continents, the OS of adult patients after relapse is disappointingly low (7%).
Only a selected group of patients who were able to get a hematopoietic stem cell transplant after relapse became long-term survivors. (Reproduced with permission from Fielding et al., 2007.)

Results with allogeneic transplant
CIBMTR data

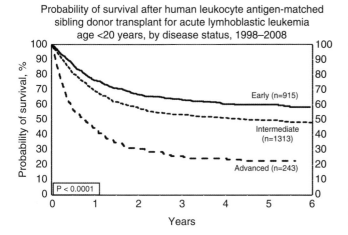

Probability of survival after human leukocyte antigen-matched sibling donor transplant for acute lymphoblastic leukemia age <20 years, by disease status, 1998–2008

Early (n=915)
Intermediate (n=1313)
Advanced (n=243)
P < 0.0001

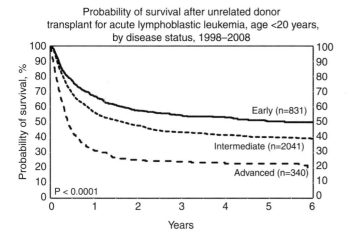

Probability of survival after unrelated donor transplant for acute lymphoblastic leukemia, age <20 years, by disease status, 1998–2008

Early (n=831)
Intermediate (n=2041)
Advanced (n=340)
P < 0.0001

Among young patients with ALL, for whom chemotherapy has a high success rate, allogeneic transplantation is generally reserved for patients with high-risk disease (i.e., high leukocyte count at diagnosis and the presence of poor-risk cytogenetic markers), who fail to achieve remission or who relapse after chemotherapy. Among the 2471 patients younger than 20 years of age receiving an HLA-matched sibling transplant, the three-year probabilities of survival were 63%±2%, 54%±2%, and 26%±3% for patients with early, intermediate, and advanced disease, respectively. The corresponding probabilities of survival among the 3212 recipients of an unrelated donor transplant were 55%±2%, 44%±1%, and 24% ±2%. (CIBMTR data and graph provided by Tanya Pedersen; reproduced with permission.)

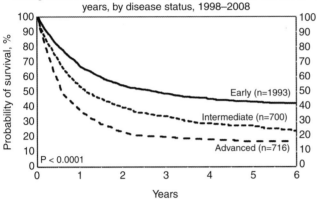

Probability of survival after human leukocyte antigen-matched sibling donor transplant for acute lymphoblastic leukemia, age ≥ 20 years, by disease status, 1998–2008

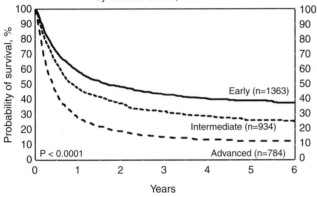

Probability of survival after unrelated donor transplant for acute lymphoblastic leukemia, age ≥20 years, by disease status, 1998–2008

Older age at disease onset is a high-risk factor in ALL. Consequently, a larger proportion of ALL patients 20 years of age or older undergo an allogeneic transplant early in the disease process. Among 3409 patients ≥20 years of age receiving an HLA-matched sibling transplant, the three-year survival probabilities were 49%±1%, 34% ±2%, and 20%±2% for patients with early, intermediate, and advanced disease, respectively. Corresponding probabilities among the 3081 recipients of an unrelated donor transplant were 43%±2%, 32%±2%, and 15%±2%. (CIBMTR data and graph provided by Tanya Pedersen; reproduced with permission.)

Chemotherapy versus HLA-identical sibling bone marrow transplants for adults with ALL in first remission

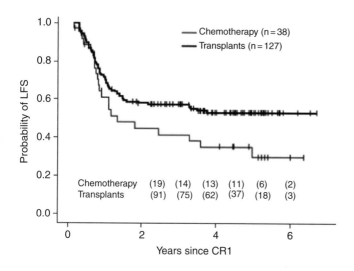

Probability of LFS for adults with ALL in first remission, mean age ≤30 years. Numbers in parentheses indicate number of patients still at risk at 1, 2, 3, 4, 5, and 6 years since first remission.

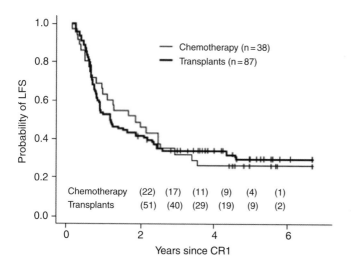

Probability of LFS for adults with ALL in first remission, age >30 years. Numbers in parentheses indicate number of patients still at risk at 1, 2, 3, 4, 5, and 6 years since first remission.
In this study from the Japanese Adult Leukemia Study Group, the OS was significantly worse in younger patients (≤30 years) treated with chemotherapy than with a matched related bone marrow transplant. In the older age group (>30 years) the results with chemotherapy were better. (Reproduced with permission from Oh et al., 1998.)

No disadvantage in outcome of using matched unrelated donors as compared with matched sibling donors for BMT in children with ALL in second remission

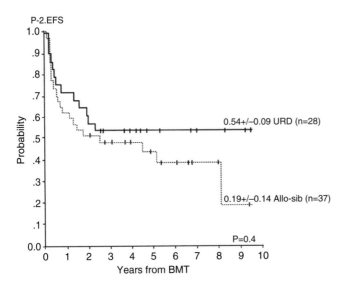

In this Scandinavian study, 65 pediatric patients with ALL in CR2 underwent allogeneic BMT. Of the allografts, 37 came from HLA-matched siblings and 28 from URD. The survival of both groups was equivalent, although higher rates of acute and chronic GVHD were observed in the URD group. (Reproduced with permission from Saarinen-Pihkala et al., 2001.)

Addendum: with improved typing techniques, the outcomes of matched unrelated transplants is comparable to matched related transplants even for adults (Sellar et al., 2011).

Better outcome of adult ALL after early genoidentical allogeneic BMT than after late high-dose therapy and autologous BMT: a GOELAMS trial

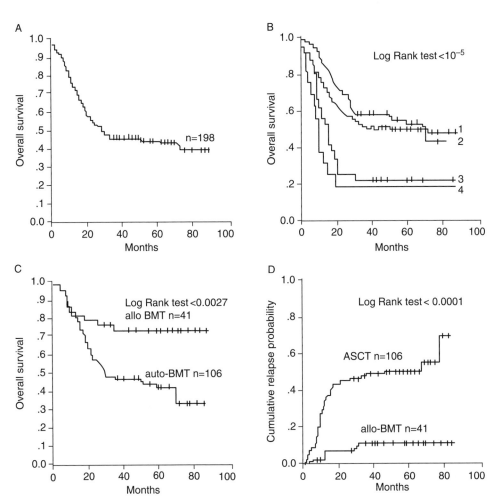

One hundred and ninety-eight patients with high-risk ALL received induction chemotherapy with vincristine, idarubicine, L-asparaginase, and steroids. High risk was defined as age >35 years, non-T-ALL, WBC >30 × 10^9/L, t(9;22), t(4;11) or t(1;19), or failure to achieve CR after one induction course. Patients who had a matched related donor received an allograft after two consolidation courses, whereas patients who did not have a donor or who were older than 50 years received an autologous transplant after one additional cycle of reinduction chemotherapy. The OS of the entire population is shown in (A); the OS according to the number of adverse prognostic factors in (B); the OS in (C); and the relapse probability between both groups in (D). (Reproduced with permission from Hunault et al., 2004.)

Comparable long-term survival after unrelated and HLA-matched sibling donor hematopoietic SCT for ALL in children younger than 18 months old

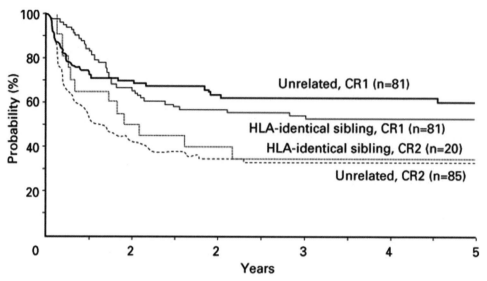

Adjusted probabilities of OS in infant leukemia. (Reproduced with permission from Eapen et al., 2006.)

Indications for transplant
HLA-identical family member transplant

Indication	DFS (%)
1. Patient older than 12 years, younger than 56 years, with ALL in CR1, if one or more adverse risk factors are present	45–75
2. ALL in CR2 or subsequent CR * (patient <56 years)	10–30
3. Primary refractory ALL (patient <56 years)	10–20
4. Ph-positive (or BCR/ABL-positive) ALL in first CR (patient <56 years)	30–40

* indication for allogeneic transplant in CR1 is controversial and will evolve as new treatments and new markers for risk become available. (See also Goldstone, 2009 and Larson, 2009.)

Autologous blood/marrow SCT

There are no general indications; autologous transplant is used only in special cases or in studies in patients younger than 66 years, for example, with CR1 cells cryopreserved, who cannot tolerate a two- to three-year maintenance therapy.

Indication	DFS (%)
1. ALL in CR1	30–40
2. ALL in CR2	10–20

HLA-identical unrelated donor transplant

Used for patients younger than 51 years, with no matched related donor available.

Indication	DFS (%)
1. Ph-positive ALL in CR1	20–40
2. ALL beyond CR1	20–40

Special aspects of transplants in children

The benefit of allogeneic SCT (matched related or matched unrelated) was demonstrated in very high-risk ALL over chemotherapy alone in CR1; the benefit in CR2 or subsequent remission was also demonstrated in most studies, but there is not sufficient data for use of auto-SCT. TBI-containing regimens are considered superior to non-TBI-containing regimens (Hahn et al., 2006b).

Contraindications to transplant

1. Patient beyond CR2.
2. General contraindications to transplant.

Pretransplant workup

1. Evaluation of PB and BM:

    - Morphology
    - Cytochemistry
    - Immune phenotype
    - Cytogenetics (and molecular testing, as appropriate)
    - Testing for minimal residual disease if available
2. See the general pretransplant workup (page 239).

Monitoring posttransplant

Do a bone marrow aspirate, with cytogenetic evaluation (and immunological and molecular evaluation of minimal residual disease, as appropriate) at 1, 3, 12, and 24 months.

Treatment algorithm for adult patients with newly diagnosed ALL

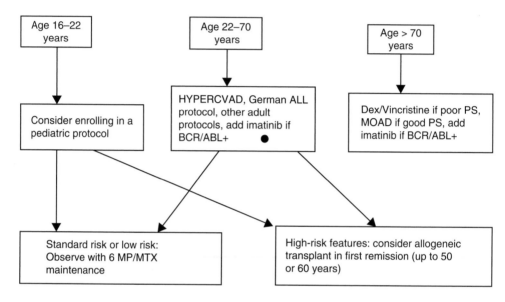

Enroll on clinical trial if eligible and informed consent is obtained

- Age 16–22 years
- Age 22–70 years
- Age > 70 years

Consider enrolling in a pediatric protocol

HYPERCVAD, German ALL protocol, other adult protocols, add imatinib if BCR/ABL+   ●

Dex/Vincristine if poor PS, MOAD if good PS, add imatinib if BCR/ABL+

Standard risk or low risk: Observe with 6 MP/MTX maintenance

High-risk features: consider allogeneic transplant in first remission (up to 50 or 60 years)

● General recommendations: reduce dose of cytarabine if patient is older than 60 years, give anthracyclines only if LVEF is appropriate, give CNS prophylaxis (8 LP if low-risk, 16 LP if high-risk)

Recent data indicate that patients with Ph+ ALL benefit from posttransplant TKIs. In older patients with ALL in CR1, a reduced-intensity condition may be a feasible option.

References and further reading

Bassan R & Hoelzer D. 2011. Modern therapy of acute lymphoblastic leukemia. *J Clin Oncol* 29: 532–543.

Bassan R, Spinelli O, Oldani E, et al. 2009. Improved risk classification for risk-specific therapy based on the molecular study of minimal residual disease (MRD) in adult acute lymphoblastic leukemia (ALL). *Blood* 113: 4153–4162.

Eapen M, Rubenstein P, Zhang MJ, et al. 2006. Comparable survival after HLA-matched sibling donor hematopoietic stem cell transplantations for acute leukemia in children younger than 18 months. *J Clin Oncol* 24: 145–151.

Fielding AK, Richards SM, Chopra R, et al. 2007. Outcome of 609 adults after relapse of acute lymphoblastic leukemia (ALL); an MRC UKALL12/ECOG 2993 study. *Blood* 109: 944–950.

Goldstone AH. 2009. Transplants adult ALL – ?
Allo for everyone. *Biol Blood Marrow
Transplant* **15**: S7–S10.

Hahn T, Wall D, Camitta B, et al. 2006a. The
role of cytotoxic therapy with hematopoietic
stem cell transplantation in the therapy of
acute lymphoblastic leukemia in adults: an
evidence-based review. *Biol Blood Marrow
Transplant* **12**: 1–30.

Hahn T, Wall D, & Camitta B. 2006b. ASBMT
position statement. The role of cytotoxic
therapy with hematopoietic stem cell
transplantation in the treatment of acute
lymphoblastic leukemia in children. *Biol
Blood Marrow Transplant* **12**: 370–371.

Hunault M, Harousseau Jl, Delain M, et al. 2004.
Better outcome of adult acute lymphoblastic
leukemia after early genoidentical allogeneic
bone marrow transplantation (BMT) than
after late high-dose therapy and autologous
BMT: a GOELAMS trial. *Blood*
104: 3028–3037.

Khaled SK, Thomas SH, & Forman SJ. 2012.
Allogeneic hematopoietic cell transplantation
for acute lymphoblastic leukemia in adults.
Curr Opin Oncol **24**: 182–190.

Larson RA. 2009. Allogeneic hematopoietic cell
transplantation is not recommended for all
adults with standard-risk acute lymphoblastic
leukemia in first complete remission. *Biol
Blood Marrow Transplant* **15**: 11–16.

Marks DI, Aversa F, & Lazarus HM. 2006.
Alternative donor transplants for adult acute
lymphoblastic leukaemia: a comparison of
the three major options. *Bone Marrow
Transplant* **38**: 467–475.

Mato AR & Luger SM. 2006. Autologous stem
cell transplant in ALL: who should we be
transplanting in first remission? *Bone
Marrow Transplant* **37**: 989–995.

Oh H, Gale RP, Zhang MJ, et al. 1998.
Chemotherapy vs HLA-identical sibling bone
marrow transplants for adults with acute
lymphoblastic leukemia in first remission.
Bone Marrow Transplant **22**:
253–257.

Pui CH & Evans WE. 2006. Treatment of acute
lymphoblastic leukemia. *N Engl J Med* **354**:
166–178.

Ramanujachar R, Richards S, Hann I, et al. 2007.
Adolescents with acute lymphoblastic
leukemia: outcome on UK National
Paediatric (ALL97) and adult (UKALLXII/
E2993) trials. *Pediatr Blood Cancer*
48: 254–261.

Saarinen-Pihkala UM, Gustafsson G, Ringdén
O, et al. 2001. No disadvantage in outcome
of using matched unrelated donors as
compared with matched sibling donors for
bone marrow transplantation in children
with acute lymphoblastic leukemia in
second remission. *J Clin Oncol*
19: 3406–3414.

Sellar R, Goldstone AH, & Lazarus HM. 2011.
Redefining transplant in acute leukemia.
Curr Treat Options Oncol **12**: 312–328.

Chapter

5 Therapeutic decision making in BMT/SCT for chronic myeloid leukemia and other myeloproliferative syndromes

Reinhold Munker, Hillard M. Lazarus, and Kerry Atkinson

Classification of chronic myeloid leukemia (CML)

Clinical variants of CML:

1. Typical CML (Philadelphia chromosome present, BCR/ABL-positive [94%])
2. Atypical CML (Philadelphia chromosome absent, BCR/ABL-positive [4%])
3. Atypical BCR/ABL negative CML (Philadelphia chromosome absent, BCR/ABL-negative [2%])

The BMT Data Book, Third Edition, ed. Reinhold Munker et al. Published by Cambridge University Press. © Cambridge University Press 2013.

Staging of CML

Chronic phase:

1. No significant symptoms
2. None of the features of accelerated phase or blastic phase
3. Sensitive to tyrosine kinase inhibitors (TKIs) (most newly diagnosed cases, see page 64)
4. Resistant to TKIs

Accelerated phase (any one or more of the following criteria):

1. WBC count difficult to control with conventional use of TKI or busulfan/hydroxyurea in terms of doses required
2. Rapid doubling of WBC count (≥ 5 days)
3. $\geq 10\%$ blasts in blood or marrow
4. $\geq 20\%$ blasts plus promyelocytes in blood or marrow
5. $\geq 20\%$ basophils plus eosinophils in blood
6. Anemia or thrombocytopenia unresponsive to TKI
7. Persistent thrombocytosis
8. Additional chromosome changes (evolving new clone)
9. Increasing splenomegaly
10. Development of chloromas or myelofibrosis
11. Patient in a second (or subsequent) chronic phase after blast crisis

Blastic phase:

1. $\geq 30\%$ blasts plus promyelocytes in blood or bone marrow

Prognostic factors for outcome with conventional chemotherapy

Historically, the following factors indicated a poor prognosis (with hydroxyurea or busulfan):

- Marked splenomegaly
- High circulating numbers of blast cells
- High platelet count ($>700 \times 10^9$/L)
- Blood or marrow basophilia (basophils plus eosinophils $>15\%$)
- Ph negativity
- Older age

EBMT risk score (based on risk factors for allogeneic SCT)

Risk factor	Score and description
Disease phase	0 if chronic phase, 1 if accelerated phase, 2 if blast crisis
Age	0 if <20 years, 1 if 20–40 years, 2 if >40 years
Interval from diagnosis	0 if ≤ 1 year; 1 if >1 year
Donor-recipient gender match	1 if female donor and male recipient; 0 for any other match

Score 0–2, low risk; score 3 or 4, intermediate; score 5–6, high risk.

Definitions of hematologic, cytogenetic, and molecular responses
Commonly used definitions of hematologic and cytogenetic responses

Term	Definition
Complete hematologic remission	WBC $<10 \times 10^9$/L; platelets $<450 \times 10^9$/L; no splenomegaly
Partial hematologic remission	Counts improved but not normal, basophils $<5\%$, no immature cells in PB
Complete cytogenetic response	Absence of Philadelphia chromosome, with at least 20 metaphases studied
Major cytogenetic response	Suppression of Philadelphia chromosome to $<35\%$ of metaphases
Minor cytogenetic response	Suppression of Philadelphia chromosome to 36%–65% of metaphases
Major molecular response	Ratio of BCR/ABL to ABL (or other housekeeping genes) $\leq 0.1\%$ on the international scale
Molecular remission	Undetectable BCR/ABL mRNA transcripts by real-time quantitative and/or nested PCR in two consecutive blood samples of adequate quality

Results with standard therapy

With the introduction of α-IFN into the conventional management of CML, it was possible to obtain cytogenetic remissions in a proportion of patients for the first time. With the introduction of imatinib (and other TKIs), it is now also possible to obtain molecular remissions in a proportion of patients. The current standard treatment is 400 mg imatinib orally. In patients who do not respond, the dose of imatinib may be increased to 600 or 800 mg, or alternative TKIs (dasatinib, nilotinib), or experimental treatments should be used. (See treatment algorithm and indication for allogeneic transplant in a subsequent section.) There are data that patients with intermediate- or high-risk benefit from a second generation TKI (nilotinib 300 mg twice daily or dasatinib 100 mg daily). The previous standard treatment (IFN-α and hydroxyurea) has no role in first-line treatment but can be used if other agents are not available or if an urgent cytoreduction is needed.

Five-year follow-up of patients receiving imatinib for CML

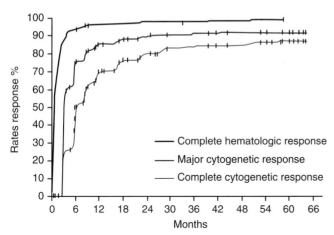

Graph showing Kaplan–Meier estimates of the cumulative best response to initial imatinib therapy. At 12 months after the initiation of imatinib, the estimated rates of having a response were: complete hematologic response, 96%; major cytogenetic response, 85%; and complete cytogenetic response, 69%. At 60 months, the respective rates were 98%, 92%, and 87%, respectively. Data for patients who discontinued imatinib for reasons other than progression, and who did not have an adequate response, were censored at the last follow-up visit. Data for patients who did not have an adequate response and who stopped imatinib because of progression were censored at maximum follow-up. In this randomized clinical trial, 553 patients were treated with imatinib and followed for at least five years. About 7% had progressed to blast crisis or accelerated phase. Patients who had a complete cytogenetic response or whose BCR/ABL transcript levels had fallen by at least 3 log had a significantly lower risk of disease progression than patients without a complete cytogenetic response. The estimated OS was 89% at five years. (Reproduced with permission from Druker et al., 2006.)

Results with allogeneic transplant
CIBMTR data

Owing to the success of TKIs, the frequency of allogeneic transplantation has significantly decreased between 1998 and 2009.

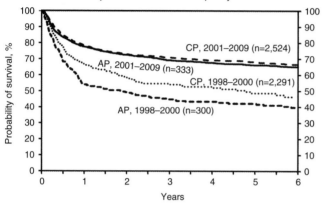

Probability of survival after human leukocyte antigen-identical sibling donor transplants for chronic myelogenous leukemia, 1998–2009
- by disease status and transplant year -

CML is no longer the most common indication for allotransplants, although it remains a curative option for patients who failed or who tolerate TKIs poorly. The CIBMTR has data for 5448 HLA-matched sibling donor allotransplants for CML, 2591 from 1998 to 2000 and 2857 from 2001 to 2009. Among patients in the chronic phase (CP), the three-year probability of survival was 69%±1% and 70%±1% for transplants performed in the periods 1998 to 2000 and 2001 to 2009, respectively. Corresponding three-year survival probabilities for patients in the accelerated phase (AP) were 45%±3% and 54%±3%. (Data kindly provided by Tanya Pedersen and Zhiwei Wang [CIBMTR, website accessed 2/18/2012].)

Results of allogeneic transplantation for CML patients who failed TKIs

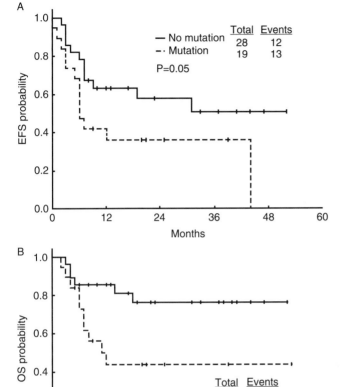

In a recent series of 47 patients who had failed imatinib and received an allogeneic stem cell transplant (allo-SCT), most (89%) responded. At the time of transplant, 34 patients were in the chronic phase, nine in the accelerated phase, and four in blast crisis. Mutations in the *BCR-ABL1* kinase domain were found in 40% of the entire group. About half of the patients received a matched related and half a matched unrelated transplant. The event-free survival (EFS) (A) and OS (B) were clearly different depending on the mutational status, with mutation positivity conferring a worse prognosis. (Reproduced with permission from Jabbour et al., 2011.)

Donor lymphocyte infusions (DLI) for relapse of CML after allogeneic transplant

DLIs are effective for relapsed CML after allogeneic transplant and can induce permanent remissions in the majority of patients relapsing in the chronic phase. DLIs can, however, be associated with significant complications (GVHD, pancytopenia, infections).

DLI for relapsed CML: prognostic relevance of the initial cell dose

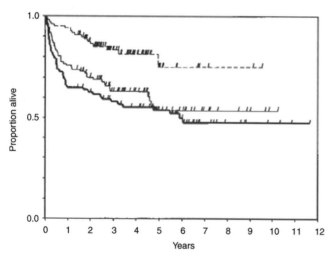

The probability of survival was studied in 344 patients treated with donor lymphocytes for relapsed CML after an allogeneic transplantation. The upper group received an initial dose of $\leq 0.2 \times 10^8$ mononuclear cells/kg, the middle group 0.21×10^8 to 2.0×10^8 mononuclear cells/kg, and the lower group $>2.0 \times 10^8$ mononuclear cells/kg. It was concluded from this study that a stepwise approach should be used, starting with a low dose and repeating DLI according to efficacy and development of GVHD. The outcome of DLI also depends to a large extent on the stage at relapse, with patients who relapse in blast crisis coming into remission less frequently than patients who relapse in the chronic phase. (Reproduced with permission from Guglielimi et al., 2002.)

The serial measurement of BCR/ABL transcripts in the PB of patients after an allo-SCT appears helpful in determining which patients are likely to relapse and need additional treatment like DLI. Kaeda et al. (2006) measured BCR/ABL transcript levels with a sensitive quantitative real-time PCR and developed four categories: (1) persistent negativity; (2) fluctuating, low-level positivity; (3) persistent low-level positivity; and (4) molecular or cytogenetic relapse. Most patients who had molecular relapse progressed further. Especially in the first six months after transplant, categories [2] and [3] do not exclude patients from being cured, whereas in category [4] other treatments (DLI, TKIs, other new agents) should be considered.

Results with allogeneic transplant for CML in children

A group of experts recently published recommendations for children with CML. As in adults, TKIs are considered as the standard approach for CML in the chronic phase. Patients who fail the "landmark" responses, are resistant to TKIs, or present in the accelerated phase or blast crisis should be evaluated for allogeneic transplantation. A full-intensity stem cell transplantation is considered as optimal in the pediatric population (Andolina et al., 2012).

Results with autologous transplant for CML

A meta-analysis of six trials evaluating autologous transplant followed by INF-α in comparison to only IFN-α showed no survival advantage (CML autografts trials collaboration,

2006). Therefore, at present, autografts for CML should not be performed outside of clinical trials. Owing to the activity of imatinib, it is now possible to harvest and store autologous stem cells in molecular remission, which then may be used in future clinical trials in molecular, cytogenetic, or clinical relapse.

Results with reduced-intensity allogeneic transplant for CML

Crawley et al. (2005) surveyed patients in the EBMT database who received a reduced-intensity transplant for CML from the EBMT database. The TRM at 100 days was 6.1%. The OS at three years was 58%, and the progression-free survival (PFS) was 37%. The best results were observed in patients in the chronic phase and in those conditioned with busulfan, fludarabine, and antithymocyte globulin (ATG). These results show that a reduced-intensity transplant is feasible in CML, but the outcome may be inferior to the results obtained with a standard allogeneic transplant in the past, because now most patients have failed TKIs and most also have a contraindication to a myeloablative transplant.

Results with allogeneic transplant for myeloproliferative syndromes (MPS) other than CML

The prognosis and clinical presentation of other myeloproliferative disorders is more variable; therefore, no universal recommendations can be given. Truly BCR/ABL-negative CML and chronic myelomonocytic leukemia generally have an aggressive clinical course and are considered as an indication for allogeneic transplantation. The rationale and results of allogeneic transplants for idiopathic myelofibrosis were reviewed by Papageorgiou et al. (2006). Selected younger patients had a high-risk myelofibrosis and a matched donor benefit from an allogeneic transplant following RIC. In a recent communication from Seattle, a d100 mortality of 13% and a seven-year actuarial survival of 61% for matched related and unrelated transplants was reported (Deeg et al., 2011).

Based on these results, Scott et al. (2012) evaluated the usefulness of the "Dynamic International Prognostic Scoring System" to predict outcome after allogeneic transplantation. This index takes age, constitutional symptoms, hemoglobin, leukocyte count, and circulating blasts into account. These data are based on 170 patients transplanted in Seattle between 1990 and 2009. Eighty-six patients were transplanted from related donors and 84 from unrelated donors. Overall, allogeneic transplant can cure idiopathic myelofibrosis, but is associated with significant toxicity, especially in the advanced stages. The following figure shows the long-term survival, relapse-free survival, and NRM among these patients (reproduced with permission). The authors recommend considering patients with high-risk and intermediate-risk 2 for allogeneic transplantation.

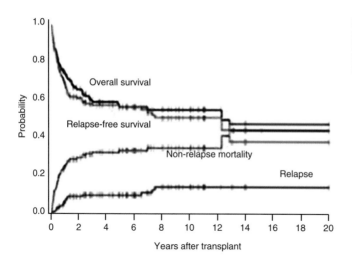

Long-term outcome of 170 patients transplanted for idiopathic myelofibrosis. (Reproduced with permission from Scott et al., 2012.)

Indications for allogeneic transplant in CML (recommendations of the European Leukemia NET)

Treatment failure of imatinib, no contraindication for allogeneic transplant, HLA-matched donor available.

Treatment failure as defined:

At 3 months: no hematologic response.

At 6 months: complete hematologic response and no cytogenetic response.

At 12 months: (defined as >35% Ph + metaphases) less than partial cytogenetic response.

At 18 months: less than a complete cytogenetic response.

If, at any point, a complete hematologic or cytogenetic response is lost or highly resistant BCR/ABL mutations appear.

Relative indication in the case of a suboptimal response, is defined as:

At 3 months: no cytogenetic response.

At 6 months: less than partial cytogenetic response.

At 12 months: less than complete cytogenetic response.

At 18 months: less than a major molecular response, and at any point if a major molecular response is lost, or other mutations or other chromosomal abnormalities appear.

(Modified from Baccarani et al., 2009.)

Algorithm for the treatment of CML

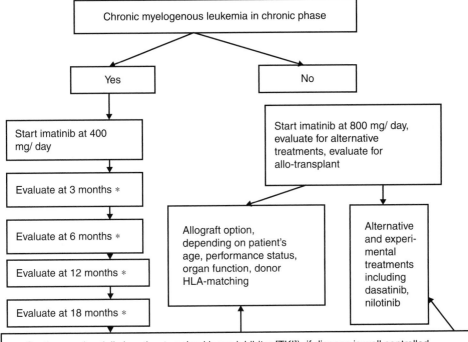

* Continue on imatinib (or other tyrosine kinase inhibitor [TKI]), if disease is well controlled (see page 64 for criteria for imatinib failure)
* Switch to other TKI if not controlled and perform allogeneic transplant if donor is available
* Evaluate for transplant if on second-line TKI and if a highly resistant mutant in BCR/ABL binding domain is identified, disease is not well controlled, and other conditions for transplant are met

Contraindications to transplant

1. Patient responding to TKIs, in molecular remission
2. Patient in uncontrolled blast crisis (poor long-term results)
3. Patient with other contraindications for transplantation (comorbid conditions)

Pretransplant workup

1. See the general pretransplant workup (page 239).
2. Bone marrow aspirate, with cytogenetic evaluation and BCR/ABL PCR testing by real-time techniques.

Monitoring posttransplant

1. Bone marrow aspirate, with cytogenetic evaluation and BCR/ABL PCR testing (standardized real-time technology), at three weeks, 12 weeks, one year, and two years posttransplant (no longer done routinely in many centers for uncomplicated transplants).
2. BCR/ABL PCR testing of blood leukocytes at 1, 3, 6, 8, 12, 16, 20, 24, 30, 36, and 48 months posttransplant with real-time quantitative PCR; longer if clinically indicated.

References and further reading

Andolina JR, Neudorf SM, & Corey SJ. 2012. How I treat: childhood CML. *Blood* **119**: 1821–1830.

Baccarani M, Cortes J, Pane F, et al. 2009. Chronic myeloid leukemia: an update of concepts and management recommendations of European Leukemia Net. *J Clin Oncol* **27**: 6041–6051.

CML Autograft Trials Collaboration. 2006. Autologous stem cell transplantation in chronic myeloid leukaemia: a meta-analysis of six randomized trials. *Cancer Treat Rev* **33**: 39–47.

Crawley C, Szydlo R, Lalancette M, et al. 2005. Outcomes of reduced intensity transplantation for chronic myeloid leukemia: an analysis of prognostic factors from the Chronic Leukemia Working Party of the EBMT. *Blood* **106**: 2969–2976.

Deeg HJ & Appelbaum FR. 2011. Indications for and current results with allogeneic hematopoietic cell transplantation in patients with myelofibrosis. *Blood* **117**: 7185.

Druker BJ, Guilhot F, O'Brien SG, et al. 2006. Five-year follow-up of patients receiving imatinib for chronic myeloid leukemia. *N Engl J Med* **355**: 2408–2417.

Guglielmi C, Arcese W, Dazzi F, et al. 2002. Donor lymphocyte infusion for relapsed chronic myelogenous leukemia. *Blood* **100**: 397–405.

Jabbour E, Cortes J, Santos FPS, et al. 2011. Results of allogeneic hematopoietic stem cell transplantation for chronic myelogenous leukemia patients who failed TKIs after developing *BCR-ABL1* kinase domain mutations. *Blood* **117**: 3641–3647.

Kaeda J, O'Shea RM, Olavarria E, et al. 2006. Serial measurement of BCR-ABL transcripts in the peripheral blood after allogeneic stem cell transplantation for CML: an attempt to define patients who may not require further therapy. *Blood* **107**: 4171–4176.

Papageorgiou SG, Castleton A, Bloor A, et al. 2006. Allogeneic stem cell transplantation as treatment for myelofibrosis. *Bone Marrow Transplant* **38**: 721–727.

Scott BL, Gooley TA, Sorror ML, et al. 2012. The dynamic international prognostic scoring system for myelofibrosis predicts outcomes after hematopoietic cell transplantation. *Blood* **119**: 2657–2664.

Therapeutic decision making in BMT/SCT for chronic lymphatic leukemia

Nebu V. Koshy, Reinhold Munker, Hillard M. Lazarus, and Kerry Atkinson

Disease staging

Rai classification

Stage	Survival (months)
Stage 0: bone marrow (40%) and blood lymphocytosis ($>4 \times 10^9$/L); no enlarged nodes	>120
Stage I: lymphocytosis with enlarged nodes	95
Stage II: lymphocytosis with enlarged spleen or liver or both	72
Stage III: lymphocytosis with anemia	30
Stage IV: lymphocytosis with thrombocytopenia	30

(Reproduced from Rai et al., 1975.)

The BMT Data Book, Third Edition, ed. Reinhold Munker et al. Published by Cambridge University Press. © Cambridge University Press 2013.

Binet classification

Stage	Survival (months)
Stage A: Hb >10/dL and platelets ≥100 × 10⁹/L; fewer than three enlarged areas[a]	>120
Stage B: Hb >10/dL and platelets ≥100 × 10⁹/L; three or more enlarged areas	61
Stage C: Hb <10/dL and/or platelets <100 × 10⁹/L; any number of enlarged areas	32

[a] the cervical, axillary, and inguinal areas (unilateral or bilateral) and the spleen and liver each count as one area; therefore, the number of enlarged areas can take any value between zero and five. (Reproduced from Binet et al., 1981.)

Immune phenotype and cytogenetic abnormalities

95% B phenotype (typical marker profile surface Ig faint, $CD3^-$, $CD5^+$, $CD10^-$, $CD19^+$, $CD20^+$ faint, $CD23^+$)

5% T-phenotype (these leukemias are no longer considered as CLL, they are classified as T-lymphoproliferative disorders.)

Cytogenetic findings
Incidence and prognostic relevance

Aberrations	Incidence	Prognosis
Total aberrations	82%	
13q deletion	55%	Favorable*
Trisomy 12	16%	Unfavorable–intermediate
11q deletion	18%	Unfavorable
17p abnormality	7%**	Unfavorable

Note: these data are based on interphase cytogenetics (fluorescence in situ hybridization [FISH]) as conventional cytogenetics does not always provide results.
* if only cytogenetic abnormality; ** incidence is 40%–50% in refractory patients.
(Reproduced from Döhner et al., 2000.)

Prognostic factors

Patients with CLL have a variable outcome with conventional treatment, ranging from a median survival of 30–40 months (Rai stage III–IV; Binet stage C) to >120 months (Rai stage 0; Binet stage A). This is important to consider when contemplating allogeneic transplantation.

Prognostic factors for outcome with conventional therapy

Better outcome	Worse outcome
Non-diffuse marrow involvement	Diffuse marrow involvement
Normal β_2 microglobulin	Elevated β_2 microglobulin
Absence of high-risk cytogenetic aberrations	Presence of high-risk cytogenetic aberrations (see previous table)
Ig V_H genes mutated	Ig V_H genes germ line ($\geq$98% IgV_H homology)
ZAP-70 negative*	ZAP-70 elevated* (>20% cells positive)
CD38 negative	CD38 positive (>30% of cells positive)
Absence of p53-mutation	Presence of mutated p53 (15% of cases)
Slower lymphocyte doubling time	Faster lymphocyte doubling time
Low miR-15a and miR-16–1	Low miR-29 and miR-181**

* ZAP-70 not universally standardized and reproducible; ** associated with high level expression of the TCL1 gene (Calin et al., 2007).

Results with conventional therapy

- Indications for treatment

Debilitating constitutional symptoms, Stages III or IV or Binet B or C, rapid disease progression even in earlier stages, progressive cytopenia, refractory autoimmune anemia or thrombocytopenia, progressive or massive hepatosplenomegaly or lymphadenopathy, recurrent infections (International Workshop on Chronic Lymphocytic Leukemia [IWCLL] criteria).

- Outcome

Treatment with alkylating agents alone has not changed the natural history; five-year survival is 68%, but newer treatments have improved the outcome.

- Chlorambucil treatment

6–8 mg/d or 15–20 mg/m^2 every two weeks or 30–40 mg/m^2 monthly (comment: alkylator treatment is now rarely used; however, chlorambucil may be the preferred treatment in elderly patients).

Chemoimmunotherapy improves PFS over chemotherapy

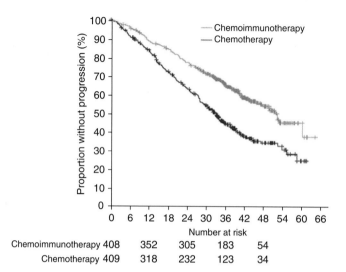

In this study, 817 untreated patients with CD20-positive CLL were randomized; 409 patients were allocated to chemotherapy (fludarabine-cyclophosphamide) and 408 patients were allocated to chemoimmunotherapy (fludarabine–cyclophosphamide–rituxan [FCR]). Chemoimmunotherapy, according to this study, improved progression-free and OS. (Reproduced with permission from Hallek et al., 2010.) (See following treatment recommendations.)

Chemoimmunotherapy 408	352	305	183	54
Chemotherapy 409	318	232	123	34

Treatment recommendations and factors used to determine first-line therapy

Important are: stage of the disease, fitness of the patient, and genetic characteristics (FISH) of the leukemic clone.

1. Patients at the early stage (Binet A and B, Rai 0-II) without symptoms usually do not require therapy; early treatment is currently tested in clinical trials for patients at high risk.

2. In patients with advanced (Binet C, Rai III-IV) or active, symptomatic disease, treatment should be initiated.

3. For patients in good physical condition ("go go"), as defined by normal creatinine clearance and low comorbidity score, FCR combination or similar chemoimmunotherapy should be offered.

4. Patients with relevant comorbidity ("slow go") may be treated with chorambucil. Alternatives are bendamustine or a dose-reduced fludarabine-containing regimen to achieve symptom control.

5. Patients with symptomatic disease and with del17p or p53 mutations respond poorly to fludarabine or FC, and show a response rate of approximately 50% to alemtuzumab monotherapy or to FCR, but these responses usually have a short duration of a few months to one or two years. These patients should be evaluated for allo-SCT in first remission.

6. New treatments like Bruton's tyrosine kinase (BTK) inhibitors are under development.

Results with allogeneic transplant

Autologous compared with allogeneic SCT for poor-risk chronic lymphatic leukemia (CLL) (overall survival)

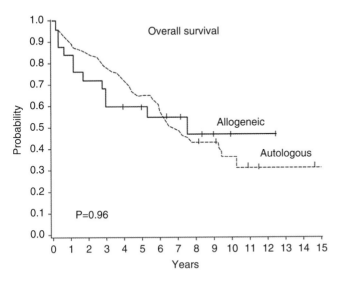

The long-term follow-up of 162 patients with high-risk CLL who underwent an auto-SCT (n=137) and T-cell depleted allo-SCT (n=25) was reported by Gribben et al. (2005). The OS of both groups was not different. Most patients treated with donor lymphocytes after relapse from an allogeneic transplant responded, demonstrating a significant graft-versus-leukemia (GVL) effect. (Reproduced with permission from Gribben et al., 2005.)

Non-myeloablative transplantation for advanced CLL
Outcome after non-myeloablative transplantation for CLL

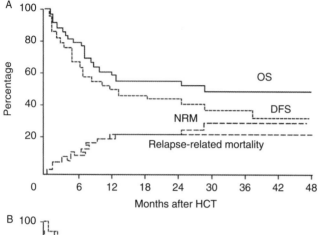

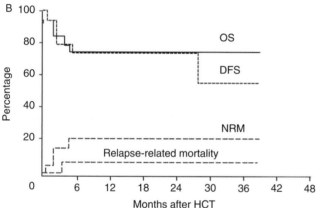

Sixty-four patients with advanced CLL were treated with non-myeloablative conditioning with or without fludarabine (n=53; n=11). Forty-four donors were related, 20 unrelated. Sixty-one patients had sustained engraftment. Among patients with measurable disease, an overall response of 67% was observed. The cumulative incidence of NRM, relapse-related mortality, and OS are shown in the figure (A: related recipients; B: unrelated recipients). (Reproduced with permission from Sorror et al., 2005.)

Results with autologous transplant

In a Finnish multicenter study (Jantunen et al., 2006), 72 patients with CLL received an autologous transplant between 1995 and 2005. No early treatment-related deaths were observed. The projected survival free from progression in this study was 48 months. Currently, autologous SCT has no established role in the treatment of CLL.

Special problems in transplantation for CLL

1. Prior fludarabine treatment can
   - Render the marrow hypocellular and impair autologous harvest. Therefore, in patients who are considered candidates for an autologous SCT, a collection should be scheduled after the first-line treatment response; however, an interval of 2–3 months after the last dose of fludarabine should be planned
   - Accentuate posttransplant T-cell deficiency

2. Autoimmune phenomena (e.g., hemolytic anemia or thrombocytopenia) may recur after autologous or allogeneic transplant despite continuing morphologic remission.
3. Richter's transformation to aggressive non–Hodgkin lymphoma (NHL) may occur after autologous transplant.
4. The time to CR posttransplant may be prolonged. Posttransplant lymphocytosis may occur but be polyclonal.
5. Consider giving weekly IV Ig at 400–500 mg/kg until day 84 posttransplant for hypogammaglobulinemic patients, to minimize infection risk due to humoral immune deficiency.

CIBMTR data for CLL

Probability of survival after autologous and HLA-matched sibling donor hematopoietic cell transplantation for chronic lymphocytic leukemia, 2000–2009 by donor type and conditioning regimen intensity

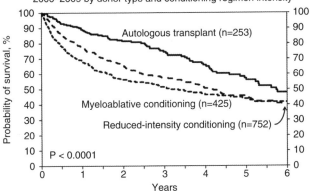

Both autologous and allogeneic transplants are treatment options for CLL patients who fail standard chemotherapy or have high-risk features (e.g., cytogenetic abnormalities, short remission intervals). The use of RIC regimens for allogeneic transplant continues to increase in this population. Among the 1430 patients who underwent transplantation for CLL, the three-year probabilities of survival were 74% ± 3% after autologous transplant, 51% ± 3% after an HLA-matched sibling transplant with a myeloablative conditioning regimen, and 57% ± 2% after an HLA-matched sibling transplant with a RIC regimen. (Data kindly provided by Tanya Pedersen and Zhiwei Wang [CIBMTR, 2/7/2012].)

Results of allogeneic transplants in different series

(Reduced-intensity conditioning, modified from Brown, 2011.)

Currently available, conventional therapies have limited efficacy in refractory or resistant patients. PFS is short even in responders. Remission needs to be consolidated. Autologous SCT is not curative. Myeloablative SCT has long-term DFS of 30%–40% but also a NRM in the range of 20%–40%. RIC SCT offers potential for cure, but has a NRM of 16%–32%. Relapse remains a problem with RIC, particularly in patients with active disease at the time of SCT. The best option is to employ RIC early in the disease course.

	Dreger et al. (2010)	Khouri et al. (2011)	Sorror et al. (2010)	Brown et al. (2008, 2011)
N	90	86	136	84
Conditioning	FC-based +/− ATG	FCR primarily	2GyTBI + F	FB
PFS	42% EFS @ 4 y	36% @ 5 y	32% @ 5 y	51% @ 4 y
OS	65% @ 4 y	51% @ 5 y	41% @ 5 y	65% @ 4 y
NRM	23% @ 4 y	17% @ 1 y	32% @ 5 y	16% @ 4 y
Relapse	40% @ 4 y	39% @ 3 y	36% @ 5 y	33% @ 4 y
Extensive cGVHD	55% @ 2 y	56% @ 5 y	51%	64% @ 2 y
Median follow-up	46 mo	37 mo	NR	57 mo
Major poor prognostic factors	Uncontrolled disease at SCT; Alem exposure	CD4 counts <100; low serum IgG	LNs≥5 cm; Alem within 12 mo	Year of SCT prior to 2004

N, number of patients; cGVHD, chronic graft-versus-host disease; F, fludarabine; FC, fludarabine–cyclophosphamide; Alem, Alemtuzumab; R, rituxan; TBI, total-body irradiation; NR, not recorded; LNs, lymph node size; FB, fludarabine–busulfan.

Indications for transplant
HLA-identical sibling transplant
1. Patient in Rai stage I–IV or Binet stage B or C and has additional risk factors (see later)
2. Patient <45 years of age for myeloablative conditioning and <65 years of age for RIC
3. Karnofsky score ≥80%
4. Presence of risk factors (as proposed by EBMT, Dreger et al., 2007)

   • Non-response or early relapse (<12 months) after purine analogs, especially if the patient is young, has not failed more than two regimens, and is in a good medical condition
   • Relapse within 24 months after having achieved a response with purine analog-based combination therapy or autologous transplantation
   • Patients with p53 abnormalities, requiring treatment

Comment: only a small proportion of patients with CLL are candidates for an allogeneic transplant, but a fraction will become long-term survivors.

Autologous blood/marrow SCT
There are no clear indications for autologous blood/marrow SCT at present; the transplant can be considered within studies for patients <65 years who relapse after initial treatment or do not consider allogeneic transplantation.

Contraindications to transplant
Transplant is contraindicated in patients in Rai stage 0 or Binet stage A not meeting the earlier mentioned indications for transplant.

Pretransplant workup

1. See the general pretransplant workup (page 239)
2. Bone marrow aspirate; to include FISH, cytogenetic evaluation, and molecular analysis of Ig gene rearrangement
3. Coombs test
4. Immune phenotyping including ZAP70

Monitoring posttransplant

1. Bone marrow aspirate, with cytogenetic and molecular evaluation at 3 weeks, 12 weeks, 1 year, and 2 years
2. Immune phenotyping at 6 weeks, 12 weeks, 1 year, and 2 years

References and further reading

Binet JL, Auquier A, Dighiero G, et al. 1981. A new prognostic classification of chronic lymphocytic leukemia derived from a multivariate survival analysis. *Cancer* **48**: 198–206.

Binet JL, Caligaris-Cappio F, Catovsky D, et al. 2006. Perspective on the use of new diagnostic tools in the treatment of chronic lymphocytic leukemia. *Blood* **107**: 859–861.

Brown JR, Stevenson K, Kim HT, et al. 2008. Comparative outcome of myeloablative and reduced intensity allogeneic stem cell transplantation for chronic lymphocytic leukemia. *Blood* **112**: 972.

Brown JR. 2011. The treatment of relapsed refractory chronic lymphocytic leukemia. *Hematology Am Soc Hematol Educ Program* **2011**: 110–118.

Calin GA, Pekarsky Y, & Croce CM. 2007. The role of microRNA and other non-coding RNA in the pathogenesis of chronic lymphocytic leukemia. *Best Pract Res Clin Haematol* **20**: 425–437.

Döhner H, Stilgenbauer S, Benner A, et al. 2000. Genomic aberrations and survival in chronic lymphocytic leukemia. *N Engl J Med* **343**: 1910–1918.

Dreger P, Corradini P, Kimby E, et al. 2007. Indications for stem cell transplantation in chronic lymphocytic leukemia: the EBMT transplant consensus. *Leukemia* **21**: 12–17.

Dreger P, Dohner H, Ritgen M, et al. 2010. Allogeneic stem cell transplantation provides durable disease control in poor-risk chronic lymphocytic leukemia: long-term clinical and MRD results of the German CLL Study Group CLL3X trial. *Blood* **116**: 2438–2447.

Gladstone DE & Fuchs E. 2012. Hematopoietic stem cell transplantation for chronic lymphocytic leukemia. *Curr Opin Oncol* **24**: 176–181.

Gribben JG, Zahrieh D, Stephans K, et al. 2005. Autologous and allogeneic stem cell transplantations for poor-risk chronic lymphocytic leukemia. *Blood* **106**: 4389–4396.

Hallek M, Fischer K, Fingerle-Rowson G, et al. 2010. Addition of rituximab to fludarabine and cyclophosphamide in patients with chronic lymphocytic leukemia: a randomized, open-label, phase 3 trial. *Lancet* **376**: 1164–1174.

Jantunen E, Itälä M, Siitonen T, et al. 2006. Autologous stem cell transplantation in patients with chronic lymphocytic leukaemia: the Finnish experience. *Bone Marrow Transplant* **37**: 1093–1098.

Keating MJ, Flinn I, & Jain V. 2002. Therapeutic role of alemtuzumab (Campath-1H) in patients who have failed fludarabine. *Blood* **99**: 3554–3561.

Khouri IF, Bassett R, Pondexter N, et al. 2011. Nonmyeloablative allogeneic stem cell transplantation in relapsed/refractory chronic lymphocytic leukemia: long-term follow up, prognostic factors, and effect of human leukocyte histocompatibility antigen subtype on outcome. *Cancer* **117**: 4679–4688.

Michallet M, Archimbaud E, Bandini G, et al. 1996. HLA-identical sibling bone marrow transplantation in younger patients with chronic lymphocytic leukemia. *Ann Intern Med* **124**: 311–315.

Rai KR & Han T. 1990. Prognostic factors and clinical staging in chronic lymphocytic leukemia. *Hematol Oncol Clin North Am* **4**: 447–451.

Rai KR, Sawitsky A, Cronkite EP, et al. 1975. Clinical staging of chronic lymphocytic leukemia. *Blood* **46**: 219–234.

Sorror ML, Maris MB, Sandmaier BM, et al. 2005. Hematopoietic cell transplantation after nonmyeloablative conditioning for advanced chronic lymphocytic leukemia. *J Clin Oncol* **23**: 3819–3829.

Sorror ML, Storer B, Sandmaier BM, et al. 2010. Impacts of cytogenetic abnormalities and prior alemtuzumab on outcomes of patients (pts) with high-risk chronic lymphocytic leukemia (CLL) given nonmyeloablative allogeneic hematopoietic cell transplantation (HCT). *Blood* **116**: 2364.

Wright SJ, Robertson LE, O'Brien S, et al. 1994. The role of fludarabine in haematological malignancies. *Blood Rev* **8**: 125–134.

Chapter

7

Therapeutic decision making in BMT/SCT for myelodysplasia

Carolina Escobar, Reinhold Munker, and Kerry Atkinson

MDS constitutes a group of clonal hematopoietic stem cell disorders occurring often in the elderly that are characterized by cytopenias and cytogenetic abnormalities, and can evolve into AML. The prevalence and incidence of MDS have increased in the last 20 years, likely as a result of increasing longevity of the population. These disorders are heterogeneous and staged and classified according to the percentage of blasts in the bone marrow, cytogenetic abnormalities, and number of cytopenias. As shown on pages 78–79, several staging systems are available. The International Prognostic Scoring System (IPSS) will divide cases of MDS into groups according to survival and risk for leukemia transformation. The disadvantage of this scoring system is that it does not take into account age, ferritin, transfusion dependence, and marrow fibrosis. There are other scoring systems like the WHO Prognostic Scoring System for OS and relapse. A revised scoring system is currently under development (Appelbaum et al., 2011).

The BMT Data Book, Third Edition, ed. Reinhold Munker et al. Published by Cambridge University Press. © Cambridge University Press 2013.

Disease staging and classification

FAB classification of MDS

Subtype	Blood myeloblasts	Bone marrow myeloblasts	Other features
Refractory anemia (RA)	<1%	<5%	
RA with ringed sideroblasts	<1%	<5%	RS>15% BM cells
RA with excess blasts (RAEB)	<5%	5%–20%	
CMML	<5%	<20%	AMC >1000/μL

CMML, chronic myelomonocytic leukemia; RS, ringed sideroblasts; BM, bone marrow; AMC, absolute monocyte count.

The WHO classification of MDS

Disease	Blood findings	Bone marrow findings
RA	Anemia, no or rare blasts <1 × 10^9/L monocytes	Erythroid dysplasia only <10% N or megas dysplastic, <5% blasts, <15% ringed sideroblasts
RA with ringed sideroblasts (RARS)	Anemia, no blasts	Erythroid dysplasia only <10% N or megas dysplastic, ≥15% ringed sideroblasts, <5% blasts
Refractory cytopenia with multilineage dysplasia (RCMD)	Cytopenias (bicytopenia or pancytopenia), no or rare blasts, no Auer rods, <1 × 10^9/L monocytes	Dysplasia in ≥10% of cells in two or more myeloid cell lines, <5% blasts in marrow, no Auer rods, <15% ringed sideroblasts
Refractory cytopenia with multilineage dysplasia and ringed sideroblasts (RCMD-RS)	Cytopenias (bicytopenia or pancytopenia), no or rare blasts, no Auer rods, <1 × 10^9/L monocytes	Dysplasia in ≥10% of cells in two or more myeloid cell lines, ≥5% ringed sideroblasts, <5% blasts, no Auer rods
RA with excess blasts–1	Cytopenias, <5% blasts, no Auer rods <1 × 10^9/L monocytes	Unilineage or multilineage dysplasia, 5%–9% blasts, no Auer rods
RA with excess blasts–2	Cytopenias, 5%–19% blasts, Auer rods, +/− <1 × 10^9/L monocytes	Unilineage or multilineage dysplasia, 10%–19% blasts, Auer rods +/−
MDS, unclassified	Cytopenias, no or rare blasts, no Auer rods	Unilineage N or mega dysplasia, <5% blasts, no Auer rods
MDS associated with isolated del (5q)	Anemia <5% blasts, platelets normal or increased	Normal to increased megakaryocytes with hypolobated nuclei, <5% blasts, no Auer rods, isolated del (5q)

N, neutrophils; megas, megakaryocytes.

International prognostic scoring system for MDS

Prognostic variable	Score value				
	0	0.5	1.0	1.5	2.0
BM blasts (%)	<5	5–10	–	11–20	21–30*
Karyotype	Good	Intermediate		Poor	
Cytopenias	0/1	2/3			

Karyotypes, good: normal, -Y, 5q-, alone 20q-; poor: complex (≥3 abnormalities) or chromosome 7 abnormalities; intermediate: other abnormalities
* cases with 21%–30% blasts are now considered as AML. (Adapted from Greenberg et al., 1997.)

Survival and risk of leukemia for IPSS risk groups

Risk group	Score	Median survival (yr)	Risk of leukemia (%)
Low	0	5.7	19
INT-1	0.5–1.0	3.5	30
INT-2	1.5–2.0	1.2	33
High	>2.0	0.4	45

Cytogenetic abnormalities

Abnormality	Incidence (%)
De novo MDS	
–5/del(5q)	6–20
–7/del(7q)	1–10
Trisomy 8	5–10
-Y	1–10
Del(20q)	2–5
Del(1q)	<1–7
Complex (≥3 abnormalities)	10–20
Normal cytogenetics	40–50
Treatment-related MDS	
–5/del(5q)	40
–7/del(7q)	40
Other karyotypic abnormalities	0–10

(Modified from Olney et al., 2007.)

Characteristics of MDS and AML secondary to prior chemotherapy

In addition to de novo presentation, MDS and AML can occur secondary to prior cytotoxic chemotherapy, in which case there is a poorer prognosis than with de novo disease.

Secondary MDS/AML has been found to be associated with use of the following agents:

1. Alkylating agents (e.g., MOPP, especially if radiotherapy is also used): MDS with abnormalities of chromosome 5 or 7
2. Epipodophyllotoxins: AML with short latency (1–3 years); M4 or M5 FAB subtype; 11q23 abnormalities
3. Anthracyclines: AML with properties similar to those of epipodophyllotoxin-induced AML
4. Taxanes/cyclophosphamide: increased risk with high-dosage regimens using these agents; AML with properties similar to those of anthracycline-induced AML

Compared with de novo AML, secondary AML (or treatment-related AML)

- Is less likely to enter CR with conventional chemotherapy
- Is more likely to show prolonged cytopenia during remission induction
- Features a shorter duration of CR1 (5–23 months in reported series studies)
- Entails shorter survival

Options for conventional treatment for MDS

Treatment	Comments
Supportive treatment	For all patients, blood transfusions, treatment of infections, bleeding, hematopoietic growth factors as needed
Demethylating agents (azacitine, decitabine)	MDS necessitating treatment, 17%–23% complete responses, delay leukemic transformation, improve performance status, both for lower- and higher-risk patients
Low-dose chemotherapy	In selected patients with increased bone marrow blasts
Intensive chemotherapy	In selected patients with a high risk of transformation
Immunosuppressive agents	In selected patients – Int-1≤60 years, or HLA–DR15+, or positive for PNH clone or hypoplastic MDS
Lenalidomide	Indicated for lower-risk patients, especially active in 5q-syndrome
New and other treatments: inhibitors of histone deacetylases, TNF-α receptors, alemtuzumab, clofarabine, sapacitabine	Role unclear at present; response in selected patients

(See Deschler et al., 2006, for decision analysis in older patients with high-risk MDS or AML.)

Results with conventional therapy and new agents

Efficacy of azacitidine compared with standard care

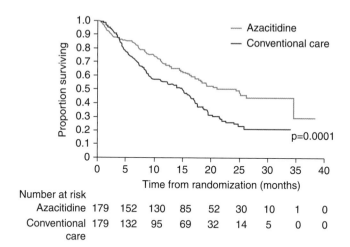

In this international study, 358 patients with MDS were randomly assigned to receive azacytidine (75 mg/m^2 per day for seven consecutive days every 28 days or conventional regimens, which includes some patients who received induction chemotherapy). The survival of both groups is shown in the graph. (Reproduced with permission from Fenaux et al., 2009.)

Number at risk

Azacitidine	179	152	130	85	52	30	10	1	0
Conventional care	179	132	95	69	32	14	5	0	0

Lenalidomide in MDS with chromosome 5q deletion

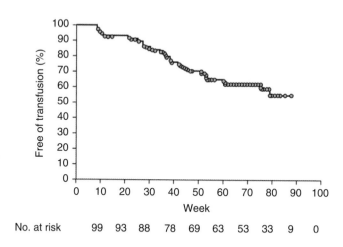

One hundred and eighty-four patients with MDS and the 5q31 deletion received 10 mg of lenalidomide for 21 days every four weeks or daily. The patients had a low or intermediate-1 risk and a transfusion-dependent anemia. Among all patients, 76% had a reduced need for transfusions with a median of 104 weeks of follow-up. The figure shows that the responses were long lasting, as at a follow-up of 80 weeks, the median duration of transfusion independence was not yet reached. (Reproduced with permission from List et al., 2006.)

No. at risk

	99	93	88	78	69	63	53	33	9	0

Results with autologous transplant
The role of stem cell source in auto-HSCT for patients with MDS

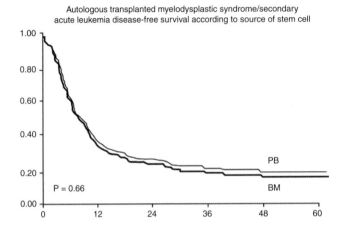

Autologous transplanted myelodysplastic syndrome/secondary acute leukemia disease-free survival according to source of stem cell

For certain patients with MDS, autologous SCT can result in long-term disease control without the toxicities of allogeneic transplantation. In a European registry study, the outcome of autologous SCT was compared with regard to the source of stem cells (bone marrow versus PB). As shown in the figure, both sources of stem cells resulted in an equivalent DFS and likelihood of relapse (survival in months). (Reproduced with permission from de Witte et al., 2006.)

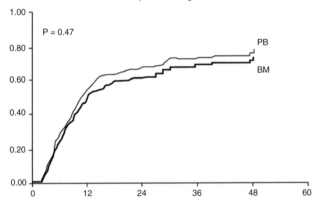

Autologous transplanted myelodysplastic syndrome/secondary acute leukemia relapse according to source of stem cell

Results with allogeneic transplant
Conditioning with targeted busulfan and cyclophosphamide for hemopoietic SCT from related and unrelated donors in patients with MDS

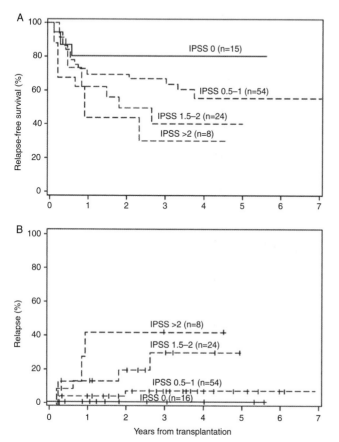

A total of 109 patients (aged 6–66 years, age median 46 years) were transplanted in Seattle following targeted busulfan and cyclophosphamide. Forty-five patients had related stem cell donors while 69 patients had unrelated stem cell donors. The Kaplan–Meier estimates of three-year relapse-free survival were 56% for related and 59% for unrelated recipients. The NRM at 100 days was 12% for related and 13% for unrelated recipients. Factors significantly correlated with relapse were the IPSS score, poor-risk cytogenetics, and treatment-related etiology. (Reproduced with permission from Deeg et al., 2002.)

A decision analysis of allogeneic BMT for MDS: delayed transplantation for low-risk myelodysplasia is associated with improved outcome

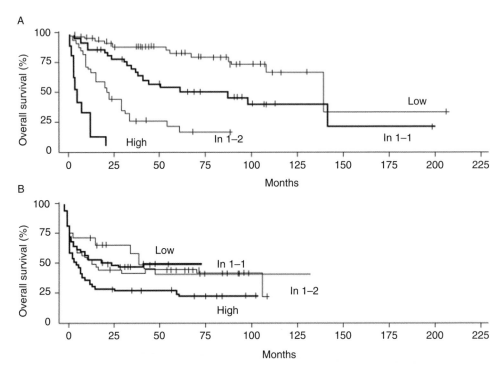

BMT can cure MDS, although transplantation carries significant risks of morbidity and mortality. Because the optimal timing of HLA-matched BMT for MDS is unknown, the authors constructed a Markov model to examine three transplantation strategies for newly diagnosed MDS: transplantation at diagnosis, transplantation at leukemic progression, and transplantation at an interval from diagnosis but prior to leukemic progression. Analyses using individual patient risk-assessment data from transplantation and nontransplantation registries were performed for all four (IPSS) risk groups, with adjustments for quality of life. For low and intermediate-1 IPSS groups, delayed transplantation maximized OS. Transplantation before leukemic transformation was associated with a greater number of life years than transplantation at the time of leukemic progression. In a cohort of patients under the age of 40 years, an even more marked survival advantage for delayed transplantation was noted. For intermediate-2 and high IPSS groups, transplantation at diagnosis maximized OS. For low- and intermediate-1-risk MDS, delayed BMT is associated with maximal life expectancy, whereas immediate transplantation for intermediate-2- and high-risk disease is associated with maximal life expectancy. In the figure, the OS of patients included in the analysis who did not undergo SCT (A), stratified by risk group, is shown. In (B) the survival of patients who underwent transplantation from the time of transplantation is shown. (Reproduced with permission from Cutler et al., 2004.)

Retrospective comparison of RIC and conventional high-dose conditioning for allogeneic hematopoietic SCT using HLA-identical sibling donors in MDS

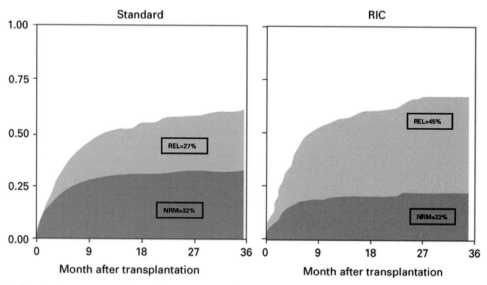

In this multicenter retrospective study, the outcome of 836 patients with MDS who underwent a matched HLA-identical sibling transplant was analyzed according to the type of conditioning used: 215 patients underwent RIC whereas 621 underwent a full myeloablative transplant. The patients in the RIC group were mainly older and had other comorbidities and risk factors. The figure shows, in a competing risk model, that the NRM is higher in the standard dose conditioning group whereas the incidence of relapse (REL) is higher in the RIC group. The three-year probability of PFS and the OS were similar in both groups (39% respectively, 45% after myeloablative conditioning versus 33% and 41% after RIC). It was concluded that lower NRM was encouraging; however, it was recommended that younger patients with no contraindications for standard dose myeloablative transplants should not receive RIC transplants outside of clinical trials. (Reproduced with permission from Martino et al., 2006.)

CIBMTR data for MDS

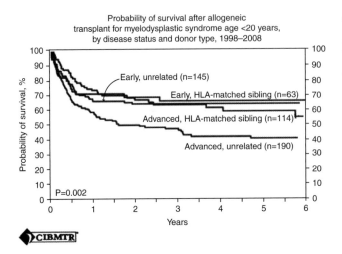

Probability of survival after allogeneic transplant for myelodysplastic syndrome age <20 years, by disease status and donor type, 1998–2008

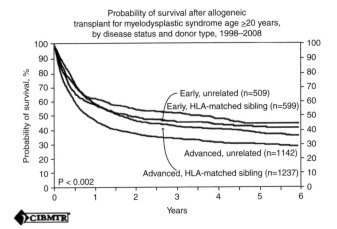

Probability of survival after allogeneic transplant for myelodysplastic syndrome age ≥20 years, by disease status and donor type, 1998–2008

Allogeneic transplant is a potentially curative treatment for MDS. Outcomes differ according to the recipient's age and disease status at the time of transplant, as well as by donor type. Among 177 recipients of an HLA-matched allogeneic transplant younger than 20 years (upper graph), the three-year probabilities of survival were 65% ± 6% and 63% ± 5% for patients with early and advanced disease, respectively. The corresponding probabilities of survival in the 331 recipients receiving an unrelated donor transplant were 63% ± 4% and 47% ± 4%. Among the 1836 patients ≥20 years receiving an HLA-matched sibling transplant (lower graph), the three-year probabilities of survival were 50% ± 2% and 41% ± 2% for early and advanced MDS, respectively. The corresponding probabilities in the 1651 older patients receiving an unrelated donor transplant were 44% ± 2% and 32% ± 2%. (Data kindly provided by Tanya Pedersen; reproduced with permission.)

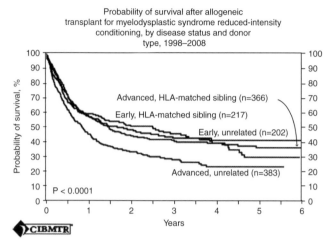

Probability of survival after allogeneic transplant for myelodysplastic syndrome reduced-intensity conditioning, by disease status and donor type, 1998–2008

The median age of patients at diagnosis with MDS is 70 years, limiting the use of myeloablative conditioning regimens for most patients with this disease. RIC regimens are increasingly used for allogeneic transplantation in MDS. Among 1168 patients who underwent RIC allogeneic transplantation for MDS from 1998 to 2008, the three-year survival probabilities for recipients of HLA-matched donor transplants (n=583) were 45% ± 4% and 41% ± 3% for early and advanced MDS, respectively. The corresponding probabilities for recipients of unrelated donor transplants (n=585) were 42% ± 4% and 28% ± 3. (Data kindly provided by Tanya Pedersen; reproduced with permission.)

Indications for transplant

The general indication for allogeneic transplant in MDS is that the patient is unlikely to be stable for a prolonged period with conventional treatment, has a matched donor, and has no contraindications to transplant. In patients with low or intermediate-1 risk, transplant should be delayed until there are signs of progression (transfusion dependence, increase in cytopenias, increase of blasts in bone marrow) but before AML transformation to maximize the survival benefit. Higher-risk MDS patients should always be considered for transplant.

HLA-identical family member transplant

	DFS
1. RA (if significant neutropenia)	60%
2. RAS (or thrombocytopenia)	60%
3. RAEB	30%–50%
4. RAEBt	30%–50%
5. AML evolved from MDS	
(a) in CR1	50%–60%
(b) in first relapse	20%–30%
(c) in CR2 or subsequent remission	20%–30%
(d) at presentation if hypocellular marrow (unlikely to remit with chemotherapy)	may do well
(e) refractory	10%–20%

HLA-partially matched (for 5/6 or 9/10 antigens) family member or matched unrelated transplant

- As for the preceding regimen, but subtract 10% from DFS

Autologous blood/marrow SCT

1. Patient with AML evolved from MDS, with • CR1 cells cryopreserved and	30%(?)
2. Patient with AML evolved from MDS in CR1	30%(?)

Contraindications to autologous transplant

Autologous blood/marrow SCT is contraindicated if there is a persistent cytogenetic or molecular abnormality in the remission marrow.

Allogeneic transplant is contraindicated if there are general contraindications, like poor performance status, significant organ dysfunction, and uncontrolled infection.

Pretransplant workup

The pretransplant workup is the same as for AML (page 39).

Monitoring posttransplant

Monitoring is the same as for AML (page 39).

References and further reading

Appelbaum FR. 2011. The role of hematopoietic cell transplantation as therapy for myelodysplasia. *Best Pract Res Clin Hematol* **24**: 541–547.

Cutler CS, Lee SJ, Greenberg P, et al. 2004. A decision analysis of allogeneic bone marrow transplantation for the myelodysplastic syndromes: delayed transplantation for low-risk myelodysplasia is associated with improved outcome. *Blood* **104**: 579–585.

Deeg HJ, Storer B, Slattery JT, et al. 2002. Conditioning with targeted busulfan and cyclophosphamide for hemopoietic stem cell transplantation from related and unrelated donors in patients with myelodysplastic syndrome. *Blood* **100**: 1201–1207.

Deschler B, de Witte T, Mertelsmann R, et al. 2006. Decision-making for older patients with high-risk myelodysplastic syndrome or acute myeloid leukemia: problems and approaches. *Haematologica* **91**: 1513–1522.

De Witte T, Brand R, van Biezen A, et al. 2006. The role of stem cell source in autologous hematopoietic stem cell transplantation for patients with myelodysplastic syndromes. *Haematologica* **91**: 750–756.

Fenaux P, Mufti GJ, Hellstrom-Lindberg E, et al. 2009. Efficacy of azacitidine compared with that of higher risk myelodysplastic syndromes: a randomized, open label phase III study. *Lancet Oncol* **10**: 223–232.

Greenberg P, Cox C, Lebeau MM, et al. 1997. International scoring system for evaluating prognosis in myelodysplastic syndromes. *Blood* **89**: 2079–2088.

Hofmann WK & Koeffler HP. 2005. Myelodysplastic syndrome. *Annu Rev Med* **56**: 1–16.

Ingram W, Lim ZY, & Mufti GJ. 2007. Allogeneic transplantation for myelodysplastic syndrome (MDS). *Blood Rev* **21**: 61–71.

List A, Dewald G, Bennett J, et al. 2006. Lenalidomide in the myelodysplastic syndrome with chromosome 5 q deletion. *N Engl J Med* **355**: 1456–1465.

Martino R, Iacobelli S, Brand R, et al. 2006. Retrospective comparison of reduced intensity conditioning and conventional high-dose conditioning for allogeneic stem cell transplantation using HLA-identical sibling donors in myelodysplastic syndromes. *Blood* **108**: 836–846.

Olney HJ & LeBeau MM. 2007. Evaluation of recurrent cytogenetic abnormalities in the treatment of myelodysplastic syndromes. *Leuk Res* **31**: 427–434.

Parmar S, de Lima M, Deeg HJ, et al. 2011. Hematopoietic stem cell transplantation for myelodysplastic syndrome: a review. *Sem Oncol* **38**: 693–704.

Platzbecker U, Wermke M, Radke J, et al. 2011. Azacitidine for treatment of imminent relapse in MDS or AML patients after allogeneic HSCT: results of the RELAZA trial. *Leukemia* **26**: 381–389.

Hematopoietic cell transplantation for non-Hodgkin lymphoma

Saurabh Chhabra and Ginna G. Laport

Classification of non-Hodgkin lymphoma (NHL)

Annually, more than 56 000 cases of NHL are diagnosed in the United States and are a common indication for allogeneic or auto-SCT. Clinically, staging is performed according to the Ann Arbor classification.

World Health Organization classification of B-cell and T-cell neoplasms (Savage & Gregory, 2010)

B-cell neoplasms	T-cell neoplasms
Precursor B-cell neoplasms	Precursor T-cell neoplasms
B-lymphoblastic leukemia/lymphoma not otherwise specified (NOS)	T-lymphoblastic leukemia/lymphoma
B-lymphoblastic leukemia/lymphoma with recurrent genetic abnormalities	

The BMT Data Book, Third Edition, ed. Reinhold Munker et al. Published by Cambridge University Press. © Cambridge University Press 2013.

(cont.)

B-cell neoplasms	T-cell neoplasms
Mature B-cell neoplasms	**Mature T-cell neoplasms**
Aggressive lymphomas	Aggressive lymphomas
DLBCL: variants, subgroups and subtypes/entities	T-cell prolymphocytic leukemia
DLBCL, NOS	Aggressive NK cell leukemia
Common morphologic variants: centroblastic, immunoblastic, anaplastic	Peripheral T-cell lymphoma, NOS
	Angioimmunoblastic T-cell lymphoma
Rare morphologic variants	ALCL, ALK positive
Molecular subgroups: germinal center B-cell like (GCB) and activated B-cell like (ABC)	ALCL, ALK negative
	Extranodal NK/T-cell lymphoma, nasal type
Immunohistochemical subgroups: CDS$^+$ DLBCL, GCB, and non-GCB	Enteropathy-type T-cell lymphoma
	Hepatosplenic T-cell lymphoma
DLBCL subtypes	Subcutaneous panniculitis-like T-cell lymphoma
T-cell/histiocyte-rich large B-cell lymphoma	Adult T-cell leukemia/lymphoma
Primary DLBCL of the CNS	Primary cutaneous γ-δ T-cell lymphoma
Primary cutaneous DLBCL, leg type	Primary cutaneous CD8$^+$ aggressive epidermotropic T-cell lymphoma
EBV-positive DLBCL of the elderly	
Other lymphomas of large B-cells	
Primary mediastinal large B-cell lymphoma	
Intravascular large B-cell lymphoma	
DLBCL associated with chronic inflammation	
Lymphomatoid granulomatosis	
ALK-positive large B-cell lymphoma	
Plasmablastic lymphoma	
Large B-cell lymphoma arising in HHV-8-associated multicentric Castleman disease	
Primary effusion lymphoma	
Borderline cases	
B-cell lymphoma, unclassifiable, with features intermediate between DLBCL and Burkitt lymphoma	

(cont.)

B-cell neoplasms	T-cell neoplasms
B-cell lymphoma, unclassifiable, with features intermediate between DLBCL and classical Hodgkin lymphoma (HL)	
Burkitt lymphoma	
MCL	
Indolent lymphomas	*Indolent lymphomas*
FL	T-cell large granular lymphocytic leukemia
Primary cutaneous follicle center lymphoma	Chronic lymphoproliferative disorders of NK cells
Extranodal marginal zone lymphoma of mucosa-associated lymphoid tissue (MALT)	Mycosis fungoides
	Sézary syndrome
Nodal marginal zone lymphoma	Primary cutaneous CD30$^+$ T-cell lymphoproliferative disorder
Splenic B-cell lymphoma/leukemia, unclassifiable	Primary cutaneous CD4$^+$ small/ medium T-cell lymphoma
Lymphoplasmacytic lymphoma	
Heavy chain disease	
Plasma cell neoplasms	
CLL/small lymphocytic lymphoma (SLL)	
B-cell prolymphocytic leukemia	
Hairy cell leukemia	

Phenotypic markers and chromosomal translocations in NHL (Savage & Gregory, 2010)

Non-Hodgkin lymphoma	Surface Ig	CD5	CD10	CD20	Other	Cyclin D1	Cytogenetics	Oncogene	Function
CLL/SLL	Weak	+	–	Weak	CD23$^+$, FMC$^-$	–	No diagnostic abnormalities	–	–
Follicular	++	–	+	+		–	t(14;18)	BCL2	Antiapoptosis
Mantle cell	++	+	–	+	CD23$^-$, FMC^{-+}	+	t(11;14)	Cyclin D1	Cell cycle regulator
Marginal zone/extranodal marginal zone lymphoma	+	–	–	+		–	t(11;18)	AP12-MALT	Resistance to *Helicobacter pylori* treatment
Lymphoplasmacytic lymphoma	++	–	–	+	CD25$^{+/-}$, CD38$^{+/}$ $^-$	–	t(9;14)	–	–
Hairy cell leukemia	++	–	–	+	CD11c$^+$, CD25$^+$, CD103$^+$	Weak	–	–	–
DLBCL	+	Rare	+/–	+		–	t(14;18), t(3;14), t(3;v)	BCL2	Antiapoptosis
							t(8;14), t(2;8), t(2;22)	BCL6	Transcription factor
							Rare	CMYC	Transcription factor
Burkitt lymphoma	+	–	+	+	TdT$^-$	–	t(8;14), t(2;8), t(2;22)	CMYC	Transcription factor
ALCL, ALK-positive	–	–	–	–	CD2$^+$, CD3$^{-/+}$, EMA$^+$	–	t(2;5)	ALK	Tyrosine kinase

Diffuse large B-cell lymphoma (DLCL)

International Prognostic Index

The IPI proposed in 1993 (Shipp et al., 1993) has been used in the risk stratification for patients with DLBCL. The age-adjusted IPI (aaIPI) has also been widely employed, particularly to tailor more intensive therapy such as an auto-HSCT.

International Prognostic Index (IPI) and age-adjusted index for aggressive lymphoma patients treated with doxorubicin-containing combination chemotherapy (Shipp et al., 1993). (Reproduced with permission.)

Risk group	Risk factors (n)	Distribution of cases (%)	CR rate (%)	5-year OS (%)
All ages				
Low (L)	0.1	35	87	73
Low-intermediate (LI)	2	27	67	51
High-intermediate (HI)	3	22	55	43
High (H)	4.5	16	44	26
Age-adjusted index (≤60)				
Low (L)	0	22	92	83
Low-intermediate (LI)	1	32	78	69
High-intermediate (HI)	2	32	57	46
High (H)	3	14	46	32

Revised IPI

The IPI remains predictive in the rituximab era, but it identifies only two risk groups (see following figure). Redistribution of the IPI factors into a revised IPI (R-IPI) provides a more clinically relevant prediction of outcome (Sehn et al., 2007). The R-IPI identifies three distinct prognostic groups with a very good (four-year PFS, 94%; OS, 94%), good (four-year PFS, 80%; OS, 79%), and poor (four-year PFS, 53%; OS, 55%) outcome, respectively (P<0.001) (see figure on page 95). The IPI (or R-IPI) no longer identifies a risk group with less than a 50% chance of survival.

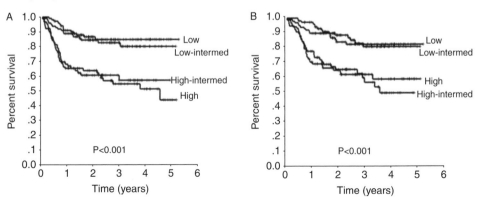

Outcome according to the standard IPI. A: PFS; B: OS, according to the standard IPI in the rituximab era (Sehn et al., 2007). (Reproduced with permission.)

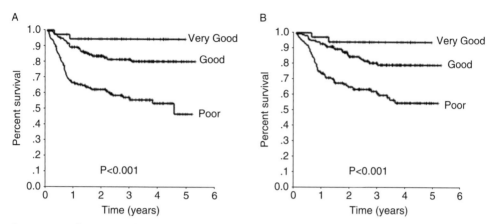

Outcome according to revised (R)-IPI. A: PFS; B: OS, according to the R-IPI. (Reproduced with permission from Sehn et al., 2007.)

Autologous HCT in the first complete remission (CR1)

Recent data supports the use of auto-HCT as consolidation in DLBCL patients with intermediate- and high-risk disease after achieving CR (Stiff et al., 2011). However, this practice is currently not standard of care.

Autologous HCT for relapsed/refractory DLBCL

Patients with relapsed DLBCL receive a second-line (or salvage) regimen followed by auto-HCT, if chemosensitive disease is demonstrated (El Gnaoui et al., 2007; Kewalramani et al., 2004; Lopez et al., 2008). Patients with primary refractory lymphoma and those with chemoresistant disease have a poor prognosis (Hamlin et al., 2003; Vose et al., 2004). A third to a half of DLBCL patients fail to achieve CR with standard induction and require salvage therapy that includes auto-HCT (Vose et al., 2001). Retrospective results have demonstrated that approximately a third of these patients can experience long-term survival. Chemoresistant disease, Karnofsky performance status (KPS) score <80, age >55 years, ≥3 prior regimens, and not receiving involved-field radiation therapy (IFRT) (pre- or posttransplant) were adverse prognostic factors for OS. The CORAL (Collaborative Trial in Relapsed Aggressive Lymphoma) trial described later in this chapter also found that prior rituximab therapy and early relapse were poor prognostic factors.

Commonly used salvage regimens prior to HCT for relapsed/refractory DLBCL
(Zelenetz et al., 2012)

- ICE: ifosfamide, carboplatin, etoposide ± rituximab
- DHAP: dexamethasone, high-dose cytarabine, cisplatin, prednisone ± rituximab
- GDP: gemcitabine, dexamethasone, cisplatin (or carboplatin) ± rituximab
- ESHAP: etoposide, methylprednisolone, high-dose cytarabine, cisplatin ± rituximab
- EPOCH: etoposide, vincristine, doxorubicin, cyclophosphamide, prednisone ± rituximab
- GemOx: gemcitabine, oxaliplatin ± rituximab
- MINE: mesna, ifosfamide, mitoxantrone, etoposide ± rituximab

The role of auto-HCT in the treatment of relapsed disease was defined by the prospective randomized PARMA trial that compared auto-HCT with nontransplant salvage therapy (Philip et al., 1995). Patients with intermediate or high-grade aggressive lymphoma in first relapse (n=215; majority had DLBCL) and who had chemosensitive disease after DHAP salvage chemotherapy were randomized to receive either further DHAP therapy or auto-HCT. Both five-year OS and EFS were significantly superior in the auto-HCT group versus the chemotherapy-only group (46% and 53%, P=0.001, and 12% and 32%, P=0.038, respectively) (see following figures).

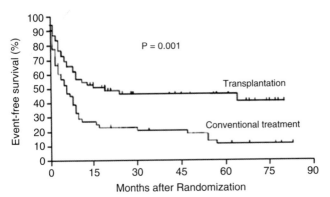

EFS of patients in the transplantation and conventional-treatment groups (Philip et al., 1995). (Reproduced with permission.)

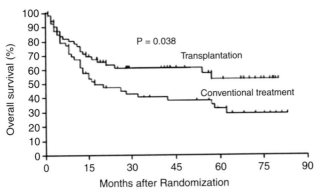

OS of patients in the transplantation and conventional-treatment groups (Philip et al., 1995). (Reproduced with permission.)

The phase II of the CORAL study evaluated two salvage regimens in DLBCL and assessed the role of rituximab maintenance after auto-HCT (Gisselbrecht et al., 2010). Patients with relapsed DLBCL or patients who had not achieved CR after CHOP or R-CHOP therapy were first randomized between R-ICE and R-DHAP. Chemoresponsive patients proceeded to auto-HCT. Patients underwent a second randomization to maintenance rituximab or observation. There was no significant difference in response rate or survival between R-DHAP and R-ICE as salvage therapy; the response rate was 63% with both regimens. Only half of the patients proceeded to auto-HCT. The response rate to salvage therapy was lower in patients previously treated with rituximab compared with rituximab-naive patients (83% vs. 51% P<0.001), which translated to a lower three-year EFS in patients pretreated with rituximab compared with no prior rituximab (21% vs. 47%).

Patients who had early relapse (<12 months) after induction therapy had poor outcomes (see following figure). In a subset analysis, patients with germinal center B (GCB)-like DLBCL had a more favorable outcome when treated with R-DHAP compared with R-ICE (three-year PFS of 100% vs. 27%, respectively). Patients with activated B-cell (ABC)-like DLBCL had a poor outcome irrespective of the regimen.

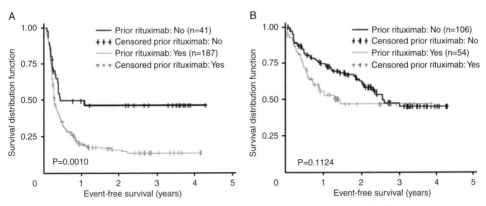

A: EFS according to prior rituximab treatment and relapse <12 months after diagnosis. B: EFS according to prior rituximab treatment and relapse >12 months after diagnosis (Gisselbrecht et al., 2010). (Reproduced with permission.)

Conditioning regimens for autologous HCT for DLBCL

There is no standard conditioning regimen for auto-HCT (Friedberg et al., 2011). Commonly used myeloablative regimens include BEAM, cyclophosphamide, BCNU, etoposide (CBV), and cyclophosphamide/TBI (Friedberg, 2011). In the absence of randomized trials, comparative studies suggest lower rates of therapy-related myeloid neoplasms (t-MDS/T-AML) (Swerdlow et al., 2008) and other long-term toxicities with chemotherapy-only conditioning regimens (Armitage et al., 2003). Thus, the BEAM or the CBV regimen is often favored, with the possible addition of localized radiation therapy at sites of persistent disease (Biswas et al., 2010). Radioimmunotherapy (RIT) is a feasible alternative to TBI, providing targeted radiotherapy while sparing normal structures (Friedberg, 2011). Although no randomized data against standard radiation therapy (TBI) is available, a few phase I–II trials have shown RIT-based conditioning to be safe with low TRM (Nademanee et al., 2005; Press et al., 2000; Vose et al., 2005). However, a large randomized multicenter trial that compared [131]iodine-tositumomab/BEAM to rituximab/BEAM for auto-HCT in relapsed DLBCL patients did not show a difference in survival or progression between the two arms (Vose et al., 2011).

Allogeneic HCT for relapsed/refractory DLBCL

Allo-SCT (allo-HCT) has generally been offered as treatment for relapsed high-risk or refractory disease or for patients who relapsed after auto-HCT. The CIBMTR study compared the outcomes of DLBCL patients undergoing first auto-HCT (n=837) and myeloablative MRD allo-HCT (n=79) that were reported between 1995 and 2003 (Lazarus et al., 2010). Allo-HCT was associated with higher NRM but with a similar risk of disease progression compared with lower-risk patients who received auto-HCT, and the allo-HCT group had more patients with intermediate-high or high-risk IPI, and extranodal or marrow involvement. For patients who relapse after auto-HCT, allo-HCT can be used as a salvage strategy. The EBMT registry published a retrospective analysis of 101 patients (van Kampen et al., 2011). About two-thirds of the patients received an RIC regimen, and 70% had a MRD. At three years, the NRM was 28%, with relapse and OS rates being 30% and 53%, respectively.

Involved field radiotherapy after transplantation

IFRT after HCT is offered to select patients based on observations that lymphoma patients frequently relapse in sites of previously bulky disease. IFRT has unequivocally demonstrated significant effect on local control in numerous published series with the sites at greatest risk of failure being those failing to achieve a CR to salvage therapy prior to HCT (Biswas et al., 2010; Ochler-Janne et al., 2008). However, the survival benefit of IFRT after HCT is equivocal despite the clear benefit of local control. Despite the lack of randomized trials, IFRT is routinely recommended due to its benefit in achieving local control and its ability to convert patients with persistent disease to CR after HCT. Post-IFRT is often administered one to three months post-HCT when blood counts have fully recovered.

Mantle cell lymphoma
Mantle cell lymphoma IPI

The mantle cell lymphoma (MCL) IPI (MIPI) is a formula-based computed index that allows separation of three well-balanced groups of patients with significantly different prognoses – low-risk (median OS not reached), intermediate-risk (median OS of 51 months), and high-risk groups (median OS of 29 months) – based on the four independent prognostic factors: age, performance status, lactate dehydrogenase (LDH), and leukocyte count (Hoster et al., 2008) (see following figure). The simplified MIPI (s-MIPI) is a more practical score-based index developed by the same authors. The s-MIPI score measured immediately prior to auto-HCT has also been reported to be predictive for OS and PFS (Thompson et al., 2011) (see the following table).

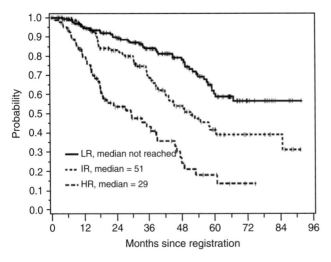

OS according to the MIPI. LR indicates low risk, MIPI <5.7; IR, intermediate risk, score 5.7–6.2; and HR, high risk, ≥6.2. MIPI is calculated as $[0.03535 \times$ age (years)$] + 0.6978$ (if ECOG >1) $+ [1.367 \times \log_{10}(LDH/ULN)] + [0.9393 \times \log_{10}($WBC count$)]$ (Hoster et al., 2008). ECOG, Eastern Cooperative Oncology Group; ULN, upper limit of normal. (Reproduced with permission.)

Simplified Mantle Cell Lymphoma International Prognostic Index

Points	Age (yr)	Eastern Cooperative Oncology Group	LDH/ULN	White blood cell count (10^9/L)
0	<50	0–1	<0.67	<6.700
1	50–59	–	0.67–0.99	6.700–9.999
2	60–69	2–4	1.000–1.49	1.000–14.999
3	≥70	–	≥1.5000	≥15000

For each prognostic factor, 0–3 points are assigned to each patient. Points are totaled to a maximum of 11. Patients with 0–3 points were low risk, 4–5 points were intermediate risk, and 6–11 were high risk. LDH was weighted according to the ratio to the ULN (Hoster et al., 2008) (Reproduced with permission.)

The Ki-67 index has also been shown to be an independent prognostic factor at diagnosis. In a series of 249 advanced-stage MCL patients, the Ki-67 index was predictive for OS (RR 1.27 for 10% higher Ki-67, P<0.001), independent of clinical prognostic factors (Determann et al., 2008). The three groups with a Ki-67 index of less than 10%, 10% to less than 30%, and 30% or more showed a significantly different OS in patients treated with CHOP (P<0.001) or R-CHOP (P=0.013).

Autologous and allogeneic HCT
Autologous transplantation for MCL
MCL comprises 5%–10% of all NHL. It is characterized by an aggressive course with a median OS of three years (Ghielmini & Aucca, 2009; Romaguera et al., 2010). MCL is chemosensitive, but responses are typically short-lived with chemotherapy. Given the poor long-term outcomes with standard chemotherapy, auto-HCT has been offered as consolidation therapy. A notable study comes from the Nordic group (the second Nordic MCL trial) that evaluated intensive induction immunochemotherapy with alternating cycles of "maxi" R-CHOP and R-cytarabine followed by auto-HCT in a phase II trial (Geisler et al., 2008). The six-year EFS and OS were 56% and 70%, respectively. No relapse was observed after five years. When compared with the previous Nordic MCL trial, the addition of rituximab and high-dose cytarabine appeared to improve outcomes (see following figure). Interestingly, it was found that the MIPI and s-MIPI were superior to the IPI in predicting survival in this Nordic study group (Geisler et al., 2010).

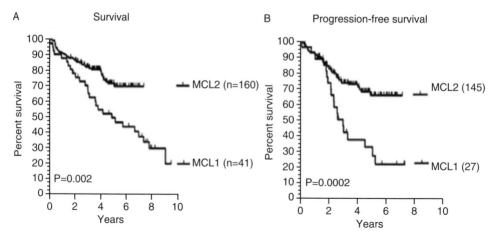

Overall survival, A: of patients of National Lymphoma Group protocols MCL-1 and MCL-2, respectively; B: PFS of protocols MCL-1 and MCL-2, respectively, of responders who completed treatment (Geisler et al., 2008). (Reproduced with permission.)

The CALGB (Cancer and Leukemia Group B) reported the results of a prospective study of 78 MCL patients of less than 70 years of age who received induction with augmented CHOP and methotrexate, followed by high-dose cytarabine and etoposide mobilization, and then auto-HCT in CR1 (Damon et al., 2009). Rituximab was a part of induction, consolidation, and high-dose therapy (HDT). With a median follow-up of 4.7 years, five-year PFS and OS rates were 56% and 64%. These results also suggested that the addition of rituximab and high-dose cytarabine, with auto-HCT in CR1, have markedly improved survival in MCL.

Allogeneic HCT for MCL

Myeloablative allo-HCT can confer long-term DFS and cures in patients who failed auto-HCT but at the cost of NRM of 30%–40% (Kroger et al., 1998; Laudi et al., 2010). Promising results have been reported with RIC allo-HCT. The Seattle group published the results of non-myeloablative allo-HCT using fludarabine/TBI (2 Gy) for relapsed/refractory MCL (n=34) (Maris et al., 2004). At two years, the DFS and OS were 60% and 65%, respectively, while the relapse and NRM rates were 9% and 24% at two years, respectively. Of note, those transplanted in CR did not relapse after a median follow-up of 24.6 months. The M.D. Anderson group reported outcomes of RIC allo-HCT using fludarabine, cyclophospham-ide, and rituximab as conditioning for relapsed/refractory MCL (n=35) (Tam et al., 2009); most had chemosensitive disease. The one-year NRM rate was 9%. With a median follow-up of 56 months, the median PFS was 60 months, while the median OS had not been reached. A plateau in the survival curves was observed in both series, suggesting that allo-HCT may eradicate MCL in a significant proportion of patients with relapsed/refractory disease (Ayala & Tomblyn, 2011).

Follicular NHL

The definitive management of advanced follicular lymphoma (FL) remains controversial due to numerous treatment options available. The natural history of FL is characterized by a continuous pattern or relapses resulting in progressively shorter remission durations.

Follicular lymphoma IPI

The FLIPI is a widely used index for prognostication in newly diagnosed FL patients (Solal-Celigny et al., 2004) (see following figure and table).

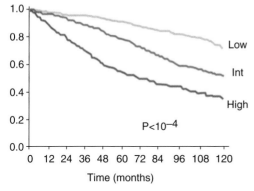

Follicular Lymphoma
International
Prognostic Index

- Age >60 yr
- Ann Arbor stage III/IV disease
- LDH > ULN
- Hemoglobin <120 g/L
- >4 nodal sites

Survival according to risk group as defined by the FLIPI.

Outcome and relative risk of death according to risk group as defined by the Follicular Lymphoma International Prognostic Index (FLIPI)

FLIPI risk group	Risk factors (n)	5-year overall survival	10-year overall survival
Low	0–1	91%	71%
Intermediate	2	78%	51%
High	≥3	53%	36%

Autologous and allogeneic HCT

There is no role for auto-HCT as early consolidation therapy as three randomized trials have shown no benefit in survival when compared to conventional therapy as front-line treatment (Gyan et al., 2009; Lenz et al., 2004; Sebban et al., 2006).

For FL patients beyond first response, retrospective analyses have shown that auto-HCT can provide benefit for patients who are not heavily pretreated prior to auto-HCT (Devetten et al., 2009). For patients with relapsed disease who demonstrate chemosensitivity to salvage therapy, one prospective randomized trial from Europe has shown that auto-HCT confers a longer EFS with a trend toward improved OS compared to salvage therapy alone.

Allo-HCT is the only known curative therapy for patients with FL. Although no randomized trials have been completed, results have consistently shown less relapse among recipients of allo-HCT compared to auto-HCT. However, the TRM associated with myeloablative allo-HCT has limited the benefits of the lower relapse rates. Therefore, the use of RIC allo-HCT is being offered increasingly to FL patients who are beyond first response. With follow-up times ranging from three to nine years, several studies utilizing various RIC regimens with related and unrelated donors have reported EFS and OS of 65%–72% and 73%–78%, respectively (Khouri et al., 2011; Piana et al., 2010; Shea et al., 2011). The Blood and Marrow Transplant Clinical Trials Network (BMT CTN) is conducting a phase

II multicenter RIC allo-HCT trial using FCR (fludarabine, cyclophosphamide, rituximab) as the conditioning regimen to confirm the efficacy of this modality in patients with relapsed FL.

Peripheral T-cell lymphomas

The peripheral T-cell lymphomas (PTCLs) generally are associated with a poor prognosis with a five-year survival of <30% and a median survival of 20–34 months (Foss et al., 2011). With the exception of ALK+ anaplastic large-cell lymphomas, the PTCLs are characterized by high remission rates after frontline chemotherapy, but relapse inevitably occurs. In light of the poor prognosis of most patients with PTCL, high-dose chemotherapy with auto-HCT is commonly offered to patients as consolidation therapy or for relapsed or refractory disease.

Autologous and allogeneic HCT

Owing to the rarity and the heterogeneity of the PTCL histologies, no randomized trials have addressed the role of auto-HCT as frontline therapy. However, several prospective trials have addressed this question and have demonstrated PFS of 30%–59% with a median follow-up of three to six years (d'Amore et al., 2011; Mercadal et al., 2008; Reimer et al., 2009) (see following figure). It should be noted that these studies are intent-to-treat analyses, and approximately one-third of the patients were induction failures and thus did not proceed to auto-HCT. Factors that predicted for a more favorable outcome included anaplastic large-cell lymphoma (ALCL) histology, low-risk IPI or PIT (Prognostic Index for PTCL-U) score at diagnosis, and most importantly, chemosensitivity (Reimer et al., 2009). Several retrospective analyses have examined the role of auto-HCT as early consolidation therapy. As compared to the prospective studies, the retrospective analyses reported generally superior survival outcomes as they only included patients who actually received auto-HCT, which indicates that all patients were chemosensitive and thus were inherently favorable risk patients. The retrospective studies report PFS of 60%–70% with median follow-up ranging from four to six years (Numata et al., 2010; Rodriguez et al., 2007).

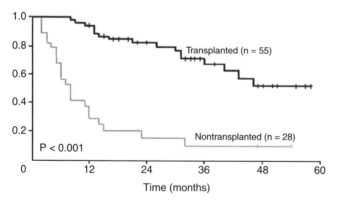

Estimated five-year OS for PTCL patients who underwent autologous HCT as first-line therapy compared with only 11% who did not undergo HCT (Reimer et al., 2009). (Reproduced with permission.)

Allo-HCT is also a reasonable option for PTCL patients with relapsed or refractory disease or as consolidation therapy for patients with more aggressive PTCL histologies such as hepatosplenic T-cell lymphoma and enteropathy-associated T-cell NHL. The existence of a graft-versus-lymphoma effect in the PTCL histologies is supported by responses seen after

DLI for relapsed disease and in observed plateaus in DFS after allo-HCT. Allo-HCT with RIC regimens have yielded more encouraging results as the TRM has been prohibitive with myeloablative conditioning regimens (Dodero et al., 2012; Goldberg et al., 2012; Jacobsen et al., 2011; Kyriakou et al., 2009).

Secondary malignancies after transplantation

Secondary malignancies after HCT are rare events, but nevertheless, all patients should be advised of the risks of secondary malignancies and be encouraged to be screened routinely for such complications long term. After auto-HCT, the risk of therapy-related myeloid neoplasms (t-MDS/t-AML) has an overall incidence of 4% at seven years with a median onset of 2.5 years. Risk factors include prior alkylator agents, long duration of prior conventional chemotherapy, and higher dose of pre-HCT radiation therapy (Metayer et al., 2003).

Recipients of allo-HCT are at risk for secondary solid cancer and posttransplant lymphoproliferative disorders (PTLD). Regarding solid tumors, there is a latency period of three to five years after allogeneic HCT with cumulative incidence rates of 1%–2% at 10 years and 3% at 20 years (Hari et al., 2010; Loren et al., 2011). The use of TBI and chronic GVHD are the strongest risk factors for the development of solid tumors. TBI exposure is associated with nonsquamous cell cancers especially of the breast, thyroid, bone, brain, and malignant melanoma and also increases the risk of basal cell skin cancer. The development of squamous cell cancers of the skin and mucosal surfaces increases with the presence of chronic GVHD (Leisenring et al., 2006).

PTLD manifests in the setting of significant immunosuppression after allo-HCT and usually occurs early or within six months after HCT. The overall incidence is 1% at 10 years after HCT, and the vast majority is associated with Epstein–Barr virus (EBV) infection. Receipt of a T-cell depleted graft, use of ATG in the conditioning regimen, and HLA disparity between recipient and donor are the strongest predictors of developing PTLD (Landgren et al., 2009). Monitoring PB EBV DNA viral load with quantitative PCR assays can identify patients at risk for developing PTLD (Reddy et al., 2011). Treatment with rituximab-based preemptive therapy can be effective in preventing EBV viremia from progressing to overt PTLD. It is recommended that rituximab therapy commences when the PB EBV DNA as measured by quantitative PCR reaches >1000 copies/mL (Baes et al., 2010; van Esser et al., 2002).

CIBMTR data

A

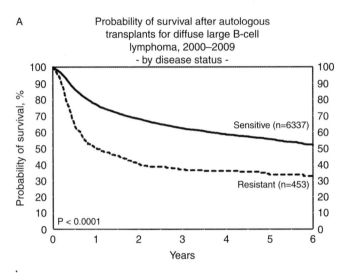

Probability of survival after autologous transplants for diffuse large B-cell lymphoma, 2000–2009 - by disease status -

Sensitive (n=6337)

Resistant (n=453)

P < 0.0001

A: autologous HCT is an accepted treatment indication for DLBCL and, similar to FL, most auto-HCTs are performed in patients with chemosensitive disease. Among the 6790 patients who received an auto-HCT for DLBCL between the years 2000 and 2009, the three-year probabilities of survival were 62% ± 1% and 37% ± 2% for patients with chemosensitive and chemoresistant disease, respectively (Pasquini & Wang, 2011).

B

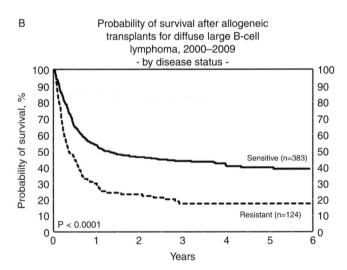

Probability of survival after allogeneic transplants for diffuse large B-cell lymphoma, 2000–2009 - by disease status -

Sensitive (n=383)

Resistant (n=124)

P < 0.0001

B: allo-HCT for treatment of DLBCL is performed less frequently than for FL and is generally used only in patients with aggressive disease that has been resistant to previous therapies, including auto-HCT. Among the 507 patients who underwent an HLA-matched sibling HCT for DLBCL from 2000 to 2009, the three-year probabilities of survival were 44% ± 3% and 17% ± 4% for patients with chemosensitive and chemoresistant disease, respectively (Pasquini & Wang, 2011).

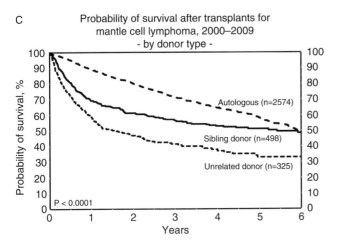

C: the optimal timing of HCT for MCL is not well defined. As with other mature B-cell lymphoproliferative disorders, auto-HCT is the most common transplant approach. Among the 2574 patients who received an auto-HCT for MCL between 2000 and 2009, the three-year probability of survival was 71% ± 1%. Among 823 patients who underwent an allo-HCT for MCL during the same period, the three-year probabilities of survival were 57% ± 2% and 41% ± 3% for sibling and unrelated donor transplants, respectively (Pasquini & Wang, 2011).

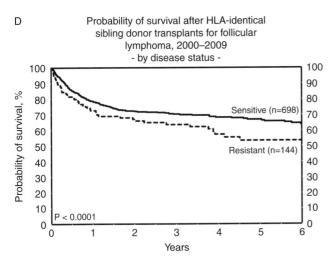

D: similar to HL, allo-HCT for FL is performed in patients who experience disease relapse after multiple lines of therapy or who have refractory disease and an available HLA-match donor. Among 842 patients receiving HLA-matched sibling donor transplants for FL between 2000 and 2009, the three-year probabilities of survival were 70% ± 2% and 64% ± 4% for patients with chemosensitive and chemoresistant disease, respectively (Pasquini & Wang, 2011).

Lymphoblastic lymphoma

LBL is a rare and highly aggressive lymphoma most commonly of precursor T-cell origin. LBL is seen most frequently in adolescents and young adults with a male predominance and typically involves the mediastinum, CNS, and bone marrow. Intensified and prolonged chemotherapy together with CNS prophylaxis similar to ALL-type regimens confer long-term DFS rates ranging from 62% to 70% (Hoelzer et al., 2002; Thomas et al., 2004). The addition of auto-HCT or allo-HCT as consolidation therapy has not improved these outcomes (Bouabdallah et al., 1998; Song et al., 2007). For patients with more advanced disease, retrospective series have shown less relapse with allo-HCT compared to auto-HCT. However, the OS between the two types of HCT is comparable due to the higher NRM seen in the allo-HCT group. A CIBMTR retrospective analysis compared the outcomes of 204 LBL patients at different stages of disease who received auto-HCT (n=128) or allo-HCT (n=76) (Levine et al., 2003). The relapse rates were 56% versus 34% in the auto-HCT and allo-HCT groups, respectively, but the survival of 44% versus 39% was comparable as the higher NRM in the allo-HCT group. Thus, for advanced disease that is chemosensitive, auto-HCT is a valid option but allo-HCT should also be considered for younger patients with a compatible donor.

Burkitt lymphoma

Burkitt lymphoma (BL) is a highly aggressive B-cell lymphoma accounting for 1%–2% of adult lymphomas in the United States and Western Europe (Linch, 2012). BL is character-ized by a high proliferation rate but is highly curable when treated with brief-duration intensive chemotherapy and aggressive intrathecal prophylaxis. Disease-free survival ranges from 70% to 100% with upfront intensive chemotherapy (Lacasce et al., 2004; Linch et al., 2012; Thomas et al., 2006). In light of these high response rates and durable remissions, auto-HCT in CR1 is not routinely recommended. A few studies have explored this question but studies are small and heterogenous and show no definitive evidence that auto-HCT improves survival as consolidation versus frontline chemotherapy alone. For BL patients with recurrent or refractory lymphoma, two retrospective registry studies showed no difference in relapse or survival between auto-HCT and allo-HCT (Peniket et al., 2003). In the CIBMTR study, the relapse rates with auto-HCT and allo-HCT groups were 65% versus 63%, and EFS were 27% versus 31%, respectively (Gross et al., 2010).

HIV-related lymphoma

NHL is an AIDS-defining diagnosis and is several-fold more common in HIV-positive individuals (Engels et al., 2008). DLBCL, BL, and Burkitt-like lymphoma are the most common types in these patients (Ayala & Tomblyn, 2011). The outcome has improved significantly in HIV patients on highly active antiretroviral therapy (HAART), and is now similar to non-HIV patients with NHL (Lim et al., 2005). Auto-HCT in patients with HIV NHL is feasible and effective with most patients continuing HAART throughout the peritransplant period (Ayala & Tomblyn, 2011). The City of Hope reported their experience of 20 HIV patients (18 NHL and 2 HL) with high-risk lymphoma (Krishnan et al., 2005). At a median follow-up of 31 months, 17 of 20 patients were disease-free. The EBMT Lymphoma Working Party presented retrospective data on 68 patients with HIV-related NHL who had auto-HCT (Balsalobre et al., 2009). The one-year NRM rate was 7.5%, mainly from bacterial infections, and the relapse rate was 30% at 24 months. At a median follow-up of 32 months, OS was 61%. Disease status at transplant and chemosensitivity were prognostic indicators of outcome.

Allo-HCT in HIV patients has challenges, including the risk of opportunistic infection, the potential effect of HIV on the bone marrow environment, and immune reconstitution following HCT (Ayala & Tomblyn, 2011). However, the availability of HAART has increased the feasibility of allo-HCT in this high-risk population. The published literature comprises mostly case reports. The BMT CTN is currently conducting a phase II allo-HCT trial for patients with HIV-related lymphoma.

Imaging and transplantation

PET is useful in the pre-therapy staging, treatment monitoring, and post-therapeutic evalu-ation of patients with lymphoma (Dodero et al., 2010). Several studies have shown that PET before auto-HCT is predictive for PFS and/or OS (Alousi et al., 2008; Filmont et al., 2007).

A retrospective analysis of NHL and HL patients undergoing auto-HCT showed that a positive pre-HCT PET scan predicted for a decreased PFS, whereas a post-HCT PET scan did not predict for EFS or OS after auto-HCT (Palmer et al., 2011).

A prospective study examining the role of PET in allo-HCT reported that, in patients with various histologies of HL and NHL, a positive PET scan pre-HCT did not impact survival or relapse (Lambert et al., 2010). However, after allo-HCT, PET surveillance appeared to add useful information to that provided by CT, allowing earlier DLI in many who relapsed post-HCT. This data suggested that allo-HCT may overcome the unfavorable prognostic effects of a positive pre-transplant PET, and PET scanning may be helpful post-HCT. However, routine PET surveillance after HCT is not currently recommended in this setting.

Guidelines for post-HCT surveillance

1. **2012 National Comprehensive Cancer Network (NCCN) Guidelines for DLBCL** recommend restaging CT scans for patients in remission every six months for up to two years, without ongoing routine surveillance, unless clinically indicated (Zelenetz et al., 2012).
2. **2010 European Society of Medical Oncology (ESMO) Guidelines for DLBCL** (Tilly & Dreyling, 2010) advocate minimal adequate radiological examinations at 6, 12, and 24 months after treatment, usually by a CT scan; there is no definitive evidence that routine imaging in patients in CR provides any outcome advantage. These guidelines specifically advise against routine PET surveillance, but recommend PET at the end of treatment. ESMO recommends minimal adequate radiological examinations every six months for two years, and then annually, for FL (Dreyling, 2010).

Pre-HCT evaluation

- Medical history and physical examination
- Complete blood count with differential
- Basic blood chemistry, including LDH and uric acid tests
- Serum protein electrophoresis/immunofixation to exclude monoclonal (M-spike) immunoglobulin peaks
- Serum IgA, IgG, and IgM
- Bone marrow aspiration and biopsy
- Immunophenotyping by flow cytometry of bone marrow
- Hepatitis B virus (HBV) and HIV serology
- Imaging study includes CT scans of the neck, thorax, abdomen, and pelvis, or a PET-CT scan
- Multigated (MUGA) scan/echocardiogram
- Pulmonary function test, including diffusion capacity for carbon monoxide

Post-HCT evaluation

- History and physical examination, and basic laboratory studies every three to six months posttransplant for five years, and then annually or as clinically indicated.

- For patients with DLBCL, NCCN guidelines recommend a CT scan no more often than every six months for two years after completion of therapy, and then only as clinically warranted (Zelenetz et al., 2012). A PET-CT is not recommended for routine surveillance, once the patient has achieved CR.

References and further reading

Alousi AM, Saliba RM, Okoroji GJ, et al. 2008. Disease staging with positron emission tomography or gallium scanning and use of rituximab predict outcome for patients with diffuse large B-cell lymphoma treated with autologous stem cell transplantation. *Br J Haematol* **142**: 786–792.

Armitage JO, Carbone PP, Connors JM, et al. 2003. Treatment-related myelodysplasia and acute leukemia in non-Hodgkin's lymphoma patients. *J Clin Oncol* **21**: 897–906.

Ayala E & Tomblyn M. 2011. Hematopoietic cell transplantation for lymphomas. *Cancer Control* **18**: 246–257.

Baes AH, Cao Q, Wagner JE, et al. 2010. Monitoring and preemptive rituximab therapy for Epstein-Barr virus reactivation after antithymocyte globulin containing nonmyeloablative conditioning for umbilical cord blood transplantation. *Biol Blood Marrow Transplant* **16**: 287–291.

Balsalobre P, Díez-Martin JL, Re A, et al. 2009. Autologous stem-cell transplantation in patients with HIV-related lymphoma. *J Clin Oncol* **27**: 2192–2198.

Biswas T, Dhakal S, Chen R, et al. 2010. Involved field radiation after autologous stem cell transplant for diffuse large B-cell lymphoma in the rituximab era. *Int J Rad Oncol Biol Phys* **77**: 79–85.

Bouabdallah R, Xerri L, Bardou VJ, et al. 1998. Role of induction chemotherapy and bone marrow transplantation in adult lymphoblastic lymphoma: a report on 62 patients from a single center. *Ann Oncol* **9**: 619–625.

Damon LE, Johnson JL, Niedzwiecki D, et al. 2009. Immunochemotherapy and autologous stem-cell transplantation for untreated patients with mantle-cell lymphoma: CALGB 59909. *J Clin Oncol* **27**: 6101–6108.

d'Amore F, Relander T, Lauritzen GF, et al. 2011. High-dose chemotherapy and autologous stem cell transplantation in previously untreated peripheral t-cell lymphoma – final analysis of a large prospective multicenter study (NLG-T-01). *Blood* **118**: 331.

Determann O, Hoster E, Ott G, et al. 2008. Ki-67 predicts outcome in advanced-stage mantle cell lymphoma patients treated with anti-CD20 immunochemotherapy: results from randomized trials of the European MCL Network and the German Low Grade Lymphoma Study Group. *Blood* **111**: 2385–2387.

Devetten MP, Hari PN, Carreras J, et al. 2009. Unrelated donor reduced-intensity allogeneic hematopoietic stem cell transplantation for relapsed and refractory Hodgkin lymphoma. *Biol Blood Marrow Transplant* **15**: 109–117.

Dodero A, Crocchiolo R, Patriarca F, et al. 2010. Pretransplantation [18-F]fluorodeoxyglucose positron emission tomography scan predicts outcome in patients with recurrent Hodgkin lymphoma or aggressive non-Hodgkin lymphoma undergoing reduced-intensity conditioning followed by allogeneic stem cell transplantation. *Cancer* **116**: 5001–5011.

Dodero A, Spina F, Narni F, et al. 2012. Allogeneic transplantation following a reduced-intensity conditioning regimen in relapsed/refractory peripheral T-cell lymphomas: long-term remissions and response to donor lymphocyte infusions support the role of a graft-versus-lymphoma effect. *Leukemia* **26**: 520–526.

Dreyling M. 2010. Newly diagnosed and relapsed follicular lymphoma: ESMO Clinical Practice Guidelines for diagnosis, treatment and follow-up. *Ann Oncol* **21**: S181–S183.

El Gnaoui T, Dupuis J, Belhadj K, et al. 2007. Rituximab, gemcitabine and oxaliplatin: an effective salvage regimen for patients with relapsed or refractory B-cell lymphoma not candidates for high-dose therapy. *Ann Oncol* **18**: 1363–1368.

Engels EA, Biggar RJ, Hall HI, et al. 2008. Cancer risk in people infected with human immunodeficiency virus in the United States. *Int J Cancer* **123**: 187–194.

Filmont JE, Gisselbrecht C, Cuenca X, et al. 2007. The impact of pre- and post-transplantation positron emission tomography using 18-fluorodeoxyglucose on poor-prognosis lymphoma patients undergoing autologous stem cell transplantation. *Cancer* **110**: 1361–1369.

Foss FM, Zinzani PL, Vose JM, et al. 2011. Peripheral T-cell lymphoma. *Blood* **117**: 6756–6767.

Friedberg JW. 2011. Relapsed/refractory diffuse large B-cell lymphoma. Hematology Am Soc Hematol Educ Program 2011: 498–501.

Geisler CH, Kolstad A, Laurell A, et al. 2008. Long-term progression-free survival of mantle cell lymphoma after intensive front-line immunochemotherapy with in vivo-purged stem cell rescue: a nonrandomized phase 2 multicenter study by the Nordic Lymphoma Group. *Blood* **112**: 2687–2693.

Geisler CH, Kolstad A, Laurell A, et al. 2010. The mantle cell lymphoma international prognostic index (MIPI) is superior to the international prognostic index (IPI) in predicting survival following intensive first-line immunochemotherapy and autologous stem cell transplantation (ASCT). *Blood* **115**: 1530–1533.

Ghielmini M & Zucca E. 2009. How I treat mantle cell lymphoma. *Blood* **114**: 1469–1476.

Gisselbrecht C, Glass B, Mounier N, et al. 2010. Salvage regimens with autologous transplantation for relapsed large B-cell lymphoma in the rituximab era. *J Clin Oncol* **28**: 4184–4190.

Goldberg JD, Chou JF, Horwitz S, et al. 2012. Long-term survival in patients with peripheral T-cell non-Hodgkin lymphomas after allogeneic hematopoietic stem cell transplant. *Leuk Lymphoma* **53**: 1124–1129.

Gross TG, Hale GA, He W, et al. 2010. Hematopoietic stem cell transplantation for refractory or recurrent non-Hodgkin lymphoma in children and adolescents. *Biol Blood Marrow Transplant* **16**: 223–230.

Gyan E, Foussard C, Bertrand P, et al. 2009. High-dose therapy followed by autologous purged stem cell transplantation and

doxorubicin-based chemotherapy in patients with advanced follicular lymphoma: a randomized multicenter study by the GOELAMS with final results after a median follow-up of 9 years. *Blood* **113**: 995–1001.

Hamlin PA, Zelenetz AD, Kewalramani T, et al. 2003. Age-adjusted international prognostic index predicts autologous stem cell transplantation outcome for patients with relapsed or primary refractory diffuse large B-cell lymphoma. *Blood* **102**: 1989–1996.

Hari PN, Majhail NS, Zhang MJ, et al. 2010. Race and outcomes of autologous hematopoietic cell transplantation for multiple myeloma. *Biol Blood Marrow Transplant* **16**: 395–402.

Hoelzer D, Gokbuget N, Digel W, et al. 2002. Outcome of adult patients with T-lymphoblastic lymphoma treated according to protocols for acute lymphoblastic leukemia. *Blood* **99**: 4379–4385.

Hoster E, Dreyling M, Klapper W, et al. 2008. A new prognostic index (MIPI) for patients with advanced-stage mantle cell lymphoma. *Blood* **111**: 558–565.

Jacobsen ED, Kim HT, Ho VT, et al. 2011. A large single-center experience with allogeneic stem-cell transplantation for peripheral T-cell non-Hodgkin lymphoma and advanced mycosis fungoides/Sezary syndrome. *Ann Oncol* **22**: 1608–1613.

Kewalramani T, Zelenetz AD, Nimer SD, et al. 2004. Rituximab and ICE as second-line therapy before autologous stem cell transplantation for relapsed or primary refractory diffuse large B-cell lymphoma. *Blood* **103**: 3684–3688.

Khouri I, Saliba RM, Valverde R, et al. 2011. Nonmyeloablative allogeneic stem cell transplantation with or without 90yttrium ibritumomab tiuxetan (90YIT) is curative for relapsed follicular lymphoma: median 9 year follow-up results. *Blood* **118**: 662.

Krishnan A, Molina A, Zaia J, et al. 2005. Durable remissions with autologous stem cell transplantation for high-risk HIV-associated lymphomas. *Blood* **105**: 874–878.

Kroger N, Hoffknecht M, Dreger P, et al. 1998. Long-term disease-free survival of patients with advanced mantle-cell lymphoma following high-dose chemotherapy. *Bone Marrow Transplant* **21**: 55–57.

Kyriakou C, Canals C, Finke J, et al. 2009. Allogeneic stem cell transplantation is able to induce long-term remissions in angioimmunoblastic T-cell lymphoma: a retrospective study from the Lymphoma Working Party of the European Group for Blood and Marrow Transplantation. *J Clin Oncol* **27**: 3951–3958.

Lacasce A, Howard O, Lib S, et al. 2004. Modified magrath regimens for adults with Burkitt and Burkitt-like lymphomas: preserved efficacy with decreased toxicity. *Leuk Lymphoma* **45**: 761–767.

Lambert JR, Bomanji JB, Peggs KS, et al. 2010. Prognostic role of PET scanning before and after reduced-intensity allogeneic stem cell transplantation for lymphoma. *Blood* **115**: 2763–2768.

Landgren O, Gilbert ES, Rizzo JD, et al. 2009. Risk factors for lymphoproliferative disorders after allogeneic hematopoietic cell transplantation. *Blood* **113**: 4992–5001.

Laudi N, Arora M, Burns L, et al. 2006. Efficacy of high-dose therapy and hematopoietic stem cell transplantation for mantle cell lymphoma. *Am J Hematol* **81**: 519–524.

Lazarus HM, Zhang MJ, Carreras J, et al. 2010. A comparison of HLA-identical sibling allogeneic versus autologous transplantation for diffuse large B cell lymphoma: a report from the CIBMTR. *Biol Blood Marrow Transplant* **16**: 35–45.

Leisenring W, Friedman DL, Flowers ME, et al. 2006. Nonmelanoma skin and mucosal cancers after hematopoietic cell transplantation. *J Clin Oncol* **24**: 1119–1126.

Lenz G, Dreyling M, Schiegnitz E, et al. 2004. Myeloablative radiochemotherapy followed by autologous stem cell transplantation in first remission prolongs progression-free survival in follicular lymphoma: results of a prospective, randomized trial of the German Low-Grade Lymphoma Study Group. *Blood* **104**: 2667–2674.

Levine JE, Harris RE, Loberiza FR Jr, et al. 2003. A comparison of allogeneic and autologous bone marrow transplantation for lymphoblastic lymphoma. *Blood* **101**: 2476–2482.

Linch DC. 2012. Burkitt lymphoma in adults. *Br J Haematol* **156**: 693–703.

Lim ST, Karim R, Nathwani BN, et al. 2005. AIDS-related Burkitt's lymphoma versus diffuse large-cell lymphoma in the pre-highly active antiretroviral therapy (HAART) and HAART eras: significant differences in survival with standard chemotherapy. *J Clin Oncol* **23**: 4430–4438.

Lopez A, Gutierrez A, Palacios A, et al. 2008. GEMOX-R regimen is a highly effective salvage regimen in patients with refractory/relapsing diffuse large-cell lymphoma: a phase II study. *Eur J Haematol* **80**: 127–132.

Loren AW, Chow E, Jacobsohn DA, et al. 2011. Pregnancy after hematopoietic cell transplantation: a report from the late effects working committee of the Center for International Blood and Marrow Transplant Research (CIBMTR). *Biol Blood Marrow Transplant* **17**: 157–166.

Maris MB, Sandmaier BM, Storer BE, et al. 2004. Allogeneic hematopoietic cell transplantation after fludarabine and 2 Gy total body irradiation for relapsed and refractory mantle cell lymphoma. *Blood* **104**: 3535–3542.

Mercadal S, Briones J, Xicoy B, et al. 2008. Intensive chemotherapy (high-dose CHOP/ESHAP regimen) followed by autologous stem-cell transplantation in previously untreated patients with peripheral T-cell lymphoma. *Ann Oncol* **19**: 958–963.

Metayer C, Curtis RE, Vose J, et al. 2003. Myelodysplastic syndrome and acute myeloid leukemia after autotransplantation for lymphoma: a multicenter case-control study. *Blood* **101**: 2015–2023.

Nademanee A, Forman S, Molina A, et al. 2005. A phase 1/2 trial of high-dose yttrium-90-ibritumomab tiuxetan in combination with high-dose etoposide and cyclophosphamide followed by autologous stem cell transplantation in patients with poor-risk or relapsed non-Hodgkin lymphoma. *Blood* **106**: 2896–2902.

Numata A, Miyamoto T, Ohno Y, et al. 2010. Long-term outcomes of autologous PBSCT for peripheral T-cell lymphoma:

retrospective analysis of the experience of the Fukuoka BMT group. *Bone Marrow Transplant* 45: 311–316.

Oehler-Janne C, Taverna C, Stanek N, et al. 2008. Consolidative involved field radiotherapy after high dose chemotherapy and autologous stem cell transplantation for non-Hodgkin's lymphoma: a case-control study. *Hematol Oncol* 26: 82–90.

Palmer J, Goggins T, Broadwater G, et al. 2011. Early post transplant (F-18) 2-fluoro-2-deoxyglucose positron emission tomography does not predict outcome for patients undergoing auto-SCT in non-Hodgkin and Hodgkin lymphoma. *Bone Marrow Transplant* 46:847–851.

Pasquini MC & Wang Z. 2011. *Current use and outcome of hematopoietic stem cell transplantation*. CIBMTR Summary Slides.

Peniket AJ, Ruiz de Elvira MC, Taghipour G, et al. 2003. An EBMT registry matched study of allogeneic stem cell transplants for lymphoma: allogeneic transplantation is associated with a lower relapse rate but a higher procedure-related mortality rate than autologous transplantation. *Bone Marrow Transplant* 31: 667–678.

Philip T, Guglielmi C, Hagenbeek A, et al. 1995. Autologous bone marrow transplantation as compared with salvage chemotherapy in relapses of chemotherapy-sensitive non-Hodgkin's lymphoma. *N Engl J Med* 333: 1540–1545.

Pinana JL, Martino R, Gayoso J, et al. 2010. Reduced intensity conditioning HLA identical sibling donor allogeneic stem cell transplantation for patients with follicular lymphoma: long-term follow-up from two prospective multicenter trials. *Haematologica* 95: 1176–1182.

Press OW, Eary JF, Gooley T, et al. 2000. A phase I/II trial of iodine-131-tositumomab (anti-CD20), etoposide, cyclophosphamide, and autologous stem cell transplantation for relapsed B-cell lymphomas. *Blood* 96: 2934–2942.

Reddy N, Rezvani K, Barrett AJ, et al. 2011. Strategies to prevent EBV reactivation and posttransplant lymphoproliferative disorders (PTLD) after allogeneic stem cell

transplantation in high-risk patients. *Biol Blood Marrow Transplant* 17: 591–597.

Reimer P, Rudiger T, Geissinger E, et al. 2009. Autologous stem-cell transplantation as first-line therapy in peripheral T-cell lymphomas: results of a prospective multicenter study. *J Clin Oncol* 27: 106–113.

Rodriguez J, Conde E, Gutierrez A, et al. 2007. The results of consolidation with autologous stem-cell transplantation in patients with peripheral T-cell lymphoma (PTCL) in first complete remission: the Spanish Lymphoma and Autologous Transplantation Group experience. *Ann Oncol* 18: 652–657.

Romaguera JE, Fayad LE, Feng L, et al. 2010. Ten-year follow-up after intense chemoimmunotherapy with rituximab-hyperCVAD alternating with rituximab-high dose methotrexate/cytarabine (R-MA) and without stem cell transplantation in patients with untreated aggressive mantle cell lymphoma. *Br J Haem* 150: 200–208.

Savage KJ & Gregory SA. 2010. *Lymphomas. American Society of Hematology-Self Assessment Program*, Chapter 18, pp. 511–554.

Sebban C, Mounier N, Brousse N, et al. 2006. Standard chemotherapy with interferon compared with CHOP followed by high-dose therapy with autologous stem cell transplantation in untreated patients with advanced follicular lymphoma: the GELF-94 randomized study from the Groupe d'Etude des Lymphomes de l'Adulte (GELA). *Blood* 108: 2540–2544.

Sehn LH, Berry B, Chhanabhai M, et al. 2007. The revised international prognostic index (R-IPI) is a better predictor of outcome than the standard IPI for patients with diffuse large B-cell lymphoma treated with R-CHOP. *Blood* 109: 1857–1861.

Shea T, Johnson J, Westervelt P, et al. 2011. Reduced-intensity allogeneic transplantation provides high event-free and overall survival in patients with advanced indolent B cell malignancies: CALGB 109901. *Biol Blood Marrow Transplant* 17: 1395–1403.

Shipp MA, Harrington DP, Andersen JR, et al. 1993. A predictive model for aggressive non-Hodgkin's lymphoma. *N Engl J Med* 329: 987–994.

Solal-Celigny P, Roy P, Colombat P, et al. 2004. Follicular lymphoma international prognostic index. *Blood* **104**: 1258–1265.

Song KW, Barnett MJ, Gascoyne RD, et al. 2007. Primary therapy for adults with T-cell lymphoblastic lymphoma with hematopoietic stem-cell transplantation results in favorable outcomes. *Ann Oncol* **18**: 535–540.

Stiff PJ, Unger JM, Cook J, et al. 2011. Randomized phase III U.S./Canadian intergroup trial (SWOG S9704) comparing CHOP ± R for eight cycles to CHOP ± R for six cycles followed by autotransplant for patients with high-intermediate (H-Int) or high IPI grade diffuse aggressive non-Hodgkin lymphoma (NHL). *J Clin Oncol* **29**: S8001.

Swerdlow SH, Campo E, Harris NL, et al. 2008. *WHO Classification of Tumors of Hematopoietic and Lymphoid Tissues*. 4th edn. Lyon: IARC Press.

Tam CS, Bassett R, Ledesma C, et al. 2009. Mature results of the M. D. Anderson Cancer Center risk-adapted transplantation strategy in mantle cell lymphoma. *Blood* **113**: 4144–4152.

Thomas DA, Faderl S, O'Brien S, et al. 2006. Chemoimmunotherapy with hyper-CVAD plus rituximab for the treatment of adult Burkitt and Burkitt-type lymphoma or acute lymphoblastic leukemia. *Cancer* **106**: 1569–1580.

Thomas DA, O'Brien S, Cortes J, et al. 2004. Outcome with the hyper-CVAD regimens in lymphoblastic lymphoma. *Blood* **104**: 1624–1630.

Thompson LA, Guthrie KA, Budde LE, et al. 2011. The pre-transplant mantle cell lymphoma international prognostic index predicts overall and progression-free survival following high-dose therapy and autologous stem cell transplant for mantle cell lymphoma. *Blood* **118**: 2026.

Tilly H & Dreyling M. 2010. Diffuse large B-cell non-Hodgkin's lymphoma: ESMO Clinical Practice Guidelines for diagnosis, treatment and follow-up. *Ann Oncol* **21**: S172–S174.

van Esser JW, Niesters HG, van der Holt B, et al. 2002. Prevention of Epstein-Barr virus-lymphoproliferative disease by molecular monitoring and preemptive rituximab in high-risk patients after allogeneic stem cell transplantation. *Blood* **99**: 4364–4369.

van Kampen RJ, Canals C, Schouten HC, et al. 2011. Allogeneic stem-cell transplantation as salvage therapy for patients with diffuse large B-cell non-Hodgkin's lymphoma relapsing after an autologous stem-cell transplantation: an analysis of the European Group for Blood and Marrow Transplantation Registry. *J Clin Oncol* **29**: 1342–1348.

Vose JM, Bierman PJ, Enke C, et al. 2005. Phase I trial of iodine-131 tositumomab with high-dose chemotherapy and autologous stem-cell transplantation for relapsed non-Hodgkin's lymphoma. *J Clin Oncol* **23**: 461–467.

Vose JM, Carter SL, Burns LJ, et al. 2011. Randomized phase III trial of 131-iodine-tositumomab (Bexxar)/carmustine, etoposide, cytarabine, melphalan (BEAM) vs. rituximab/BEAM and autologous stem cell transplantation for relapsed diffuse large B-cell lymphoma (DLBCL): no difference in progression-free (PFS) or overall survival (OS). *Blood* **118**: 661.

Vose JM, Rizzo DJ, Tao-Wu J, et al. 2004. Autologous transplantation for diffuse aggressive non-Hodgkin lymphoma in first relapse or second remission. *Biol Blood Marrow Transplant* **10**: 116–127.

Vose JM, Zhang MJ, Rowlings PA, et al. 2001. Autologous transplantation for diffuse aggressive non-Hodgkin's lymphoma in patients never achieving remission: a report from the Autologous Blood and Marrow Transplant Registry. *J Clin Oncol* **19**: 406–413.

Zelenetz A, Abramson JS, Advani A, et al. 2012. *NCCN Clinical Practice Guidelines in Oncology: Non-Hodgkin's Lymphomas*. NCCN, Ver 2. Available at: http://www.nccn.org/professionals/physician_gls/pdf/nhl.pdf.

Chapter 9
Therapeutic decision making in BMT/SCT for Hodgkin lymphoma

Reinhold Munker, Hillard M. Lazarus, and Kerry Atkinson

Disease classification

(A) Nodular lymphocyte predominant HL	5%
(B) Classical HL	
I. Lymphocyte-rich	5%–8%
II. Nodular sclerosis	35%–55%
III. Mixed cellularity	20%–35%
IV. Lymphocyte depletion	3%–4%

The BMT Data Book, Third Edition, ed. Reinhold Munker et al. Published by Cambridge University Press. © Cambridge University Press 2013.

Disease staging

Modified Ann Arbor Staging System:

Stage I: involvement of a single lymph node region (I) or of a single extralymphatic organ or site (I_E).

Stage II: involvement of two or more lymph node regions on the same side of the diaphragm (II) or localized involvement of an extralymphatic organ or site and of one or more lymph node regions on the same side of the diaphragm (II_E).

Stage III: involvement of lymph node regions on both sides of the diaphragm (III), which may also be accompanied by localized involvement of an extralymphatic organ or site (III_E).

Stage IV: diffuse or disseminated involvement of one or more extralymphatic organs in tissues with or without associated lymph node enlargement.

Systemic symptoms: each stage is subdivided into A and B categories; B for patients with defined symptoms, and A for those without. The B classification is for patients with: (1) unexplained weight loss of more than 10% of body weight in the six months before admission; (2) unexplained fever, with temperatures above 38°C; or (3) night sweats.

Prognostic factors for outcome with conventional therapy

Factor	Better prognosis	Worse prognosis
Stage	Stage I–II	Stage III–IV
Histology	Nodular lymphocyte predominant	Lymphocyte depleted
System symptoms	None	Fevers, night sweats, weight loss
Age	<40 years	>40 years
Gender	Female	Male

Risk factors for early-stage Hodgkin lymphoma (HL)

(Modified from Tubiana et al., 1989.)

- Large mediastinal mass
- B symptoms
- Elevated erythrocyte sedimentation rate
- Involvement of ≥4 lymph node areas
- Age >50 years

Risk factors for advanced HL

(International Prognostic Score; Hasenclever & Diehl, 1998.)

- Serum albumin <40 g/L
- Hb <105 g/L

- Male
- Age >45 years
- Stage IV
- WBC $>15 \times 10^9$/L
- Lymphocyte count $<0.6 \times 10^9$/L

Results with conventional therapy in adult patients

Long-term treatment results in limited-stage HL (data from Milan, Vancouver, and German Hodgkin Study Group, using brief ABVD chemotherapy followed by radiation or chemotherapy only)

OS	95%–98%
DFS	93%–96%

Long-term treatment results in advanced HL (data of German Hodgkin Study Group, protocol HD9, results at five years)

COPP/ABVD + RT	
OS	79%
Freedom from treatment failure	67%
Standard BEACOPP + RT	
OS	84%
Freedom from treatment failure	75%

(Modified from Connors, 2005.)

Results with autologous transplant

Autologous SCT is a standard treatment for patients who relapse after multiagent chemotherapy and offers a chance of long-term remission or cure. Currently, the results of autologous transplantation are better and the toxicity is lower than in the past; therefore, patients should not proceed to second- or third-line salvage regimens. A recent review article reports a five-year PFS of 50%–60% after auto-SCT (Colpo et al., 2012).

Autotransplants are quite effective in primary refractory disease

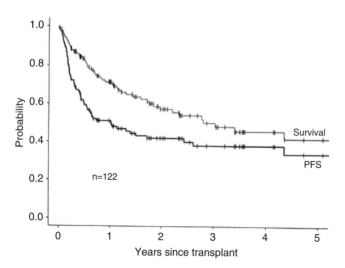

Probability of OS and PFS after autotransplantation for Hodgkin disease in patients never achieving remission. (Reproduced with permission from Lazarus et al., 1999.)

CIBMTR data

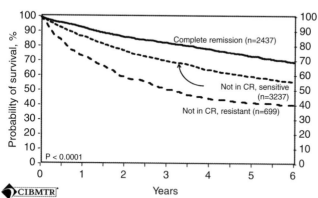

Probability of survival after autologous transplant for Hodgkin lymphoma, by disease status, 1998–2008

Transplantation for HL patients who have failed initial chemotherapy or radiation therapy. Survival after transplant depends on the disease response to previous salvage therapy. Among the 6373 patients receiving an autologous transplant for Hodgkin disease between 1998 and 2008, the three-year probabilities of survival were 82% ± 1%, 70% ± 1%, and 51% ± 2% for patients in CR, in partial remission (PR), and with chemoresistant disease, respectively. (Graph kindly provided by Tanya Pedersen [CIBMTR].)

Prognostic factors affecting long-term outcome after SCT in HL autografted after a first relapse (357 patients; Spanish data).

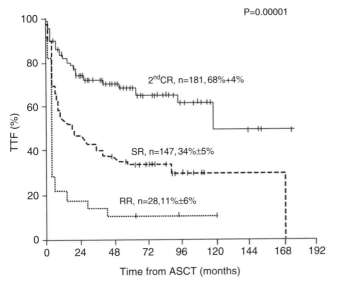

In this study, the OS was 57% ± 3% at five years. At five years, 49% ± 3% had not failed their treatment (were in remission). Risk factors for an adverse outcome were advanced stage at diagnosis, additional radiotherapy before auto-SCT, a short CR1, and detectable disease before transplantation. In this Kaplan–Meier plot, the treatment results (TTF, time-to-treatment failure) are differentiated according to the disease status at the auto-SCT. SR, sensitive relapse; RR, resistant relapse. (Reproduced with permission from Sureda et al., 2005.)

Results with myeloablative allogeneic transplant
Results of standard conditioning allogeneic transplant are not better than autologous transplant

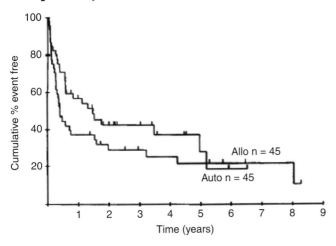

Probability of OS, comparing autologous (auto) and allogeneic (allo) transplants. (Reproduced with permission from Milpied et al., 1996.)

In this EBMT registry study, 45 patients who had an allogeneic transplant were matched with 45 patients who underwent an autologous transplant. The treatment results at four years were as follows:

Allogeneic versus autologous	
OS	25% vs. 37%
PFS	15% vs. 24%
Relapse	61% vs. 61%
NRM	48% vs. 27%

Results with non-myeloablative allogeneic transplant

Because standard conditioning allogeneic transplant has a high TRM, no survival advantage compared to autologous transplant could be demonstrated. More recently, attempts were made to treat relapsed HL with salvage chemotherapy followed by reduced-intensity allogeneic transplant, potentially demonstrating a graft-versus-lymphoma effect (Porter et al., 2003).

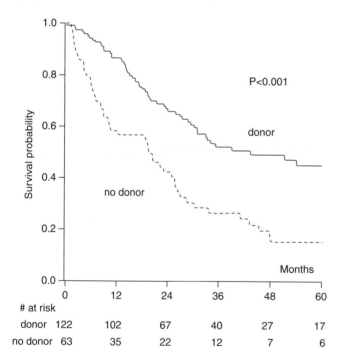

This retrospective study from Italy demonstrates that patients who relapse after an autologous transplant have a better prognosis if they find a matched related or unrelated donor. The survival curve shows OS of 185 patients in whom a donor search was initiated immediately after an autologous transplant had failed. (Reproduced with permission from Sarina et al., 2010.) The transplanted patients had different types of RIC transplants. The overall prognosis and role of reduced-intensity transplants for HL patients is also illustrated by the CIBMTR data.

CIBMTR data

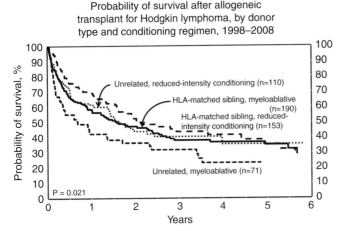

Probability of survival after allogeneic transplant for Hodgkin lymphoma, by donor type and conditioning regimen, 1998–2008

HL is an infrequent indication for allogeneic transplant and generally performed only in patients who experience disease relapse after receiving multiple lines of therapy or who have refractory disease and an available HLA-matched donor. The use of RIC regimens in these heavily pretreated patients allows for a graft-versus-lymphoma effect with less regimen-related toxicity. Among 343 patients receiving HLA-matched transplant for Hodgkin disease between 1998 and 2008, the three-year probabilities of survival were 38% ± 4% with a myeloablative conditioning regimen and 43% ± 5% with a RIC regimen. The corresponding probabilities of survival in the 181 recipients of an unrelated donor transplant were 32% ± 6% and 41% ± 6%, respectively. (Graph kindly provided by Tanya Pedersen [CIBMTR].)

Comment: the current salvage regimens and conditioning protocols for HL were reviewed recently by Colpo et al., 2012.

Indications for autologous transplant

1. Untreated first relapse, especially if CR1 is <1 year. Exceptions are relapse after initial radiotherapy (may be salvaged by chemotherapy) and localized relapse after initial chemotherapy (may be salvaged by combined modality treatment). All other patients should be investigated for auto-SCT.

2. Subsequent chemosensitive relapse or CR.

3. Primary induction failure with MOPP/ABVD (this may be recognized early; for example, progression after two cycles of induction chemotherapy, or by PET positivity after four cycles of chemotherapy).

Recommendations for salvage chemotherapy

Most experts agree that 2–3 cycles of salvage chemotherapy should be administered once the indication for an autologous transplant is given. Commonly used regimens are ICE, ESHAP, DHAP, GDP, and mini-BEAM. The combination of gemcitabine, dexamethasone, and cisplatin (GDP) was described as a relatively nontoxic and effective salvage regimen (Kuruvilla et al., 2006). Of special importance is that more patients completed the stem cell collection after one apheresis (73%) in comparison with a historic group of patients treated with the mini-BEAM regimen (36%). Up to one-third of patients with relapsed HL are poor mobilizers and may need a bone marrow harvest or other strategies. This is often related to stem cell-toxic chemotherapy, extended field irradiation, and other factors. Commonly used regimens for the transplant conditioning are CVB and BEAM. Regimens incorporating TBI are used less frequently because many patients previously underwent large-field radiation (especially mantle field irradiation). PET negativity has been found to prognosticate stable remissions before and after autologous transplants. Patients with limited stage relapse, residual PET positivity, and initial bulky sites of disease should be considered for involved field radiotherapy either before or after auto-SCT.

Contraindications to autologous transplant

1. Resistant relapse (relative contraindication)
2. CR1
3. Usual contraindications for autologous transplant (poor organ function, uncontrolled infection)

Indications for allogeneic transplant

If an HLA-identical family member donor is available, consider allogeneic transplant in the presence of any of the following:

1. Relapse after autologous transplant
2. Autologous transplant not feasible
3. Younger patient

However, allogeneic transplant is experimental and for most patients should be performed as a reduced-intensity transplant (in chemosensitive relapse).

In addition, most patients failing an autologous transplant have a poor long-term outcome (mainly due to relapses) whatever strategy is used; therefore, new strategies should be developed. Interesting responses with a conjugated CD30 antibody (brentuximab vedotin) were seen in patients who had failed autologous transplants. Other agents like histone deacetylase inhibitors or bendamustine are in clinical trials (Colpo et al., 2012; Kuruvilla et al., 2011).

Monitoring posttransplant

1. Physical examination, CT scans every three months for two years, then every six months for five years, may be supplemented or replaced by PET imaging
2. Complete laboratory status including LDH at same intervals, thyroid stimulating hormone (TSH) if neck and/or mediastinum were irradiated
3. Additional tests if clinical suspicion of relapse
4. After five years, annual health examination including screening and counseling for second malignancies

References and further reading

Colpo A, Hochberg E, & Chen YB. 2012. Current status of autologous stem cell transplantation in relapsed and refractory Hodgkin's lymphoma. *Oncologist* **17**: 80–90.

Connors JM. 2005. State-of-the-art therapeutics: Hodgkin's lymphoma. *J Clin Oncol* **23**: 6400–6408.

Hasenclever D & Diehl V. 1998. A prognostic score for advanced Hodgkin's disease. International Prognostic Factors Project on Advanced Hodgkin's Disease. *N Engl J Med* **339**: 1506–1514.

Kuruvilla J, Keating A, & Crump M. 2011. How I treat relapsed and refractory Hodgkin lymphoma. *Blood* **117**: 4208–4217.

Kuruvilla J, Nagy T, Pintilie M, et al. 2006. Similar response rates and superior early progression-free survival with gemcitabine, dexamethasone, and cisplatin salvage therapy compared with carmustine, etoposide, cytarabine, and melphalan salvage therapy prior to autologous stem cell transplantation for recurrent or refractory Hodgkin lymphoma. *Cancer* **106**: 353–360.

Lazarus HM, Rowlings PA, Zhang MJ, et al. 1999. Autotransplants for Hodgkin's disease in patients never achieving remission: a report from the autologous blood and marrow transplant registry. *J Clin Oncol* **17**: 534–545.

Milpied N, Fielding AK, Pearce RM, et al. 1996. Allogeneic bone marrow transplant is not better than autologous transplant for patients with relapsed Hodgkin's disease. *J Clin Oncol* **14**: 572–578.

Porter DL, Stadtmauer EA, & Lazarus HM. 2003. "GVHD": graft-versus-host disease or graft-versus-Hodgkin's disease? An old acronym with new meaning. *Bone Marrow Transplant* **31**: 739–746.

Sarina B, Castagna L, Farina L, et al. 2011. Allogeneic transplantation improves the overall and progression-free survival of Hodgkin lymphoma patients relapsing after autologous transplantation: a retrospective study based on the time of HLA typing and donor availability. *Blood* **115**: 3671–3677.

Sureda A, Constans M, Iriondo A, et al. 2005. Prognostic factors affecting long-term outcome after stem cell transplantation in Hodgkin's lymphoma autografted after a first relapse. *Ann Oncol* **16**: 625–633.

Tubiana M, Henry-Amar M, Cardé P, et al. 1989. Toward comprehensive management tailored to prognostic factors of clinical stages I and II in Hodgkin's disease. The EORTC lymphoma group controlled clinical trials: 1964–87. *Blood* **73**: 47–56.

Chapter

10
Therapeutic decision making in hematopoietic SCT for multiple myeloma

Reinhold Munker, Hillard M. Lazarus, and Kerry Atkinson

Diagnosis
Differential diagnosis of plasma cell disorders

Monoclonal gammopathy of undetermined significance (MGUS)	
Multiple myeloma variants	Smoldering multiple myeloma Symptomatic (active) multiple myeloma Osteosclerotic myeloma (POEMS syndrome) Plasma cell leukemia Non-secretory myeloma
Solitary plasmacytoma	Osseous plasmacytoma Extraosseous plasmacytoma
Amyloid light-chain (AL) amyloidosis	

Minimal diagnostic criteria

MGUS	M-protein <10% plasma cells in BM	Risk of progression to myeloma of 25% after 20 years
	Asymptomatic	
	No evidence of end-organ damage	
Smoldering multiple myeloma	M-protein 10%–20% plasma cells in bone marrow (BM)	Progression to symptomatic myeloma at a median of 2–4 years
	Asymptomatic No evidence of end-organ damage	
Symptomatic multiple myeloma	M-protein, >10% plasma cells in BM or histologically documented plasmacytoma. Evidence of end-organ damage (CRAB): calcium (serum) >0.25 mmol/L. Renal insufficiency: serum creatinine >2.75 mmol/L. Anemia: hemoglobin 2 g/dL below normal. Bone lesions: lytic or compression fractures. Other: hyperviscosity, amyloidosis, recurrent infections	Requires immediate therapy

International staging system for multiple myeloma

Stage	Criteria	Median survival
I	Serum β2-microglobulin <3.5 mg/dL *and* serum albumin ≥ 3.5 g/dL	62 months
II	Serum β2-microglobulin <3.5 mg/dL but serum albumin <3.5 g/dL *or* serum β2-microglobulin >3.5 mg/dL but <5.5 mg/dL	44 months
III	Serum β2-microglobulin >5.5 mg/dL	29 months

(Reproduced from Greipp et al., 2005.)

Myeloma is a heterogeneous disease in terms of expected outcomes. The International Staging System (ISS) provides a simple prognostic profile (based on measurements in serum of albumin and β2-microglobulin) (Durie et al., 2006). The ISS can identify patients with expected survivals ranging from <2.5 years to >5 years. Whether high-risk patients should benefit from more aggressive approaches, such as up-front allogeneic HSCT, has not been evaluated in formal clinical trials. A molecular genetic profile is a promising approach to identify patients who may or may not respond to specific drugs/drug combinations. It may be possible in the future to predict the drugs and the intensity of the therapy that should be used in an individual patient. The prognosis of multiple myeloma overall has improved because of the widespread use of autologous transplantation, new agents, and improved supportive care (Kristinsson et al., 2007; Kumar et al., 2008; see also graph on page 12).

Adverse prognostic factors

Age >65 years

Advanced stage

Plasma cell leukemia

Low serum albumin, elevated serum β2-microglobulin level, high serum LDH levels

Elevated C-reactive protein

Renal failure

Extensive bone disease (more than three osteolytic lesions), high plasma cell labeling index

Cytogenetic abnormalities: del 13q, t(4;14), del 17p13 (by FISH, p53 locus), amplification of 1q21 (detected by FISH), t(14;16) by FISH, complex karyotypes, hypodiploidy

Note: FISH studies should be performed on CD138 selected cells

Molecular signature of aggressive disease

The International Uniform Response Criteria for multiple myeloma

Stringent complete response: sCR	CR plus: normal FLC ratio and no clonal cells in BM (immunochemistry or flow cytometry)
Complete response: CR	Negative immunofixation in serum and urine. BM <5% plasma cells
Very good partial response: VGPR	M-protein detectable on immunofixation but not on electrophoresis, or >90% serum M-protein reduction, urine M-protein <200 mg/24 hrs
Partial response: PR	>50% M-protein reduction in serum, >90% in urine to less than 200 mg/24 hrs
Stable disease: SD	Not meeting criteria for CR, VGPR, PR, or PD
Progressive disease: PD	>25% increase in serum and/or urine M-protein, % BM plasma cells. New bone lesions or soft tissue plasmacytoma, hypercalcemia

FLC, free light chains. (From Durie et al., 2006).

Several studies have identified CR as a meaningful predictor of patient outcome. Patients achieving CR after standard-dose chemotherapy or HSCT would have a clear benefit in terms of EFS and OS compared to those who do not. Short of CR, the level of clinical response does not correlate with discernible different outcomes. It is assumed that CR achieved by standard-dose chemotherapy is comparable to CR achieved after HSCT, but this issue has not been formally studied. The meaning of stringent CR has not been validated to date.

Up-front treatment of multiple myeloma: autologous transplant as standard in transplant eligible patients

From a historical perspective, clinical trials comparing various standard-dose chemotherapy regimens have failed to show a significant superiority of any of them in terms of OS. As illustrated by a recent review of SWOG (South West Oncology Group) experience, the use of alkylating agents singly or in combination, steroids, anthracyclines, and vinca alkaloids resulted in outcomes similar to those previously achieved with melphalan and prednisone (Durie et al., 2006b). The median survival in the various trials ranges from 31 to 38 months.

HDT with autologous transplant support has been the only therapy modality shown to improve PFS and OS compared to the outcomes achieved with standard-dose chemotherapy regimens.

To date, up-front therapy with the new generation of targeted therapies (thalidomide, lenalidomide, and bortezomib) has shown significant improvements in response rates and PFS in patients who were not candidates for transplantation. An interesting new combination is oral melphalan, prednisone, and lenalidomide. Among 54 elderly patients, 81% achieved at least a partial response (Palumbo et al., 2007). More recently the new therapies were introduced into the up-front treatment of multiple myeloma. These new treatment protocols can be administered as a three-drug induction (bortezomib–dexamethasone plus cyclophosphamide or doxorubicin or lenalidomide for 3–6 cycles). An alternative is a two-drug induction (bortezomib–dexamethasone or lenalidomide–dexamethasone). Most induction regimens are given for 3–6 cycles followed by a stem cell collection and an auto-SCT (Palumbo & Anderson, 2011). Patients with renal failure should receive bortezomib-containing induction.

When should an autologous transplant be performed? Most experts agree that it should be part of the initial treatment; however, a prospective randomized study and to a large extent a U.S. intergroup study found similar OS for up-front transplant versus delayed HSCT (at first relapse). In countries where the new agents are not available, an induction with VAD or similar protocols is recommended. Melphalan should be avoided as part of the induction regimen because of its stem cell toxicity. At the Mayo Clinic, patients with standard risk myeloma have stem cells collected after four cycles of an induction regimen, but are offered either auto-SCT or the continuation of treatment (lenalidomide–dexamethasone) until a maximum response is reached, with the option of a later SCT (Kumar, 2011).

Survival has improved in multiple myeloma, both at diagnosis and after the relapse

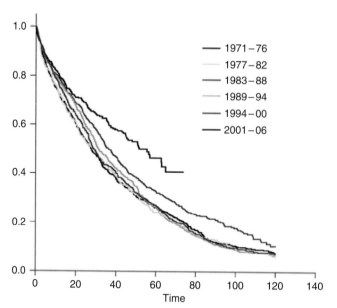

The Kaplan–Meier curves show that survival of patients has improved, especially after 2001. This correlates with the introduction of auto-SCT and novel agents. (These data are from the Mayo Clinic; Kumar et al., 2008, and were reproduced with permission.)

Effect on OS of a second autologous transplant according to the response of a first auto-SCT

A Very good partial response after first transplantation

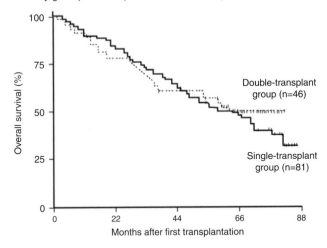

A significant improvement in DFS and OS was noted only in patients who have failed to achieve at least a VGPR (B), while no effect was seen in patients who have achieved a CR or VGPR after the first transplant (A). (Reproduced with permission from Attal et al., 2003.)

B Absence of very good partial response after first transplantation

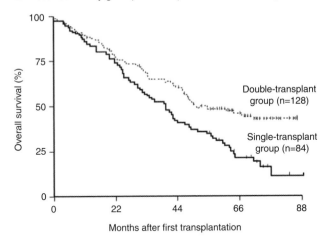

Concept of total therapy

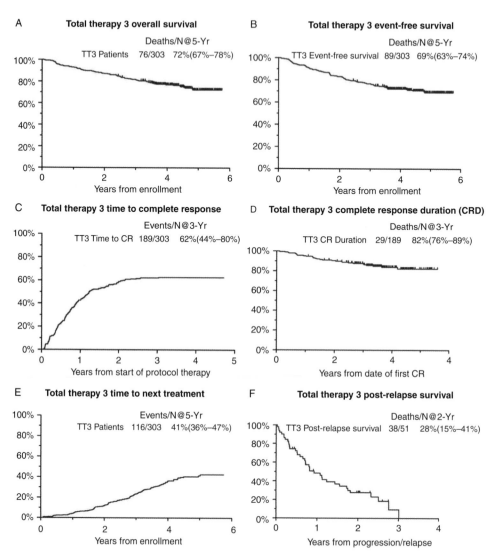

In the concept of total therapy 3 (TT3) (developed by the Myeloma Institute for Research and Therapy at the University of Arkansas), two cycles of VTD-PACE* were given as induction followed by a melphalan-based tandem transplant, and at reduced doses, a consolidation treatment was given. Subsequently, the patients were maintained for one year with VTD* and for two years with TD.* The clinical outcome of TT3 is shown in the figure. (Reproduced with permission by van Rhee et al., 2010.) In this protocol, the premature discontinuation of bortezomib was a significant adverse prognostic factor. * V, bortezomib; T, thalidomide; D, dexamethasone; P, continuous infusion cisplatin; A, doxorubicin; C, cyclophosphamide; E, etoposide.

Allogeneic transplant

In a consensus statement of the International Myeloma Working Group, the role of allo-SCT was reviewed (Lokhorst et al., 2010). The participants concluded that the introduction of RIC lowers the toxicity and mortality associated with myeloablation, but they saw no convincing evidence that allo-RIC improves survival compared with autologous transplantation. Despite earlier positive results by Bruno et al. (2007), the concept of auto-allotransplants could not improve survival in most studies compared with double autologous transplants. The following figure shows the results of a large study organized by the BMT CTN.

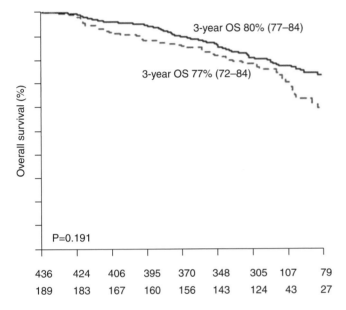

The upper curve (solid line) shows the OS in the double autologous group; the lower curve (dashed line) shows the survival in the auto-allo group. (Reproduced with permission from Krishnan et al., 2011.)

The outcome of unrelated SCT for multiple myeloma was reviewed recently by Kröger (2010). There are limited data, but the OS may be comparable to transplants from siblings.

CIBMTR data for multiple myeloma

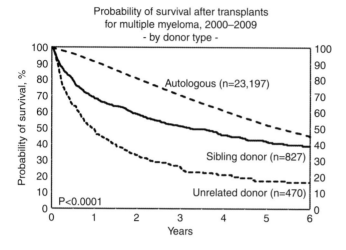

Probability of survival after transplants
for multiple myeloma, 2000–2009
- by donor type -

Autologous (n=23,197)

Sibling donor (n=827)

Unrelated donor (n=470)

P<0.0001

Years

Multiple myeloma (MM) is the most common indication for autologous HCT. Among 23 197 patients who received an autotransplant for MM between 2000 and 2009, the three-year probability of survival was 70% ± 1%. Allogeneic transplantation for MM is reserved for patients with high-risk disease and the majority performed after an autologous HCT with RIC or non-myeloablative conditioning regimens. Among the patients who received an allogeneic HCT from 2000 to 2009, the three-year probabilities of survival were 51% ± 2% for the 827 recipients of HLA-matched sibling donor grafts and 26% ± 2% for the 470 recipients of unrelated donor grafts. (Reproduced with permission from Pasquini MC & Wang, 2011. Available at: www.cibmtr.org/. Accessed 4/22/2011.)

Conclusions from recent studies

1. Auto-HSCT improves the outcome of patients with multiple myeloma when used as part of the up-front therapy. Similar OS is observed when auto-HSCT is used as rescue for first relapse/progression.
2. A second auto-HSCT (tandem transplants) improves the outcomes of single transplants. In particular, it benefits the subset of patients who fail to achieve a VGPR or CR after a first auto-HSCT.
3. Novel agents (thalidomide, lenalidomide, or bortezomib) used as maintenance or as part of the up-front therapy result in higher CR rates and improved PFS of patients treated with autologous transplants as part of their up-front therapy. The full impact of these drugs still has to be realized. Further new agents (carfilzomib, pomalidomide, elotuzumab) are under development.
4. MEL 200 mg/m^2 is a superior conditioning regimen compared to MEL 100 (100 mg/m^2) and to MEL/TBI.
5. Selected patients may benefit from an allogeneic transplant, especially if they have a matched related donor.

Indications for transplantation

Autologous: most patients with multiple myeloma, up to age 70 years, having undergone induction regimen and having collected PB stem cells.

Preferred sequence: induction regimen, followed by auto-SCT and planned second autologous transplantation for patients who do not reach CR or VGPR.

Allogeneic: selected patients with certain risk factors indicating aggressive disease, up to age 65 years, being in good performance status or aggressive relapse after autologous transplant in young patients in good performance status.

Contraindications to transplantation

Usual contraindications, like severe infections, heart failure, end-stage lung disease, resistant relapse

Renal failure is not a contraindication, but a risk factor for autologous transplantation (for a review see Pineda-Roman et al., 2007)

Pretransplant workup

1. Skeletal survey
2. Magnetic resonance imaging (MRI) of spine and other major bones
3. PET imaging (especially for clinically aggressive disease)
4. BM aspiration and biopsy
5. Quantitative serum immunoglobulins and immunoelectrophoresis/immunofixation, serum β_2-microglobulin
6. Quantitative Bence Jones protein determination, urine and serum
7. Free light-chain (FLC) determination (urine and serum) (important to determine remission)
8. If clinically indicated, investigation for amyloidosis (risk factor for poor outcome)
9. See also general pretransplant workup

Monitoring posttransplant

1. Quantitative serum immunoglobulins and immunoelectrophoresis/immunofixation, serum β_2-microglobulin at 1, 3, 6, 9, 12, 18, 24, 30, 36, and 48 months
2. Quantitative Bence Jones protein determination and FLC determination (urine and serum) at same time points
3. Skeletal survey/MRI (if abnormal findings before transplant, or if clinically indicated) at 6, 12, 24, and 36 months
4. PET imaging if positive before transplant at three months posttransplant
5. BM aspirate/biopsy at 3, 12, and 24 months or increase in paraprotein or new cytopenia
6. Chimerism studies (at 1, 3, 6, 12 months) for allogeneic transplants

Maintenance posttransplant

Maintenance therapy can be administered as low-dose thalidomide, or thalidomide–prednisone, or as low-dose lenalidomide. Most studies show that maintenance with these agents increases PFS but not OS. Most experts advocate maintenance especially in high-risk disease (Kumar, 2011; Palumbo et al., 2011). In a recent multicenter study, lenalidomide significantly lengthened PFS post auto HCT. However, toxicities including second malignancies (8% vs. 3% in the placebo arm) were observed (McCarthy et al., 2012).

References and further reading

Attal M, Harousseau JL, Facon T, et al. 2003. Single versus double autologous stem-cell transplantation for multiple myeloma. *N Engl J Med* **349**: 2495–2502.

Bladé J, Rosiñol L, Cibeira MT, et al. 2010. Hematopoietic stem cell transplantation for multiple myeloma beyond 2010. *Blood* **115**: 3655–3663.

Bruno B, Rotta M, Patriarca F, et al. 2006. A comparison of allografting with autografting for newly diagnosed myeloma. *N Engl J Med* **356**: 1110–1120.

Bruno B, Rotta M, Patriarca F, et al. 2007. A comparison of allografting with autografting for newly diagnosed myeloma *N Engl J Med* **356**: 2434–2441.

Durie BGM, Harousseau JL, Miguel JS, et al. 2006a. International uniform response criteria for multiple myeloma. *Leukemia* **20**: 1467–1473.

Durie BGM, Harousseau JL, Miguel JS, et al. 2006b. Magnitude of response with myeloma frontline therapy does not predict outcome: importance of time to progression in Southwest Oncology Group chemotherapy trials. *J Clin Oncol* **22**: 1857–1863.

Greipp PR, San Miguel J, Crowley JJ, et al. 2005. International staging system for multiple myeloma. *J Clin Oncol* **23**: 3412–3420.

Krishnan A, Pasquini MC, Logan B, et al. 2011. Autologous haematopoietic stem-cell transplantation followed by allogeneic or autologous haemopoietic stem-cell transplantation in patients with multiple myeloma (BMT CTN 0102): a phase 3 biological assignment trial. *Lancet Oncol* **12**: 1195–1203.

Kristinsson SY, Landgren O, Dickman PW, et al. 2007. Patterns of survival in multiple myeloma: a population-based study of patients diagnosed in Sweden from 1973 to 2003. *J Clin Oncol* **25**: 1993–1999.

Kröger N. 2010. Unrelated stem cell transplantation for patients with multiple myeloma. *Curr Opin Hematol* **17**: 538–543.

Kumar SK, Rajkumar SV, Dispenzieri A, et al. 2008. Improved survival in multiple myeloma and the impact of novel therapies. *Blood* **111**: 2516–2520.

Kumar S. 2011. Treatment of newly diagnosed multiple myeloma in transplant-eligible patients. *Curr Hematol Malig Rep* **6**: 104–112.

Lokhorst H, Einsele H, Vesole D, et al. 2010. International myeloma working group consensus statement regarding the current status of allogeneic stem-cell transplantation for multiple myeloma. *J Clin Oncol* **28**: 4521–4530.

McCarthy PL, Owzar K, Hofmeister CC, et al. 2012. Lenalidomide after stem cell transplantation for multiple myeloma. *N Eng J Med* **366**: 1770–1781.

Moreau P, Avet-Loiseau H, Harousseau JL, et al. 2011. Current trends in autologous stem cell transplantation in the era of novel therapies. *J Clin Oncol* **29**: 1898–1906.

Palumbo A & Anderson K. 2011. Multiple myeloma. *N Engl J Med* **364**: 1046–1060.

Palumbo A, Falco P, Corradini P, et al. 2007. Melphalan, prednisone, and lenalidomide treatment for newly diagnosed myeloma: a report from the GIMEMA-Italian multiple myeloma network. *J Clin Oncol* **25**: 4459–4465.

Pasquini MC & Wang Z. 2011. Current use and outcome of hematopoietic stem cell transplantation: CIBMTR summary slides 2011/2012. Available from http://www.cibmtr.org

Pineda-Roman M & Tricot G. 2007. High-dose therapy in patients with plasma cell dyscrasias and renal dysfunction. *Contrib Nephrol* **153**: 182–194.

Van Rhee F, Szymonifka J, Anaissie E, et al. 2010. Total therapy 3 for multiple myeloma: prognostic implications of cumulative dosing and premature discontinuation of VTD maintenance components, bortezomib, thalidomide, and dexamethasone, relevant to all phases of therapy. *Blood* **116**: 1220–1227.

Chapter

11

Therapeutic decision making in SCT for amyloidosis

Reinhold Munker, Hillard M. Lazarus, and Kerry Atkinson

Definition

Amyloidosis results from altered protein folding, leading to the deposit of insoluble amyloid fibrils in possibly every organ or organ system of the body. Untreated, systemic amyloidosis is generally fatal.

Disease classification

Disease	Pathogenic principle	Clinical syndromes
AA amyloidosis	Serum amyloid A protein	Reactive systemic amyloidosis associated with chronic inflammatory diseases
AL amyloidosis	Monoclonal immunoglobulin light chains	Systemic amyloidosis associated with monoclonal immunoglobulins or immunoglobulin fragments
Other rare inherited forms of amyloidosis	Pathologic proteins deposited in various organs	Neurological and visceral manifestations

---

The BMT Data Book, Third Edition, ed. Reinhold Munker et al. Published by Cambridge University Press. © Cambridge University Press 2013.

In this chapter, only the most common form of amyloidosis, amyloid light-chain (AL) amyloidosis will be discussed. Primary AL amyloidosis is caused by the proliferation of malignant B-cell clones in the absence of a frank plasma cell dyscrasia–like multiple myeloma. Common target organs of AL amyloidosis are the kidneys (nephrotic syndrome, kidney failure), the heart (cardiomyopathy), the liver (hepatomegaly), and the gastrointestinal (GI) tract (malabsorption or unexplained diarrhea). Other typical manifestations include macroglossia and peripheral neuropathy. Secondary AL amyloidosis is observed in at least 15% of patients with multiple myeloma.

Results of conventional therapy

The survival of untreated patients with AL amyloidosis is short. In older studies, a median survival time of 7–8 months was reported. Later, the treatment with alkylating agents was introduced, which stabilizes the disease, but rarely results in remissions. Conventional treatment consists of cycles of oral prednisone, and melphalan extends the median period of survival to about 12–18 months. Recently, combinations of lenalidomide and dexamethasone, bortezomib and dexamethasone, and other drugs were introduced and appear to have promising activity (Palladini & Merlini, 2011). A staging system was proposed on the basis of N-terminal pro-brain natriuretic peptides (NT-proBNP) and cardiac troponins T or I (c-TnT or c-TnI). Based on this staging system, high-, low-, and intermediate-risk patients can be discriminated (see following table; Dispenzieri et al., 2004).

Proposed staging system for systemic AL amyloidosis

Stage	Criteria	Median survival
I	Values low for all three markers	27.2 (26.4) months
II	Values elevated for only one marker	11.1 (11.1) months
III	Values elevated for two or three markers	4.1 (3.5) months

Definitions of normal or low: NT-proBNP <332 ng/L, c-TnT <0.035 µg/L, c-TnI <0.1 µg/L.

Results of autologous transplantation

Analogous to the treatment of multiple myeloma, auto-SCT was introduced in the mid-1990s for patients with AL amyloidosis. Initially, a high frequency of remissions was noted, but later unacceptably high complication rates (up to 40% TRM) were observed. It became clear that patient selection as well as optimal supportive treatment was of utmost importance to improve the outcome for patients with AL amyloidosis receiving autologous transplants.

In a multicenter study in Great Britain, 92 patients with systemic amyloidosis were transplanted between 1994 and 2004 (Goodman et al., 2006). The median age of these patients was 53 years and a median of two organs (mainly kidneys, but also heart, liver, and GI tract) were involved. If all causes of death are considered, the mortality rate related to the transplant was 23% at day 100. During the earlier period (1994–1998) the mortality was

32%, but decreased to 13% during the later period (1999–2004). Risk factors for TRM were the number of affected organs, poor performance status, low serum albumin, and advanced age. A disease response, defined as a ≥50% reduction in the pathological light-chain protein present in AL amyloidosis, was observed in 83% of evaluable patients. The overall median survival of the transplanted patients was 5.3 years. Patients who survived the autologous transplant beyond day 100 had a median survival of 8.5 years. In many centers, a high incidence of transplant-related complications has dampened the interest in autologous transplantation for treatment of AL amyloidosis. However, in experienced centers and in carefully selected patients a lower rate of complications can be observed. One center reported a series of 15 patients treated over seven years and observed no transplant-related deaths (Chow et al., 2005).

Long-term outcome of AL amyloidosis after high-dose melphalan and auto-SCT

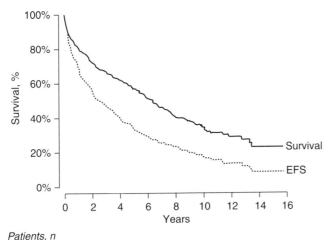

In this long-term follow-up study from Boston, 421 consecutive patients with AL amyloidosis were treated with high-dose melphalan and auto-SCT. In the entire group, the TRM was 11.4%. By intention to treat, 34% of patients reached a CR (negative serum and urine immunofixation and normal free-light chain ratio). The overall median survival was 6.3 years and the median EFS was 2.6 years. (Reproduced with permission from Cibeira et al., 2011.)

Patients, n								
Survival :	421	291	210	143	93	49	22	6	0
EFS :	421	291	167	94	65	23	11	3	0

In an earlier review article, Comenzo & Gertz (2002) discussed the risk factors involved in transplanting patients with amyloidosis and, on the basis of these, established risk categories. For stem cell mobilization, lower doses of cyclophosphamide or G-CSF alone are generally recommended. Special care should be taken to prevent edema accumulation in patients with nephrotic syndrome. A higher dose of collected stem cells is preferable (e.g., 5×10^6 CD34$^+$ cells/kg). GI toxicity, especially bleeding, mucositis, and nausea are frequent problems after transplant. During the posttransplant period, many patients are hypotensive. The hypotension may be caused by volume depletion, autonomic neuropathy, bleeding, sepsis, and/or adrenal insufficiency. Cardiac conduction disturbances are common and in patients with significant arrhythmias or bradycardias, a pacemaker is indicated. All patients should be referred to a cardiologist before transplant, as the echo-cardiographic finding, a septal thickness of >12 mm, is highly suggestive of cardiac involvement by amyloidosis.

In selected younger patients, a reduced-intensity allogeneic transplant can offer a chance of remission or cure for AL amyloidosis. Imamura et al. (2006) describe the case of a 43-year-old patient with amyloidosis who presented with orthostatic hypotension, diarrhea, nephrotic syndrome, and cardiac involvement. The patient received a reduced-intensity transplant from his HLA-identical sister following conditioning with fludarabine 25 mg/m^2 for five days and melphalan 90 mg/m^2 on day -2. The monoclonal paraprotein disappeared within two months and the patient had an improved performance status 20 months after the transplant.

In a recent publication from the Mayo Clinic, data on 270 patients who underwent auto-SCT for systemic amyloidosis were reviewed (Gertz et al., 2007). The median age was 57 years. Nephrotic range proteinuria was observed in more than half of the patients. Overall, 69% of patients had renal involvement, 51% cardiac involvement, 11% peripheral nerve involvement, and 16% hepatic involvement. Most patients required three aphereses. After transplantation, most patients engrafted between day 14 and day 16. The overall mortality at day 100 was 11%. The intensity of conditioning was correlated with outcome, which may reflect a bias in patient selection. Among the 213 patients surviving six months, 86 patients had a hematologic CR, 91 had PR, and 36 had no response. A randomized study comparing auto-SCT with standard nontransplant treatment has been initiated in the United States. In a French randomized study (high-dose melphalan versus melphalan plus dexamethasone), no survival advantage could be found for the high-dose group (median OS 22.2 months for the high-dose group versus 56.9 months for the melphalan–dexamethasone group) (Jaccard et al., 2007).

Amyloidosis secondary to multiple myeloma is not a contraindication to transplant, but special risk factors have to be considered (Bahlis & Lazarus, 2006). Induction chemotherapy before stem cell collection may not be necessary, especially in cases with a low plasma cell infiltration of the BM. If required, a short course of dexamethasone is considered optimal. Cardiotoxic, neurotoxic, and nephrotoxic drugs should be avoided. The melphalan dose should be adjusted according to the risk group as recommended for primary amyloidosis. Multiple specialists should be involved (multidisciplinary approach).

Indications for transplantation

Indications for autologous transplantation include biopsy-proven AL amyloidosis, age up to 65 or 70 years, and good performance status.

Contraindications to transplantation

Contraindications for transplantation include advanced cardiac involvement and involvement of three or more organs.

Eligibility criteria and follow-up

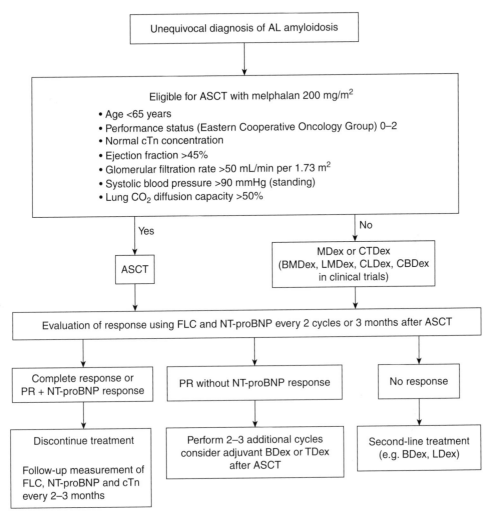

ASCT, autologous stem cell transplantation; cTn, cardiac troponins; MDex, oral melphalan plus dexamethasone; CTDex, combination of cyclophosphamide, thalidomide, and dexamethasone; BMDex, combination of bortezomib, melphalan, and dexamethasone; LMDex, combination of lenalidomide, melphalan, and dexamethasone; CLDex, combination of cyclophosphamide, lenalidomide, and dexamethasone; CBDex, combination of cyclophosphamide, bortezomib, and dexamethasone; FLC, circulating free light chains; NT-proBNP, N-terminal natriuretic peptide type B; PR, partial hematologic response; BDex, bortezomib plus dexamethasone; LDex, lenalidomide plus dexamethasone. (Modified from Palladini & Mellini, 2011.)

Follow-up after transplantation

- Serum/urine monoclonal paraprotein concentration, FLC concentration
- Organ function (kidney, heart, other involved organs)
- Troponin, NT-proBNP

References and further reading

Bahlis NJ & Lazarus HM. 2006. Multiple myeloma-associated AL amyloidosis: is a distinctive therapeutic approach warranted? *Bone Marrow Transplant* **38**: 7–15.

Chow LQM, Bahlis N, Russell J, et al. 2005. Autologous transplantation for primary systemic AL amyloidosis is feasible outside a major amyloidosis referral center. *Bone Marrow Transplant* **36**: 591–596.

Cibeira MT, Sanchorawala V, Seldin DC, et al. 2011. Outcome of AL amyloidosis after high-dose melphalan and autologous stem cell transplantation: long-term results in a series of 412 patients. *Blood* **118**: 4346–4352.

Comenzo RL & Gertz MA. 2002. Autologous stem cell transplantation for primary systemic amyloidosis. *Blood* **99**: 4276–4282.

Dispenzieri A, Gertz MA, Kyle RA, et al. 2004. Serum cardiac troponins and N-terminal pro-brain natriuretic peptide: a staging system for primary systemic amyloidosis. *J Clin Oncol* **22**: 3751–3757.

Dispenzieri A, Lacy MQ, Zeldenrust SR, et al. 2007. The activity of lenalidomide with or without dexamethasone in patients with primary systemic amyloidosis. *Blood* **109**: 465–470.

Gertz MA, Lacy MQ, Dispenzieri A, et al. 2007. Transplantation for amyloidosis. *Curr Opin Oncol* **19**: 136–141.

Goodman HJB, Gillmore JD, Lachman HJ, et al. 2006. Outcome of autologous stem cell transplantation for AL amyloidosis in the UK. *Br J Haematol* **134**: 417–425.

Imamura T, Ogata M, Kohno K, et al. 2006. Successful reduced intensity allogeneic stem cell transplantation for systemic AL amyloidosis. *Am J Hematol* **81**: 281–283.

Jaccard A, Moreau P, Leblond V, et al. 2007. High-dose melphalan versus melphalan plus dexamethasone for AL amyloidosis. *N Engl J Med* **357**: 1083–1093.

Palladini G & Merlini G. 2011. Transplantation vs. conventional-dose therapy for amyloidosis. *Curr Opin Oncol* **23**: 214–220.

Sanchorawala V, Wright DG, Seldin DC, et al. 2001. An overview of the use of high-dose melphalan with autologous stem cell transplantation for the treatment of AL amyloidosis. *Bone Marrow Transplant* **28**: 637–642.

12

Therapeutic decision making in BMT/SCT for nonseminomatous germ cell tumor of testis

Reinhold Munker, Hillard M. Lazarus, and Kerry Atkinson

Introduction

Nearly 80% of newly diagnosed and approximately 25% of relapsed testicular cancer patients can be cured using conventional combination chemotherapy with or without resection (Einhorn, 1997; Sonneveld et al., 2001).

Disease classification

Germ cell tumors (GCT) of the testis

Type	Frequency (%)
Seminoma	40%
Nonseminomatous GCT	
Teratoma (mature/immature)	5%
Teratocarcinoma	25%
Embryonal carcinoma	25%
Choriocarcinoma	1%
Yolk sac tumor	<1%

The BMT Data Book, Third Edition, ed. Reinhold Munker et al. Published by Cambridge University Press. © Cambridge University Press 2013.

Disease staging and rationale for high-dose therapy (HDT)

For diagnostic workup, staging, and treatment recommendations, we refer to the NCCN Practice guidelines, version 2/2012, section *Testicular Cancer*, accessible at www.nccn.org.

For some germ cell cancer patients, the five-year survival rates are considerably less than 50%. Use of increased dose intensity and alternating chemotherapy regimens may improve outcome. Alternatively, auto-SCT has been used successfully. The treatment of advanced GCT including high-dose chemotherapy was discussed in several recent review articles (Connolly & McCaffrey, 2009; de Giorgi et al., 2003; Jones & Vasey, 2003; Sonpavde et al., 2007).

Prognostic factors for outcome with conventional therapy

Prognosis	Nonseminoma	Seminoma
Good	Testis/retroperitoneal primary, no nonpulmonary visceral metastases, AFP <1000 ng/mL, HCG <5000 IU/L, LDH 1.5 × ULN	Any primary site No nonpulmonary visceral metastases Normal AFP Any HCG, any LDH
Intermediate	Testis/retroperitoneal primary, no nonpulmonary visceral metastases, AFP ≥1000 and <10,000 ng/mL or HCG ≥5000 and <50,000 IU/L, or LDH ≥ 1.5 × ULN and <10 × ULN	Any primary site Nonpulmonary visceral metastases Normal AFP Any HCG, any LDH
Poor	Mediastinal primary or nonpulmonary visceral metastases or AFP >10,000 ng/mL or HCG >50,000 IU/L or LDH >10 × ULN	No patients classified as poor prognosis

AFP, α-fetoprotein; HCG, human chorionic gonadotropin. (Markers measured post-orchiectomy.) (Modified from IGCCCG, 1997.)

In addition to radical orchidectomy, treatment of nonseminomatous (NS) GCT may involve retroperitoneal lymph node dissection (RPLND), conventional-dose cytotoxic chemotherapy, or high-dose chemotherapy supported by auto-SCT.

Results with autologous transplant
Phase III randomized trial of conventional-dose chemotherapy with or without high-dose chemotherapy and autologous hematopoietic stem cell rescue as first-line treatment for patients with poor prognosis metastatic GCT

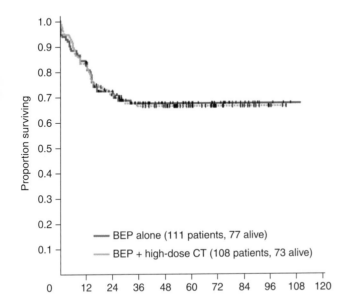

OS for patients randomly assigned to four cycles of bleomycin–etoposide–cisplatin (BEP) compared with two cycles of BEP followed by two cycles of high-dose carboplatin–etoposide–cyclophosphamide plus autologous hematopoietic stem cell rescue (CT). (Reproduced with permission from Motzer et al., 2007.)

— BEP alone (111 patients, 77 alive)

— BEP + high-dose CT (108 patients, 73 alive)

In this study, in 219 patients with high-risk features, no difference in survival and complete response rates could be found. However, in the subset of patients with an unsatisfactory tumor marker decline, the one-year durable complete response rate was different: 61% in the patients who received high-dose chemotherapy versus 34% in the patients who received only four cycles of BEP.

High-dose chemotherapy compared with standard-dose BEP in patients with poor-risk GCT

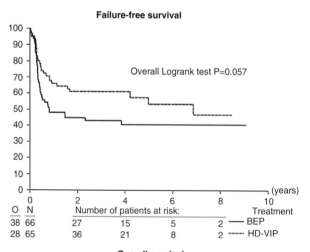

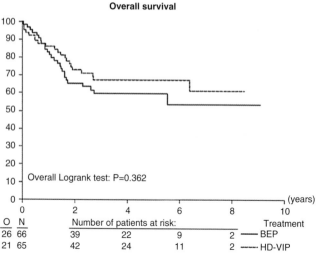

In this study (which was stopped early due to poor recruitment) patients with poor-prognosis feature germ cell tumors were randomized to receive either four cycles of BEP or one cycle of standard-dose cisplatin–etoposide–ifosfamide (VIP) followed by three cycles of high-dose VIP then stem cell infusion. Overall the outcome in this phase III study was not different. The high-dose arm tended to show a better failure-free survival (upper graph); however, the OS was comparable (lower graph). (Reproduced with permission from Daugaard et al., 2011.)

High-dose chemotherapy and stem cell rescue for metastatic GCT

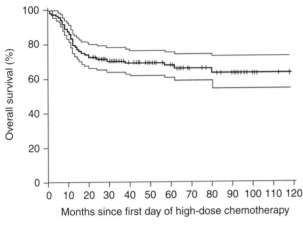

No. at risk   184 161 128 103 80 61   49 27 23 17 7   4

In this large, single center study, 184 consecutive patients with metastatic testicular cancer were treated with two cycles of HDT (carboplatin 700 mg/m^2 and etoposide 750 mg/m^2, each for three consecutive days). All patients had progressed after cisplatinum-containing combination chemotherapy. Thirty-five patients had seminomas while 149 had nonseminomatous GCT. The figure shows the Kaplan–Meier estimates of OS and the 95% confidence intervals (CI). Of the 135 patients who received HDT as second-line treatment, 94 were disease free during follow-up compared with 22 of 49 patients who received HDT as third-line or later treatment. The DFS differed according to a risk score that included a third-line treatment, platinum refractoriness, and advanced IGCCCG stage. (Reproduced with permission from Einhorn et al., 2007.)

Risk factors before autologous transplantation

- Resistance to cisplatinum-containing regimens
- Primary mediastinal GCT
- Progressive disease
- Serum β-HCG >1000 mU/mL (Beyer et al., 1996)

Tandem versus single autologous transplantation

Several centers have used two consecutive or tandem autotransplant procedures rather than a single autotransplant. It was estimated that 30% of all transplants for GCT patients are tandem transplants. The CIBMTR (Lazarus et al., 2007) recently reported that tandem autotransplants are associated with less TRM than a planned single transplant with no differences in disease-related outcomes or OS at three years. It was concluded that patient selection may have influenced the results of this observational study and that a randomized, prospective trial is needed to determine which approach, if either, is better.

Possible indications for autologous transplant

1. Progression during BEP remission induction chemotherapy; indication unclear at present; should be performed only within controlled clinical trials.
2. Incomplete response to salvage chemotherapy; relapse after salvage chemotherapy. Most experts agree with this indication; however, should be performed preferably within clinical trials.

Pretransplant workup

1. Serum β-HCG, which is elevated in
   - 100% of choriocarcinomas
   - 50% of embryonal carcinomas
   - 5%–10% of seminomas
2. Serum α-fetoprotein, which can be produced by
   - embryonal carcinoma
   - teratocarcinoma
   - yolk sac tumor
   - combined tumors, but not pure seminoma
3. Serum LDH
4. CT scan of chest, abdomen, pelvis, and brain
5. Also see the general pretransplant workup (page 239)

Monitoring posttransplant

1. β-HCG, α-fetoprotein, and LDH at 1, 2, and 3 weeks, and then at 1, 2, 3, 6, 12, and 24 months
2. CT scan chest, abdomen, and pelvis at 3, 12, and 24 months

References and further reading

Beyer J, Kramar A, Mandanas R, et al. 1996. High-dose chemotherapy as salvage treatment in germ cell tumors: a multivariate analysis of prognostic variables. *J Clin Oncol* 14: 2638–2645.

Connolly RM & McCaffrey JA. 2009. High-dose chemotherapy plus stem cell transplantation in advanced germ cell cancer: a review. *Eur Urol* 56: 57–64.

Daugaard G, Skoneczna I, Aass N, et al. 2011. A randomized phase III study comparing standard dose BEP with sequential high-dose cisplatin, etoposide, and ifosfamide (VIP) plus stem-cell support in males with poor-prognosis germ cell cancer. An intergroup study of EORTC, GTCSG, and Grupo Germinal (EORTC 30974). *Ann Oncol* 22: 1054–1061.

De Giorgi U, Papiani G, Severini G, et al. 2003. High-dose chemotherapy in adult patients with germ cell tumors. *Cancer Control* 10: 48–56.

Einhorn EH. 1997. Testicular cancer: an oncological success story. *Clin Cancer Res* 3: 2630–2632.

Einhorn LH, Williams SD, Chamness A, et al. 2007. High-dose chemotherapy and stem cell rescue for metastatic germ-cell tumor. *N Engl J Med* 357: 340–348.

IGCCCG: 1997. International Germ Cell Consensus classification: a prognostic factor-based staging system for metastatic germ cell cancers. *J Clin Oncol* 15: 594–603.

Jones RH & Vasey PA. 2003. Testicular cancer-management of advanced disease. *Lancet Oncol* 4: 738–747.

Lazarus HM, Stiff PJ, Carreras J, et al. 2007. Utility of single versus tandem autotransplants for advanced testes/germ cell cancer: a Center for International Blood and Marrow Transplantation Research (CIBMTR) analysis. *Biol Blood Marrow Transplant* **13**: 778–789.

Motzer RJ, Nichols CJ, Margolin KA, et al. 2007. Phase III randomized trial of conventional-dose chemotherapy with or without high-dose chemotherapy and autologous hematopoietic stem-cell rescue as first-line treatment for patients with poor-prognosis metastatic germ cell tumors. *J Clin Oncol* **25**: 247–256.

Sonneveld DJ, Hoekstra HJ, van der Graaf WT, et al. 2001. Improved long term survival of patients with metastatic nonseminomatous testicular germ cell carcinoma in relation to prognostic classification systems during the cisplatin era. *Cancer* **91**: 1304–1315.

Sonpavde G, Hutson TE, Roth BJ. 2007. Management of recurrent testicular germ cell tumors. *Oncologist* **12**: 51–61.

Chapter

13

Therapeutic decision making in BMT/ SCT for renal cell cancer

Richard W. Childs and Reinhold Munker

Introduction: scientific rationale

Kidney cancer accounts for approximately 3%–4% of all malignancies in adults. The major histological type of RCC is clear cell carcinoma, which makes up about 70% of all spontaneous cases. Less frequent histological types are papillary RCC and chromophobe RCC. The clear cell type of RCC has a high frequency of mutations in the von Hippel–Lindau (VHL) gene, which functions as a tumor suppressor. As a consequence of VHL inactivation, a large number of genes that contribute to the tumorigenicity of clear cell carcinoma may be overexpressed, including vascular endothelial growth factor (VEGF). Metastatic RCC has a poor prognosis (mean survival between six and 24 months), and unlike many other solid tumors, is largely unresponsive to cytotoxic chemotherapy. Over the last seven years, there has been a dramatic increase in the number of therapies available to treat this malignancy, largely composed of drugs that target specific angiogenic pathways and mammalian target of rapamycin pathways. These agents can improve PFS and OS but result in tumor regression in only a minority of patients, with drug resistance and tumor progression ultimately occurring.

Unlike most solid tumors, RCC appears to be immunogeneic, expressing antigens that may be a target for the immune system, including but not limited to GP75, RAGE1, PRAME, CAIX, and antigenic molecules derived from a human endogenous retrovirus type E (HERV-E). In rare instances, spontaneous remissions are observed. In 10%–20% of patients, immunotherapy with IL-2 and IFN-α leads to remissions or the regression of metastatic lesions. The observation that this tumor is immunoresponsive led to studies exploring the susceptibility of RCC to a graft-versus-tumor (GVT) effect following allogeneic HSCT (Bregni et al., 2011; Childs et al.,

The BMT Data Book, Third Edition, ed. Reinhold Munker et al. Published by Cambridge University Press. © Cambridge University Press 2013.

1999; Tykodi et al., 2011). Here the outcome and status of studies investigating allogeneic hematopoietic SCT as immunotherapy for RCC are discussed.

Results of conventional treatment

Until recently, immunotherapy utilizing high-dose IL-2 or IFN-α (9 MU s.c. t.i.w.) was considered a standard of care for patients with metastatic RCC. Both cytokines can have considerable toxicity, are not tolerated by all patients, and lead to objective responses in only 10%–20% of all patients. Although some patients have durable responses with these therapies, including a rare minority of patients who achieve CR that are curative, the low overall response rate probably prolongs survival for only 4–6 months.

Over the eight years, several new agents that target specific angiogenic and/or growth and proliferation pathways were approved for the treatment of metastatic RCC. These agents (sunitinib, sorafenib, pazopanib, axitinib, bevacizumab, temsirolimus, and everolimus) now represent the mainstay of therapy to treat patients with metastatic RCC, with many having been shown to result in an improvement in PFS and OS compared to the placebo or IFN-α (Pal et al., 2012; Ravaud & Wallerand, 2009; Schöffski et al., 2006). The multi-kinase inhibitor sorafenib targets Raf-1, B-raf, c-kit, Flt3, and other kinases and inhibits angiogenesis. In patients with advanced RCC not treated with cytokines (cytokine-naïve), sorafenib doubled the PFS to 25 weeks (compared with 12 weeks in placebo-treated patients). Sunitinib is another oral multi-targeted TKI. In a trial in cytokine-refractory metastatic RCC patients, responses were observed in approximately 40% of patients. In another study, responses were observed in 45% of patients. The average duration of response was 9.9 months. Overall, these and other TKIs appear to improve survival and induce more objective responses than does IFN. Axitinib was recently shown to improve PFS as compared with sorafenib in patients with previously treated metastatic RCC. Despite their activity against this tumor, CR with these agents are rarely observed and disease progression ultimately occurs in most treated patients.

Temsirolimus and everolimus inhibit the mammalian target of rapamycin (mTOR) and disrupt mTOR-dependent signaling pathways. Both drugs have been shown to significantly improve the OS and PFS in patients with advanced RCC compared to IFN-α alone, leading to their approval by the U.S. Food and Drug Administration (FDA). Although therapeutics inhibiting VEGF and mTOR have advanced the field for the treatment of this malignancy, inevitable disease progression and death from tumor occurs, highlighting the need for therapies that explore alternative therapeutic targets. Albeit rare, the observation that RCC can be cured by immunotherapy has maintained research interest in exploring new methods to target the human immune system against this cancer.

Results of allogeneic transplantation

Transplanted donor T-cells mediating GVL effects have the ability to cure patients with a number of different hematological malignancies. Until the late 1990s, little data existed as to whether solid tumors might like-wise be susceptible to allogeneic immunotherapy. The recent paradigm shift in the field of HSCT that GVT effects could be powerful enough to eradicate malignant diseases while avoiding toxicities associated with myeloablative conditioning led to the exploration of allogeneic immunotherapy to treat metastatic RCC and other solid tumors incurable with conventional therapy. Case reports about 13 years ago and small case series describing regression of metastatic RCC, ovarian cancer, pancreatic cancer, breast cancer, and colon cancer following allo-SCT established the notion that tumors of epithelial origin might likewise be susceptible to killing by transplanted donor immune cells (the table on pages 150–151 summarizes the data on RCC).

At present, RCC remains the solid tumor in which allogeneic GVT responses have been best characterized. The first case report of a GVT effect resulting in complete remission of metastatic RCC after allogeneic transplantation was reported in 1999 (Childs et al., 1999). Subsequently, a series of 19 patients treated at the National Heart, Lung, and Blood Institute (NHLBI) with treatment-refractory metastatic RCC who received a non-myeloablative PB SCT was reported (Childs et al., 2000). All patients were transplanted from matched sibling donors, 17 had full matches, two had 5/6 antigen matches. Cyclophosphamide (60 mg/kg on days 6 and 7) and fludarabine (25 mg/m^2 on days 5 to 1) were used as the conditioning regimen. To enhance GVT effects, cyclosporin was withdrawn early in patients with mixed T-cell chimerism or disease progression. Patients who did not respond received up to three infusions of donor lymphocytes. Overall, 10/19 patients (53%) responded with regression of metastases observed radiographically (three patients had a complete response, seven a partial response). (See the following figure for survival curves.)

Regression of RCC after non-myeloablative PB SCT

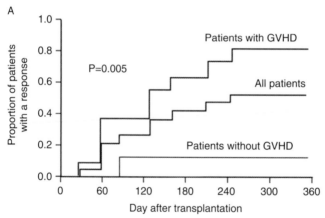

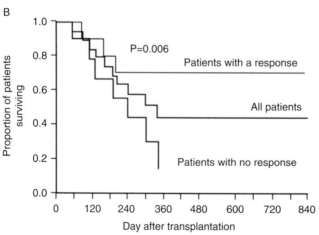

Outcome in 19 patients with metastatic RCC who received an allogeneic SCT. A: shows the Kaplan–Meier estimate of the cumulative probability of a response in all 19 patients and in patients with and without acute GVHD of grade II, III, or IV. Patients in whom acute GVHD developed after transplantation had a significantly higher probability of a response (P=0.005). B: shows the Kaplan–Meier estimate of survival in all patients and in patients with and without a response after transplantation. (Trend toward statistical significance [P=0.06].) (Reproduced with permission from Childs et al., 2000.)

The regression of metastases was delayed, occurring for a median of 129 days after transplantation, and often followed the withdrawal of cyclosporin and the establishment of complete donor-T-cell chimerism. This study prompted a number of subsequent studies in which generally, despite careful patient selection, a lower response rate and in some cases higher toxicity were observed. Considerable variability in selection criteria for potential transplant candidates, varying GVHD prophylaxis regimens, and differences in transplant strategies used to enhance GVT effects (i.e., how aggressively immunosuppression is withdrawn posttransplant) may in part account for differences in transplant outcome (Storb et al., 2003; Yang et al., 2006). (In the following table, the results of more recent studies are summarized [Bregni et al., 2011; Gommersall et al., 2004].) Subsequent to the NHLBI study, two trials of fludarabine-based transplantation regimens confirmed the observation of GVT effects with disease regression occurring in 57% (4/7) (Bregni et al., 2002) and 33% (4/12) (Rini et al., 2002) patients, with all responses occurring more than 100 days after transplantation.

Published series of allogeneic HCT for RCC*

Ref.[a]	Number of patients	Conditioning	GVHD Prophylaxis	Percentage of patients				Response post-DLI/IFN
				aGVHD (II–IV)	cGVHD	TRM	Response (CR + PR)	
U.S. centers								
[18,26][‡]	74	Flu + Cy	CSP	55	47	11	39	Yes
[19,20][‡]	18	Flu + Cy	Tac + MMF	18	58	28	22	No
[21,22][‡]	23	Flu + Mel	Tac + MTX	65	No data	39	26	No
[23]	8	Flu + TBI	CSP + MMF	50	50	13	13	Yes
[24]	22	Flu + Cy	Tac + MTX	50	23	9	0	N/A
[25]	16	Flu + Cy or Flu + TBI	CSP + MMF	44	43	13	31	Yes
International centers								
[27]	7	Flu + Cy	CSP + MTX	0[†]	No data	29[†]	0[†]	N/A
[28,29][‡]	25	TT + Flu + Cy	CSP + MTX or sirolimus	48	36	24	20	Yes
[30]	10	Flu + TBI ± ATG	CSP + MMF	50	43	30	0	N/A
[31]	25	Flu + Bu + ATG	CSP	42	44	9	8[†]	No
[32]	9	Flu/Cla + Bu + ATG	CSP	44	50	0	11	No
[33]	7	Flu + Cy + ATG	CSP ± MMF	29	67	14	29	Yes

[34]	5	Flu + Cy	CSP + MTX	60	75	0	0	N/A
[35]	7	Flu + TBI	CSP + MMF	29[†]	67[†]	0[†]	14[†]	No
[36][‡]	124	Flu + variable	CSP ± variable	39	40	16	29[¶]	Yes
[37]	11	Flu + Cy/Me/Bu ± ATG	CSP ± MTX	30	86	27	9	No
[38]	7	Flu + Cy/Bu ± TBI ± ATG	CSP or Tac	57	43	43	57	No

[a] references are from the report by Tykodi et al., 2011; *published series with more than three patients and reported in English are listed; [‡]reference includes previously reported patients; [†]percentages for RCC subset of patients.
[¶]Response rate calculated for 98/124 patients surviving >90 days posttransplant.
a, acute; c, chronic; Flu, fludarabine; Cy, cyclophosphamide; Mel, melphalan; TT, thiotepa; Cla, cladribine; Bu, busulfan; CSP, cyclosporin; Tac, tacrolimus; MMF, mycophenyate mofetil; MTX, methotrexate; N/A: not applicable.
(Reproduced from Tykodi et al., 2011, with permission).

Artz et al. (2005) published a follow-up to the Rini study in which four PR were observed among 19 patients with five transplant-related deaths. As expected, the responders lived longer than non-responders. In an intergroup study involving 14 institutions and 22 patients, no objective responses and two treatment-related deaths were observed (Rini et al., 2006). In a report from Seattle, eight patients had a non-myeloablative SCT for metastatic RCC (Tykodi et al., 2004). The patients were conditioned with fludarabine and low-dose TBI. Only one patient had a PR following DLIs and IFN-α. Interestingly, CD8+ cytotoxic T-lymphocyte (CTL) clones recognizing minor histocompatibility antigens (mHCa) could be isolated from five patients studied. In a large study from Europe, 124 patients from 21 different centers received a non-myeloablative transplant for metastatic RCC. One hundred and six patients had a matched related, five a partially matched related, and 13 an unrelated transplant. As immunosuppression, cyclosporin alone or cyclosporin combined with methotrexate or mycophenolate mofetil was given. All but three patients engrafted and the cumulative incidence of moderate to severe acute GVHD was 40% (33% for chronic GVHD). The TRM was 16% at one year. A tumor response was observed in 28 of 98 evaluable patients (cumulative incidence 32%; CI, 18%–46%) including 24 PR and four CR. CR occurred at a median 265 days after HCT (range 180–365 days) while PR occurred at a median 135 days post-HCT (range 42–600 days). Responses were associated with a shorter time from diagnosis, and partial mismatched and acute GVHD. Factors associated with survival included chronic GVHD, DLI, >3 metastatic sites, and a Karnofsky index >70%. Patients with chronic GVHD and given donor lymphocytes experienced a two-year survival of 70% (Barkholt et al., 2006).

Allogeneic SCT for metastatic RCC in Europe (multicenter data on 124 patients)

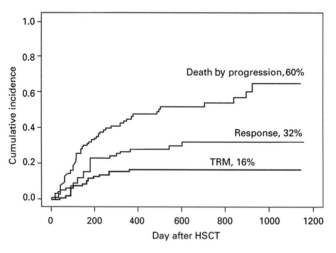

Cumulative incidence of patients with tumor response and death after allogeneic hematopoietic SCT for metastatic RCC. A patient was defined as evaluable concerning tumor response if she/he survived more than three months. Time to and cumulative incidence of TRM and time to and cumulative incidence of death by progressive disease are given. (Reproduced with permission from Barkholt et al., 2006.)

In a follow-up to their initial report, investigators from the NHLBI at the National Institutes of Health (NIH) reported the outcome of the first 75 patients transplanted following fludarabine and cyclophosphamide-based conditioning (Takahashi et al., 2008); 74/75 patients achieved durable engraftment with acute and chronic GVHD developing in approximately 50% of patients. Although 8% of patients died from transplant-related complications, 38% of patients had an objective disease response including 27% who had a PR and 9% who had a CR, with responses occurring at a median of 160 days following transplant (range 30–425 days). A subgroup analysis showed patients who had clear cell carcinoma with lung only disease had the highest response rate (55%; see following figure). Remarkably, responses were only seen again in patients with the clear cell variant of RCC, with 0/10 non-clear cell tumors showing a disease response. Recently the Milano group updated their long-term results on 25 patients with metastatic RCC that underwent allogeneic transplantation; at a median 65 months follow-up, five patients were alive including one in CR, one in PR, and three with stable disease (Bregni et al., 2011).

Jointly, these studies have established that metastatic RCC, which is resistant to IFN-α and high-dose IL-2 immunotherapy, may in some cases be responsive to allogeneic immunotherapy following RIC, with survival being prolonged in responding compared to nonresponding patients.

Overall disease response to allogeneic transplant for RCC and response based on RCC histology (clear cell RCC versus non-clear cell RCC)

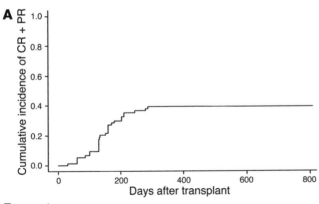

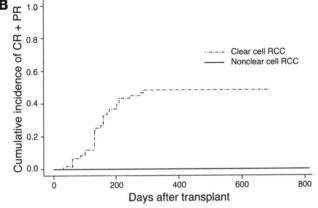

A: the cumulative incidence of disease response (combined CR + PR) following non-myeloablative allogeneic HSCT. Onset of disease regression was delayed by a median of 133 days (range, 30–287 days) following HSCT. **B**: disease responses (CR plus PS) were only observed in RCC patients with clear-cell histology (48% versus 0% cumulative incidence of a disease response; P=0.0018). (From Takahashi et al., 2008, reproduced with permission.)

Tumor responses are often substantially delayed after transplantation, highlighting the importance of careful selection of potential candidates for this approach, where pretransplant life expectancy of at least four months may be required for patients to have a chance of benefiting from this approach. Two studies which failed to show GVT effects in RCC reported tumor progression-related death occurred at three and 5.5 months, respectively, highlighting the need for not utilizing this approach as a "last ditch effort" in patients with treatment refractory and rapidly progressive disease who have an extremely short anticipated survival.

These pilot trials have been promising, establishing proof of principle of RCC's susceptibility to transplanted donor immune cells after allogeneic transplantation and have further shown that long-term disease control can be established using this approach in a fraction of transplanted patients. It must be noted that recent advances in the treatment of metastatic RCC with "targeted" drug therapies have dramatically reduced the number of transplants being performed for RCC over the past eight years. However, targeted therapy is not devoid of side effects, is costly, and only results in partial responses that are inevitably followed by disease progression. The observation that partial and sometimes complete and durable regression of metastatic RCC can occur following HCT has provided the impetus to refine this treatment approach further.

Mechanisms accounting for graft-versus-renal cell carcinoma (RCC) responses after transplantation

The mechanisms leading to regression of RCC following allogeneic transplantation are not well characterized, although clinical observations suggest donor immune cells mediate these effects (Ishiyama et al., 2009). The identification of the mechanisms through which graft-versus-RCC effects occur and the antigens expressed on RCC cells that serve as targets for donor immune cells remains an active area of investigation (Conrad et al., 2006; Takahashi et al., 2004). In some responding patients, T-cells with in vitro tumor cytotoxicity patterns consistent with recognition of mHCa and tumor-restricted antigens have been identified (Tykodi et al., 2004).

Using an ELISPOT analysis, we have recently established the presence of RCC reactive donor T-cells in the blood of patients who have had a disease response following allogeneic transplantation (Takahashi et al., 2008). Furthermore, we have successfully generated donor CD8+ T-cell clones from lymphocytes obtained from responding patients that have direct cytotoxicity against patients' RCC cells. Using cDNA expression cloning, we recently identified a new RCC tumor antigen recognized by donor T-cells isolated from a patient at the time of tumor regression; the genes encoding this antigen were found to be derived from a HERV, which is overexpressed in >50% of clear cell carcinomas but not in any normal tissues. Antigens derived from this virus were found to be highly immunogenic, stimulating cytotoxic T-cells that kill RCC cells in vitro and in vivo.

Most studies have reported that GVT effects appear limited to the clear cell variant of RCC (see B in previous figure, page 153). This observation as well as the observation that IL-2 responses occur most commonly against clear cell carcinoma suggest the dominant immunogenic antigens targeted by the human immune system might be limited to this tumor histology. Remarkably, we recently observed that HERV-E expression is restricted to the clear cell subtype of RCC (ccRCC) characterized by an inactivation of the von Hippel–

Lindau tumor suppressor gene (*VHL*) with subsequent stabilization of hypoxia-inducible transcription factors HIF-1α and -2α (Cherkasova et al., 2011). The transcriptional up-regulation of HERV-E was subsequently found to be related to three critical events: (i) *VHL* inactivation, (ii) HIF-2α overexpression, and (iii) hypomethylation of the HERV-E 5'LTR. The HERV-E expression in ccRCC was found to linearly correlate with HIF-2α levels and could be silenced in tumor cells by either transfection of normal *VHL* or siRNA inhibition of HIF-2α. Subsequently, HIF-2α was found to serve as a transcriptional factor for HERV-E by binding with an HIF response element localized in the proviral 5'LTR. Remarkably, the LTR was found to be hypomethylated only in HERV-E-expressing ccRCC, while other tumors and normal tissues possessed a hypermethylated LTR preventing proviral expression. Taken altogether, these studies have provided insight into the mechanisms by which RCC regresses following transplantation, showing that GVT effects against this malignancy may be associated with non-tumor-specific immune targeting of minor antigens and tumor-specific immune responses to antigens expressed on RCC.

The identification of RCC reactive T-cells in a patient who had a durable regression of RCC following an allogeneic transplant has provided valuable insights into potential mechanisms through which GVT effects occur after transplantation. Importantly, these insights could be used for translational research aimed at boosting human immunity against antigenic components of this HERV-E.

Enhancing graft-versus-RCC: what is next?

The identification of RCC tumor-restricted antigens targeted by donor immune cells could lead to the development of transplant approaches that enhance GVT effects through posttransplant tumor vaccination or the adoptive infusion of donor T-cells with tumor antigen specificity. Another approach to bolster donor immunity against RCC would be to incorporate the use of alloreactive killer IgG-like receptor (KIR)-incompatible NK cells into the transplant regimen. In vitro, allogeneic KIR-incompatible NK cells are more cytotoxic against RCC cells compared to autologous NK cells (Igarashi et al., 2004). Indirect evidence suggests alloreactive donor NK cells may play a role in mediating GVT effects in some patients following allogeneic transplantation. A recent analysis of metastatic RCC patients transplanted at the NHLBI from a sibling donor following non-myeloablative conditioning showed KIR incompatibility between the patient and donor predicted response and survival (Srinivasan et al., 2006). In this study, KIR incompatibility (defined as the presence of one or more KIR genotypes in donor cells where the corresponding MHC Class I inactivating ligand was absent in the recipient) predicted for a higher response rate as well as improved OS. This effect was most pronounced in patients lacking HLA-Bw4 who received a transplant from donors with genotypic evidence of KIR3DL1. A murine model of allogeneic transplantation for RCC has also provided evidence that alloreactive donor NK cells can enhance GVT effects against RCC resulting in a prolongation of survival (Lundqvist et al., 2007). The adoptive infusion of LY49-incompatible alloreactive donor NK (analogous to human KIR-incompatible NK cells) cells significantly reduced the risk of acute GVHD and enhanced graft-versus-murine RCC effects, resulting in a significant improvement in survival. Whether adoptively infused alloreactive NK cells will potentiate GVT effects in humans undergoing HCT for metastatic RCC will be evaluated in a clinical transplant trial to be conducted at the NHLBI at the NIH.

The identification of target antigens potentially mediating GVT effects following allogeneic transplantation holds the potential for the development of transplant trials that specifically target the donor immune system against RCC-specific antigens. Although novel and previously identified mHCa expressed on RCC cells may be a target for a GVT effect, broad tissue distribution occurs commonly, which could lead to GVHD if such antigens were targeted to bolster a GVT effect (Tykodi et al., 2011). Identification of antigens restricted to RCC cells, such as HERV-E antigens and mHCa such as HA-1, could lead to the rational development of trials that specifically target the donor immune system against targets not expressed on normal tissues, through actions such as pretransplant vaccination of the donor or by stimulating donor T-cells to these antigens in vitro for subsequent adoptive infusion after transplantation.

Future directions

Metastatic RCC remains one of the most deadly malignant tumors. The rapid development of new therapeutic options to treat this malignancy has led to drugs that improve OS and PFS, although complete responses and the possibility of cure do not yet appear possible with non-immunotherapy-based treatments. The results of allogeneic treatment for metastatic RCC have established proof of principle that this approach can be used as a successful form of immunotherapy in this disease. In a setting of transplantation preceded by RIC for patients who had failed conventional immunotherapy, objective and durable responses have been observed in a minority of patients. Patient selection and experience by the transplant center is critical, as some centers have observed fewer or no responses and the success of allogeneic immunotherapy has to be weighed against the toxicity of GVHD. In most studies, a small proportion of patients (10%–20%) became long-term survivors.

The development of regimens that incorporate maneuvers to cytoreduce tumor bulk might also be used to improve transplant outcome. Identification of tumor antigens restricted to RCC cells could lead to trials that specifically target the donor immune system against RCC by pretransplant vaccination of the donor or by stimulating donor T-cells to these antigens in vitro for subsequent adoptive infusion after transplantation. Future studies might benefit from combining the new targeted drug therapies with allogeneic transplantation and other immunotherapy approaches such as posttransplant use of vaccines directed against RCC-associated antigens or the adoptive infusion of tumor antigen-specific T-cells and/or NK cells (Liu et al., 2012). It is critical that methods are developed that enhance the specificity of the graft-versus-tumor (GVT) effect and lessen the severity of GVHD. Until these approaches are proven successful, the application of allogeneic transplantation for RCC will remain investigational and limited.

References and further reading

Artz AS, Van Besien K, Zimmerman T, et al. 2005. Long-term follow-up of nonmyeloablative allogeneic stem cell transplantation for renal cell carcinoma: The University of Chicago experience. *Bone Marrow Transplant* **35**: 253–260.

Barkholt L, Bregni M, Remberger M, et al. 2006. Allogeneic haematopoietic stem cell transplantation for metastatic renal cell carcinoma in Europe. *Ann Oncol* **17**: 1134–1140.

Bregni M, Dodero A, Peccatori J, et al. 2002. Nonmyeloablative conditioning followed by hematopoietic cell allografting and donor lymphocyte infusions for patients with metastatic renal and breast cancer. *Blood* **99**: 4234–4236.

Bregni M, Herr W, & Blaise D, 2011. Allogeneic stem cell transplantation for renal cell carcinoma. *Expert Rev Anticancer Ther* **11**: 901–911.

Cherkasova E, Malinzak E, Rao S, et al. 2011. Inactivation of the von Hippel-Lindau tumor suppressor leads to selective expression of a human endogenous retrovirus in kidney cancer. *Oncogene* **30**: 4697–4706.

Childs R, Chernoff A, Contentin N, et al. 2000. Regression of metastatic renal-cell carcinoma after nonmyeloablative peripheral-blood stem-cell transplantation. *N Engl J Med* **343**: 750–758.

Childs RW, Clave E, Tisdale J, et al. 1999. Successful treatment of metastatic renal cell carcinoma with a nonmyeloablative allogeneic peripheral-blood progenitor-cell transplant: evidence for a graft-versus-tumor effect. *J Clin Oncol* **17**: 2044–2049.

Conrad R, Remberger M, Cederlund K, et al. 2006. Inflammatory cytokines predominate in cases of tumor regression after hematopoietic stem cell transplantation for solid cancer. *Biol Blood Marrow Transplant* **12**: 346–354.

Gommersall L, Hayne D, Lynch C, et al. 2004. Allogeneic stem-cell transplantation for renal cell cancer. *Lancet Oncol* **5**: 561–567.

Igarashi T, Wynberg J, Srinivasan R, et al. 2004. Enhanced cytotoxicity of allogeneic NK cells with killer immunoglobulin-like receptor ligand incompatibility against melanoma and renal cell carcinoma cells. *Blood* **104**: 170–177.

Ishiyama K, Takami A, Suzuki S, et al. 2009. Relationship between tumor-infiltrating T lymphocytes and clinical response after reduced-intensity allogeneic hematopoietic stem cell transplantation for advanced renal cell carcinoma: a single center prospective study. *Jpn J Clin Oncol* **39**: 807–812.

Liu L, Zhang W, Qi, X, et al. 2012. Randomized study of autologous cytokine-induced killer cell immunotherapy in metastatic renal carcinoma. *Clin Cancer Res* **18**: 1751–1759.

Lundqvist A, McCoy JP, Samsel L, et al. 2007. Reduction of GVHD and enhanced anti-tumor effects after adoptive infusion of alloreactive NK-cells from MHC matched donors. *Blood* **109**: 3603–3606.

Pal SK, Williams S, Josephson DY, et al. 2012. Novel therapies for metastatic renal cell carcinoma: efforts to expand beyond the VEGF/mTOR signaling paradigm. *Mol Cancer Ther* **11**: 526–537.

Ravaud A & Wallerand H. 2009. Molecular pathways in metastatic renal cell carcinoma: the evolving role of mammalian target of rapamycin inhibitors. *Eur Urol Suppl* **8**: 793–798.

Rini BI, Campbell SC, & Rathmell WK. 2006. Renal cell carcinoma. *Curr Opin Oncol* **18**: 289–296.

Rini BI, Halabi S, Barrier R, et al. 2006. Adoptive immunotherapy by allogeneic stem cell transplantation for metastatic renal cell carcinoma: a CALGB intergroup phase II study. *Biol Blood Marrow Transplant* **12**: 778–785.

Rini BI, Zimmerman T, Stadler WM, et al. 2002. Allogeneic stem-cell transplantation of renal cell cancer after nonmyeloablative chemotherapy: feasibility, engraftment, and clinical results. *J Clin Oncol* **20**: 2017–2024.

Schöffski P, Dumez H, Clement P, et al. 2006. Emerging role of tyrosine kinase inhibitors in the treatment of advanced renal cell cancer: a review. *Ann Oncol* **17**: 1185–1196.

Srinivasan R, Carrington M, Suffredini D, et al. 2006. Impact of KIR and HLA genotypes on outcome in nonmyeloablative hematopoietic cell transplantation (HCT) using HLA matched related donors. *Blood* **108**: 323a.

Storb RF, Lucarelli G, McSweeney PA, et al. 2003. Hematopoietic cell transplantation for benign hematological disorders and solid tumors. *Hematology Am Soc Hematol Educ Program* 2003: 372–397.

Takahashi Y & Childs RW. 2004. Nonmyeloablative transplantation: an allogeneic-based immunotherapy for renal cell carcinoma. *Clin Cancer Res* **10**: 6353S–6359S.

Takahashi Y, Harashima N, Kajigaya S, et al. 2008. Regression of human kidney cancer following allogeneic stem cell transplantation is associated with recognition of an HERV-E antigen by T cells. *J Clin Invest* **118**: 1099–1109.

Tykodi SS, Warren EH, Thompson JA, et al. 2004. Allogeneic hematopoietic cell transplantation for metastatic renal cell carcinoma after nonmyeloablative conditioning: toxicity, clinical response, and immunological response to minor histocompatibility antigens. *Clin Canc Res* **10**: 7799–7811.

Tykodi SS, Sandmaier B, Warren EH, et al. 2011. Allogeneic hematopoietic cell transplantation for all renal cell carcinoma: ten years after. *Expert Opin Biol Ther* **11**: 763–773.

Yang JC & Childs R. 2006. Immunotherapy for renal cell cancer. *J Clin Oncol* **24**: 5576–5583.

Chapter

14

Therapeutic decision making in BMT/SCT for soft tissue sarcomas

Reinhold Munker, Vishwas Sakhalkar, Hillard M. Lazarus, and Kerry Atkinson

Disease classification

Ewing sarcoma

Neuroblastoma

Osteosarcoma

Malignant fibrous histiocytoma

Liposarcoma

Fibrosarcoma

Rhabdomyosarcoma

Schwannoma

Other types of soft tissue sarcomas

Guidelines about the staging and treatment of soft tissue sarcomas can be found in the recommendations of the National Comprehensive Cancer Network (www.nccn.org) and the specialized pediatric oncologic literature (for neuroblastomas, Ewing sarcomas, and osteosarcomas).

Results with HDT followed by autologous SCT

Owing to the multiple types of soft tissue sarcomas and because of the different prognosis of adult versus pediatric sarcomas, few concrete data exist to validate the role of HDT. Theoretically, patients with relapsed disease or high-risk metastatic disease would benefit from an increased dose intensity by overcoming drug resistance to standard-dose therapy.

The BMT Data Book, Third Edition, ed. Reinhold Munker et al. Published by Cambridge University Press. © Cambridge University Press 2013.

In pediatric soft tissue sarcomas, the published studies do not show a clear benefit for consolidation with HDT. The recommendation was given that future trials of HDT must define rigorous eligibility criteria; must have an appropriate, preferably randomized, control group; and must be designed with sufficient power to evaluate the hypothesis that HDT results in a better outcome than standard chemotherapy (Meyers, 2004). The only exception to this statement is neuroblastoma where two randomized studies showed an advantage for HDT (Berthold et al., 2005; Matthay et al., 1999). Pedrazolli et al. (2006) gave an extensive review about the BMT trials for solid tumors in adults (excluding breast cancer).

Neuroblastoma

High-risk neuroblastoma is one of the most frequent indications for an autologous transplant in the pediatric age group. The current standard of care is: 5–6 cycles of induction chemotherapy, surgery, radiation (to the tumor bed and beyond), auto-SCT, followed by six months of oral retinoic acid. Using such an approach, 30%–50% long-term survival can be expected in high-risk neuroblastoma. The practical and research issues concerning SCT for neuroblastoma were discussed by Fish & Grupp (2008) and Grupp et al. (2012). In a large study in patients with high-risk neuroblastoma, it was shown that high-dose chemotherapy with stem cell support improved the PFS but not the OS (Matthay et al., 1999). The improvement was especially clear for patients who received 13-*cis* retinoic acid. A more recent study also found an advantage for HDT versus oral consolidation (Berthold et al., 2005). In extension of the earlier studies, Matthay et al. (2007) treated 148 patients suffering from progressive, refractory or relapsed high-risk neuroblastoma with 18 mCi/kg of ^{131}I-MIBG (targeted radiation therapy) followed by BMT with cryopreserved hematopoietic stem cells (because of significant BM toxicity of MIBG). At one year, EFS for all patients was 18% and OS was 49%, while OS at two years was 29%.

Long-term outcome in children with high-risk neuroblastoma treated with auto-SCT

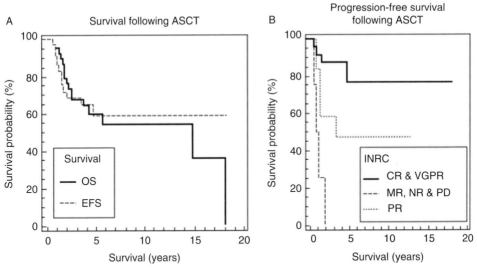

Survival following autologous stem cell transplantation (ASCT) for high-risk neuroblastoma. (A): OS and PFS following ASCT. (B): PFS according to the International Neuroblastoma Response Criteria before ASCT. OS at five years was estimated at 60.2% and at 10 years at 54.7%. The long-term survivors had significant late effects (related both to chemotherapy and SCT). Growth delay and pubertal failure were common. Many patients had hearing problems, orthopedic complications, and renal impairment, and some had thyroid dysfunction. The long-term outcomes for 40 children with neuroblastoma are given. With an improved prognosis, the problems of late toxicity have to be addressed. (Reproduced with permission from Trahair et al., 2007.) ASCT, autologous stem cell transplantation; INRC, International Neuroblastoma Response Criteria; CR, complete recovery; VGPR, very good partial response; MR, minor response; NR, no response; PD, progressive disease; PR, partial recovery.

Indications for autologous transplantation in neuroblastoma

First-line high-risk: neuroblastoma patients older than one year, if stage 4 at diagnosis, or having amplification of N-MYC. INSS (International Neuroblastoma Staging System) stages 2 to 4 at any age.

Relapse: any metastatic relapse (over age one year); any relapsed patient with N-MYC amplification.

Ewing sarcoma and other soft tissue sarcomas

In Europe, a group of pediatric oncologists performed a randomized study of Ewing sarcomas (comparing standard chemotherapy with high-dose chemotherapy; the EURO-EWING study). In cases with primary disseminated multifocal Ewing sarcoma, high-dose chemotherapy with stem cell rescue was given as consolidation treatment (administered only to 60% of patients). Preliminary results show that in the entire group of 281 patients, the EFS at three years was 27% ± 3%, the OS was 34% ± 4% (Ladenstein et al., 2010). In a previous, nonrandomized single-institution study, 36 patients with high-risk Ewing sarcoma and other pediatric solid tumors underwent an SCT. The age median at the time of transplant was 11.5 years with a range of 2–26 years. The OS at one year was 63%. At three years, the survival had dropped to 33%. A better survival was observed in patients with Ewing sarcoma and desmoplastic small round cell tumor compared to that in other pediatric solid tumors treated in the same cohort. A potential benefit was seen for patients treated with a busulfan-containing regimen (Fraser et al., 2006). In a different study including mainly young adults with metastatic or primary localized Ewing sarcoma, a five-year OS of 63% and a PFS of 47% was observed (Laurence et al., 2005). High-dose chemotherapy (based on melphalan and other alkylators) was given as consolidation following induction chemotherapy, radiation, surgery, and maintenance chemotherapy. In another recent publication, the results were reported for 33 patients treated at a single institution for recurrent or progressive Ewing sarcomas (McTiernan et al., 2006). The conditioning regimen consisted mainly of busulfan and melphalan and the age median of the patients was 19 years (range 7–33 years). One patient died from a treatment-related complication (neutropenic colitis). The two-year EFS was 42.5% and the five-year EFS was 38.2%. A Kaplan–Meier plot for EFS and OS from the time of transplant is shown in the following figure.

Long-term outcome following SCT for Ewing sarcoma

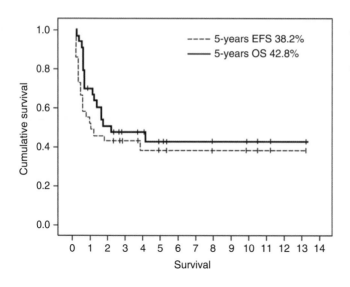

EFS and OS for patients transplanted for recurrent or progressive Ewing sarcoma. (Reproduced with permission from Mc Tiernan et al., 2006.)

Based on these and other case series, many investigators have the impression that high-dose chemotherapy should play a role in the treatment of aggressive or relapsed soft tissue sarcomas (Kasper et al., 2004). However, at present, randomized controlled clinical trials are lacking.

References and further reading

Berthold F, Boos J, Burdach S, et al. 2005. Myeloablative megatherapy with autologous stem cell rescue versus oral maintenance chemotherapy as consolidation treatment in patients with high-risk neuroblastoma: a randomized controlled trial. *Lancet Oncol* **6**: 649–658.

Fish JD & Grupp SA. 2008. Stem cell transplantation for neuroblastoma. *Bone Marrow Transplant* **41**: 159–165.

Fraser CJ, Weigel BJ, Perentesis JP, et al. 2006. Autologous stem cell transplantation for high-risk Ewing's sarcoma and other pediatric solid tumors. *Bone Marrow Transplant* 37: 175–181.

Grupp SA, Asgharzadeh S, & Yanik GA. 2012. Neuroblastoma: issues in transplantation. *Biol Blood Marrow Transplant* 18: S92–S100.

Kasper B, Ho AD, & Egerer G. 2005. Is there an indication for high-dose chemotherapy in the treatment of bone and soft tissue sarcoma? *Oncology* 68: 115–121.

Ladenstein R, Pötschger U, Le Deley MC, et al. 2010. Primary disseminated multifocal Ewing sarcoma: results of the Euro-Ewing 99 trial. *J Clin Oncol* 28: 3284–3291.

Laurence V, Pierga JY, Barthier S, et al. 2005. Long-term follow-up of high-dose chemotherapy with autologous stem cell rescue in adults with Ewing tumor. *Am J Clin Oncol* 28: 301–309.

Matthay KK, Villablanca JG, Seeger RC, et al. 1999. Treatment of high-risk neuroblastoma with intensive chemotherapy, radiotherapy, autologous bone marrow transplantation, and 13-cis-retinoic acid. *N Engl J Med* 341: 1165–1173.

Matthay KK, Yanik G, Messina J, et al. 2007. Phase II study on the effect of disease sites, age, and prior therapy on response to iodine-131-metaiodobenzylguanidine therapy in refractory neuroblastoma. *J Clin Oncol* 25: 1054–1060.

Mc Tiernan A, Driver D, Michelagnoli MOP, et al. 2006. High dose chemotherapy with bone marrow or peripheral stem cell rescue is an effective treatment option for patients with relapsed or progressive Ewing's sarcoma family of tumours. *Ann Oncol* 17: 1301–1305.

Meyers PA. 2004. High-dose therapy with autologous stem cell rescue for pediatric sarcomas. *Curr Opin Oncol* 16: 120–125.

Pedrazzoli P, Ledermann JA, Lotz JP, et al. 2006. High dose chemotherapy with autologous hematopoietic stem cell support for solid tumors other than breast cancer in adults. *Ann Oncol* 17: 1479–1488.

Trahair TN, Vowels MR, Johnston K, et al. 2007. Long-term outcomes in children with high-risk neuroblastoma treated with autologous stem cell transplantation. *Bone Marrow Transplant* 40: 741–746.

Therapeutic decision making in BMT/SCT for severe aplastic anemia

Reinhold Munker, Anna Locasciulli, and Kerry Atkinson

Etiology

1. Idiopathic (most frequent type of aplastic anemia)
2. Chemical and physical agents

   (a) Agents that regularly produce aplasia if dose is sufficient

   cytotoxic drugs
   ionizing radiation
   benzene and related agents
   inorganic arsenic

   (b) Agents that occasionally produce aplasia (idiosyncratic)

   chloramphenicol
   sulfonamides, penicillins, tetracyclines
   quinacrine
   diphenylhydantoin
   tolbutamide
   phenylbutazone, indomethacin
   carbamazepine
   acetylsalicylic acid
   chlorpromazine
   gold compounds
   penicillamine
   hair dyes

---

solvents, DDT
cimetidine

3. Infections (e.g., viral hepatitis, EBV, HIV)
4. Congenital
   Fanconi anemia
   Shwachman–Diamond syndrome
   Amegakaryocytic thrombocytopenia

Disease staging

Parameter	Severe aplastic anemia*	Very severe aplastic anemia
Blood		
Neutrophils	$<0.5 \times 10^9$/L	$<0.2 \times 10^9$/L
Platelets	$<20 \times 10^9$/L	
Reticulocytes	<1% (corrected)	
Marrow	Severe hypocellularity (<25% normal cellularity) or moderate hypocellularity with hemopoietic cells <30% of residual cells	

* any two of the three blood parameters or either marrow criteria.

Results with conventional therapy

The two main therapeutic options for patients with severe aplastic anemia are combination immune suppressive treatment or allogeneic transplantation, if a suitable donor is available.

A protocol for combination immune suppressive treatment is as follows (Frickhofen et al., 2003):

1. Methylprednisolone, 5 mg/kg on days 1–8 (single oral dose or IV infusion over 30 minutes); then prednisolone, 1 mg/kg/day for days 9–14; then taper the dose until day 29. The incorporation of steroids is important as it prevents or ameliorates serum sickness. The dose used in EBMT protocols is somewhat lower: 1–2 mg/kg/day for two weeks, 0.5 mg/kg during the third week, tapering to zero during the fourth week.
2. Antithymocyte globulin (ATG) (e.g., ATGAM, Pharmacia & Upjohn/Pfizer, produced in horses), 20 mg/kg IV over six hours on days 1–8. Some centers also give 40 mg/kg/day over four days. Administer in normal saline at a concentration of no more than 1 mg/mL. Perform a skin test before infusion: give a dose of 0.1 mL of a 1/1000 dilution (5 μg) intradermally; use normal saline, as a control, on the other arm. If wheal or erythema of >10 mm develops within an hour, particular caution is recommended. A systemic reaction precludes use.

   - Use a high-flow vein, as phlebitis is common. Alternatively, use a CVC
   - Use an in-line filter of 0.2- to 1.0-μm mesh
   - Have a tray containing epinephrine (adrenaline) 1/1000 (0.3 mL SC initially if anaphylaxis), antihistamines, and an airway device within reach

3. Cyclosporin, 12 mg/kg/day, in two divided doses orally. A lower dose is recommended by the EBMT (5 mg/kg/d). Continue for at least six months. Keep trough levels 200–300 ng/mL for the first four weeks, then 150–200 ng/mL. If there is marked toxicity, cease for 1–4 days, and then re-institute at two-thirds of the former dose.
4. ATG produced in horses can be substituted by ATG produced in rabbits (Thymoglobulin, Genzyme), which is administered IV at a dose of 3.5 mg/kg/day over five days; however, it was recently shown in a randomized trial that rabbit ATG is inferior to horse ATG (Scheinberg et al., 2011).

Note: immunosuppressive therapy has fewer acute complications and less TRM than allogeneic transplantation, but has significant long-term adverse events (relapse, secondary cytogenetic abnormalities, development of MDS, evolution to AML, development of paroxysmal nocturnal hemoglobinuria [PNH]). Recently, a high incidence of subclinical EBV reactivation was described following rabbit-ATG in combination with cyclosporin (Scheinberg et al., 2007). Information about current European studies for severe aplastic anemia is available at the website of the EBMT (www.ebmt.org/5workingparties).

Triple immune suppressive therapy for severe aplastic anemia (multicenter study)

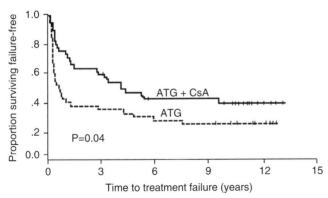

In this long-term follow-up study, patients treated with cyclosporin (CsA) + ATG had longer failure-free survival than patients treated without CsA. A response was observed in 70% of patients treated with CsA + ATG versus only in 41% treated with ATG alone. Most patients treated with CsA needed only one course of immunosuppression whereas many patients treated without CsA needed several courses. The relapse rate, projected at 38% after 11.3 years, was similar between the two treatment groups. In 26% of the patients responding to a CsA-containing regimen, the remissions were dependent on CsA. Clonal or malignant diseases developed in 26% of all patients. (Reproduced with permission from Frickhofen et al., 2003.)

Other treatment options (especially for patients with nonsevere aplastic anemia) include the following:

- Initial therapy with cyclosporin alone (not recommended)
- Use of androgens
- Use of hemopoietic growth factors (not recommended as a single agent)
- High-dose cyclophosphamide (50 mg/kg/day over four consecutive days) without stem cell support is a salvage treatment for patients who fail to respond to ATG (Brodsky et al., 2004), but has significant toxicities

Results with allogeneic transplant
HLA-identical sibling transplant (Seattle, Stanford, and City of Hope data)

In a study from Seattle and other centers with long-term follow-up, the 8–12-year survival was close to 90% (Storb et al., 2004). Ninety-four consecutive patients received HLA-matched related marrow grafts and were conditioned with cyclophosphamide IV 50 mg/kg on each of four successive days. Twelve hours after the first, second, and third dose of cyclophosphamide, patients were given horse ATG (Atgam) at 30 mg/kg IV over 10–12 hours. Among these patients, 87 had received multiple transfusions and 38 had failed immunosuppressive therapy. Their ages ranged from 2–59 years (median age 26 years). After transplantation, 89 patients received a methotrexate/cyclosporin regimen for GVHD prevention. Cyclosporin with or without prednisone was given in four patients, and no immunosuppression was given in one patient. Ninety-six percent of patients had sustained engraftment, whereas 4% rejected grafts between two and seven months after transplantation. Of the four patients who rejected, three are alive with successful second grafts. Acute grade II GVHD was seen in 32% of patients, grade III in 7% , and grade IV in 1%. Chronic GVHD occurred in 32% of patients, most of whom responded completely to immunosuppressive therapy.

Comment 1: the outcome of matched sibling allogeneic transplantation has improved over the last 10 years. The addition of ATG to the conditioning with cyclophosphamide may have a lesser role than previously thought, because a randomized study comparing cyclophosphamide to the combination of cyclophosphamide with ATG did not clearly improve the outcome with the combined treatment (Champlin et al., 2007).

Comment 2: most experts prefer BM as a stem cell source for severe aplastic anemia as PB stem cells lead to a somewhat higher incidence of chronic GVHD and a poorer long-term outcome. The superiority of BM over PB stem cells was recently confirmed for unrelated donors (Eapen et al., 2011). In younger patients with severe aplastic anemia, a screening for Fanconi anemia should be performed, because such patients are hypersensitive to alkylating agents and require a different conditioning protocol (low-dose cyclophosphamide, fludarabine-based regimens).

The standard conditioning with related matched donors for severe aplastic anemia is cyclophosphamide/ATG (see page 284); in some centers fludarabine-based conditioning is used.

HLA-identical unrelated donor transplant (multicenter study, EBMT data)

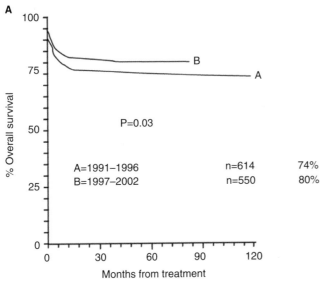

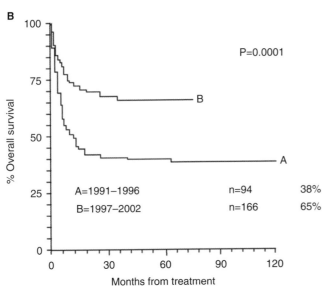

In this large EBMT study, the outcome of transplant for acquired severe aplastic anemia was compared for two time periods (1991–1996 and 1997–2002) and for HLA-identical sibling transplants (A) and for alternative donors (B). The prognosis (OS) improved significantly, especially for alternative donor transplants. (Reproduced with permission from Locasciulli et al., 2007.)

Pediatric data for matched related and alternative SCT (single institution study)

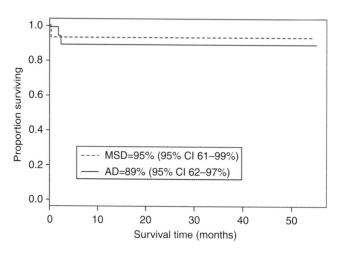

In this pediatric, single-center, nonrandomized study, the survival of matched sibling donor (MSD) transplants was comparable to alternative donor (AD) transplants. The median age of all patients was 9.4 years (range 1.3–18.4 years). (Reproduced with permission from Kennedy-Nasser et al., 2006.)

Legend in figure:
- - - - MSD=95% (95% CI 61–99%)
—— AD=89% (95% CI 62–97%)

Indications for allogeneic transplant

1. If an HLA-identical sibling or syngeneic donor is available and the recipient is less than 40 years of age:

   • Severe or very severe aplastic anemia

2. If there is a partially HLA-matched (9 of 10 antigens) family member donor or an HLA-identical unrelated donor available:

   • Immune suppressive treatment (generally two courses) has failed
   • Some centers transplant first-line with a molecularly matched unrelated donor if the patient is young (<30 years), but this is not a standard approach
   • Owing to improvements in molecular typing, recent studies recommend a somewhat earlier use of unrelated donors for severe aplastic anemia (Meyers & Maziarz, 2010)

Pretransplant workup

1. See the general pretransplant workup (page 239)
2. BM biopsy, aspirate, and cytogenetics (to exclude myelodysplasia)

Caveat: 5%–15% of patients with aplastic anemia may have cytogenetic abnormalities at diagnosis (e.g., monosomy 7, deletion 5q). The prognostic relevance is unclear at present.

3. Flow cytometry for CD55 and CD59 (to exclude PNH)

Caveat: PNH clones may be observed in severe aplastic anemia.

4. In younger patients, exclude inherited BM failure syndromes
5. Hepatitis and HIV screen (to determine possible viral etiology)

Monitoring posttransplant

1. BM aspirate and cytogenetic evaluation at three and 12 weeks and one year
2. ABO status at 1, 3, 6, and 12 months if there was a pretransplant donor–recipient difference

3. Monitoring for long-term complications of allogeneic transplant especially chronic GVHD, second malignancies
4. Monitoring for relapse and secondary clonal evolution if not full chimera

References and further reading

Brodsky RA, Chen AR, Brodsky I, et al. 2004. High-dose cyclophosphamide as salvage therapy for severe aplastic anemia. *Exp Hematol* **32**: 435–440.

Champlin RE, Perez WS, Passaweg JR, et al. 2007. Bone marrow transplantation for severe aplastic anemia: a randomized controlled study of conditioning regimes. *Blood* **109**: 4582–4585.

Eapen M, Rademacher JK, Antin JH, et al. 2011. Effect of stem cell source on outcomes after unrelated donor transplantation in severe aplastic anemia. *Blood* **118**: 2618–2621.

Frickhofen N, Heimpel H, Kaltwasser JP, et al. 2003. Antithymocyte globulin with or without cyclosporine A: 11-year follow-up of a randomized trial comparing treatments of aplastic anemia. *Blood* **101**: 1236–1242.

Kennedy-Nasser AA, Leung KS, Mahajan A, et al. 2006. Comparable outcomes of matched-related and alternative donor stem cell transplantation for pediatric severe aplastic anemia. *Biol Blood Marrow Transplant* **12**: 1277–1284.

Locasciulli A, Oneto R, Bacigalupo A, et al. 2007. Outcome of patients with acquired aplastic anemia given first-line bone marrow transplantation or immunosuppressive treatment in the last decade: a report from the European Group for Blood and Marrow Transplantation. *Haematologica* **92**: 11–18.

Marsh JW. 2007. Treatment of acquired aplastic anemia. *Haematologica* **92**: 2–5.

Meyers G & Maziarz RT. 2010. Is it time for a change? The case for early application of unrelated allo-SCT for severe aplastic anemia. *Bone Marrow Transplant* **45**: 1479–1488.

Scheinberg P, Fischer SH, Li L, et al. 2007. Distinct EBV and CMV reactivation patterns following antibody-based immunosuppressive regimens in patients with severe aplastic anemia. *Blood* **109**: 3219–3224.

Scheinberg P, Nunez O, Weinstein B, et al. 2011. Horse versus rabbit antithymocyte globulin in acquired aplastic anemia. *N Engl J Med* **365**: 430–438.

Storb R, Blume KG, O'Donnell MR, et al. 2004. Cyclophosphamide and antithymocyte globulin to condition patients with aplastic anemia for allogeneic transplantation: the experience in four centers. *Biol Blood Marrow Transplant* **7**: 39–44.

Young NS, Calado RT, & Scheinberg P. 2006. Current concepts in the pathophysiology and treatment of aplastic anemia. *Blood* **108**: 2509–2519.

Therapeutic decision making in BMT/SCT for congenital immunodeficiencies

Vishwas Sakhalkar, Reinhold Munker, and Kerry Atkinson

Introduction

Among the early successes of allogeneic BMT were those achieved in the area of congenital immunodeficiencies. In certain diseases and certain donor–recipient combinations, over 90% of patients can be cured by allogeneic transplantation. Worldwide, over 3000 patients with congenital immunodeficiencies have been treated by allogeneic transplantation. The following table gives a list of the current indications. Patients with congenital immunodeficiencies generally manifest as severe infections within the first year of life. In the absence of a hematopoietic SCT or BMT, most severe immunodeficiencies are fatal. The European Society for Immunodeficiencies (ESID) in collaboration with the EBMT provides guidelines for the conditioning regimens in use for primary immunodeficiencies (www.esid.org and www.ebmt.org). For reviews related to BMT and congenital immunodeficiencies, see Buckley, 2003; Buckley et al., 1999; and Steward and Jarisch, 2005. Szabolcs et al. (2010) gave a very detailed overview of the primary immunodeficiencies treated by BMT/SCT.

With the advent of genetic mapping, SCID is now increasingly classified on a genetic basis. This gives a more precise characterization of the immunological defects. Thus, it is becoming clear which types have the best cure rate, allowing the stratification of therapy. For example, patients with a mutation in the antigen receptor gene *Artemis* (resulting in a T-B- NK+ phenotype) were described as having a worse prognosis.

Estimations of the incidence of immune deficiency syndromes vary widely. On the basis of registry reports, an incidence of 1:70 000 to 1:1 000 000 live births is suggested.

The BMT Data Book, Third Edition, ed. Reinhold Munker et al. Published by Cambridge University Press. © Cambridge University Press 2013.

The screening for SCID could result in a large benefit to affected individuals, making screening cost-effective in spite of the low incidence of the disease, would lead to an early diagnosis, and would increase the success rate of BMT for immune deficiency (McGhee et al., 2005). This screening could be performed with a T- and B-cell assay in addition to the family history.

Immune deficiency syndromes are examples of disorders that primarily affect a single lineage, such as the lymphoid or myeloid lineages, and can be cured with BMT. For most immune deficiencies, the goal of BMT is to restore sufficient numbers of normal cells of the affected lineage(s); reconstitution of an unaffected lineage is not required for cure of the disease.

Current indications for SCT for congenital immunodeficiencies

SCID (mutations in at least 13 different genes)
  SCID with absence of T- and B-cells (autosomal recessive)
  SCID with absence of T-cells (X-linked recessive)
  Reticular dysgenesis

Non-SCID immunodeficiencies (also designated as "leak" SCID/CID syndromes)
  Severe T-cell deficiencies (Omenn's syndrome, ZAP-70 deficiency, PNP deficiency, MHC Class II deficiency, bare lymphocyte syndrome and others)
  Hyper-IgM syndrome
  Hereditary lymphohistiocytosis
  X-linked proliferation syndrome
  Wiskott–Aldrich syndrome
  Certain disorders of phagocyte number and function
  CD95 deficiency (lymphoproliferative syndrome with autoimmunity)

PNP, purine nucleoside phosphorylase.

Results of BMT/SCT for severe combined immunodeficiency (SCID)

In SCID, a cure rate of more than 90% is observed if HLA-identical donors are used, especially if patients are transplanted before six months of age. This cure rate is remarkable considering the heavy infectious load of many patients before transplant. The results have steadily improved because of better transplant regimes and supportive care. In many instances, no conditioning is given. A low incidence of GVHD is observed. In SCID with only T-cell defects, B-cells of the recipient often coexist with donor-derived T-cells. If mismatched family members are used as donors, the success or cure rate is lower (60%–70%). The problem of GVHD can be reduced by T-cell depletion or CD34 selection. However, this procedure delays the restoration of T-cell immunity. If unrelated donors or mismatched family members are used, a conditioning regimen is necessary (a reduced dose of busulfan and cyclophosphamide). If no conditioning is given (for matched sibling donors), B-cell defects may persist in some patients, thus requiring long-term immunoglobulin replacement.

The poorest BMT results are still seen among patients with absent T- and B-cells but maintained NK cell function (T-B-NK+). A unique yet significant transplant issue in immune deficiency patients is the presence of infection at the time of BMT. Some SCID patients have multiple and severe infections at the time of transplant, especially when identified at an older age. Their presence can significantly lower the chances of a cure by the transplant. On the other hand, these infections are extremely unlikely to be eradicated by the patient's virtually nonexistent immune system without reconstitution of the immune system by BMT. In many developing countries, the BCG vaccine is routinely administered at birth. Therefore, disseminated BCG infection is a well-documented mode of presentation of severe immune deficiency. Recently, it was found that BMT combined with antituberculous therapy is a promising approach for cure in these countries (Jaing at al., 2006). The pattern of infection both in SCID and non-SCID patients is related to the defective T- and B-cell lines. A wide variety of viral, fungal, and bacterial infections (often disseminated) is observed.

Testing for the presence of maternal chimerism is important when performing pre-transplant compatibility assessment and has a bearing on donor/host compatibility and the ultimate outcome of the transplant in cases of SCID. It was shown as early as 1980 that maternal cells engraft and persist in the circulation of infants with SCID. In normal individuals, microchimerism by maternal cells is observed in up to 42% of UCB samples. The survival of these maternal cells is limited; on the contrary, in SCID patients, a long-term engraftment of maternal T-cells may occur in up to 40% of patients and contribute to graft rejection and worsening GVHD.

Results of BMT/SCT for non-SCID

Non-SCID are more heterogeneous in their presentation and prognosis. As conditioning, busulfan–cyclophosphamide is generally given. Considerable experience has been accumulated with allo-SCT for Wiskott–Aldrich syndrome (WAS) (Filipovich et al., 2001). This syndrome is characterized by thrombocytopenia, eczema, immune deficiency, and an increased risk for the development of lymphomas. WAS is X-linked and results from mutations in the *WASP* gene. It is recommended (as in most other congenital immuno-deficiencies) that transplants be performed as early as possible. The International Bone Marrow Transplant Registry (IBMTR) and the National Marrow Donor Program (NMDP) reported the outcome for 170 patients with WAS. Most transplant recipients were younger than five years old, had a pretransplant performance score greater than 90%, and received conditioning regimens without radiation as well as non-T-cell-depleted grafts. The five-year probability of survival was 70% for all patients. HLA-identical sibling transplants had a survival probability of 87%, as compared to 52% and 71% for other related and unrelated donors, respectively (see following figure). In particular, boys receiving an unrelated transplant had a survival similar to those receiving a transplant from HLA-identical siblings.

Impact of donor type on outcome of BMT for WAS: collaborative study of the International Bone Marrow Transplant Registry and the National Marrow Donor Program

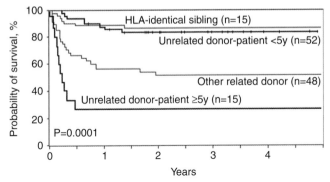

Probabilities of survival for 170 patients receiving BMT for WAS with respect to donor type and age. There was no significant difference in the risk of mortality after HLA-matched sibling transplants as compared to unrelated donor transplants in children younger than five years old. Significantly worse survival rates were associated with use of related donors other than HLA-identical siblings, regardless of recipient age, and with use of unrelated donors in patients older than five years. (Reprinted with permission from Filipovich et al., 2001.)

In immunodeficiency diseases other than SCID, results tend to be poorer, probably because patients tend to present later when they are significantly infected. In WAS, for example, results are best in those transplanted before five years of age. Selection of appropriate patients is often difficult. Transplantation would cure a majority of those affected if performed at an early age before onset of significant complications. However, because of the risk of early death following SCT, it is conventional to use more conservative treatments (e.g., prophylactic antibiotics, intravenous immunoglobulin), withholding SCT until complications ensue. Unfortunately, this greatly increases the risks associated with SCT at that stage. An excellent example of this dilemma is provided by chronic granulomatous disease, where prophylactic approaches are improving, but many patients still eventually develop serious infective complications. At present, the indication for SCT in granulocyte disorders remains restricted to patients with significant complications, especially when matched sibling donors are not available (Goldblatt, 2002).

The European experience with SCT for immunodeficiencies between 1968 and 1999 was published by Antoine et al. (2003) (see page 176). Altogether, 919 patients received 1082 transplants (475 SCID patients and 444 non-SCID patients). In SCID, the three-year survival was significantly better after HLA-identical transplantation than after mismatched transplantation (77% vs. 54%; P=0.002). In HLA-mismatched SCT, SCID without B-cells had a worse prognosis than SCID with residual B-cells. In non-SCID, three-year survival after genotypically HLA-matched, phenotypically HLA-matched, HLA-mismatched related, and unrelated donor transplantation was 71%, 42%, 42%, and 59%, respectively. Acute GVHD predicted a poor prognosis regardless of the origin of the donor, except for HLA-identical sibling transplants in SCID. Overall, the transplant results have improved over the last 20–35 years because of better treatment and prophylaxis of transplant- and disease-related complications.

Long-term survival and transplantation of hemopoietic stem cells for immunodeficiencies: report of the European experience 1968–1999

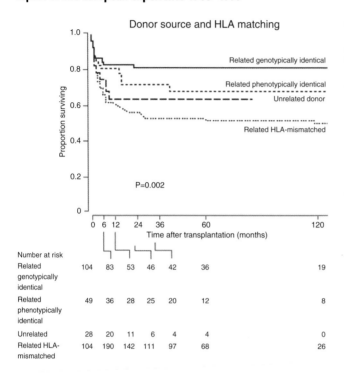

Cumulative probability of survival in SCID patients, according to donor source (related or unrelated donor) and HLA matching. (Reproduced with permission from Antoine et al., 2003.)

Number at risk							
Related genotypically identical	104	83	53	46	42	36	19
Related phenotypically identical	49	36	28	25	20	12	8
Unrelated	28	20	11	6	4	4	0
Related HLA-mismatched	104	190	142	111	97	68	26

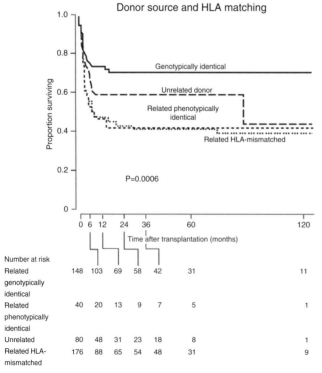

Cumulative probability of survival in non-SCID patients, according to donor source (related or unrelated donor) and HLA matching. (Reproduced with permission from Antoine et al., 2003.)

Number at risk							
Related genotypically identical	148	103	69	58	42	31	11
Related phenotypically identical	40	20	13	9	7	5	1
Unrelated	80	48	31	23	18	8	1
Related HLA-mismatched	176	88	65	54	48	31	9

Reduced-intensity conditioning (RIC) for congenital immunodeficiencies

In a single institutional study, the results of 82 transplants following RIC of 81 children with congenital immunodeficiencies were recently reported (Veys et al., 2005). The immunological disorders included SCID (20) and non-SCID (61). The majority of donors were unrelated (matched unrelated 40, unrelated mismatched 21), 71 patients received BM stem cells and 10 received PB stem cells. The conditioning included fludarabine and melphalan (combined with alemtuzumab [51 patients] or ATG [24 patients]). The transplants were generally well tolerated and 84% of the patients survived with no significant differences with regard to donor types or between SCID and non-SCID diseases. The immune reconstitution appeared comparable to conventional SCT. The incidence of severe GVHD was low, but unexpectedly, EBV reactivation was common. In conclusion, RIC appears to be a valid alternative to standard transplant regimens.

Indications for allogeneic transplant

Diagnosis of a severe congenital immunodeficiency (as outlined in the table on page 173) and availability of a matched related (or unrelated) donor are absolute indications in SCID and relative indications in some non-SCID disorders.

Contraindications to allogeneic transplant

Severe, uncontrolled infection.

Gene therapy for primary immunodeficiency

Gene therapy using autologous progenitor and stem cells is an alternative for patients who do not find an appropriate donor. Booth et al. (2011) recently described the successes and challenges of gene therapy for primary immunodeficiency. Diseases treated so far include X-linked SCID, SCID caused by adenosine deaminase deficiency, chronic granulomatous disease, and WAS.

References and further reading

Antoine C, Müller S, Cant A, et al. 2003. Long-term survival and transplantation of haematopoietic stem cells for immunodeficiencies: report of the European experience 1968–99. *Lancet* **361**: 553–60.

Booth C, Gaspar HB, & Thrasher AJ. 2011. Gene therapy for primary immunodeficiency. *Curr Opin Pediatr* **23**: 659–666

Buckley RH. 2003. Treatment options for genetically determined immuno-deficiency. *Lancet* **361**: 541–42.

Buckley RH, Schiff SE, Schiff RI, et al. 1999. Hematopoietic stem-cell transplantation for the treatment of severe combined immunodeficiency. *N Engl J Med* **340**: 508–16.

Filipovich AH, Stone JV, Tomany SC, et al. 2001. Impact of donor type on outcome of bone marrow transplantation for Wiskott-Aldrich syndrome: collaborative study of the International Bone Marrow Transplant Registry and the National Marrow Donor Program. *Blood* **97**: 1598–603.

Fischer A. 2004. Allogeneic hematopoietic stem cell transplantation for congenital immune deficiencies. In Atkinson K, Champlin R, Ritz J, et al., eds. *Clinical Bone Marrow and Blood*

Stem Cell Transplantation. Cambridge: Cambridge University Press, pp. 947–962.

Goldblatt D. 2002. Current treatment options for chronic granulomatous disease. *Expert Opin Pharmacother* **3**: 857–63.

Jaing T-H, Lee W-I, Lin T-Y, et al. 2006. Successful unrelated mismatched cord blood transplantation in an infant with severe combined immunodeficiency and *Mycobacterium bovis* bacillus Calmette-Gue'rin disease. *Pediatr Transplantation* **10**: 501–04.

McGhee SA, Stiehm ER, & McCabe ER. 2005. Potential costs and benefits of newborn screening for severe combined immunodeficiency. *J Pediatr* **147**: 603–608.

Parkman R. 2000. Hematopoietic stem cell transplantation for primary immunodeficiency and metabolic diseases. *Hematology Am Soc Hematol Educ Program* **2000**: 319–323.

Steward CG & Jarisch A. 2005. Haemopoietic stem cell transplantation for genetic disorders. *Arch Dis Child* **90**: 1259–1263.

Szabolcs P, Cavazzana-Calvo M, Fischer A, et al. 2010. Bone marrow transplantation for primary immunodeficiency diseases. *Pediatr Clin N Am* **57**: 207–237.

Veys P, Rao K, & Amrolia P. 2005. Stem cell transplantation for congenital immunodeficiencies using reduced-intensity conditioning. *Bone Marrow Transplant* **35**: S45–S47.

Chapter

17

Therapeutic decision making in BMT/SCT for hemoglobinopathies

Shalini Shenoy, Reinhold Munker, and Kerry Atkinson

β-Thalassemia syndromes

Syndrome	Main characteristics	Clinical features
Thalassemia major	Severe anemia, life-limiting iron overload from transfusions	Hb <7 g/dL, marked splenomegaly, skeletal changes, jaundice
Thalassemia intermedia	Less severe anemia, chronic transfusions not required, survival to adult life	Hb 7–10 g/dL, moderate splenomegaly, mild or no skeletal changes
Thalassemia minor	Asymptomatic, abnormal red cell morphology, little or no anemia	Hb >10 g/dL, mild or no splenomegaly
Thalassemia minima	Undetectable except by inference from family studies	No abnormal clinical features

The BMT Data Book, Third Edition, ed. Reinhold Munker et al. Published by Cambridge University Press. © Cambridge University Press 2013.

Complications of sickle cell disease (SCD)

Pain crises

Severe anemia

Chest syndrome

Infection

Stroke

Leg ulcers

Retinopathy

Pulmonary hypertension

Sickle cell nephropathy

Results with conventional therapy for thalassemia

The two main therapeutic options for patients with thalassemia major are transfusion/chelation therapy or allogeneic transplant, if a suitable donor is available.

Outcome with transfusion/chelation therapy

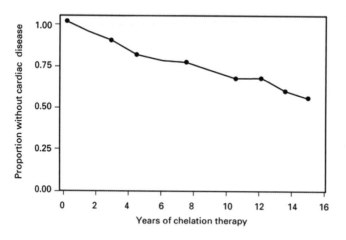

Survival without cardiac disease during chelation therapy in 97 patients with thalassemia major. (Reproduced with permission from Olivieri et al., 1994.)

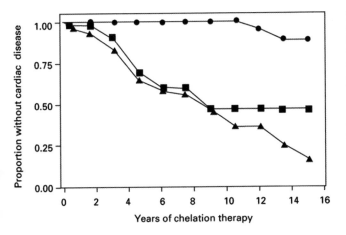

Survival without cardiac disease, according to the proportion of serum ferritin measurements greater than 2500 ng/mL. The circles show cardiac disease-free survival among patients in whom fewer than 33% of ferritin measurements exceeded 2500 ng/mL. Squares show survival among patients in whom 33%–67% of ferritin measurements exceeded 2500 ng/mL. Triangles show survival among patients in whom more than 67% of ferritin measurements exceeded 2500 ng/mL. (Reproduced with permission from Olivieri et al., 1994.)

Chelation for iron overload

Drugs	Application	Dosage	Side effects	Comments
Deferoxamine (desferal)	Subcutaneous (8 hr via pump)	25–50 mg/kg	Inflammation at infusion sites, ototoxicity	Longest experience for effectiveness
Deferasirox	Oral once daily	5–30 mg/kg	GI toxicity, increased creatinine	Shorter experience, better compliance
Deferiprone	Oral three times daily	75 mg/kg total daily dose	GI discomfort, arthralgia, increased liver enzymes	Shorter experience

Results with conventional therapy for SCD

Outcome of sickle cell anemia: a four-decade observational study of 1056 patients in Los Angeles

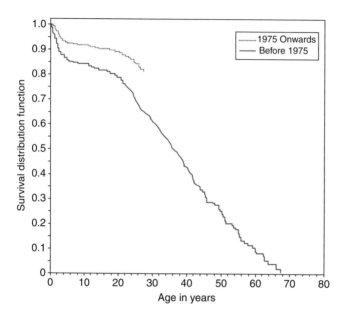

Survival curves before and after 1975: Cox regression survival curves comparing the 884 Hb SS patients born before or after January 1, 1975, demonstrating a significant improvement in those born after 1975. In this prospective study, the median survival of patients with SCD was between 35 and 40 years. Having a clearly identified condition like leg ulcer, osteonecrosis, and retinopathy predicted the development of more severe end-organ damage and early death. By age 40 years and above, nearly half of the surviving patients had developed irreversible organ damage. (Reproduced with permission from Powars et al., 2005.)

Survival and reasons for mortality in SCD in recent years (2000–2005)

Survival age and causes of death for deceased subjects

Median survival age[a]	Years (95% CI)
Total	40 (35,53)
Males	40 (34,48)
Females	39 (33,56)
Age at death (Years)	Number of patients
20–29	8
30–39	15
40–49	8
50–59	7
≥60	5
Cause of death	Numbers diagnosed
Cardiac	
Pulseless electrical activity arrest	5

(cont.)

Cause of death	Numbers diagnosed
Congestive heart failure	3
Myocardial infarction	3
Pulmonary	
Pulmonary embolus	4
Pulmonary hypertension	1
Respiratory disorder	1
Other complications of SCD	
Stroke	4
Multiorgan failure	3
Liver failure	2
Chronic renal failure	1
Anoxic brain injury	1
Sickle cell anemia	3
Other	6[b]
Unknown	6

[a] Median survival age and 95% CI are calculated from the Cox model.
[b] Foreign body aspiration (2), intestinal disorder (1), complications after fall (1), narcotic overdose (1), assault (1). These data outline the predominantly cardiopulmonary causes of sudden death that still prevail in patients with SCD resulting in median survival rates of 40 years despite significant advances in supportive care such as hydroxyurea therapy, extended phenotype matched blood transfusions, erythrocytapheresis, etc. (Reproduced with permission from Fitzhugh et al., 2010.)

As the natural history of SCD was tracked, as many as 45% of children with initial strokes developed second strokes or progressive silent cerebral infarcts despite adequate chronic transfusion therapy; a surprisingly high rate of CNS disease progression despite supportive care (Hulbert et al., 2011).

Results with allogeneic transplant for thalassemia major

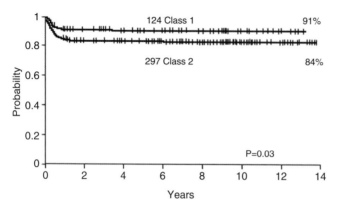

Probability of thalassemia-free survival in pediatric patients with thalassemia (update of the Pesaro data, HLA-identical related donors).
Thalassemia-free survival in 321 patients with thalassemia (Class 1 and Class 2 according to Pesaro criteria, see page 189 for details). These patients underwent myeloablative conditioning with Bu14-CY200. All donors were HLA-identical family members. (Reproduced with permission from Gaziev et al., 2003.)

Results of unrelated SCT in young adults with thalassemia

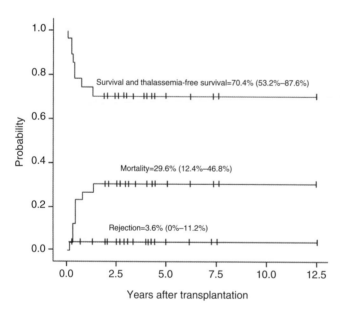

Kaplan–Meier probabilities of survival, thalassemia-free survival, mortality, and rejection in 27 adult Class 3 thalassemia patients transplanted from HLA-matched unrelated donors (between parenthesis: 95% confidence limits). (Reproduced with permission from La Nasa et al., 2005.)

Results of related CBT in patients with thalassemia and SCD

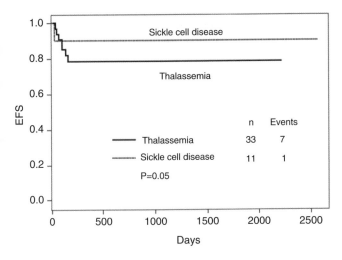

Kaplan–Meier estimate of the probability of EFS according to the original disease. A total of 44 patients had a related UCB transplant (33 with thalassemia, 11 with SCD). The median age was five years and the age range 1–20 years. No patient died and 36 of the 44 patients remained free of disease with a median follow-up of 24 months. (Reproduced with permission from Locatelli et al., 2003.)

Reduced toxicity BMT for thalassemia

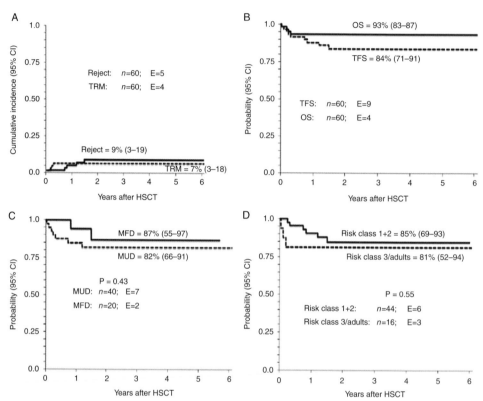

Outcomes of the study population. A: Cumulative incidence of transplantation-related mortality (TRM) and graft rejection (Reject). B: Five-year Kaplan–Meier estimate of overall survival (OS) and thalassemia-free survival (TFS) for the whole cohort of patients. C: Five-year Kaplan–Meier estimate of thalassemia-free survival (TFS) according to the type of donor used (MFD indicates matched family donor; and MUD, matched unrelated donor). D: Five-year Kaplan–Meier estimate of thalassemia-free survival (TFS) according to the patient's class of risk.

A modified reduced toxicity myeloablative regimen consisting of treosulfan, fludarabine, and thiotepa was reported to have 84% thalassemia-free survival in 60 patients with related (20) and unrelated (40) donor marrow transplants with graft failure of 9% and mortality of 7%. (Reproduced with permission from Bernardo et al., 2012.)

Unrelated donor reduced-intensity transplantation for children with transfusion-dependent thalassemia

The Thalassemia Clinical Research Network and the Pediatric Blood and Marrow Transplant Consortium have recently completed a 20-patient phase II trial of reduced-intensity unrelated BM and UCB transplants for thalassemia using hydroxyurea, alemtuzumab, fludarabine, melphalan, and thiotepa for conditioning (the URTH trial). The regimen was well tolerated and follow-up is in progress (personal communication, Shenoy).

Results with allogeneic transplant for SCD
Results of conventional full dose allotransplantation in pediatric patients

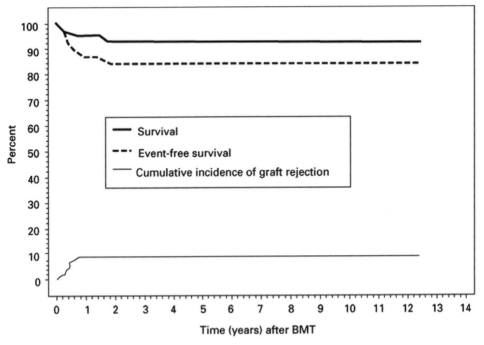

Survival and EFS after BMT for SCD. The Kaplan–Meier probabilities of survival and EFS among 59 patients who received HLA-identical sibling BM allografts are shown. In addition, the cumulative incidence of graft rejection and recurrent SCD is shown. An event was defined as death, graft rejection, or return of SCD. (Reproduced with permission from Walters et al., 2005.)

Registry data from the CIBMTR was similar. Following sibling donor myeloablative transplantation in 67 patients (median age 10 years), OS was 97%; DFS was 85% (Panepinto et al., 2007).

Results of mobilized PB SCT from matched sibling donors following very low intensity conditioning

Long-term mixed donor chimerism was reported in 10 patients (adults and children) following matched sibling donor PB SCT after very low intensity conditioning consisting of alemtuzumab and low-dose (300 cGy) radiation. Nine of the ten engrafted donor cells maintained mixed donor–recipient chimerism. Sirolimus was used as posttransplant GVHD prophylaxis for extended periods to maintain T-cell tolerance and chimerism (Hsieh et al., 2009).

Unrelated donor BMT for severe SCD using an RIC regimen (BMT CTN–the SCURT trial)

This trial is ongoing to evaluate the feasibility of matched unrelated donor marrow transplantation after alemtuzumab, fludarabine, and melphalan-based RIC (Shenoy et al., 2005). Children younger than 19 years of age are eligible if they have stroke, acute chest syndrome, or severe pain. The cord arm of the trial was closed for increased risk of graft rejection in five of eight patients (Kamani et al., 2012).

Indications for transplant

1. If an HLA-identical sibling donor is available:
   - Thalassemia major (transplant preferably in childhood, CBT feasible)
   - SCD: stroke, elevated transcranial Doppler velocity, recurrent acute chest syndrome, veno-occlusive crisis or priapism, pulmonary hypertension, tricuspid regurgitation, osteonecrosis, red cell alloimmunization, silent stroke especially with cognitive impairment, sickle nephropathy (Shenoy, 2011)
2. If no HLA-identical sibling donor is available (less than 14% of SCD patients will have matched sibling donors):
   - Unrelated donor transplant from HLA-matched donor (limited experience); best available stem cell source (BM or UCB)
   - Adequate cell dose essential for success of donor UCB transplantation is associated with significant morbidity and risks of graft rejection and is best done in a study setting. Registry data from the CIBMTR, Eurocord-Netcord and the New York Blood Center in 51 hemoglobinopathy patients that underwent unrelated UCB transplants showed DFS of 21% and 50% in thalassemia and SCD, respectively (Ruggeri et al., 2011)
3. If no suitable unrelated cord or marrow product is available (approximately 50% of SCD patients will have suitable matched cord or BM products available):
   - Experimental haploidentical transplantation trials may be considered after careful consideration of the pros and cons of transplant. One ongoing trial uses a novel approach of posttransplant cyclophosphamide for GVHD prevention (Brodsky et al., 2008)

Contraindications to transplant

1. If an HLA-identical sibling donor is available:
   - In thalassemia, impaired cardiac function or hepatic cirrhosis (result in poor transplant outcomes). Contraindications to transplant for SCD include poor functional status following severe cerebrovascular disease; significantly lowered cardiac, renal, or pulmonary function; pulmonary hypertension; and hepatic cirrhosis

Red cell alloimmunization is not a contraindication to transplant but may result in increased rates of graft rejection.

Pretransplant workup

1. See the general pretransplant workup (page 239)
2. Hb electrophoresis with Hb A_2, S, and F quantitation
3. Genetic confirmation of diagnosis of thalassemia
4. Family studies, especially on marrow donor, as in the preceeding item 2
5. Serum ferritin and iron-binding capacity
6. Ejection fraction and pulmonary arterial pressure
7. Pulmonary function testing

8. Fasting blood sugar
9. Liver biopsy to assess for hepatic siderosis, chronic active hepatitis, chronic persistent hepatitis, and portal fibrosis (except in children, three years of age without hepatomegaly)
10. Assessment of risk category (Pesaro score, applies for thalassemia)
    - Class 1: no risk factors
    - Class 2: 1 to 2 risk factors
    - Class 3: all three risk factors

    Risk factors:
    - hepatomegaly
    - portal fibrosis in pretransplant liver biopsy
    - inadequate quality of pretransplant chelation therapy

    Assessment of chelation therapy:
    - Adequate if desferrioxamine was initiated within 18 months of first transfusion and was administered subcutaneously for 8–10 hours, continuously, five or more days per week
    - Inadequate if there was any deviation from that protocol
11. Assessment of growth and development and pubertal assessment using Tanner growth charts

Myeloablative conditioning or RIC regimen for hemoglobinopathy transplants

Traditionally, transplants for hemoglobinopathies have utilized myeloablative conditioning with the busulfan/cyclophosphamide-based regimen to achieve donor cell engraftment. This has been a successful approach in sibling donor transplants using either BM or UCB as the source of stem cells. In SCD, DFS was 85% in children. The rate of graft rejection in these studies was 10%, and the mortality was 7%. The disadvantages include late toxicities such as ovarian failure and poorer outcomes in the unrelated donor setting and in older patients. Myeloablative transplants have been successful in young thalassemia patients (<17 years old) with matched siblings. Graft rejection was lowered from 30% to 8% in the related donor setting by the addition of hydroxyurea, fludarabine, and azathioprine to increase the intensity of pretransplant suppression (Sodani et al., 2004). The Italian transplant group used thiotepa to improve donor engraftment in related CBT and unrelated BMT (Locatelli et al., 2003). Unrelated donor transplant outcomes in thalassemia were improved by extended haplotype matching when feasible.

Myeloablative transplantation for SCD has been shown to ameliorate pain successfully and prevent ongoing CNS and pulmonary damage, thus providing a cure in SCD (Walters et al., 2010). As before, the disadvantages include late toxicities such as ovarian failure; poor tolerability in the unrelated donor setting and in older patients; and also effects on growth, gonadal, and neurocognitive functions; and the risk of second malignancies (Fitzhugh et al., 2008). The toxicities (early and late) of myeloablative preparative regimen in all patients and higher mortality following unrelated donor transplantation led to studies of RIC regimen for hemoglobinopathy transplants. The transplant regimen using a lowered dose of busulfan or low-dose irradiation to improve tolerability resulted in higher rates of graft rejection (e.g., Jacobsohn et al., 2004). A more immunosuppressive approach based on profound recipient immunosuppression with alemtuzumab was well tolerated and resulted in stable donor engraftment (Shenoy et al., 2005). Reduced-intensity transplants may yet be successful in achieving donor cell engraftment with newer more immunosuppressive approaches. Their goal would be to increase tolerability and reduce the morbidity associated with a myeloablative regimen in hemoglobinopathy patients and are being tested in larger hemoglobinopathy-specific trials, as previously mentioned. Reduced-intensity transplant approaches for older patients with SCD are in development. If a stable engraftment is reached, a mixed chimerism even at low levels of 20%–50% can be tolerated after a transplant for hemoglobinopathies and does not lead to relapse (Hsieh et al., 2011; Walters et al., 2001).

Disease-specific (SCD) precautions during transplant

1. Reduce Hb S to <45% before beginning conditioning therapy.
2. Maintain seizure prophylaxis during and after transplant until patient is off calcineurin inhibitors.
3. Strict control of hypertension; maintain BP within 10% of baseline to avoid cerebrovascular events.
4. Maintain Hb level at 10 gm/dL; a higher Hb level may result in increased viscosity and promote cerebrovascular events.
5. Maintain platelet counts at >50 000/dL to avoid cerebrovascular hemorrhagic complications.
6. SCD patients are at a higher risk of developing PRES (posterior reversible encephalopathy syndrome) and should be monitored carefully especially with the use of calcineurin inhibitors for GVHD prophylaxis.

Monitoring posttransplant

1. Bone marrow aspiration and chimerism evaluation at 1, 3, 6, 12, 18, and 24 months posttransplant. Additional analyses as needed during withdrawal of immunosuppression
2. ABO status (blood type analysis) at 1, 3, 6, 12, 18, and 24 months if there was a pretransplant donor–recipient difference
3. Hb electropheresis at 1, 3, 6, 12, 18, and 24 months posttransplant
4. Serum ferritin (monthly venesection beginning three months posttransplant may be required to lower serum ferritin); alternately, chelation therapy may be considered following engraftment to achieve ongoing iron chelation

References and further reading

Bernardo ME, Piras E, Vacca A, et al. 2012. Allogeneic hematopoietic stem cell transplantation in thalassemia major: results of a reduced-toxicity conditioning regimen based on the use of treosulfan. *Blood* **120**: 473–476.

Brodsky RA, Luznik L, Bolaños-Meade J, et al. 2008. Reduced intensity HLA-haploidentical BMT with post transplantation cyclophosphamide in nonmalignant hematologic diseases. *Bone Marrow Transplant* **42**: 523–527.

Fitzhugh CD, Lauder N, Jonassaint JC, et al. 2010. Cardiopulmonary complications leading to premature deaths in adult patients with sickle cell disease. *Am J Hematol* **85**: 36–40.

Fitzhugh CD, Perl S, Hsieh MM. 2008. Late effects of myeloablative bone marrow transplantation (BMT) in sickle cell disease (SCD). *Blood* **111**: 1742–1743.

Gaziev J & Lucarelli G. 2003. Stem cell transplantation for hemoglobinopathies. *Curr Op Pediatr* **15**: 24–31.

Hsieh MH, Fitzhugh CD, & Tisdale JF. 2011. Allogeneic hematopoietic stem cell transplantation for sickle cell disease: the time is now. *Blood* **118**: 1197–1207.

Hsieh MM, Kang EM, Fitzhugh CD, et al. 2009. Allogeneic hematopoietic stem-cell transplantation for sickle cell disease. *N Engl J Med* **361**: 2309–2317.

Hulbert ML, McKinstry RC, Lacey JL, et al. 2011. Silent cerebral infarcts occur despite regular blood transfusion therapy after first strokes in children with sickle cell disease. *Blood* **117**: 772–779.

Jacobsohn DA, Duerst R, Tse W, et al. 2004. Reduced intensity haematopoietic stem-cell transplantation for treatment of non-malignant diseases in children. *Lancet* **364**: 156–162.

Kamani NR, Walters MC, Carter S, et al. 2012. Unrelated donor cord blood transplantation for children with severe sickle cell disease: results of one cohort from the phase II study from the Blood and Marrow Transplant Clinical Trials Network (BMT CTN). *Biol Blood Marrow Transplant* **18**: 1265–1272.

La Nasa G, Caocci G, Argiolu F, et al. 2005. Unrelated donor stem cell transplantation in adult patients with thalassemia. *Bone Marrow Transplant* **36**: 971–975.

Locatelli F, Rocha V, Reed W, et al. 2003. Related umbilical cord transplantation in patients with thalassemia. *Blood* **101**: 2137–2143.

Olivieri NF, Nathan DG, MacMillan JH, et al. 1994. Survival in medically treated people with homozygous beta-thalassemia. *N Engl J Med* **331**: 574–578.

Panepinto JA, Walters MC, Carreras J, et al. 2007. Matched-related donor transplantation for sickle cell disease: report from the Center for International Blood and Transplant Research. *Br J Haematol* **137**: 479–485.

Powars DR, Chan LS, Hiti A, et al. 2005. Outcome of sickle cell anemia. A 4 decade observational study of 1056 patients. *Medicine* **84**: 363–376.

Ruggeri A, Eapen M, Scaravadou A, et al. 2011. Umbilical cord blood transplantation for children with thalassemia and sickle cell disease. Eurocord Registry; Center for International Blood and Marrow Transplant Research; New York Blood Center. *Biol Blood Marrow Transplant* **17**: 1375–1382.

Shenoy S. 2011. Hematopoietic stem cell transplantation for sickle cell disease: current practice and emerging trends. *Hematology Am Soc Hematol Educ Program* 2011: 273–279.

Shenoy S, Grossman WJ, di Persio J, et al. 2005. A novel reduced-intensity stem cell transplant regimen for non-malignant disorders. *Bone Marrow Transplant* **35**: 345–352.

Sodani P, Gaziev D, Polchi P, et al. 2004. New approach for bone marrow transplantation in patients with class 3 thalassemia aged younger than 17 years. *Blood* **104**: 1201–1203.

Walters MC. 2005. Stem cell therapy for sickle cell disease: transplantation and gene therapy. *Hematology Am Soc Hematol Educ Program* 2005: 66–73.

Walters MC, Hardy K, Edwards S, et al. 2010. Pulmonary, gonadal, and central nervous system status after bone marrow transplantation for sickle cell disease. Multicenter Study of Bone Marrow Transplantation for Sickle Cell Disease. *Biol Blood Marrow Transplant* **16**: 263–272.

Walters MC, Patience M, Leisenring W, et al. 2001. Stable mixed hematopoietic chimerism after bone marrow transplantation for sickle cell anemia. *Biol Blood Marrow Transplant* **7**: 665–673.

Chapter

18 HSCT for inborn errors of metabolism and neurodegenerative disorders

Robert F. Wynn, Jaap J. Boelens, and Muhammad A. Saif

Basic principles and rationale for allogeneic HSCT in inborn errors of metabolism (IEM)

The IEM are a group of genetic disorders in which a multisystem progressive disorder arises from enzyme deficiency and accumulation of products of metabolism within the cells and tissues. After successful engraftment following HSCT, the donor cells not only reconstitute the lymphohematopoietic system but also, more slowly, replace tissue macrophages such as Kupfer cells in the liver and microglial cells in the CNS of the host. In most IEM, the beneficial effect of HSCT on disease outcome is mediated by a process called cross correction. This was first shown in vitro, over three decades ago, in fibroblast cell cultures of Hurler syndrome (MPSIH) and Hunter syndrome (MPSII) patients (Neufeld, 1983). In HSCT, the enzyme produced and secreted by the engrafted donor cells is taken up by the enzyme-deficient host cells, leading to the correction of the underlying disease phenotype in the patient (Krivit, 1983).

The first allogeneic HSCT for MPSIH was performed in the U.K. in 1981 (Hobbs et al., 1981). To date, over two thousand HSCTs have been carried out for metabolic disorders, mostly in MPSIH patients. Other metabolic disorders treated with HSCT include MPSII, Maroteaux Lamy syndrome (MPSVI), Sly syndrome (MPSVII), α-mannosidosis, and X-linked adrenoleukodystrophy (X-ALD). In a successful allogeneic HSCT in IEM, the enzyme delivered by the donor cells should be adequate to prevent substrate accumulation within a given disease and stop or reverse the disease progression. However, in certain lysosomal storage diseases (LSDs) such as San Filippo disease (MPSIII), normalization of enzyme levels is not sufficient to halt the disease progression (Sivakumur & Wraith, 1999). This reflects the complex pathogenesis and the difficulty in treating this group of illnesses. The reason for apparent HSCT failure in some IEMs remains unclear. Another important consideration of HSCT efficacy in these disorders is the selective response in some organs after HSCT (Masterson et al., 1996), particularly if the transplant is performed late after the diagnosis or in the presence of advanced disease. This makes it imperative to plan the transplant at the right time, preceded by a thorough evaluation of the disease complications in the patients under consideration for the HSCT.

The two most common indications for HSCT in IEM are MPSIH and X-ALD. However, the mechanism by which the transplant corrects the underlying disease pathology is completely different in these two prototype disorders. Therefore, these are briefly discussed separately.

Hurler syndrome (MPSIH)

Deficiency of the lysosomal enzyme alpha-L-iduronidase results in failure to degrade macromolecular glycosaminoglycans within the lysosome. This results in accumulation of heparan sulfate and dermatan sulfate within the cells, which disrupts the normal structure and physiology of the cells and tissue, leading to a progressive multisystem disorder. The severity of the disease manifestation depends upon the underlying genetic mutation. The genotype-phenotype correlation is complex, which explains the heterogeneous presentation and variable course of illness in patients suffering from similar gene mutations. The most severe form of this disorder is MPSIH. The mildest presentation is described as Scheie syndrome (MPSIS) and an intermediate severity illness also exists, which is known as Hurler–Scheie syndrome (MPSIHS). Usually, more severe forms of disease present early during childhood and can progress rapidly, leading to premature death. Milder phenotypes are often diagnosed later in life and may be associated with near normal life expectancy. The somatic manifestations include hepatic and splenic enlargement and soft tissue deposition resulting in coronary artery disease, heart valve dysfunction, and airway problems. Cardiac manifestations can be fatal if left untreated. The CNS manifestations are more pronounced in MPSIH and include loss of acquisition of new skills and subsequent loss of acquired skills (dementia). Musculoskeletal abnormalities can present as thoracolumbar kyphotic gibbus, hip and knee joint dysplasias, and poor mobility. Collectively they are known as dysostosis multiplex.

X-linked adrenoleukodystrophy (X-ALD)

X-ALD is the most common peroxisomal disorder. This is caused by defective ALD protein, which results in accumulation of fatty acids within the tissues and body fluids. Four distinct clinical phenotypes result from this genetic disorder. The spectrum of illness ranges from asymptomatic individuals to a rapidly progressive severe inflammatory cerebral demyelinopathy (cerebral ALD) (Moser et al., 1992). The HSCT results in excellent short-term and long-term outcome in this disorder (Loes et al., 1994b; Shapiro et al., 2000), but the exact mechanism by which the transplantation reverses the cerebral demyelination remains unknown. The HSCT is usually offered to the patients with cerebral X-ALD who have early disease. Serial brain MRI is used to monitor boys, as this is an X-linked disorder, known to be at risk of this disorder so that patients are offered HSCT as soon as there are any MRI features of disease progression based on a validated MRI scoring system (Loes et al., 1994a).

Outcome of HSCT in IEM

Most of the data available on the outcome of transplant comes from MPSIH patients. In 2008, Moore et al. published data on long-term survival of mucopolysaccharidosis type I (MPSI) patients in the U.K. OS of the patients who received the HSCT was superior to those who did not receive the transplant (see following figure) and the probability of survival after transplantation was 68%, 66%, and 64% at two, five, and ten years, respectively (Moore et al., 2008). GVHD, graft rejection, and infection were the major causes of mortality and significant morbidity. In various studies over the last two decades, the OS of HSCT in MPSIH patients has been reported to be around 40%–70% (Peters et al., 1996, 1998a; Souillet et al., 2003).

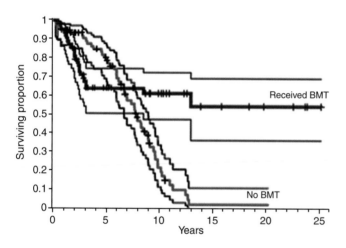

Survival of BMT/HSCT recipients with MPSI compared to those who did not receive HSCT. (Reproduced with permission from Moore et al., 2008.)

A number of studies have shown consistently that HSCT improves the clinical outcome including organomegaly and functional and neuropsychological outcome, particularly if done earlier in asymptomatic patients (Peters et al., 1998b). Despite an excellent clinical outcome in some IEMs, it is important to remember that in some tissues and organs, the response to HSCT is inconsistent and the improvement may be patchy; for example, musculoskeletal abnormalities are less responsive to HSCT (Weisstein et al., 2004). Over the last two decades, the outcome of HSCT in MPSIH has improved steadily (Prasad et al., 2008; Staba et al., 2004), with some centers reporting the OS to be around 90% in the patients transplanted after 2004 (Wynn et al., 2009a). The Eurocord and Duke University reported the OS and EFS of 74% and 63%, respectively, in 258 MPSI patients (see following figures).

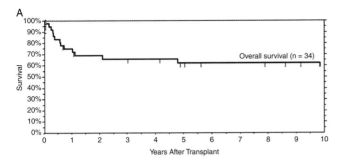

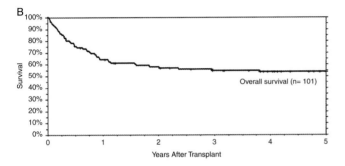

A: OS; allogeneic HSCT with matched related donors for MPSIH (University of Minnesota experience). B: OS; allogeneic HSCT with matched unrelated donors for MPDIH (based on data from the National Marrow Donor Program). (Reproduced with permission from Orchard et al., 2007.)

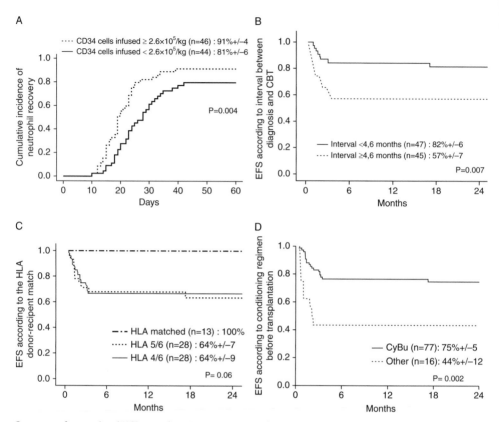

Outcomes after unrelated UCB transplantation in patients with MPSIH. A: Kaplan–Meier curves for neutrophil recovery according to the number of CD34 cells infused/kg; B: EFS according to the delay between diagnosis and transplantation; C: EFS according to the HLA donor–recipient match; D: EFS according to the conditioning regimen before transplantation. (Reproduced with permission from Boelens et al., 2009.)

Factors determining disease outcome after HSCT in Hurler syndrome and other IEM

The following factors have contributed to the improved outcome of HSCT in IEM:

1. Use of full-intensity preparative regimen

The use of full intensity conditioning regimens is associated with a lower risk of graft rejection. In the recently revised guidelines, the Inborn Error Working Party of the European Group for Blood and Marrow Transplantation (EBMT) has recommended fludarabine and busulfan as the preferred conditioning regimens for MPSIH patients. Serotherapy is based on the donor cell source and the relationship between donor and recipient.

2. Busulfan with pK-guided dosing

Busulfan with pK monitoring is important in allogeneic HSCT for IEM to ensure delivery of myeloablative levels of busulfan in conditioning regimens, particularly those that utilize single agent busulfan for myeloablation. Despite logistic challenges in monitoring the busulfan levels, increasing numbers of transplantation centers are moving toward busulfan monitoring.

3. Absence of in vitro T-cell depletion of the donor BM

The use of T-cell-replete grafts has reduced transplant rejection. An increase in successful engraftment has in turn contributed to improvement in the outcome of HSCT (see the following figure).

4. Use of UCB as a source of stem cells

Owing to the better engraftment, superior enzyme delivery, safety, and quick availability, UCB is increasingly being utilized as a source of stem cells. The outcome is particularly good in well-matched cords. The swift availability results in reduction of time from diagnosis to transplantation, which is very important in a progressive degenerative disorder. For these reasons, UCB may be considered an optimal donor cell source for this condition (see following figure).

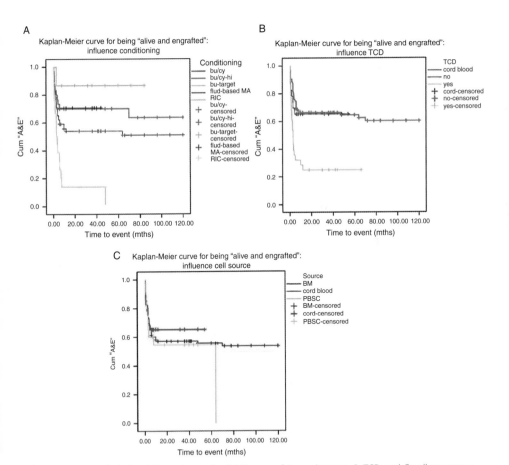

Kaplan–Meier curves for being "alive and engrafted." Influence of A: conditioning; B: TCD; and C: cell source are shown. A&E, alive and engrafted; Flud-MA, fludarabine-based myeloablative; PBSC, PB stem cell; TCD, T-cell depletion. (Reproduced with permission from Boelens et al., 2007.)

Planning HSCT in IEMs

Based on the current understanding of HSCT in MPSIH, six factors have been described that influence the outcome of transplantation in these disorders (Wynn, 2011). Understanding these factors is important for the transplant physician and may help in the decision of when to proceed with the HSCT.

1. Underlying disease

The outcome of HSCT is different in various IEMs. Some disorders respond less to the HSCT despite apparent correction of enzyme levels, and hence HSCT is not recommended in these disorders. In future, it may become possible to achieve a better outcome by delivering supraphysiological levels of enzyme by graft manipulation or gene therapy, but at present HSCT cannot be justified for all IEMs.

2. Genotype of disease

Even though the genotype–phenotype relationship is not straightforward in IEM, some genotypes lead to more severe phenotypes that have a worse outcome. Premature stop and frameshift mutations are described in a number of IEMs, which predict severe phenotypes and result in very low levels of baseline functional enzyme.

3. Age of the patient and disease severity at presentation

Most of the IEMs are progressive illnesses. Early diagnosis (prior to development of significant complications) results in a better outcome of the HSCT. This underlines the need to develop tools for early diagnosis, such as newborn screening programs.

4. Efficacy of applied therapy

Historically these illnesses were managed by symptomatic treatment only. More recently, a number of therapeutic options have become available or are under development. Enzyme replacement therapy (ERT) is available as a therapeutic option in six LSDs. Substrate reduction therapy (SRT), chaperon-mediated therapy (CMT), and gene therapy are under development, but some of these treatments such as CMT and SRT are not meant to cure the disease and are likely to be beneficial as adjuvant therapy. It is important to understand the mechanism of action, therapeutic efficacy, and the limitations of all available treatments prior to making any decision about the HSCT. CNS involvement in some IEMs precludes the use of pharmacological enzyme therapy in contrast to HSCT where cellular therapy can be delivered into the brain parenchyma by engrafted donor-derived microglial cells.

5. Complications of treatment and comorbidities at the time of HSCT

A transplantation procedure performed in severely morbid patients will predict a poor outcome regardless of the underlying disorder. Advanced cardiac and respiratory disease at the time of HSCT will inevitably carry high TRM (see figure). Optimization of clinical status, such as by the infusion of ERT, prior to undertaking the transplant, has been shown to improve the outcome of HSCT.

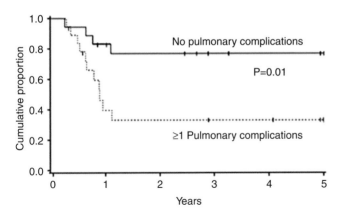

Effect of pretransplant pulmonary complications in younger patients with MPSIH. OS of patients with MPSIH transplanted before 18 months of age, stratified on the basis of a history of any pulmonary complications, is shown. (Reproduced with permission from Orchard et al., 2010.)

6. Multidisciplinary care

Even after HSCT, the patients are likely to require a multidisciplinary team approach (MDTA) toward future management of the patients. This is particularly important because certain complications of IEMs are less responsive to treatment and progress during the course of illness despite a successful HSCT. This MDTA should involve a team of clinicians including metabolic physicians, transplant clinicians, orthopedic/spinal surgeons, physical therapists, occupational health services, and psychiatrists.

Indications for HSCT in IEM

As discussed earlier, a successful HSCT should result in an acceptable and meaningful quality of life. OS as a measure of success is no longer acceptable. At present, much of the evidence on efficacy of HSCT in IEM is weak due to rarity of these illnesses and a lack of prospective studies in this area. Most of the transplantation experience is limited to small case series. There is considerable variation in practices among physicians and various centers across the world. There is no general consensus for the indications of HSCT in IEMs. A number of attempts have been made to provide a working list of metabolic diseases for which HSCT should be offered. The following table provides a list of transplant indications based on a recent communication involving the transatlantic consensus and current U.K. consensus. This list was originally prepared to guide the commissioners and purchasers of transplantation services.

Current U.K. Paediatric Bone Marrow Transplant Group indications for HSCT in children with IEM

Standard indication	Hurler syndrome
	Sly syndrome
	α-mannosidosis
	X-linked adrenoleukodystrophy
Clinical options	Aspartylglucosaminuria
	Wolman disease
	Late infantile metachromatic leukodystrophy
	Niemann–Pick disease type C2

(*cont.*)

Indications under development	Scheie syndrome, Hurler syndrome/Scheie syndrome, Hunter syndrome, Maroteaux Lamy syndrome in conjunction with ERT or where alloantibodies attenuate efficacy of ERT Pompe disease where alloantibodies attenuates efficacy of ERT Juvenile Sandhoff disease Juvenile Tay Sachs disease Early diagnosis fucosidosis Presymptomatic or milder forms of globoid cell leukodystrophy (infantile Krabbe disease when newborn and asymptomatic)
No evidence that BMT/SCT is helpful	Fabry disease Infantile Tay Sachs disease Infantile Sandhoff disease GM1 gangliosidosis Morquio syndrome Niemann–Pick disease type B Niemann–Pick disease type C

A summary of the transplant practice and practical recommendations based on our practice are described as follows:

Donor selection (donor hierarchy)

- Sibling (non-carriers of the disorder)
- MUD cord rather than MUD if equivalent match
- 6/6 cord >10/10 MUD >5/6 cord >9/10 MUD

ERT (if available)

- From diagnosis to SCT and during SCT until donor cell engraftment
- Longer if specific; e.g., cardiac pretransplant comorbidities
- Monitor the quantitative and functional immune response

Conditioning

- Busulfan
  - High-dose oral with pK monitoring
  - IV busulfan
  - 16 doses

- Fludarabine
  - 50 mg/m^2 × 4

- Serotherapy
  - Follow local practices for T-cell depletion for cord and MUD HSCT
  - None if sibling

GVHD prophylaxis

- Follow local practices according to donor source and cell source

Assessment of graft

- Chimerism analysis at day 30, 60, 90, and then every three months for two years or when clinically indicated
- Assessment of graft function; i.e., enzyme levels and disease biomarkers.

Some presentations of IEM such as cross-reactive immunological material (CRIM)-negative infantile forms of metachromatic leukodystrophy, Tay Sachs disease, and Sandhoff and globoid cell leukodystrophy (Krabbe disease) lead to rapid disease progression, and hence the window of opportunity for HSCT is very narrow. However, in some of these disorders, if the diagnosis is made on neonatal screening, the HSCT could be utilized as an effective therapeutic option (Martin et al., 2006).

Alternative strategies and their limitations

Other currently available therapeutic options include ERT and SRT.

The concept of ERT was first introduced in the 1960s by De Duve. The success of the first commercial product (Ceredase), developed by Genzyme for Gaucher diseases, led to a rapid development of ERTs for a number of other LSDs. Currently, ERT is available for six different LSDs. However, presently available ERTs cannot penetrate an intact blood–brain barrier, making this treatment ineffective in neurodegenerative IEMs. Therefore, in IEMs involving the CNS, HSCT is considered superior to ERT due to its ability to deliver the enzyme into the brain of the host. Furthermore, the efficacy of ERT may be attenuated by alloantibodies, and it has been shown recently that nearly all patients with MPSIH who received ERT develop high titer alloantibodies, but these antibodies disappear after a successful transplant (Saif et al., 2012). Analysis of urinary substrate reduction following ERT shows that it is less pronounced than that following HSCT, suggesting–at least for the kidney–that HSCT and engrafted leukocytes is a better enzyme delivery system than pharmacological ERT.

SRT works by altering the metabolic pathways and thus slowing the accumulation of metabolic end products. SRT such as miglustat is cheap and easy to administer, but has relatively limited efficacy. Chaperons are small molecular weight substances that are capable of activating the nonfunctional mutated protein, resulting in their functional activation. However, CMT and other therapies such as gene therapy are under development and are not available for clinical use as yet.

In the future, optimal outcomes for patients may involve combining different treatment modalities. Thus in many institutions now, ERT may be given prior to HSCT to improve the somatic performance of patients; for example, improving their cardiac function so they are better able to tolerate the transplant procedure.

Future perspectives

In MPSIH patients, delivery of two normal gene copies by unrelated donor HSCT results in a higher level of enzyme delivered to the recipient and leads to a better metabolic outcome when compared to those who receive either a single normal gene (by affected sibling transplant) or pharmacological enzyme replacement therapy (Wynn et al., 2009b), as shown in the following figure. This important observation, coupled with the initial reports of gene-augmented SCT in animals (Biffi et al., 2011), is clear evidence that graft manipulation to express higher copies of genes in stem cells may make HSCT more effective and a viable therapeutic option in IEMs not amenable to this type of treatment at present.

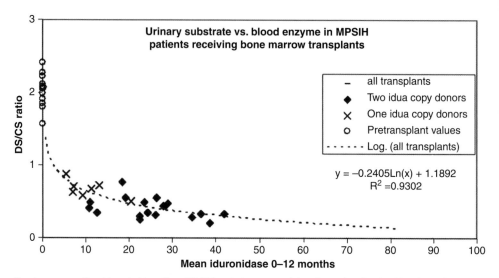

The dermatan sulfate/chondroitin sulfate (DS/DC) ratio in urine and the iduronidase level in blood significantly improves after allogeneic transplant (especially from donors with two normal iduronidase genes). (Reproduced with permission from Wynn et al., 2009b.)

The availability of alternative treatment options such as pharmacological enzyme replacement therapy and steady improvement in OS in transplantation has resulted in a greater emphasis now being placed on quality of life after the delivered treatment. Even though some of the new therapies are associated with relatively low short-term risks, they have certain limitations that compromise their efficacy. Currently, pharmacological ERT is a standard of care in some LSDs, including milder MPSI, milder MPSII, MPSVI, and Pompe disease. However, efficacy of such ERT might be attenuated by the development of alloantibodies against the enzyme, particularly in severe forms of disease that are CRIM negative. In this context, the HSCT has been shown to tolerize the recipient to the replaced enzyme (Saif et al., 2012). The alloimmune response in attenuated diseases is likely to be less severe due to the presence of CRIM, which tolerizes the recipients to the infused ERT. However, if established, the immune response has a potential to neutralize ERT even in milder forms of disease, and hence HSCT could be used as a source of enzyme and an immune tolerance mechanism simultaneously.

References and further reading

Biffi A, Aubourg P, & Cartier N. 2011. Gene therapy for leukodystrophies. *Hum Mol Genet* 20: R42–R53.

Boelens JJ, Rocha V, Aldenhoven M, et al. 2009. Risk factor analysis of outcomes after unrelated cord blood transplantation in patients with Hurler syndrome. *Biol Blood Marrow Transplant* 15: 618–625.

Boelens JJ, Wynn RF, O'Meara A, et al. 2007. Outcomes of hematopoietic stem cell transplantation for Hurler's syndrome in Europe: a risk factor analysis for graft failure. *Bone Marrow Transplant* 40: 225–233.

Hobbs JR, Hugh-Jones K, Barrett AJ, et al. 1981. Reversal of clinical features of Hurler's disease and biochemical improvement after treatment by bone-marrow transplantation. *Lancet* 2: 709–712.

Krivit W. 1983. Correction of inborn errors of metabolism by bone marrow transplant. *Basic Life Sci* 25: 63–76.

Loes DJ, Hite S, Moser H, et al. 1994a. Adrenoleukodystrophy: a scoring method for brain MR observations. *AJNR Am J Neuroradiol* 15: 1761–1766.

Loes DJ, Stillman AE, Hite S, et al. 1994b. Childhood cerebral form of adrenoleukodystrophy: short-term effect of bone marrow transplantation on brain MR observations. *AJNR Am J Neuroradiol* 15: 1767–1771.

Martin PL, Carter SL, Kernan NA, et al. 2006. Results of the cord blood transplantation study (COBLT): outcomes of unrelated donor umbilical cord blood transplantation in pediatric patients with lysosomal and peroxisomal storage diseases. *Biol Blood Marrow Transplant* 12: 184–194.

Masterson EL, Murphy PG, O'Meara A, et al. 1996. Hip dysplasia in Hurler's syndrome: orthopaedic management after bone marrow transplantation. *J Pediatr Orthop* 16: 731–733.

Moore D, Connock MJ, Wraith E, et al. 2008. The prevalence of and survival in mucopolysaccharidosis I: Hurler, Hurler-Scheie and Scheie syndromes in the UK. *Orphanet J Rare Dis* 3: 24.

Moser HW, Moser AB, Smith KD, et al. 1992. Adrenoleukodystrophy: phenotypic variability and implications for therapy. *J Inherit Metab Dis* 15: 645–664.

Neufeld EF. 1983. The William Allan Memorial Award address: cell mixing and its sequelae. *Am J Hum Genet* 35: 1081–1085.

Orchard PJ, Blazar BR, Wagner J, et al. 2007. Hematopoietic cell therapy for metabolic disease. *J Pediatr* 151: 340–346.

Orchard PJ, Milla C, Braunlin E, et al. 2010. Pre-transplant risk factors affecting outcome in Hurler syndrome. *Bone Marrow Transplant* 45: 1239–1246.

Peters C, Balthazor M, Shapiro EG, et al. 1996. Outcome of unrelated donor bone marrow transplantation in 40 children with Hurler syndrome. *Blood* 87: 4894–4902.

Peters C, Shapiro EG, Anderson J, et al. 1998a. Hurler syndrome: II. Outcome of HLA-genotypically identical sibling and HLA-haploidentical related donor bone marrow transplantation in fifty-four children.

The Storage Disease Collaborative Study Group. *Blood* 91: 2601–2608.

Peters C, Shapiro EG, & Krivit W. 1998b. Neuropsychological development in children with Hurler syndrome following hematopoietic stem cell transplantation. *Pediatr Transplant* 2: 250–253.

Prasad VK, Mendizabal A, Parikh SH, et al. 2008. Unrelated donor umbilical cord blood transplantation for inherited metabolic disorders in 159 pediatric patients from a single center: influence of cellular composition of the graft on transplantation outcomes. *Blood* 112: 2979–2989.

Saif MA, Bigger BW, Brookes KE, et al. 2012. Hematopoietic stem cell transplantation ameliorates the high incidence of neutralizing allo-antibodies observed in MPSI-Hurler after pharmacological enzyme replacement therapy. *Haematologica* 97: 1320–1328.

Shapiro E, Krivit W, Lockman L, et al. 2000. Long-term effect of bone-marrow transplantation for childhood-onset cerebral X-linked adrenoleukodystrophy. *Lancet* 356: 713–718.

Sivakumur P & Wraith JE. 1999. Bone marrow transplantation in mucopolysaccharidosis type IIIA: a comparison of an early treated patient with his untreated sibling. *J Inherit Metab Dis* 22: 849–850.

Souillet G, Guffon N, Maire I, et al. 2003. Outcome of 27 patients with Hurler's syndrome transplanted from either related or unrelated haematopoietic stem cell sources. *Bone Marrow Transplant* 31: 1105–1117.

Staba SL, Escolar ML, Poe M, et al. 2004. Cord-blood transplants from unrelated donors in patients with Hurler's syndrome. *N Engl J Med* 350: 1960–1969.

Weisstein JS, Delgado E, Steinbach LS, et al. 2004. Musculoskeletal manifestations of Hurler syndrome: long-term follow-up after bone marrow transplantation. *J Pediatr Orthop* 24: 97–101.

Wynn R. 2011. Stem cell transplantation in inherited metabolic disorders. *Hematology Am Soc Hematol Educ Program* 2011: 285–291.

Wynn RF, Mercer J, Page J, et al. 2009a. Use of enzyme replacement therapy (Laronidase) before hematopoietic stem cell transplantation for mucopolysaccharidosis I: experience in 18 patients. *J Pediatr* **154**: 135–139.

Wynn RF, Wraith JE, Mercer J, et al. 2009b. Improved metabolic correction in patients with lysosomal storage disease treated with hematopoietic stem cell transplant compared with enzyme replacement therapy. *J Pediatr* **154**: 609–611.

Chapter 19

Therapeutic decision making in BMT/SCT for autoimmune disorders

Reinhold Munker

Introduction

Severe autoimmune disorders often have a chronic relapsing course characterized by flare-ups, remissions, further progression, and finally incapacitation. Autoimmune disorders may target many different organ systems. Multiple sclerosis is characterized by inflammation and an autoimmune attack on myelin fibers, resulting in demyelination and later axonal loss. Rheumatoid arthritis is characterized by an autoimmune attack against the synovial membrane, resulting in chronic inflammation and joint destruction. In severe cases, autoimmune disorders may cause death from multiorgan involvement. A common principle for the treatment of most autoimmune disorders is immunosuppression. The evidence for the value of high-dose chemotherapy with stem cell support comes from three lines of evidence: (a) it was speculated that higher dose immunosuppression or immuno-ablation could eliminate the pathogenic autoreactive cells more thoroughly; (b) in a number of case reports, patients who underwent a BMT/SCT for a hematologic malignancy and had a coincidental autoimmune disorder came into remission of both diseases (Drachman & Brodsky, 2005); and (c) it could be demonstrated in animal experiments that the transfer of syngeneic stem cells following immunoablation may cure several autoimmune disorders (Sykes & Nikolic, 2005).) In the European data base, 900 patients underwent an auto-SCT between 1996 and 2007 for a variety of autoimmune conditions (Farge et al., 2010). In this chapter I will review the treatment results for multiple sclerosis, rheumatoid arthritis, and systemic lupus erythematosus (SLE), as well as discuss future developments.

Multiple sclerosis

Altogether, more than 300 patients have undergone autologous SCT for multiple sclerosis. Most patients were transplanted with peripheral stem cells, but a few patients were transplanted with BM. The conditioning regimens were variable, with BEAM (BCNU,

The BMT Data Book, Third Edition, ed. Reinhold Munker et al. Published by Cambridge University Press. © Cambridge University Press 2013.

etoposide, cytarabine, and melphalan) being the most frequently used. In many patients, the stem or progenitor cells were selected for CD34 positivity, and in many cases, the conditioning regimen included ATG. Both procedures lead to a T-cell depletion, which is supposed to remove cells involved in the pathogenesis of multiple sclerosis. A large earlier study involved 85 patients with multiple sclerosis transplanted at 20 centers in Europe (Fassas et al., 2002). Of the patients, 61% were female and the median age was 39 years (with a range of 20–58 years). All patients had severe disease. Most patients (70%) suffered from secondary progressive multiple sclerosis, 26% from primary progressive multiple sclerosis, and 4% from relapsing remitting multiple sclerosis. In this series, seven patients died (five from complications and toxicity of the transplant). Overall, 74% (±12%) of the patients survived free from progression at three years.

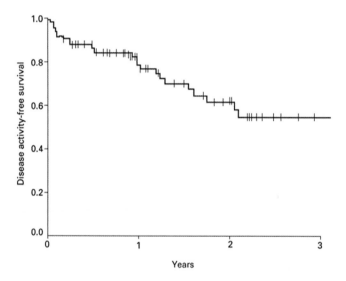

Survival free from disease activity in patients with multiple sclerosis, who underwent an auto-SCT. (Reproduced with permission from Fassas et al., 2002.)

The results of the study by Fassas et al. (2002) were considered encouraging and are in line with other, smaller case series (Drachman & Brodsky, 2005). In addition to the clinical stabilization, a reduction in the volume of lesions of multiple sclerosis ("plaques" as seen as hyperintense signals on MRI scans) and a clear reduction of active lesions, as demonstrated by gadolinium uptake, occurred. In many instances, the brain volume continued to shrink, which is consistent with the degeneration involved in progressive multiple sclerosis. In multiple sclerosis, as in other autoimmune diseases, all patients underwent multiple immunosuppressive treatments before being considered for transplantation. Therefore, opportunistic infections deserve special attention. Some centers give prophylactic immunoglobulins to all patients. Special issues in multiple sclerosis patients are engraftment syndrome and hemorrhagic cystitis after high-dose cyclophosphamide. The safety, patient selection, and ethical issues were discussed in recent review articles (Atkins, 2010; Silani & Cova, 2008). Autologous SCT is especially effective in malignant multiple sclerosis, where it lessens disability, as well as in early progressive multiple sclerosis.

Rheumatoid arthritis

It is estimated that worldwide more than 100 patients with severe rheumatoid arthritis had undergone stem cell transplantation (de Buys et al., 2005; Farge et al., 2010; Jantunen & Luosujärvi, 2005). The indication was severe disease refractory to conventional and disease-modifying agents. Most patients reported an improvement of their symptoms or of the inflammatory activity. This response was transient in many cases (months to years). In several series, the observation that patients refractory to conventional treatment before the SCT, even at relapse, responded again to "disease-modifying" antirheumatic drugs was made. In a large series, a TRM of 1.4% was reported. Since new treatments like TNF-receptor antagonists have become available, there is little evidence that autologous transplantation should, at present, be offered to patients with rheumatoid arthritis outside of a clinical trial.

Systemic lupus erythematosus

A series of 50 cases of severe and treatment-refractory SLE was published in 2006 (Burt et al., 2006). All patients had either organ- or life-threatening visceral involvement. Peripheral blood stem cells were mobilized with cyclophosphamide and G-CSF and selected for CD34 positivity. The conditioning involved high-dose cyclophosphamide (200 mg/kg) and horse ATG. In an intent-to-treat analysis, a mortality of 4% related to the transplant was observed. With a mean follow-up of 29 months, the OS following the transplant was 84% at five years and the probability of being disease free at five years was 50%. Accordingly, a significant improvement was seen in the SLE disease activity score, in the titer of anti-nuclear antibodies and of antibodies to double-stranded DNA, in complement levels and in the pulmonary diffusion capacity. These data are considered as encouraging and provide the justification for a definite randomized clinical trial.

Other autoimmune diseases (like systemic sclerosis, juvenile idiopathic arthritis) and less common diseases also received SCT and came into remission or stabilized their disease. Recently, a report was published that patients with severe, anti-TNF refractory Crohn's disease benefitted from autologous non-myeloablative SCT (91% being relapse-free at one year, 63% relapse-free at two years) (Burt et al., 2010). A similar approach was taken for patients with severe systemic sclerosis. In a randomized phase 2 study, 10/19 patients treated with SCT stabilized or improved their skin and pulmonary function (Burt et al., 2011).

Future perspectives

Autologous SCT offers hope for patients with refractory autoimmune disorders like multiple sclerosis, lupus erythematosus, and others. In different case series, response rates of 30%–50%, some of which were complete, were observed. However, the true value of and the indications for auto-SCT for autoimmune disorders should be established by randomized clinical trials. Therefore, auto-SCT cannot be considered a standard treatment at present. The value of allo-SCT for autoimmune disorders is even more controversial (Marmont, 2006). The potential benefit of a graft-versus-autoimmunity effect mediated by a healthy immune system has to be balanced against the potentially deleterious complications of GVHD. A new type of stem cell treatment involving the replacement of neurons and glial cells derived from adult or embryonic stem cells will be tested in the coming years in several neurodegenerative and autoimmune disorders. Neural stem cells may stimulate regeneration and prevent the death of neurons in the CNS (Lindvall & Kokaia, 2006).

References and further reading

Atkins H. 2010. Hematopoietic SCT for the treatment of multiple sclerosis. *Bone Marrow Transplant* 45: 1671–1681.

Burt RK, Craig RM, Milanetti F, et al. 2010. Autologous nonmyeloablative hematopoietic stem cell transplantation in patients with severe anti-TNF refractory Crohn disease: long-term follow-up. *Blood* 116: 6123–6132.

Burt RK, Shah SJ, Dill K, et al. 2011. Autologous non-myeloablative haematopoietic stem-cell transplantation compared with pulse cyclophosphamide once per month for systemic sclerosis: an open-label randomized phase 2 trial. *Lancet* 378: 498–506.

Burt RK, Traynor A, Statkute L, et al. 2006. Nonmyeloablative hematopoietic stem cell transplantation for systemic lupus erythematosus. *JAMA* 295: 527–535.

De Buys P, Khanna D, & Furst DE. 2005. Hemopoietic stem cell transplantation in rheumatic diseases – an update. *Autoimmun Rev* 4: 442–449.

Drachman DB & Brodsky RA. 2005. High-dose therapy for autoimmune neurologic diseases. *Curr Opin Oncol* 17: 83–88.

Farge D, Labopin M, Tyndall A, et al. 2010. Autologous stem cell transplantation for autoimmune diseases: an observational study on 12 years' experience from the European Group for Blood and Marrow Transplantation Working Party on autoimmune diseases. *Haematologica* 95: 284–292.

Fassas A, Passweg JR, Anagnostopoulos A, et al. 2002. Haematopoietic stem cell transplantation for multiple sclerosis. A retrospective multicenter study. *J Neurol* 249: 1088–1097.

Jantunen E & Luosujärvi R. 2005. Stem cell transplantation in autoimmune diseases: an update. *Ann Med* 37: 533–541.

Lindvall O & Kokaia Z. 2006. Stem cells for the treatment of neurological disorders. *Nature* 441: 1094–1096.

Marmont AM. 2006. Allogeneic haematopoietic stem cell transplantation for severe autoimmune diseases: great expectations but controversial evidence. *Bone Marrow Transplant* 38: 1–4.

Silani V & Cova L. 2008. Stem cell transplantation in multiple sclerosis: safety and ethics. *J Neurol Sci* 265: 116–121.

Sykes M & Nikolic B. 2005. Treatment of severe autoimmune disease by stem-cell transplantation. *Nature* 435: 620–627.

Cellular therapy

Hans-Jochem Kolb, Kerry Atkinson, and Reinhold Munker

Basic principles

In this chapter, established cellular therapies (mainly DLI) as well as novel cellular therapies (regulatory T-cells, NK cells, cytokine-induced killer cells, dendritic cells, mesenchymal stem cells, induced pluripotent stem cells, and genetically modified T-cells) will be reviewed. A survey in Europe in 2008 showed that more than 1000 patients (about 60% autologous and 40% allogeneic) were treated with such novel cellular therapies. The major indications were cardiovascular, hematologic, neurological, and musculoskeletal. Here we will discuss cellular therapies relevant to blood disorders and SCT, and will exclude stem cells delivered for cardiovascular, orthopedic, or neurological indications.

BM contains several lines of cells including: hematopoietic stem cells, progenitor cells, and mature cells, such as B- and T-lymphocytes, monocytes, dendritic cells, and NK cells. Hematopoietic stem cells are valuable for rescuing hematopoiesis after high-dose chemotherapy and radiotherapy, which are toxic to stem cells. This high-dose therapy can be used for

The BMT Data Book, Third Edition, ed. Reinhold Munker et al. Published by Cambridge University Press. © Cambridge University Press 2013.

the treatment of leukemia and other malignant diseases. However, in the treatment of leukemia, the role of lymphocytes has already been described in the literature (Barnes & Loutit, 1957). Allogeneic SCT was seen as a form of adoptive immunotherapy (Mathé et al., 1965). In human patients, lower relapse rates were seen in patients who developed GVHD (Weiden et al., 1979), and the depletion of T-cells for prevention of GVHD was associated with an increased relapse rate (Goldman et al., 1988). The effect of T-cell depletion on the relapse rate was greatest in CML, less in AML, and least in ALL (Horowitz et al., 1990).

Depletion of T-cells from the graft was highly effective in the prevention of acute GVHD (Goldman et al., 1986; Rodt et al., 1977, 1983); early withdrawal of immunosuppressive treatment in order to improve leukemia control was deleterious (Sullivan et al., 1986). Similarly, the early transfusion of donor lymphocytes after transplantation induced acute GVHD (Sullivan et al., 1989) without improving leukemia control. In experiments with dogs, donor lymphocytes could be transfused without inducing GVHD two months and later after T-cell depleted marrow transplantation (Kolb et al., 1997). Subsidence of the cytokine storm produced by the conditioning treatment and establishment of transplantation tolerance to non-hematopoietic organs may have contributed to the absence of GVHD after lymphocyte transfusions. Nevertheless mixed chimerism converted to complete chimerism after transfusion of the donor lymphocytes. It was also found that immunity to tetanus could be transferred with the lymphocytes, and reactivity to diphtheria toxoid as neoantigen was improved. Similarly, delayed transfusion of donor cells failed to produce GVHD in SCT mice (Johnson et al., 1993).

Graft-versus-host and graft-versus-leukemia reactions

Graft-versus-leukemia (GVL) reactions may be part of the graft-versus-host (GVH) reactions directed against widely distributed histocompatibility antigens or against antigens with expression restricted to hematopoietic tissue, or they may be directed at leukemia-specific antigens of proteins that are encoded by the altered genes. Another possibility is the reaction against differentiation antigens presented on immature cells and normally only expressed during ontogenesis. Blood transfusions may cause marrow aplasia in patients with severe immune deficiency, mainly caused by T-cells of the transfusion against hematopoietic cells of the patient (Anderson & Weinstein, 1990). In this manner, a GVH reaction may exert GVL effects as long as leukemia cells express histocompatibility antigens. Similarly, mixed chimerism could be converted into complete chimerism by donor lymphocyte transfusions (Marks et al., 2002). Several mHCa are predominantly expressed on hematopoietic cells (HA-1, HA-2, HB-1, BCL2a1, etc.); they may mediate strong GVL effects (Goulmy, 1997; Marijt et al., 2003; Rutten et al., 2008; Warren et., 1998). Unfortunately, the frequency of these mHCa differences is rather low, and only a minority of patients could potentially benefit. Moreover, in HLA-identical sibling transplants, differences in HA-1 increased the risk of GVHD (Goulmy et al., 1996), while in matched unrelated donor transplants, mHCa had no impact on transplant outcome (Spellman et al., 2009). In matched unrelated transplantation, many more differences may be involved including different alleles of HLA-antigens, and immunosuppressive treatment may suppress reactions. In contrast, immunosuppressive treatment is not given regularly with donor lymphocyte transfusions. Transplants from female donors into male patients are associated with strong GVL effects and chronic GVHD indicating strong immune reactivity against Y-chromosome encoded antigens (Gratwohl et al., 1998; Miklos et al., 2005; Vogt et al., 2002). These are also expressed on tissues other than hematopoiesis cells, and they may produce GVHD. Leukemia cells may over-express differentiation antigens of immature cells like Wilms tumor antigen 1 (WT-1) and PR-1 of proteinase 3 (Greiner et al., 2006; Mailander et al., 2003; Moldrem et al., 2002). These antigens are self antigens, and they may induce tolerance. Tolerance can be avoided, if these antigens are presented by foreign HLA-antigens because the same peptides may become immunogenic. In order to circumvent tolerance induction, allogeneic T-cell receptors can be transferred into autologous T-cells (Gao et al., 2003; Morgan et al., 2006).

T-cells are primarily immunized by dendritic cells of the host that present antigens professionally with HLA Class II and Class I antigens supported by costimulatory molecules and proinflammatory cytokines like IL-6 and TNF-α (Ferrara et al., 1996). An acute reaction that resembles acute GVHD can be observed even in patients transplanted from identical twins and after autologous transplantation (Teshima et al., 2002). This reaction, however, vanishes after a short course of corticosteroids and never comes back. In the allogeneic situation, histocompatibility antigens are recognized and the reaction is sustained. Conditioning treatment with TBI and chemotherapy may release proinflammatory cytokines that stimulate donor T-cells from host dendritic cells. These immune cells produce IFN-γ, IL-2, and granulocyte–macrophage colony-stimulating factor (GM-CSF), and thereby stimulate dendritic cells, further leading to the vicious circle of a "cytokine storm" (Ferrara et al., 1996). This cytokine storm can be tempered by prophylactic treatment with TNF-antibody or conditioning treatment with reduced intensity; in these cases acute GVHD can be diminished and/or delayed (Holler et al., 1995).

Activation and stimulation of dendritic cells leads to sensitization of CD8-positive T-cells against mHCa presented by Class I. This way CD8-positive cells can attack epithelial cells that do not present Class II antigens. Dendritic cells devoid of MHC Class I antigens are not able to produce GVHD (Shlomchik et al., 1999); "cross presentation" of antigens by dendritic cells of the transplant can compensate only partially. In a murine model of CML, cross presentation of host antigens by donor dendritic cells has no impact on the GVL reaction (Eibl et al., 1997; Matte et al., 2004). There is clear evidence that patients with CML (Chen et al., 2000; Eibl et al., 1997; Smit et al., 1996), AML (Mittermueller et al., 1986; Schmetzer et al., 2007; Woiciechowsky et al., 2001), and MDS (Kufner et al., 2005) can produce dendritic cells of leukemia origin. These cells can be induced in vitro, and most likely also in vivo, by treatment with GM-CSF and IL-4 or IFN-α (Schmetzer et al., 2007). Patients with a high proportion of dendritic cells of leukemia origin have a better response to donor lymphocyte transfusions (unpublished data).

The risk of GVHD in human patients is higher than in animals (Kolb et al., 1995); the rate of patients with GVHD requiring immunosuppressive treatment was 35%. The reasons for the higher incidence of GVHD after DLI are not known, but older age and immunity to alloantigens and to common viral antigens by prior exposure may contribute. The median age of the patients was 40 years, an age when the thymic function is low and tolerance is maintained by peripheral mechanisms. It is most likely that regulatory T-cells (Johnson et al., 1999) are involved in the down-regulation of dendritic cells; down-regulated dendritic cells in turn make naïve T-cells tolerant. Depletion of T-cells prior to DLI increases the risk in man (Miller et al., 2007) and in mice (Johnson et al., 1999). Chemo- and radiotherapy increase the risk of GVHD after DLI not only by lymphocyte depletion, but also by releasing cytokines that activate dendritic cells. Infections may increase the risk of GVHD by activating toll-like receptors (Elmaagacli et al., 2006; Heimesaat et al., 2010; Zeiser et al., 2011) and NOD-like receptors (Holler et al., 2004) via the same mechanisms.

Peripheral tolerance is maintained by regulatory T-cells, but they may not interfere with the GVL reaction (Edinger et al., 2003). Dendritic cells of leukemia origin can keep a GVL reaction against hematopoietic cells going. In the HLA-incompatible situation, a mixed chimerism can maintain a GVL reaction without necessarily causing GVHD (Mapara & Sykes, 2005). Presumably, expression of HLA Class II on hematopoietic cells plays a major role, because they can activate donor T-cells directly and start a GVL reaction (Sykes et al., 1999). In the HLA-identical situation, activation of donor lymphocytes requires dendritic cells as professional antigen presenting cells to recognize mHCa. According to the tissue distribution of mHCa, the reaction of donor lymphocytes can be directed against every organ or against only hematopoietic tissue including leukemia cells. Leukemia-specific antigens may exist as new proteins produced by an altered gene or gene fusions such as BCR/ABL in Philadelphia-positive CML and ALL; they can induce immune reactivity (Cathcart et al., 2004), but the effect of vaccination has been weak.

In recent years, the role of NK cells in HLA-haploidentical transplantation has been described (Ruggeri et al., 1999). Normally they are killing cells that lack self HLA-antigens (Karre et al., 1986). This may be due to a viral infection or malignancy. In the transplant setting and across HLA-differences, hematopoietic cells of the patient may miss the antigens inhibiting NK activity, and donor NK cells can kill the hematopoietic cells of the host. The HLA Class I determinants inhibit NK cells via KIR, the strongest inhibitor being HLA-C associated determinants, but there are also HLA-A and -B and CD94/NKG2A determinants. Inhibition is dominant, but activation has also occurred via KIR2DS1, KIR2DS4, and CD94/NKG2C to allow killing by NK cells. Donor NK cells can be transfused, and they survive in the patient (Curti et al., 2011). Their efficacy remains to be shown (see also page 220). Another promising approach is the use of cytokine-induced killer (CIK) cells (Schmidt-Wolf et al., 1991); these cells are induced by the anti-CD3 antibody, IFN-γ, and IL-2 stimulation, they are mainly NK T-cells and CD8-positive cells that kill HLA-unrestricted via NKG2D (see later).

Most likely it is not just one line of cells that eliminates leukemia, but a concert of immune competent cells including B-cells and macrophages. Successful control of myeloma was associated with antibody production against antigens of the tumor (Bellucci et al., 2004). Extramedullary infiltrates are less sensitive to immunotherapy; infiltration and activation of phagocytic cells may be missing. In the first of the following tables, an overview is given for the efficacy of DLI in different studies and different disease entities. The second to sixth tables give recommendations as to how donor lymphocytes should be administered in different clinical scenarios.

Disease/study cohorts	Number of patients	Overall response rate	% CCR (years)	Reference
CML				
Molecular/cytogenetic relapse				
EBMT	50	80%	80% (4)	Kolb et al., 1995
CIBMTR	3	100%		Collins et al., 1997

(cont.)

Disease/study cohorts	Number of patients	Overall response rate	% CCR (years)	Reference
Hematologic/chronic phase				
EBMT	114	77%	60% (4)	Kolb et al., 1995
CIBMTR	34	74%		Collins et al., 1997
Japan	12	92%	82% (3)	Shiobara et al., 2000
London Hammersmith	57	74%		Dazzi et al., 2000
Genova San Martino	42	86%		Raiola et al., 2003
Baltimore Johns Hopkins	17	77%		Huff et al., 2006
Boston 1	12	58%		Porter et al., 2000
Boston 2	19	63%		Alyea et al., 1998
New York	17	82%		Mackinnon et al., 1995
Transformed phase				
EBMT	36	36%	20% (4)	Kolb et al., 1995
CIBMTR	18	28%		Collins et al., 1997
Japan	11	27%	0% (3)	Shiobara et al., 2000
Genova San Martino	14	36%		Raiola et al., 2003
Boston	12	33%		Porter et al., 2000
AML/MDS				
EBMT	58	26%	15% (4)	Kolb et al., 1995
EBMT 2	171	38%	21% (2)	Schmid et al., 2007
CIBMTR	44	18%		Collins et al., 1996
US prospective	51	49%	19% (2)	Levine J et al., 2002
Japan	32	40%	AML 7% (3) MDS 33% (3)	Shiobara et al., 2000
Baltimore Johns Hopkins	13	46%	AML	Huff et al., 2006
	12	15%	MDS	
Korean MDS (G-CSF mobilized)	17	59%	31% (2)	Choi et al., 2004
Lille/France MDS	14	14%	14% (4)	Depil et al., 2004

(cont.)

Disease/study cohorts	Number of patients	Overall response rate	% CCR (years)	Reference
ALL				
EBMT	20*	15%	0%	Kolb et al., 1995
US	44*	31%	18% (1.5)°	Collins et al., 2000; Picker et al., 1993
Japan	23	25%	5% (2)°	Shiobara et al., 2000
Korea	10*	70%	20% (2)°	Choi et al., 2005
	*Most patients had chemotherapy; °overall survival			
Lymphoma/CLL				
London UC	21	53%	n.a.	Morris et al., 2004
Dutch study indolent	7	86%	57% (>3.5)	Mandigers et al., 2003
London UC				
FL	6	100%		Bloor et al., 2008
tFL	5	80%	60%	
MCL	3	100%		
CLL	3	33%	66%	
Bethesda NCI DLBCL	5	60%	60% (>3.5)	Bishop et al., 2008
German CLL Group				
minimal residual disease	9	78%	78%	Ritgen et al., 2004
London UC Hodgkin L	9	78%	56%	Peggs et al., 2004
MD Anderson Houston Hodgkin	9	44%	11%	Anderlini et al., 2004
Myeloma				
Persistent, progressive				
EBMT	17	29%	12% (2)	Kolb et al., 1995
CIBMTR	4	50%		Collins et al., 1996
CIBMTR	22	32%	18% (>1)	Salama et al., 2000
Dutch Study	27	52%	18.5%	Lokhorst et al., 2000
Johns Hopkins	20	50%	15% (>3 mo)	Huff et al., 2006
EBMT multicenter	63	38%	7,5% (>1)	van de Donk et al., 2006

(cont.)

Disease/study cohorts	Number of patients	Overall response rate	% CCR (years)	Reference
London UC				
residual	11	45%	27%	Peggs et al., 2004
progressive	8	50%	0	
Dutch study preemptive	10 CR/VGPR/ PR	100%	70% (5 yrs)	Levenga et al., 2007a

Favorite regimen for CML relapse after allogeneic transplant

Discontinue immunosuppression

Start IFN-α ≤1 Mio units per day 1–2 weeks prior to DLI

Transfuse donor lymphocytes in escalating doses starting with 1×10^6 CD3 cells/kg body weight

Increase dose to 5×10^6/kg and 1×10^7/kg after 30–60 days; if there is no GVHD, then give the rest

In HLA-mismatched start with 1×10^5/kg and escalate accordingly

Discontinue IFN-α after two negative nested PCR for bcr/abl 4 weeks apart

In case of non-response within two months, add GM-CSF 150 μg daily for 10 days every month until molecular remission

Favorite regimen for AML/MDS relapse

Discontinue immunosuppression:

In late relapse (>180 days post transplant), start low-dose cytosine arabinoside 10–20 mg subcutaneously twice a day, continue for 28 days unless there is vomitus and/or diarrhea

In case of non-response after 3–4 weeks, initiate more intensive chemotherapy including clofarabine or similar; more intensive chemotherapy is also indicated in patients with early relapse, extramedullary chloromas, or granulocytic sarcomas

After 4 weeks of low-dose Ara-C, transfuse G-CSF mobilized blood cells from the stem cell donor without further conditioning or post-grafting immunosuppression

In HLA-mismatched transplanted patients and patients given intensive chemotherapy, a short course of methotrexate 10–15 mg/kg may be given on days 1, 3, and 6 in order to prevent fulminant GVHD

GM-CSF 150 μg daily should be given day 1–10, in patients treated with methotrexate on days 14–24

(cont.)

On day 28 posttransfusion, control of blood and marrow for residual blasts and chimerism; in case of no GVHD, transfuse donor CD3+ T-cells: 1×10^6/kg body weight (preferably collected after prior stimulation with G-CSF)

Further transfusion of CD3+ T-cells can be given as clinically indicated

Favorite regimen for preemptive DLI in high-risk AML/MDS

Taper immunosuppression, day 90 posttransplantation, check for minimal residual disease by PCR (NPM1, FLT-3 ITD, MLL), FACS for leukemia-associated immune phenotype (LAIP)

Start transfusions, if there is

1. 30 days off immune suppression

2. No GVHD

3. Evidence of chimerism

4. No severe infections

Transfusions are given every 30 days in escalating doses, prophylactic antibiotics (+ antimycotics, antivirals) may be given during the treatment period

Favorite regimen for relapse of ALL/lymphoma/CLL

Patients have to be in remission for DLI

MRD of CLL may be treated successfully with donor lymphocytes

In clinical relapse, consider intensive chemotherapy including radioimmunotherapy and retransplantation from the same donor in late relapses, from a different (haploidentical?) donor in early relapses

Favorite regimen for residual or persistent myeloma

Preemptive treatment as in previous table with the addition of IFN-α (≤1 Mio units daily) and/or vaccination with dendritic cells

In persistent and progressive disease, chemotherapy with bortezomib, lenalidomide, dexamethasone, or thalidomide should be combined with donor lymphocyte transfusions (CAVE GVHD after lenalidomide!)

Chronic myelogenous leukemia

Based on promising animal experiments, the first patients were treated for relapse of CML in 1988 (Kolb et al., 1990). Two of the three patients treated are still in molecular remission; one patient had a cytogenetic relapse 20 years after treatment. Several larger studies have shown long-lasting and beneficial results in CML patients with recurrent leukemia after transplantation (see table on page 212) (Bacigalupo et al., 1997; Bar et al., 1993; Collins et al., 1997; Kolb et al., 1995; Mackinnon et al., 1995; Shiobara et al., 2000). Most patients received IFN-α prior to donor lymphocytes without success, and large numbers of donor lymphocytes were transfused. In patients given T-cell depleted transplants, the response to donor lymphocyte transfusions was better than in patients given unmodified transplants (Kolb et al., 1995). In many patients the response to donor lymphocytes was not immediate, in some patients the disease progressed for up to two months. Molecular remissions were achieved in a median time of six months, and in some patients it only occurred after more than a year had passed. Continuous immune reactivity stimulated by spontaneous differentiation of dendritic cells of leukemia origin has been postulated as a mechanism of prolonged and long-lasting response (Kolb, 2008). In contrast to the results in animals treated with donor lymphocytes, acute and chronic GVHD were observed in human patients, and some required immunosuppressive treatment. In the EBMT study, 35% of patients required treatment. Another complication was severe myelosuppression observed in about 20% of patients, predominantly patients with a large burden of leukemia. Transfusion of marrow from the donor without further conditioning was effective in these cases. Patients with myeloid aplasia in the course of chronic GVHD did not recover following infusion of donor stem cells.

Prevention of GVHD has been attempted by depletion of CD8-positive cells from the transfusion with some success (Alyea et al., 1998; Champlin et al., 1992). A most interesting approach is the transduction of a suicide gene into the T-cells so that T-cells engaged in GVHD could be killed (Bonini et al., 1998). However, cytotoxic T-cells involved in GVHD may be recruited in vivo. The simplest and most widely used approach for prevention of GVHD is the application of T-cells in escalating doses (Mackinnon et al., 1995).

Donor lymphocytes in combination with IFN-α and GM-CSF

The treatment of choice in patients with recurrent CML is the combination of donor lymphocytes in escalating doses with a treatment of low doses of IFN-α. A daily dose of ≤1 Mio units is given SQ days to weeks prior to the first transfusion. Most centers start with a dose of 10^6/kg CD3-positive cells and escalate at 30–60 day intervals to 5×10^6/kg and 10^7/kg. In patients with an HLA-mismatched donor or with a history of GVHD, the start may be with 10^5/kg CD3-positive T-cells. The response may not start immediately and some patients show even progression of the disease for weeks or months before the disease responds. The median time until molecular remission has been six months, and some patients respond only after more than a year of treatment. As a rule, patients treated for cytogenetic relapse do not develop GVHD. After the achievement of a molecular response, we preferred to wait for two negative results in the nested PCR at an interval of four weeks until we discontinued IFN-α.

Some patients do not respond to the treatment with IFN-α and donor lymphocytes; these patients may respond to the combination of GM-CSF and donor lymphocytes. The GM-CSF was given in a dose of 150 µg daily for 2–4 weeks; responses again were slow, but lasting. Higher doses put patients at risk for pulmonary complications. The GM-CSF was used with some success post-autografting for CML (Gladstone et al., 1999).

Donor lymphocytes and tyrosine kinase inhibitors

Imatinib is a selective TKI that has revolutionized the treatment of CML. Relapses of CML after transplantation could be treated with imatinib and other TKIs (Kantarjian et al., 2002; Olavarria et al., 2002), but most patients experienced a relapse after discontinuation of imatinib. The combined treatment with donor lymphocytes and imatinib has been advocated by some groups (Savani et al., 2005), but imatinib may also inhibit the effect of allogeneic lymphocytes at least in vitro (Cwynarski et al., 2004). In retrospective analysis, treatment of relapse with donor lymphocytes was superior to imatinib (Weisser et al., 2006), and excellent results were obtained in patients with advanced phase CML treated with TKI and transplanted in subsequent remission (Weisser et al., 2007).

Acute myeloid leukemia and myelodysplastic syndrome

In the EBMT study, donor lymphocyte transfusions were better in myeloid malignancies, such as CML, AML, MDS, and MPS than in lymphatic malignancies, such as ALL, CLL, and lymphoma. The response may be related to the immunogenicity favoring malignancies with spontaneous production of dendritic cells of myeloid origin. In CML, dendritic cells of leukemia origin are produced spontaneously; in AML and MDS/MPS dendritic cells are not produced spontaneously. They may be produced in vivo and in vitro by stimulation with GM-CSF (Schmetzeret al., 2007; Schuster et al., 2008).

Donor lymphocyte transfusion for relapse

In contrast to CML, a relapse of AML usually progresses more rapidly and requires chemotherapy, and leukemia blasts do not differentiate toward dendritic cells without additional treatment. A retrospective study of the EBMT showed that donor lymphocyte transfusions were beneficial in the treatment of relapse (Schmid et al., 2007), and that best results were seen in patients with late relapses (more than six months after transplantation) and with low tumor burden. We prefer a mild chemotherapy with low-dose cytosine arabinoside for four weeks prior to the transfusion of mobilized blood stem cells and GM-CSF for two weeks in order to differentiate leukemia blasts toward dendritic cells. Unmobilized T-cells are given on day 30, if there is no GVHD (Schmid et al., 2004). Some patients have experienced long-lasting and ongoing remissions using this technique. Other investigators have used azacytidine (Graef et al., 2007) or decitabine (Giralt et al., 1997) for the treatment of relapses and subsequent donor lymphocyte transfusions with some success. However, long-lasting remissions are not frequent, and some patients have experienced a relapse after more than 10 years, mostly in the form of extramedullary granulocytic sarcomas. In these patients, particular attention should be given to leukemia foci in immunologically privileged sites, such as the CNS, gonads, and eyes.

Preemptive donor lymphocyte transfusion

The better way to treat AML may be preemptive treatment either in high-risk AML as prophylaxis or guided by the demonstration of MRD (Buccisano et al., 2012). Patients with high-risk AML may be given donor lymphocytes preemptively for the prevention of relapse, if they have survived at least 120 days, are off immunosuppressive treatment for at least 30 days, and have neither GVHD nor infections. Survival was longer in patients given donor lymphocytes than in historical controls. This is true both for patients transplanted in remission and patients transplanted with active disease. Similar results were obtained in a matched case study involving patients transplanted in German centers (Kolb, 2008). However, the relapse incidence was not significantly lower than that in the control group; a selection bias may have favored patients with better survival chances. Moreover, the relapse incidence of patients given donor lymphocytes was not inferior to that of patients with GVHD that were not given donor lymphocytes. Therefore, donor lymphocytes may have prevented relapse without necessarily inducing GVHD.

Other disease entities

Myeloma

Allogeneic SCT has been used for the treatment of high-risk myeloma. Allogeneic SCT adds an immune effect against the tumor that was first shown by the transfusion of donor lymphocytes (Tricot et al., 1996; Verdonck et al., 1996). Treatment of relapse and persistent disease with donor lymphocytes has been successful in 20%–50% of patients (van de Donk et al., 2006), but most remissions are not durable (Alyea et al., 2001; Bellucci et al., 2002, 2004; Salama et al., 2000). Most responding patients develop some degree of GVHD, but the development of GVHD does not guarantee a response to donor lymphocytes. The best results are obtained through the preemptive treatment of patients with chemosensitive disease (CR, VGPR, PR) (Beitinjanch et al., 2012; Kroger et al., 2001, 2004, 2009; Levenga et al., 2007a). Several attempts have been made to increase the durability of donor lympho-cyte transfusions in myeloma: vaccination with dendritic cells of the patient (Levenga et al., 2007b), or posttransplant treatment with thalidomide (Kroger et al., 2004) or lenalidomide (Lioznov et al., 2010). However, lenalidomide increases the risk of severe GVHD, and it should be combined with bortezomib or dexamethasone in these patients.

Acute lymphoblastic leukemia/lymphoma

There are single cases with relapse of ALL that respond to donor lymphocyte transfusions, but most patients require intensive chemotherapy prior to DLI. In most patients with B-ALL, remissions are short lived; in some patients a progressive relapse is observed in the presence of severe acute GVHD. The B-ALL cells escape immune control by several mechanisms (Cardosa et al., 1996; Nijmeijer et al., 2005). The resistance may be overcome by using HLA-haploidentical donors, taking advantage of stronger histoincompatibility and NK activity (Kolb et al., 2008). In Philadelphia chromosome-positive ALL, the combination of imatinib or another TKI together with DLI may be useful (Ram et al., 2011). A new possibility is the combination of bispecific antibodies against CD20 and CD3 (Bushmann et al., 2009) or single chain antibodies CD19 × CD3 (Bargou et al., 2008) with donor lymphocytes. In contrast to B-ALL, the treatment of T-ALL may be more effective and achieve durable responses (Passweg et al., 1998) (HJK, own observation, unpublished).

There are several reports on the successful treatment of relapses of low-grade lymph-omas, CLL, and HL with donor lymphocytes (Anderlini et al., 2004; Bloor et al., 2008; Gribben et al., 2005; Mandigers et al., 2003; Morris & Mackinnon, 2005; Peggs et al., 2007; Ritgin et al., 2004). Single reports have shown evidence for a GVL effect in high-grade lymphomas (Bishop et al., 2008). The best chance of a GVL effect is seen in patients with MRD (Ritgen et al., 2004) and in patients achieving remission by radiochemotherapy. The role of antibodies and targeted therapy for durability of responses remains to be defined.

Do donor lymphocytes eliminate leukemia stem cells?

Late relapses of leukemia may occur; they are seen in CML and acute leukemia. In the latter, extramedullary relapses may occur many years after transplantation, particularly in immunologically privileged sites, such as the CNS and gonads. Therefore, control and preventive measures like CNS prophylaxis are indicated. The survival of leukemia cells in these sites without producing immediate disease is an interesting question without convincing explanation.

In some patients with indolent lymphoma, residual disease can be found without clinical symptoms and progression. It is therefore conceivable that allogeneic cells can establish an immune surveillance similar to latent viral infections, but the immunogenicity of malignant cells is inferior to that of virally infected cells and not constant. Therefore, the activity of allogeneic cells has to be stimulated by either cytokine treatment, prior chemotherapy, the combination of bispecific antibodies (Bargou et al., 2008; Bushmann et al., 2009), or T-cells engineered with allogeneic T-cell receptors (Gao et al., 1999; Morgan et al., 2006) or chimeric antigen receptors (Porter et al., 2011). Finally, histocompatibility antigens are highly immunogenic, and it would be desirable to take advantage of the donor's immune repertoire.

Novel cellular therapies
Regulatory T-cells

Regulatory T-cells (Treg) are activated T-cells that suppress autoreactive lymphocytes and control endogenous and adaptive immune responses. Treg comprise about 5%–10% of peripheral CD4+ T-lymphocytes and are defined by the expression CD4, CD25, and the transcription factor FoxP3. Treg control immune responses in many conditions like asthma and infections and may block antitumor responses. IL-2 is an essential cytokine for the development, function, and survival of Treg. It was shown that peripheral tolerance in persistent mixed chimeras is maintained via Treg. In chronic GVHD, the number of Treg is generally reduced. It was shown recently that the daily subcutaneous administration of IL-2 ameliorated chronic GVHD in 12/23 patients refractory to steroids (Koreth et al., 2011). The authors showed that this treatment increased both the absolute number of Treg and also the ratio of Treg to conventional T-cells. Furthermore, the authors could demonstrate that Treg induced under these conditions inhibited the activation of conventional T-cells. As a measure of clinical efficacy, the dose of glucocorticoids could be tapered on average by 60%. The issues of tolerance and inducible graft versus tumor effects were discussed in a recent review article (Rager & Porter, 2012). In the situation of a haploidentical transplant, the infusion of Treg may prevent GVHD and promote immune reconstitution (Di Ianni et al., 2011).

NK cells

NK cells kill nonspecifically; that is, they do not need to be sensitized to the target antigen. In normal physiology, NK cells play a role in the surveillance against tumor cells and virally infected cells. According to several studies, NK cell mismatch (activating receptors on NK cells lead to tumor cell killing in vivo) protected against leukemia relapse. This effect was seen especially in the situation of maximum immunosuppression after haploidentical SCT. For details about NK cell physiology and the hypothesis that an NK mismatch has antileukemia activity, see page 17. For a recent review about NK effects in allogeneic transplantation, see Patil et al. (2009). In the situation of lesser immunosuppression (for fully matched allogeneic NK cells) or in the autologous setting, the antitumor effects of NK cells are less obvious. Problems are targeting to tumor cells and the maintenance of an activation state. In a recent study, Bachanova et al. (2010) treated six patients with advanced NHL with activated haploidentical NK cells and observed a transient clinical response in four patients. The authors found a substantial increase in Treg, which may have limited the expansion and activity of the transfused NK cells (Bachanova et al., 2010).

Cytokine-induced killer (CIK) cells

CIK cells are generated from PB leukocytes of normal individuals or patients with cancer. They are incubated with IFN-γ, IL-2, and an activating CD3 antibody for 21–28 days. Under these culture conditions, with a regular replacement of media, the number of T-cells increases at least 10-fold, whereas the number of NK T-cells increases 30- to 1000-fold. Virtually all cells in the final product are CD3-positive and about half in different studies express CD314, an activating receptor for NK cells and a co-stimulatory receptor for T-cell activation. CIK cells kill tumor cells while sparing normal tissues and are not restricted by MHC recognition. CIK cells are active against autologous and allogeneic tumor cells and induce less GVHD than do classical donor lymphocytes. In a recently published phase I study, 18 patients with recurrent malignancies (after allogeneic transplantation) were treated with CIK cells from their donors. The dose of CIK cells was escalated up to 1×10^8 cells/kg recipient body weight. Only two patients developed grade II acute GVHD, and only one patient developed limited chronic GVHD. In five of seven patients who had measurable disease, some clinical activity of CIK cells was observed. Current research focuses on whether CIK cells can be given earlier to generate a more effective graft-versus-malignancy reaction and if they can be targeted to tumor cells by administering monospecific or bispecific antibodies (Martin, 2011). The technical aspects of CIK cells were discussed in a recent review article (Linn & Hui, 2010).

Dendritic cells

Dendritic cells are derived from both common myeloid and common lymphoid progenitors. The first step to generate dendritic cells is to culture monocytes or BM cells with GM-CSF and IL-4, which results in immature dendritic cells. Mature dendritic cells are then obtained by further culturing in media containing TNFα, IL-1β, IL-6, and prostaglandin E2. In a different approach, dendritic cells are cultured with TNFα, IL-1β, poly (I:C), IFN-α, and IFN-γ. This prevents the expansion of immunoregulatory T-cells.

Dendritic cells have the capacity to ingest toxins and pathogens and regulate the immune system. Upon challenge, dendritic cells process antigens and present them to T-lymphocytes, which subsequently mount an appropriate immune response. Under certain circumstances, dendritic cells can induce immune tolerance, silencing or modulating dangerous immune responses preventing autoimmunity or excessive reactions. Dendritic cells have been used to generate vaccines against infectious agents and cancer.

In experimental studies, dendritic cells can be used to strengthen GVT reactions, while reducing deleterious graft–host reactions. For reviews about dendritic cells in allogeneic transplantation see Hashimoto & Merad, 2011 and Kalantari et al., 2011.

Mesenchymal stem cells

The generation of MSCs and some properties were described on pages 20–23. For recent reviews and clinical applications, see Cristan et al., 2008; Le Blanc et al., 2008; Ren et al., 2012; and Sacchetti et al., 2007.

- Mesenchymal stem cells exist but are very rare. For use in clinical trials, they need to be expanded ex vivo. This results in the generation of what are predominantly progenitor cells, or transit amplifying cells, known as mesenchymal stromal cells (MSCs).
- MSCs are present in every organ in the body as they form part of the endothelium. Their traditional source is the bone marrow (frequency $1:10^5$ to $1:10^6$), but they are easily derived from gestational products including placenta and adipose tissue.
- They are large (>20 μm), spindle-shaped, fibroblastoid cells.
- The human cell surface is characteristic but not unique: $CD44^+$, $CD73^+$, $CD90^+$, $CD105^+$, $CD146^+$, HLA Class I^+, $CD11b^-$, $CD34^-$, $CD45^-$, and HLA Class II^-; HLA Class II cell surface expression can be upregulated by pre-incubation of MSCs with IFN-γ.
- MSCs secrete many proteins including hepatocyte growth factors (HGFs), angiopoietin-1, ILs, VEGF, TGFβ, ILGF-1, bFGF, and LIF.
- MSCs are immunomodulatory and mediate this through a variety of mechanisms including suppression of T-cell alloreactivity, suppression of B-cell function, suppression of NK-cell function, induction of a tolerogenic phenotype in dendritic cells, secretion of indolamine 2,3-dioxygenase (IDO), which results in the starvation of T-cells of tryptophan and increase in regulatory T-cell activity.
- MSCs are multipotent: they can differentiate into cells of mesodermal lineage – bone, cartilage, tendon, muscle, and fat – but their differentiation outside the mesodermal lineage is controversial. They can be considered the stem and progenitor cells of the skeletal system.
- MSCs have a propensity to migrate to inflamed tissue when injected intravenously due to interaction with cell adhesion molecules including P-selectin and VCAM1, chemokines, and their receptors including CXCL12, CCL2, CXCR4, and CCR2, and matrix metalloproteinases.
- They can be used to repair damage to skeletal system tissue – in some cases by producing new tissue such as bone in nonhealing bone fractures, and in some cases by immunomodulatory mechanisms through their secretion of anti-inflammatory mediators such as TSG-6.
- In HSCT, they have been reported to be useful by direct intravenous administration for treatment-refractory acute GVHD. They may also be useful in expanding HSCs from UCB by culturing the HSCs on a monolayer of MSCs prior to infusion into the recipient.
- In humans, they have also been reported to be effective in Crohn's disease, acute myocardial infarction, liver failure, hepatic cirrhosis, diabetic critical limb ischemia and foot ulceration, osteogenesis imperfecta, and periodontal tissue defects.

- In preclinical animal models of disease, they have been reported to be effective in SLE, rheumatoid arthritis, Type I diabetes mellitus, spinal cord injury, liver fibrosis, lung injury, corneal abrasion, and skin wounds.
- Most of these effects are mediated by paracrine mechanisms – the secretion of proteins at or near the site of disease.
- MHC matching between the MSC donor and the MSC recipient is not required: MSCs have been successfully transplanted across MHC barriers in large outbred immune competent animals without need for immunosuppression.
- MSCs that are HLA-matched, HLA-haploidentical, or HLA-unmatched (mismatched) with the recipient have been used successfully in clinical trials. Thus, MSCs are unique for nucleated mammalian cells in that they can be manufactured from volunteer unrelated (i.e., allogeneic) donors, cryopreserved, and shipped to healthcare facilities for use in acute or chronic medical settings, which make them the nucleated cell equivalent of Group O Rhesus-negative red blood cells.
- MSCs can be transduced readily with vectors carrying genes and this renders them a viable candidate for a gene therapy cell delivery system.

Ringden and Le Blanc (2011) published the recent experience with MSCs for complications of allogeneic transplantation. MSCs are immunomodulatory, have low toxicity, and do not require HLA compatibility. The dose of MSCs given in most studies is $1–2 \times 10^6$ cells/kg, although higher doses were given without toxicity. When MSCs were given for refractory acute GVHD, about half of the patients improved, some showing a complete response. Children tended to respond better than adults. Positive responses were also observed in chronic GVHD. MSCs also contribute to wound healing and can improve severe hemorrhagic cystitis (Wu & Hochedlinger, 2011).

Induced pluripotent stem cells

Induced pluripotent stem (IPS) cells are generated from terminally differentiated cells like skin fibroblasts or blood lymphocytes. Using a cocktail of four transcription factors (Oct4, Sox2, c-myc, and Klf4), any differentiated cell can be reprogrammed into an embryonic-like state. Human differentiated cells are reprogrammed to IPS cells using a slightly different cocktail of factors (Oct4, Sox2, Nanog, and Lin28). Originally, the transcription factors were delivered by viral integration into the genome. Later, other methods like transient transfection, nonintegrating viral methods and protein transduction were developed. From the IPS state, cells can be differentiated into any cell of the body, including hematopoietic cells. The generation of IPS cells generally relies on feeder layers, and extracellular and other growth factors. At present, many problems remain unsolved (rejection from immunogenicity, tumor formation from viral integration, oncogenicity in the host), but if IPS cells were available in unlimited quantities, many applications can be envisioned. Among these are toxicity testing and tissue replacement in patients with heart or liver failure or severe aplastic anemia (Hanley et al., 2010; Raya et al., 2009).

As a proof of principle, Raya et al. (2009) corrected the genetic defect in cells from patients with Fanconi anemia, and generated IPS cells. These cells were indistinguishable from embryonic stem cells as well as from IPS cells from normal individuals. The patients' somatic cells were reprogrammed, either directly or after genetic correction with lentiviral vectors encoding FANCA or FANCD2. The corrected IPS cells from these patients were able to differentiate into normal hematopoietic progenitors of erythroid and myeloid lineages. The corrected IPS cells from patients with Fanconi anemia could be passaged for at least 20 times and had a normal karyotype. Another disease, sickle cell anemia, would benefit if the genetic defect can be corrected in differentiated tissues and these tissues (like skin fibroblasts) can then be propagated as IPS cells or directly differentiated into red cell precursors (Jena et al., 2010).

Adoptive immunotherapy with T-cells with a modified antigen receptor

T-lymphocytes are capable of recognizing and eliminating tumor cells in patients. However, in many situations, especially in advanced cancers, the T-lymphocytes have become tolerant to tumor antigens. To circumvent tolerance, investigators have developed and expanded T-cells with modified and transgenic antigen receptors. These receptors are designated as chimeric antigen receptors (CARs) and have a new specificity. Such modified T-cells can be further activated by cytokines. The T-cells can be further modified by providing costimulatory signals. CARs are constructed by gene technology and have three domains: an exodomain that recognizes tumor-associated antigens, a transmembrane domain, and an intracellular endodomain. The endodomain has one or several signaling components of the T-cell receptor. In a recent report, a patient with refractory chronic lymphoid leukemia was treated with modified autologous T-cells (CAR with specificity for CD19 and coupled to CD137 and CD3-zeta), and cleared his tumor cells with a low dose of his T-cells (approximately 1.5×10^5/kg). The side effects of tumor lysis syndrome, lymphopenia, and hypogammaglobulinemia were observed. The modified T-cells expanded 1000-fold and persisted for more than six months in blood and BM (Porter et al., 2011). Jena et al. (2010) and Ngo et al. (2011) recently reviewed the rationale and first clinical studies of ex vivo modified T-cells for the immunotherapy of cancer. The safety aspects and technical issues of the adoptive transfer of modified T-cells were discussed in a recent symposium of the Recombinant DNA Advisory Committee (Ertl et al., 2010).

Adoptive immunotherapy with tumor-infiltrating lymphocytes (TILs) has been successful for the treatment of some patients with metastatic melanoma (for a review, see Rosenberg, 2011). In case reports, responses were observed in patients with synovial sarcoma, neuroblastoma, and refractory lymphoma. Using genetically modified TILs, patients with other solid tumors may also benefit (Rosenberg, 2011).

Di Stasi et al. (2011) developed a "safety switch" by which unwanted T-cell reactivity can be turned off when the transfected cells are exposed in vivo to a small-molecule dimerizing drug (Di Stasi et al., 2011). In the setting of a haploidentical transplant, five patients with relapsed acute leukemia were treated with genetically modified T-cells, which incorporated caspase-9 and a modified human FK-binding protein. When finally GVHD developed in four patients, the modified T-cells were ablated with a single dose of the dimerizing drug, and subsequently, the GVH reaction resolved. In the following graph, the response of a patient given modified T-cells (day 0) and the dimerizing drug (AP1903, given on day 15) is shown.

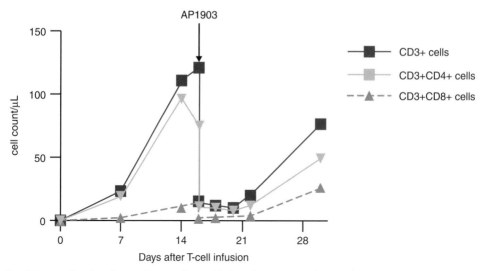

T-cell kinetics after the infusion of genetically modified T-cells. (Reproduced with permission from Di Stasi, 2011.)

Taken together, cellular therapy for blood disorders is an area of active research and development. In the next few years, it can be expected that the specificity of and the indications for cellular therapy will be expanded.

References and further reading

Alyea EP, Soiffer RJ, Canning C, et al. 1998. Toxicity and efficacy of defined doses of CD4 (+) donor lymphocytes for treatment of relapse after allogeneic bone marrow transplant. *Blood* **91**: 3671–3680.

Alyea E, Weller E, Schlossman R, et al. 2001. T-cell-depleted allogeneic bone marrow transplantation followed by donor lymphocyte infusion in patients with multiple myeloma: induction of graft-versus-myeloma effect. *Blood* **98**: 934–939.

Anderlini P, Acholonu SA, Okoroji GJ, et al. 2004. Donor leukocyte infusions in relapsed Hodgkin's lymphoma following allogeneic stem cell transplantation: CD3+ cell dose, GVHD and disease response. *Bone Marrow Transplant* **34**: 511–514.

Anderson KC & Weinstein HJ. 1990. Transfusion-associated graft-versus-host disease. *N Engl J Med* **323**: 315–321.

Bachanova V, Burns LJ, McKenna DH, et al. 2010. Allogeneic natural killer cells for refractory lymphoma. *Cancer Immunol Immunother* **59**: 1739–1744.

Bacigalupo A, Soracco M, Vassallo F, et al. 1997. Donor lymphocyte infusions (DLI) in patients with chronic myeloid leukemia following allogeneic bone marrow transplantation. *Bone Marrow Transplant* **19**: 927–932.

Bar BMAM, Schattenberg A, Mensink EJBM, et al. 1993. Donor leukocyte infusions for chronic myeloid leukemia relapsed after allogeneic bone marrow transplantation. *J Clin Oncol* **11**: 513–519.

Bargou R, Leo E, Zugmaier G, et al. 2008. Tumor regression in cancer patients by very low doses of a T cell-engaging antibody. *Science* **321**: 974–977.

Barnes DHW & Loutit JF. 1957. Treatment of murine leukaemia with X-rays and homologous bone marrow. *Br J Haematol* **3**: 241–252.

Beitinjaneh AM, Saliba R, Bashir Q, et al. 2012. Durable responses after donor lymphocyte infusion for patients with residual multiple myeloma following non-myeloablative allogeneic stem cell transplantation. *Leuk Lymphoma* **53**: 1525–1529.

Bellucci R, Alyea EP, Weller E, et al. 2002. Immunologic effects of prophylactic donor lymphocyte infusion after allogeneic marrow transplantation for multiple myeloma. *Blood* **99**: 4610–4617.

Bellucci R, Wu CJ, Chiaretti S, et al. 2004. Complete response to donor lymphocyte infusion in multiple myeloma is associated with antibody responses to highly expressed antigens. *Blood* **103**: 656–663.

Bishop MR, Dean RM, Steinberg SM, et al. 2008. Clinical evidence of a graft-versus-lymphoma effect against relapsed diffuse large B-cell lymphoma after allogeneic hematopoietic stem-cell transplantation. *Ann Oncol* **19**: 1935–1940.

Bloor AJ, Thomson K, Chowdhry N, et al. 2008. High response rate to donor lymphocyte infusion after allogeneic stem cell transplantation for indolent non-Hodgkin lymphoma. *Biol Blood Marrow Transplant* **14**: 50–58.

Bonini C, Ciceri F, Marktel S, et al. 1998. Suicide-gene-transduced T-cells for the regulation of the graft-versus-leukemia effect. *Vox Sang* **74**: S341–S343.

Buccisano F, Maurillo L, Del Principe MI, et al. 2012. Prognostic and therapeutic implications of minimal residual disease detection in acute myeloid leukemia. *Blood* **119**: 332–341.

Buhmann R, Simoes B, Stanglmaier M, et al. 2009. Immunotherapy of recurrent B-cell malignancies after allo-SCT with Bi20 (FBTA05), a trifunctional anti-CD3 x anti-CD20 antibody and donor lymphocyte infusion. *Bone Marrow Transplant* **43**: 383–397.

Cardoso AA, Schultze JL, Boussiotis VA, et al. 1996. Pre-B acute lymphoblastic leukemia cells may induce T-cell anergy to alloantigen. *Blood* **88**: 41–48.

Cathcart K, Pinilla-Ibarz J, Korontsvit T, et al. 2004. A multivalent bcr-abl fusion peptide vaccination trial in patients with chronic myeloid leukemia. *Blood* **103**: 1037–1042.

Champlin R, Giralt S, Przepiorka D, et al. 1992. Selective depletion of CD8-positive T-lymphocytes for allogeneic bone marrow transplantation: engraftment, graft-versus-

host disease and graft-versus leukemia. *Prog Clin Biol Res* **377**: 385–398.

Chen X, Regn S, Raffegerst S, et al. 2000. Interferon alpha in combination with GM-CSF induces the differentiation of leukaemic antigen-presenting cells that have the capacity to stimulate a specific anti-leukaemic cytotoxic T-cell response from patients with chronic myeloid leukaemia. *Br J Haematol* **111**: 596–607.

Choi SJ, Lee JH, Lee JH, et al. 2004. Treatment of relapsed acute myeloid leukemia after allogeneic bone marrow transplantation with chemotherapy followed by G-CSF-primed donor leukocyte infusion: a high incidence of isolated extramedullary relapse. *Leukemia* **18**: 1789–1797.

Choi SJ, Lee JH, Lee JH, et al. 2005. Treatment of relapsed acute lymphoblastic leukemia after allogeneic bone marrow transplantation with chemotherapy followed by G-CSF-primed donor leukocyte infusion: a prospective study. *Bone Marrow Transplant* **36**: 163–169.

Collins RH, Shpilberg O, Drobyski WR, et al. 1997. Donor leukocyte infusions in 140 patients with relapsed malignancy after allogeneic bone marrow transplantation. *J Clin Oncol* **15**: 433–444.

Crisan M, Yap S, Casteilla L, et al. 2008. A perivascular origin for mesenchymal stem cells in multiple human organs. *Cell Stem Cell* **3**: 301–313.

Curti A, Ruggeri L, D'Addio A, et al. 2011. Successful transfer of alloreactive haploidentical KIR ligand-mismatched natural killer cells after infusion in elderly high risk acute myeloid leukemia patients. *Blood* **118**: 3273–3279.

Cwynarski K, Laylor R, Macchiarulo E, et al. 2004. Imatinib inhibits the activation and proliferation of normal T lymphocytes in vitro. *Leukemia* **18**: 1332–1339.

Dazzi F, Szydlo RM, Cross NC, et al. 2000. Durability of responses following donor lymphocyte infusions for patients who relapse after allogeneic stem cell transplantation for chronic myeloid leukemia. *Blood* **96**: 2712–2716.

Depil S, Deconinck E, Milpied N, et al. 2004. Donor lymphocyte infusion to treat relapse after allogeneic bone marrow transplantation for myelodysplastic syndrome. *Bone Marrow Transplant* 33: 531–534.

Di Ianni M, Falzetti F, Carotti A, et al. 2011. Tregs prevent GVHD and promote immune reconstitution in HLA-haploidentical transplantation. *Blood* 117: 3921–3928.

Di Stasi A, Tey SK, Dotti G, et al. 2011. Inducible apoptosis as a safety switch for adoptive cell therapy. *N Engl J Med* 365: 1673–1683.

Edinger M, Hoffmann P, Ermann J, et al. 2003. CD4+CD25+ regulatory T cells preserve graft-versus-tumor activity while inhibiting graft-versus-host disease after bone marrow transplantation. *Nat Med* 9: 1144–1150.

Eibl B, Ebner S, Duba Ch, et al. 1997. Philadelphia-chromosome positive dendritic cells (DC) of chronic myelocytic leukemia (CML) patients induce primary cytotoxic T-cell responses to CML cells. *Bone Marrow Transplant* 19: S33.

Elmaagacli AH, Koldehoff M, Hindahl H, et al. 2006. Mutations in innate immune system NOD2/CARD 15 and TLR-4 (Thr399Ile) genes influence the risk for severe acute graft-versus-host disease in patients who underwent an allogeneic transplantation. *Transplantation* 81: 247–254.

Ertl HCJ, Zaia J, Rosenberg SA, et al. 2011. Considerations for the clinical application of chimeric antigen receptor T cells: observations from a recombinant DNA advisory committee symposium held June 15, 2010. *Cancer Res* 71: 3175–3181.

Ferrara JL, Cooke KR, Pan L, et al. 1996. The immunopathophysiology of acute graft-versus-host-disease. *Stem Cells* 14: 473–489.

Gao L, Xue SA, Hasserjian R, et al. 2003. Human cytotoxic T lymphocytes specific for Wilms' tumor antigen-1 inhibit engraftment of leukemia-initiating stem cells in non-obese diabetic-severe combined immunodeficient recipients. *Transplantation* 75: 1429–1436.

Gao L, Yang TH, Tourdot S, et al. 1999. Allo-major histocompatibility complex-restricted cytotoxic T lymphocytes in bone marrow transplant recipients without causing graft-versus-host disease. *Blood* 94: 2999–3006.

Giralt S, Davis M, O'Brien S, et al. 1997. Studies of decitabine with allogeneic progenitor cell transplantation. *Leukemia* 11: S32–S34.

Gladstone DE, Bedi A, Miller CB, et al. 1999. Philadelphia chromosome-negative engraftment after autologous transplantation with granulocyte-macrophage colony-stimulating factor for chronic myeloid leukemia. *Biol Blood Marrow Transplant* 5: 394–399.

Goldman JM, Apperley J, Jones L, et al. 1986. Bone marrow transplantation for patients with chronic myeloid leukemia. *N Engl J Med* 314: 202.

Goldman JM, Gale RP, Horowitz MM, et al. 1988. Bone marrow transplantation for chronic myelogenous leukemia in chronic phase: increased risk of relapse associated with T-cell depletion. *Ann Intern Med* 108: 806–814.

Goulmy E. 1997. Human minor histocompatibility antigens: new concepts for marrow transplantation and adoptive immunotherapy. *Immunol Rev* 157: 125–130.

Goulmy E, Schipper R, Pool J, et al. 1996. Mismatches of minor histocompatibility antigens between HLA-identical donors and recipients and the development of graft-versus-host disease after bone marrow transplantation. *N Engl J Med* 334: 281–285.

Graef T, Kuendgen A, Fenk R, et al. 2007. Successful treatment of relapsed AML after allogeneic stem cell transplantation with azacitidine. *Leuk Res* 31: 257–259.

Gratwohl A, Hermans J, Goldman JM, et al. 1998. Risk assessment for patients with chronic myeloid leukaemia before allogeneic blood or marrow transplantation. Chronic Leukemia Working Party of the European Group for Blood and Marrow Transplantation. *Lancet* 352: 1087–1092.

Greiner J, Schmitt M, Li L, et al. 2006. Expression of tumor-associated antigens in acute myeloid leukemia: implications for specific immunotherapeutic approaches. *Blood* 108: 4109–4117.

Gribben JG, Zahrieh D, Stephans K, et al. 2005. Autologous and allogeneic stem cell transplantations for poor-risk chronic lymphocytic leukemia. *Blood* **106**: 4389–4396.

Hanley J, Rastegarli G, & Nathwani AC. 2010. An introduction to induced pluripotent stem cells. *Br J Haematol* **151**: 16–24.

Hashimoto D & Merad M. 2011. Harnessing dendritic cells to improve allogeneic hematopoietic cell transplantation outcome. *Sem Immunol* **23**: 50–57.

Heimesaat MM, Nogai A, Bereswill S, et al. 2010. MyD88/TLR9 mediated immunopathology and gut microbiota dynamics in a novel murine model of intestinal graft-versus-host disease. *Gut* **59**: 1079–1087.

Holler E, Kolb HJ, Mittermüller J, et al. 1995. Modulation of acute graft-versus-host disease after allogeneic bone marrow transplantation by tumor necrosis factor (TNF) release in the course of pretransplant conditioning: role of conditioning regimens and prophylactic application of a monoclonal antibody neutralizing human TNF (MAK 195F). *Blood* **86**: 890–899.

Holler E, Rogler G, Herfarth H, et al. 2004. Both donor and recipient NOD2/CARD15 mutations associate with transplant-related mortality and GvHD following allogeneic stem cell transplantation. *Blood* **104**: 889–894.

Horowitz MM, Gale RP, Sondel PM, et al. 1990. Graft-versus-leukemia reactions after bone marrow transplantation. *Blood* **75**: 555–562.

Huff CA, Fuchs EJ, Smith BD, et al. 2006. Graft-versus-host reactions and the effectiveness of donor lymphocyte infusions. *Biol Blood Marrow Transplant* **12**: 414–421.

Jena B, Dotti G, & Cooper LJN. 2010. Redirecting T-cell specificity by introducing a tumor-specific chimeric antigen receptor. *Blood* **116**: 1035–1044.

Johnson BD, Becker EE, LaBelle JL, et al. 1999. Role of immunoregulatory donor T cells in suppression of graft-versus-host disease following donor leukocyte infusion therapy. *J Immunol* **163**: 6479–6487.

Johnson BD, Drobyski WR, & Truitt RL. 1993. Delayed infusion of normal donor cells after MHC-matched bone marrow transplantation provides an antileukemia reaction without graft-versus-host disease. *Bone Marrow Transplant* **11**: 329–336.

Kalantari T, Kamali-Sarvestani E, Ciric B, et al. 2011. Generation of immunogenic and tolerogenic clinical-grade dendritic cells. *Immunol Res* **51**: 153–160.

Kantarjian HM, O'Brien S, Cortes JE, et al. 2002. Imatinib mesylate therapy for relapse after allogeneic stem cell transplantation for chronic myelogenous leukemia. *Blood* **100**: 1590–1595.

Karre K, Ljunggren HG, Piontek G, et al. 1986. Selective rejection of H-2-deficient lymphoma variants suggests alternative immune defence strategy. *Nature* **319**: 675–678.

Kolb HJ. 2008. Graft-versus-leukemia effects of transplantation and donor lymphocytes. *Blood* **112**: 4371–4383.

Kolb HJ, Bigalke I, Termeer D, et al. 2008. Graft-vs-leukemia effects of allogeneic stem cell transplantation from HLA-haploidentical family members as compared to HLA-identical sibling donors. *ASH Annual Meeting Abstracts* **112**: 3009.

Kolb HJ, Günther W, Schumm M, et al. 1997. Adoptive immunotherapy in canine chimeras. *Transplantation* **63**: 430–436.

Kolb HJ, Mittermuller J, Clemm C, et al. 1990. Donor leukocyte transfusions for treatment of recurrent chronic myelogenous leukemia in marrow transplant patients. *Blood* **76**: 2462–2465.

Kolb HJ, Schattenberg A, Goldman JM, et al. 1995. Graft-versus-leukemia effect of donor lymphocyte transfusions in marrow grafted patients. *Blood* **86**: 2041–2050.

Koreth J, Matsuoka K, Kim HT, et al. 2011. Interleukin-2 and regulatory T cells in graft-versus-host disease. *N Engl J Med* **365**: 2055–2066.

Kroger N, Badbaran A, Lioznov M, et al. 2009. Post-transplant immunotherapy with donor-lymphocyte infusion and novel agents to upgrade partial into complete and molecular remission in allografted patients with multiple myeloma. *Exp Hematol* **37**: 791–798.

Kroger N, Kruger W, Renges H, et al. 2001. Donor lymphocyte infusion enhances remission status in patients with persistent disease after allografting for multiple myeloma. *Br J Haematol* **112**: 421–423.

Kroger N, Shimoni A, Zagrivnaja M, et al. 2004. Low-dose thalidomide and donor lymphocyte infusion as adoptive immunotherapy after allogeneic stem cell transplantation in patients with multiple myeloma. *Blood* **104**: 3361–3363.

Kufner S, Zitzelsberger H, Kroell T, et al. 2005. Leukaemia-derived dendritic cells can be generated from blood or bone marrow cells from patients with myelodysplasia: a methodological approach under serum-free culture conditions. *Scand J Immunol* **62**: 75–85.

Le Blanc K, Frassoni F, Ball L, et al. 2008. Mesenchymal stem cells for treatment of steroid-resistant severe acute graft-versus-host disease: a phase II study. *Lancet* **371**: 1579–1586.

Levenga H, Levison-Keating S, Schattenberg AV, et al. 2007. Multiple myeloma patients receiving pre-emptive donor lymphocyte infusion after partial T-cell-depleted allogeneic stem cell transplantation show a long progression-free survival. *Bone Marrow Transplant* **40**: 355–359.

Levenga H, Woestenenk R, Schattenberg AV, et al. 2007. Dynamics in chimerism of T cells and dendritic cells in relapsed CML patients and the influence on the induction of alloreactivity following donor lymphocyte infusion. *Bone Marrow Transplant* **40**: 585–592.

Levine JE, Braun T, Penza SL, et al. 2002. Prospective trial of chemotherapy and donor leukocyte infusions for relapse of advanced myeloid malignancies after allogeneic stem cell transplantation. *J Clin Oncol* **15**: 405–412.

Linn YC & Hui KM. 2010. Cytokine-induced NK-like T cells: from bench to bedside. *J Biomed Biotechn* doi 10.1155/2010/4335745.

Lioznov M, El-Cheikh J Jr, Hoffmann F, et al. 2010. Lenalidomide as salvage therapy after allo-SCT for multiple myeloma is effective and leads to an increase of activated NK (NKp44(+)) and T (HLA-DR(+)) cells. *Bone Marrow Transplant* **45**: 349–353.

Lokhorst HM, Wu K, Verdonck LF, et al. 2004. The occurrence of graft-versus-host disease is the major predictive factor for response to donor lymphocyte infusions in multiple myeloma. *Blood* **103**: 4362–4364.

Mackinnon S, Papadopoulos EB, Carabasi MH, et al. 1995. Adoptive immunotherapy evaluating escalating doses of donor leukocytes for relapse of chronic myeloid leukemia after bone marrow transplantation: separation of graft-versus-leukemia responses from graft-versus-host disease. *Blood* **86**: 1261–1268.

Mailander V, Scheibenbogen C, Thiel E, et al. 2003. Complete remission in a patient with recurrent acute myeloid leukemia induced by vaccination with WT1 peptide in the absence of hematological or renal toxicity. *Leukemia* **18**: 165–166.

Mandigers CM, Verdonck LF, Meijerink JP, et al. 2003. Graft-versus-lymphoma effect of donor lymphocyte infusion in indolent lymphomas relapsed after allogeneic stem cell transplantation. *Bone Marrow Transplant* **32**: 1159–1163.

Mapara MY & Sykes M. 2005. Induction of mixed vs full chimerism to potentiate GVL effects after bone-marrow transplantation. *Methods Mol Med* **109**: 469–474.

Marijt WA, Heemskerk MH, Kloosterboer FM, et al. 2003. Hematopoiesis-restricted minor histocompatibility antigens HA-1 or HA-2-specific T cells can induce complete remissions of relapsed acute leukemia. *Proc Natl Acad Sci USA* **100**: 2742–2747.

Marks DI, Lush R, Cavenagh J, et al. 2002. The toxicity and efficacy of donor lymphocyte infusions given after reduced-intensity conditioning allogeneic stem cell transplantation. *Blood* **100**: 3108–3114.

Martin PJ. 2011. CIK: a path to GVL without GVHD? *Biol Blood Marrow Transplant* **17**: 1569–1570.

Mathé G, Amiel JL, Schwarzenberg L, et al. 1965. Adoptive immunotherapy of acute leukemia: experimental and clinical results. *Cancer Res* **25**: 1525–1530.

Matte CC, Cormier J, Anderson BE, et al. 2004. Graft-versus-leukemia in a retrovirally induced murine CML model: mechanisms of T-cell killing. *Blood* **103**: 4353–4361.

Miklos DB, Kim HT, Miller KH, et al. 2005. Antibody responses to H-Y minor histocompatibility antigens correlate with chronic graft-versus-host disease and disease remission. *Blood* **105**: 2973–2978.

Miller JS, Weisdorf DJ, Burns LJ, et al. 2007. Lymphodepletion followed by donor lymphocyte infusion (DLI) causes significantly more acute graft-versus-host disease than DLI alone. *Blood* **110**: 2761–2763.

Mittermueller J, Kolb HJ, Gerhartz HH, et al. 1986. In vivo differentiation of leukemic blasts and effect of low dose ara-c in a marrow grafted patient with leukemic relapse. *Brit J Haematol* **62**: 757–762.

Molldrem JJ, Komanduri K, & Wieder E. 2002. Overexpressed differentiation antigens as targets of graft-versus-leukema reactions. *Curr Opin Hematol* **9**: 503–508.

Morgan RA, Dudley ME, Wunderlich JR, et al. 2006. Cancer regression in patients after transfer of genetically engineered lymphocytes. *Science* **314**: 126–129.

Morris E & Mackinnon S. 2005. Outcome following alemtuzumab (CAMPATH-1H)-containing reduced intensity allogeneic transplant regimen for relapsed and refractory non-Hodgkin's lymphoma (NHL). *Transfus Apheresis Sci* **32**: 73–83.

Morris E, Thomson K, Craddock C, et al. 2004. Outcomes after alemtuzumab-containing reduced-intensity allogeneic transplantation regimen for relapsed and refractory non-Hodgkin lymphoma. *Blood* **104**: 3865–3871.

Ngo MC, Rooney CM, Howard JM, et al. 2011. Ex vivo gene transfer for improved adoptive immunotherapy of cancer. *Hum Mol Genet* **20**: R93–R99.

Nijmeijer BA, van Schie ML, Verzaal P, et al. 2005. Responses to donor lymphocyte infusion for acute lymphoblastic leukemia may be determined by both qualitative and quantitative limitations of antileukemic T-cell responses as observed in an animal model for human leukemia. *Exp Hematol* **33**: 1172–1181.

Olavarria E, Craddock C, Dazzi F, et al. 2002. Imatinib mesylate (STI571) in the treatment of relapse of chronic myeloid leukemia after allogeneic stem cell transplantation. *Blood* **99**: 3861–3862.

Passweg JR, Tiberghien P, Cahn JY, et al. 1998. Graft-versus-leukemia effects in T lineage and B lineage acute lymphoblastic leukemia. *Bone Marrow Transplant* **21**: 153–158.

Patil S & Schwarer T. 2009. Natural killer cells – new understanding of basic biology may lead to more effective allogeneic haematopoietic stem cell transplantation. *Int Med J* **39**: 639–647.

Peggs KS, Sureda A, Qian W, et al. 2007. Reduced-intensity conditioning for allogeneic haematopoietic stem cell transplantation in relapsed and refractory Hodgkin lymphoma: impact of alemtuzumab and donor lymphocyte infusions on long-term outcomes. *Br J Haematol* **139**: 70–80.

Peggs KS, Thomson K, Hart DP, et al. 2004. Dose-escalated donor lymphocyte infusions following reduced intensity transplantation: toxicity, chimerism, and disease responses. *Blood* **103**: 1548–1556.

Picker LJ, Treer JR, Ferguson Darnell B, et al. 1993. Control of lymphocyte recirculation in man. I. Differential regulation of the peripheral lymph node homing receptor L-selection on T cells during the virgin to memory cell transition. *J Immunol* **150**: 1105–1121.

Porter DL, Collins RH Jr, Hardy C, et al. 2000. Treatment of relapsed leukemia after unrelated donor marrow transplantation with unrelated donor leukocyte infusions. *Blood* **95**: 1214–1221.

Porter DL, Levine BL, Kalos M, et al. 2011. Chimeric antigen receptor-modified T cells in chronic lymphoid leukemia. *N Engl J Med* **365**: 725–733.

Rager A & Porter DL. 2012. Cellular therapy following allogeneic stem-cell transplantation. *Therap Adv Hematol* **2**: 409–428.

Raiola AM, van Lint MT, Valbonesi M, et al. 2003. Factors predicting response and graft-versus-host disease after donor lymphocyte infusions: a study on 593 infusions. *Bone Marrow Transplant* **31**: 687–693.

Ram R, Storb R, Sandmaier BM, et al. 2011. Non-myeloablative conditioning with allogeneic hematopoietic cell transplantation for the treatment of high-risk acute lymphoblastic leukemia. *Haematologica* **96**: 1113–1120.

Raya A, Rodriguez-Piza I, Guenechea G, et al. 2009. Disease-corrected haematopietic progenitors from Fanconi anaemia induced pluripotent stem cells. *Nature* **460**: 53–59.

Ren G, Chen X, Dong F, et al. 2012. Concise review: mesenchymal stem cells and translational medicine: emerging issues. *Stem Cells Transl Med* **12**: 51–58.

Ringden O & Le Blanc K. 2011. Mesenchymal stem cells for treatment of acute and chronic graft-versus-host disease, tissue toxicity and hemorrhages. *Best Pract Res Clin Haematol* **24**: 65–72.

Ritgen M, Stilgenbauer S, von Neuhoff N, et al. 2004. Graft-versus-leukemia activity may overcome therapeutic resistance of chronic lymphocytic leukemia with unmutated immunoglobulin variable heavy-chain gene status: implications of minimal residual disease measurement with quantitative PCR. *Blood* **104**: 2600–2602.

Rodt H, Netzel B, Niethammer D, et al. 1977. Specific absorbed antithymocyte globulin for incubation treatment in human marrow transplantation. *Transplant Proc* **9**: 187–191.

Rodt H, Thierfelder S, Bender-Gotze C, et al. 1983. Serological inhibition of graft versus host disease: recent results in 28 patients with leukemia. *Haematol Blood Transfus* **28**: 92–96.

Rosenberg SA. 2011. Cell transfer immunotherapy for metastatic solid cancer – what clinicians need to know. *Nature Rev Clin Oncol* **8**: 577–585.

Ruggeri L, Capanni M, Casucci M, et al. 1999. Role of natural killer cell alloreactivity in HLA-mismatched hematopoietic stem cell transplantation. *Blood* **94**: 333–339.

Rutten CE, van Luxemburg-Heijs SA, Griffioen M, et al. 2008. HLA-DP as specific target for cellular immunotherapy in HLA class II-expressing B-cell leukemia. *Leukemia* **22**: 1387–1394.

Sacchetti B, Funari A, Michienzi S, et al. 2007. Self-renewing osteoprogenitors in bone marrow sinusoids can organise a hematopoietic microenvironment. *Cell* **131**: 324–336.

Salama M, Nevill T, Marcellus D, et al. 2000. Donor leukocyte infusions for multiple myeloma. *Bone Marrow Transplant* **26**: 1179–1184.

Savani BN, Montero A, Kurlander R, et al. 2005. Imatinib synergizes with donor lymphocyte infusions to achieve rapid molecular remission of CML relapsing after allogeneic stem cell transplantation. *Bone Marrow Transplant* **36**: 1009–1015.

Schmetzer HM, Kremser A, Loibl J, et al. 2007. Quantification of ex vivo generated dendritic cells (DC) and leukemia-derived DC contributes to estimate the quality of DC, to detect optimal DC-generating methods or to optimize DC-mediated T-cell-activation-procedures ex vivo or in vivo. *Leukemia* **21**: 1338–1341.

Schmid C, Labopin M, Nagler A, et al. 2007. Donor lymphocyte infusion in the treatment of first hematological relapse after allogeneic stem-cell transplantation in adults with acute myeloid leukemia: a retrospective risk factors analysis and comparison with other strategies by the EBMT Acute Leukemia Working Party. *J Clin Oncol* **25**: 4938–4945.

Schmid C, Schleuning M, Aschan J, et al. 2004. Low dose ara-c, donor cells and GM-CSF for treatment of recurrent acute myeloid leukemia after allogeneic stem cell transplantation: a pilot study. *Leukemia* **18**: 1430–1433.

Schmidt-Wolf IG, Negrin RS, Kiem HP, et al. 1991. Use of a SCID mouse/human lymphoma model to evaluate cytokine-induced killer cells with potent antitumor cell activity. *J Exp Med* **174**: 139–149.

Schuster FR, Buhmann R, Reuther S, et al. 2008. Improved effector function of leukemia-specific T-lymphocyte clones trained with AML-derived dendritic cells. *Cancer Genomics Proteomics* **5**: 275–286.

Shiobara S, Nakao S, Ueda M, et al. 2000. Donor leukocyte infusion for Japanese patients with relapsed leukemia after allogeneic bone marrow transplantation: lower incidence of acute graft-versus-host disease and improved outcome. *Bone Marrow Transplant* **26**: 769–774.

Shlomchik WD, Couzens MS, Tang CB, et al. 1999. Prevention of graft versus host disease by inactivation of host antigen-presenting cells. *Science* **285**: 412–415.

Smit WM, Rijnbeck M, van Bergen CAM, et al. 1996. Dendritic cells generated from FACS sorted chronic myeloid leukemia (CML) precursor cells express BCR/ABL, and are potent stimulators for allogeneic T cells. *Br J Haematol* **93**: 313 (abstr.1186).

Spellman S, Warden MB, Haagenson M, et al. 2009. Effects of mismatching for minor histocompatibility antigens on clinical outcomes in HLA-matched, unrelated hematopoietic stem cell transplants. *Biol Blood Marrow Transplant* **15**: 856–863.

Sullivan KM, Deeg HJ, Sanders J, et al. 1986. Hyperacute graft-v-host disease in patients not given immunosuppression after allogeneic marrow transplantation. *Blood* **67**: 1172–1175.

Sullivan KM, Storb R, Buckner CD, et al. 1989. Graft-versus-host disease as adoptive immunotherapy in patients with advanced hematologic neoplasms. *N Engl J Med* **320**: 828–834.

Sykes M, Preffer F, McAfee S, et al. 1999. Mixed lymphohaemopoietic chimerism and graft-versus-lymphoma effects after non-myeloablative therapy and HLA-mismatched

bone-marrow transplantation. *Lancet* **353**: 1755–1759.

Teshima T, Ordemann R, Reddy P, et al. 2002. Acute graft-versus-host disease does not require alloantigen expression on host epithelium. *Nat Med* **8**: 575–581.

Tricot G, Vesole DH, Jagannath S, et al. 1996. Graft-versus-myeloma effect: proof of principle. *Blood* **87**: 1196–1198.

van de Donk NW, Kroger N, Hegenbart U, et al. 2006. Prognostic factors for donor lymphocyte infusions following non-myeloablative allogeneic stem cell transplantation in multiple myeloma. *Bone Marrow Transplant* **37**: 1135–1141.

Verdonck LF, Lokhorst HM, Dekker AW, et al. 1996. Graft-versus-myeloma effect in two cases. *Lancet* **347**: 800–801.

Vogt MH, van den Muijsenberg JW, Goulmy E, et al. 2002. The DBY gene codes for an HLA-DQ5-restricted human male-specific minor histocompatibility antigen involved in graft-versus-host disease. *Blood* **99**: 3027–3032.

Warren EH, Greenberg PD, & Riddell SR. 1998. Cytotoxic T-lymphocyte-defined human minor histocompatibility antigens with a restricted tissue distribution. *Blood* **91**: 2197–2207.

Weiden PL, Flournoy N, Thomas ED, et al. 1979. Antileukemic effects of graft versus host disease in human recipients of allogeneic marrow grafts. *N Eng J Med* **300**: 1068–1070.

Weisser M, Schleuning M, Haferlach C, et al. 2007. Allogeneic stem-cell transplantation provides excellent results in advanced stage chronic myeloid leukemia with major cytogenetic response to pre-transplant imatinib therapy 11. *Leuk Lymphoma* **48**: 295–301.

Weisser M, Tischer J, Schnittger S, et al. 2006. A comparison of donor lymphocyte infusions or imatinib mesylate for patients with chronic myelogenous leukemia who have relapsed after allogeneic stem cell transplantation 53. *Haematologica* **91**: 663–666.

Woiciechowsky A, Regn S, Kolb H-J, et al. 2001. Leukemic dendritic cells generated in the presence of FLT3 ligand have the capacity to stimulate an autologous leukaemia-specific cytotoxic T cell response from patients with acute myeloid leukaemia. *Leukemia* **15**: 246–255.

Wu SM & Hochedlinger K. 2011. Harnessing the potential of induced pluripotent stem cells

for regenerative medicine. *Nat Cell Biol* **13**: 497–505.

Zeiser R, Penack O, Holler E, et al. 2011. Danger signals activating innate immunity in graft-versus-host disease. *J Mol Med (Berl)* **89**: 833–845.

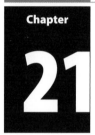

Practical aspects and procedures, including conditioning protocols and haploidentical transplantation

Reinhold Munker, Hillard M. Lazarus, and Kerry Atkinson

The BMT Data Book, Third Edition, ed. Reinhold Munker et al. Published by Cambridge University Press. © Cambridge University Press 2013.

Age limits and exclusion criteria for transplantation

Autologous blood stem cell/BM transplant	65–70 years
HLA-identical sibling transplant, myeloablative conditioning	55 years
HLA-identical sibling transplant, RIC	65–75 years
Unrelated donor transplant, myeloablative conditioning	50–55 years

Commonly used upper age limits for transplantation

In special situations, for example, biological functioning of a patient and using special conditioning protocols, these age limits can be extended. (See Klepin & Hurd (2006) for a discussion of these issues in myeloma patients.) Mineishi (2011) discussed the issues related to nonmyeloablative transplants in patients between the ages of 60 and 75 years in an editorial. In this age group, a long-term survival (5+ years) of 35% included most of these patients who survived without disease. (See also p. 5.)

Exclusion criteria for transplantation

Exclusion criteria for transplantation may include the following:

1. Severe organ dysfunction:

   - Kidney failure (serum creatinine >0.25 mmol/L [>2.8 mg/dL])
   - Liver failure (serum bilirubin >40 μmol/L [>3 mg/dL])
   - Respiratory failure (PaO_2 at room air <70 mm Hg)
   - Heart failure (left ventricular ejection fraction <40%–45%)

2. Active infection

In certain cases, patients who had hepatitis B or C can be considered for transplantation (for details, see page 343). Patients with well-controlled HIV-infection can also be considered under certain circumstances for (autologous) transplantation (for details, see page 106).

3. Poor performance status (e.g., ≤70% Karnofsky score)
4. Florid relapse of underlying malignancy
5. Refractoriness to platelet transfusion

Note: exclusion from transplant should not be based on a single test but should be discussed with the patient and an appropriate specialist. In some cases, patients who do not qualify for a myeloablative transplant may qualify for a reduced-intensity transplant.

SCT-specific comorbidity index

Other than age, multiple comorbidities influence the outcome of HSCT. With increasing use of RIC, more patients with comorbidities are considered for allogeneic transplantation. Sorror et al. (2005) modified and validated the Charlson Comorbidity Index for use in patients who undergo allogeneic SCT. The criteria for entering into the "HCT-CI" are as follows. This index can be used for the counseling of patients and to make studies comparable.

Hematopoietic cell transplantation comorbidity index (HCT-I)

Comorbidities	Definitions	HCT-CI weighted scores
Arrhythmia	Artial fibrillation or flutter, sick sinus syndrome, or ventricular arrhythmias	1
Cardiac	Coronary artery disease, congestive heart failure, myocardial infarction, or EF of $\leq$50%	1
Inflammatory bowel disease	Crohn's disease or ulcerative colitis	1
Diabetes	Requiring treatment with insulin or oral hypoglycemic, but not controlled with diet alone	1
Cerebrovascular disease	Transient ischemic attacks or cerebrovascular accident	1
Psychiatric disturbance	Depression/anxiety requiring psychiatric consult and/or treatment at the time of HCT	1
Hepatic – mild	Chronic hepatitis, bilirubin >ULN - 1.5XULN, or AST/ALT >ULN - 2.5XULN	1
Obesity	Patients with a BMI of >35 for adullts or with BMI-for-age percentile of $\geq$95th percentile for children	1
Infection	Documented infection or fever of unknown etiology requiring antimicrobial treatment before, during, and after the start of the conditioning regimen	1
Rheumatologic	SLE, rheumatoid arthritis, polymyositis, mixed connective tissue disease, and polymyalgia rheumatica	2
Peptic ulcer	Requiring treatment	2
Moderate/ severe renal	Serum creatinine >2 mg/dL, on dialysis, or prior renal transplantation	2
Moderate pulmonary	DLCO and/or FEV1 66%–80% or dyspnea on slight activity	2
Prior solid malignancy	Treated at any time in the patient's past history, excluding non-melanoma skin cancer	3
Heart valve disease	Except asymptomatic mitral valve prolapse	3
Severe pulmonary	DLCO and/or FEV1 $\leq$65% or dyspnea at rest or requiring oxygen	3
Moderate/ severe hepatic	Liver cirrhosis, bilirubin >1.5 × ULN, or AST/ALT >2.5 × ULN	3
		Total Score = …

Reproduced with permission, Sorror et al. (2005).

Prediction of NRM and OS according to the HCT-CI

Score	NRM at 2 years (%)	Survival at 2 years (%)
0	14	71
1–2	21	60
3 or more	41	34

Seattle data, modified from Sorror et al. (2005).

General pretransplant workup

1. See also the workup for each specific disease
2. Review of original pathology
3. Full blood count
4. Serum urea, electrolytes, creatinine, calcium, phosphate, uric acid, liver function tests (LFTs), C-reactive protein, and blood sugar
5. Coagulation tests (PT, APTT, fibrinogen)
6. Serology for CMV, HSV, varicella zoster virus (VZV), HIV-1, HIV-2, hepatitis B virus (HBV), hepatitis C virus (HCV), EBV (VCA, EBNA, EBV IgM), toxoplasma, human T-lymphotropic virus (HTLV)-I and HTLV-II, HHV-6, HHV-8, syphilis, adenovirus, influenza (as appropriate)
7. ABO/Rh typing with subgroups
8. HLA typing (by serological and molecular methods, for allogeneic transplantation, as appropriate)
9. Determination of chimerism markers (for allogeneic transplantation, as appropriate)
10. Creatinine clearance rate (24-hour urine collection)
11. Chest X-ray, electrocardiogram (ECG), left ventricular ejection fraction
12. Microbiology screening
13. Throat swab, nose swab, CVC exit site swab (to detect organisms such as methicillin-resistant *Staphylococcus aureus* (MRSA), methicillin-resistant *S. epidermis* (MRSE), pseudomonas, rectal swab (vancomycin-resistant enterococci [VRE])
14. Cerebrospinal fluid examination:
    - For patients with ALL, aggressive NHL, or lymphoid transformation of CML
    - Of doubtful value in patients with AML
15. BM examination (morphology, cytogenetics, MRD determination, immune phenotyping)
16. Determination of chemosensitivity of underlying disease (as appropriate)
17. Cryopreservation of autologous stem cells (as appropriate)
18. Delineation of platelet support strategy (as appropriate)
19. Dental check
20. Assessment by social worker
21. Sperm banking/embryo storage/in vitro fertilization (IVF) counseling
22. Removal of any foreign bodies (e.g., biliary stents), if possible
23. Family conference and signing of consent forms

24. Initiation of prophylactic medications (e.g., co-trimoxazole), as described later (pages 244, 345)
25. Other consultants (neurology, psychiatry), as appropriate

Definition of disease chemosensitivity

1. Achievement of CR or PR lasting at least two months after two to four courses of salvage chemotherapy
2. PR is defined as a 50% reduction in tumor diameter, although sometimes this may be difficult to evaluate (e.g., a mediastinal mass in a patient with lymphoma, in which fibrosis may prevent complete radiological resolution: use positron emission tomography (PET) imaging and fine-needle aspiration for accurate assessment

Mobilization of autologous blood stem cells

Mobilization protocols

A multitude of protocols utilizing chemotherapy alone, hemopoietic growth factor (HGF) alone, or a combination of the two have been utilized for mobilizing blood stem cells. A protocol (Jones et al., 1994) that is usually successful in mobilizing sufficient stem and progenitor cells with a single leukapheresis is as follows:

- Day 1: cyclophosphamide, 1.5 g/m^2
- Days 2–12: G-CSF, 10 μg/kg/day
- Days 10–12: leukapheresis (on first day post-nadir that WBC count reaches 8.0×10^9/L)
- Other protocols have used doses of cyclophosphamide up to 7 g/m^2, with leukapheresis being initiated when the WBC count reaches $\geq 1.0 \times 10^9$/L

When to start leukapheresis

1. If using HGF alone for mobilization: when WBC $\geq 10.0 \times 10^9$/L (usually after a daily dose of G-CSF for 4 days)
2. If using chemotherapy ± HGF for mobilization: when WBC count reaches 1.0×10^9/L on recovery after nadir
3. If monitoring PB on day of leukapheresis for CD34$^+$ cells: when CD34$^+$ cells reach 10/μL ($= 0.01 \times 10^9$/L)

Venous access for leukapheresis

Access	Advantage	Disadvantage
Peripheral veins	No central line (infection risk, etc.)	Discomfort; may have poor flow
Hickman-type central catheter	Provides access for return flow from machine	Insufficiently stiff to cope with outflow pressure to machine; can become infected
Dialysis-type central catheter (e.g., Vascath)	Provides access for both outflow and return flow (i.e., no needles); can be used as central line for subsequent transplant	Can become infected

How many cells to collect

Suggested minimum:

- CD34$^+$ cells: 2×10^6/kg
- CFU-GM: 5×10^4/kg (most centers no longer perform colony assays on the harvested or thawed collection product)

A relationship has been demonstrated between the number of CD34$^+$ cells infused and the time taken to reach an unsupported platelet count of $\geq 20 \times 10^9$/L post-autograft.

Alternative cytokines/chemokines for stem cell mobilization

- GM-CSF (Comment: at higher doses potential for serious side effects)
- Pegylated G-CSF (Comment: feasible, no clear superiority over G-CSF)
- Stem cell factor, flt3-ligand (Comment: experimental, inferior yield as single agent)
- Parathormone (Comment: experimental)
- Plerixafor (Mozobil®) (Comment: inferior or same yield as single agent, short-acting, few side effects such as bloating, injection site reactions)
- G-CSF + plerixafor (Comment: useful for poor mobilizers or patients at risk for being poor mobilizers, recommended approach: start G-CSF as usual for stem cell mobilization; on day 4 give plerixafor at a dose of 160–240 µg/kg IV or IM 6–12 hours before the intended harvest). Jantunen and Lemoli (2012) recently discussed the preemptive use of plerixafor to shorten the time for stem cell harvests
- For single agent mobilization, plerixafor was administered at a dose of 240 µg/kg subcutaneously in normal donors at 8AM and leukopheresis started at 12PM. This was repeated until the target dose of CD34+ cells was reached

Reasons for poor leukapheresis yields

- Multiple courses of combination chemotherapy
- Previous radiotherapy
- Previous rituximab or lenalidomide
- Histology of underlying malignancy
- Older age (only in some studies)

Approach to patients who are poor mobilizers

1. Remobilization (preferably after one month, using the same or a different mobilization protocol, consider combination with plerixafor)
2. BM harvest (preferably after stimulation with cytokines–"primed marrow")
3. Perform alternative treatment, instead of autologous transplantation

Cryopreservation technique used at the Fred Hutchinson Cancer Research Center, Seattle

Cell processing	Buffy coat or light-density cells
Cell concentration	2×10^7 cells/mL, final concentration
Storage container	Blood storage bag tolerant of cryogenic temperature
Sample volume	Dependent on bag size, generally 40–60 mL per bag
Cryoprotectant	10% (vol/vol) dimethylsulfoxide, final concentration
Protein	20% autologous plasma
Electrolytes	Tissue culture medium
Rate of cooling	1°C/min to −40° C, with compensation for heat of fusion, then 10°C/min to −80°C
Storage temperature	Below −135°C in nitrogen vapor-phase refrigerators or mechanical freezers
Rate of thawing	Rapidly (>100°C/min) in a 37°C water bath
Post-thaw manipulation	Addition of ACD (20% [vol/vol] of product volume), then infusion immediately after thawing without further processing; filtration through blood administration set (170-μm mesh) if clumped after thawing

(Reproduced with permission from Rowley, 1992.)

Advantages and disadvantages of blood SCT
Advantages and disadvantages of PB SCT as compared with BMT

Advantages	Disadvantages
• To recipient	• To recipient
Faster neutrophil recovery	More chronic GVHD (most studies, applies to allotransplants)
Faster platelet recovery	
Faster immunological recovery	
Fewer IV antibiotics	
Less fever ≥38.5°C	
Shorter hospitalization	
Lower cost	
More GVL? (allotransplants)	
• To donor	• To donor
No general anesthesia	Venipuncture or central IV catheter for leukapheresis
No BM harvest	
No hospitalization	Side effects from G-CSF

Allogeneic donor workup

1. History and physical examination (best done by anesthetist at anesthesia clinic preoperatively if BM is to be harvested)
2. Full blood count; blood chemistry screen, including urea, electrolytes, creatinine, blood sugar, calcium, phosphate, LFTs
3. Serology for CMV, HIV, HBV, HCV, HTLV-I and II as appropriate, HSV, VZV, EBV, *Toxoplasma*, trypanosomiasis
4. ABO/Rh typing
5. Coagulation tests (PT, APTT)
6. ECG, chest X-ray, as appropriate (see following note 1)
7. Pregnancy test for female donors

- Note 1: chest X-ray probably should be avoided in healthy young adult donors because of its possible teratogenicity
- Note 2: HIV (and HTLV) positivity is a contraindication to BM or stem cell donation. HBV or HCV positivity is a relative contraindication to donation

Serious medical conditions that preclude general anesthesia or administration of HD growth factors (e.g., SCD) or active cancer within the last five years are a contraindication to the donation of allogeneic stem cells.

Choice of allogeneic donor

If there is a choice of HLA-identical sibling donors

- Use a nontransfused male or nulliparous, nontransfused female donor (less risk for GVHD)
- Use a younger donor (less risk for GVHD)
- Use a CMV-seronegative donor (if recipient is seronegative, less risk for CMV disease)
- Use an ABO-compatible donor (less risk of hemolysis)

If there is a choice between an HLA-identical sibling donor and an identical twin donor

- For nonmalignant disease (e.g., severe aplastic anemia), use the identical twin donor
- For malignant disease, especially if the patient is less than 30 years of age and/or if there is advanced disease at the time of transplant, use the HLA-identical sibling, not twin (to obtain GVL effect)

For unrelated transplants, the National Donor Program (NMDP) and similar organizations at an international level provide a search algorithm and outcome data. (For a review, see Karanes et al., 2008.)

According to W. Navarro (NMDP workshop at ASH 2011) (personal communication) most transplant centers prefer young, male, and newly recruited (better typed) donors (a drawback is some of these donors may also be temporarily unavailable, especially donors recruited in the military). The NMDP tries to predict with a computer algorithm based on HLA haplotypes (HapLogic) which donor is likely to be a match. This algorithm reduces cost for repeated confirmatory testing of potential donors and speeds up the search for potential donors

Commonly used prophylactic medications

Drug	Timing	Purpose
1. Co-trimoxazole, 1 double strength tablet BID (800 mg sulfamethoxazole, 160 mg trimethoprim)	Daily for 2 weeks before transplant until day −1; then twice weekly from day +28 until 3–6 months after cessation of immunosuppressive medications[a]	*Pneumocystis carinii* (*jirovecii*) pneumonia (PCP) prophylaxis
2. Trimethoprim, 300 mg PO daily, plus dapsone, 150 mg PO daily	As for co-trimoxazole	PCP prophylaxis if there is a low blood count or other contraindication to co-trimoxazole
OR Pentamidine, 4 mg/kg IV, up to 300 mg per dose • Do not exceed a total pentamidine dose of 3 g • Breakthrough cases of PCP have been seen during inhaled pentamidine prophylaxis; inhalation is not recommended	Monthly	PCP prophylaxis if there is a contraindication to co-trimoxazole or trimethoprim/dapsone
3. Ganciclovir, 5 mg/kg IV	Daily from day of admission until day −1; then 3 days/week from day +28 to day +84[a]	CMV prophylaxis
4. Foscarnet, 90 mg/kg IV	If full blood count (FBC) satisfactory, as for ganciclovir	CMV prophylaxis if patient cannot tolerate ganciclovir
5. Fluconazole 100 mg BID PO or IV	Day −8 to day +15 or +25	Candida prophylaxis
6. Acyclovir, 200 mg TID PO or 250 mg TID IV if patient cannot tolerate PO	Day 180 to day 360 or according to institutional guidelines	HSV prophylaxis
7. Norfloxacin, 400 mg BID PO[b]	Day 0 to day + 21	Prophylaxis against Gram-negative bacteria
8. Allopurinol, 300 mg PO daily	Day −8 to day −1	Prophylaxis for urate nephropathy

In high-risk patients, posaconazole may be used as prophylaxis against fungal infections and ursodeoxydiotic acid as prophylaxis against hepatic veno-occlusive disease.
[a]other similar protocols available; [b]other gyrase-inhibitors available.

Treatment of CNS leukemia pretransplant

Treat with intrathecal methotrexate, 12.5 mg, and/or cytosine arabinoside, 50 mg, giving one of the drugs every four days until the disease is eliminated, depending on patient tolerance; usually twice weekly for about three weeks. Try to clear the CSF (cerebrospinal fluid) of leukemic cells before starting conditioning regimen. These drugs can be given with hydrocortisone, 50 mg, to reduce arachnoiditis risk. All drugs should be in preservative-free diluent.

- Methotrexate, 10 mg/m^2 ($\leq$15 mg total dose) (usually either 12.5 or 15 mg), leucovorin rescue after IT MIX (optional), begin after 24 hours, PO 5–10 mg, total of six doses every six hours
- Cytosine arabinoside, 30 mg/m^2 (usually 50 mg). Use Cytosar powder with preservative-free diluent–not cytarabine liquid, which is hypertonic. Avoid giving at the same time as systemic cytosine arabinoside, which may increase toxicity
- Hydrocortisone, 50 mg, dissolved in preservative-free normal saline
- Liposomal cytosine arabinoside, 50 mg intrathecally (should be combined with steroid, repeat in two weeks, possibly more effective, but also more toxic than standard cytosine arabinoside)

Procedure

- Perform lumbar puncture (LP) in standard fashion
- Measure pressure
- Take samples for culture, biochemistry (glucose, protein), and cytology
- Attach the syringe containing the drug to the hub of the LP needle. Inject slowly. Aspirate back gently at regular intervals to confirm that the CSF will flow back freely
- At conclusion, remove the needle, apply a local dressing, and ensure that the patient lies flat for 6–24 hours
- Use extreme care to ensure that the drugs to be given are the correct drugs. Fatalities have been reported from administration of the wrong drug or dose intrathecally

Posttransplant

- Give six intrathecal injections of methotrexate or cytosine arabinoside at the previously described dosages every two weeks, starting at week 5 posttransplant

Platelet count

- As for all invasive procedures, the platelet count should be $\geq$50 $\times$10^9/L at the time of lumbar puncture

Central venous catheter (CVC) management
Triple-, double-, and single-lumen right atrial catheters

Single-, double-, and triple-lumen catheters are available. A single-lumen catheter is rarely used for BMT/SCT patients; double-lumen catheters are the most commonly used, and triple-lumen catheters are advised for mismatched family member or matched unrelated donor transplants. The specifications from one manufacturer are given as an example:

- Single lumen: 9.6 FR with Vitacuff, 90 cm in length, 1.6 mm in internal diameter; 1.8 mL priming volume

- Double lumen: 12 FR with Vitacuff, 90 cm in length, 1.6 mm in internal diameter; 1.8 mL priming volume
- Triple lumen: 12.5 FR with Vitacuff, 90 cm in length, two lumens 1.0 mm in internal diameter; one lumen 1.5 mm in internal diameter; two lumens 0.7-mL priming volume, one lumen 1.6-mL priming volume

Each of these catheters has a Luer lock connector at the external end and a Dacron cuff attached 30 cm from the catheter's external end that, when *in situ*, lies approximately midway in the subclavian tunnel. The purpose of the Dacron cuff is to facilitate the growth of fibrous tissue to prevent catheter dislodgement and to serve as a barrier to ascending infection. The tip of the catheter should lie within the superior vena cava, in close proximity to the right atrium. The catheter may be inserted via the cephalic, subclavian, or external jugular vein, and it exits via a subcutaneous tunnel on the anterior chest wall.

Right atrial catheters provide semipermanent venous access and allow

- Blood sampling for laboratory tests
- Administration of all intravenous fluids, medications, blood products, and total parenteral nutrition
- Monitoring of central venous pressure

Insertion of the catheter

The catheter may be inserted in the operating theater under general anesthesia or in the procedure room under local anesthesia, using an image intensifier.

Preoperative/local anesthetic preparation

1. A consent form should be completed, indicating the use of a single-, double-, or triple-lumen catheter.
2. The patient should shower or wash with antibacterial lotion 3–4 hours before operation.
3. The general preoperative care is the same as for any other surgery case.
4. Record the results of the current FBC and coagulation studies on the form for the preoperative checklist.
5. If the platelet count is less than 50×10^9/L, a platelet transfusion should be given as close to the time of operation as possible.
6. An antibiotic such as cefazolin, 1 g IV, should be given by the anesthetist or surgeon just before the procedure.

Postoperative care

1. Routine observations.
2. Chest X-ray to confirm the position of the catheter.
3. IV fluids as required; otherwise, lumens can be flushed and capped.
4. The dressing should remain intact until the first day postinsertion, unless there is excessive bleeding from the neck incision or the exit site.
5. Place a small piece of tape (with tabs) around the catheter so that a cannula clamp can be placed on the tab. The catheter thus can be clamped to the patient's clothes to reduce the "drag" on the catheter and prevent possible dislocation.

Safe management of the catheter

1. Ensure that each patient with a CVC has a cannula clamp.
2. When a patient is attached to a line for IV fluids, the catheter must be clamped to the patient's clothes using the cannula clamp and Transpore tape over the catheter.

If the patient is not attached to a line for IV fluids, the catheter can be secured to the patient's clothing in the same way.

3. When a patient goes to the shower, the catheter can be secured either by taping the ends to the chest wall or by attaching the catheter to a piece of tape tied around the neck.
4. A catheter should not be allowed to hang "free," as this may result in its dislodgement.
5. Safety pins should NEVER be used to attach the catheter to clothing, because of the risk of piercing the catheter.

Management of a dislodged catheter

1. If the catheter is accidentally pulled completely out, place the patient in bed (lying left side down), apply pressure to the neck incision site, and treat for air embolism (see page 253).
2. If the catheter becomes dislodged but is not pulled completely out (i.e., the cuff is completely exposed), place the patient in bed, with instructions to lie still, clamp the catheter. Cover the site with a sterile clear adhesive dressing and tape the catheter ends to the chest wall to minimize "drag." Subsequently, the catheter can be removed under optimal conditions. *Stop any infusions.*
3. If the catheter cuff is only half exposed, a chest X-ray should be taken to determine if the catheter remains in the correct position. The cuff should be observed daily for further exposure, and the catheter should be secured at all times to prevent complete dislodgement. Place a sterile adhesive dressing around the catheter at completion of dressing, before applying Primapore for added security.

Dressing the catheter exit site

Purpose
- Daily reduction in skin flora
- Daily inspection of exit site for signs of infection
- Daily observation for signs of dislodgement

Equipment
- One dressing pack
- Primapore dressing
- Two Betadine swabs
- Hydrogen peroxide (3%)
- Sterile would swab

Procedure
1. Wash hands and prepare the equipment.

2. Remove the old dressing. Observe the exit site for any signs of dislodgement. Observe for any signs of infection at the exit site or along the subcutaneous tunnel. If the exit site is reddened and/or tender, take a swab for culture and sensitivity.

3. Repeat hand wash. Drape the patient using a sterile dressing towel.

4. Using hydrogen peroxide (3%), clean the skin around the catheter, working in a circular motion from the inner area to the outer area to a diameter of approximately 10 cm. On the first postoperative day, clean the neck incision.

5. Using a Betadine swab, and working in a circular motion, swab the skin around the site. On the first postoperative day, swab the neck incision and leave it exposed. Allow the Betadine to dry on the skin.

6. Place a sterile dressing over exit site, rotating its position daily.

7. Using a cannula clamp and tape tabs, clamp the catheter to the patient's clothing to prevent traction or accidental pulling on the catheter. The piece of tape should be changed every week (more often if soiled). Some brands have clamps; these clamps should also have their positions changed regularly, for the same reason.

8. If sutures are present, they can be removed 7–10 days after insertion of the catheter (for a single-lumen catheter) or after 14 days (for double- and triple-lumen catheters).

9. All intravenous lines should be changed every Monday, Wednesday, and Friday, preferably to coincide with the daily dressing procedure to minimize handling of the catheter. If any contamination of the lines occurs, and after blood products have been infused, the lines should be changed. Aseptic technique must be used when changing lines; a sterile plastic sheet and sterile gloves should be used.

10. Before discharge from hospital, the patient and a family member will need instruction regarding daily dressing of the exit site. The demonstration and instruction should emphasize the need for asepsis and also include information regarding possible risks associated with the catheter. Instruction should begin as soon as possible after insertion of the catheter, to allow the patient and family member sufficient time to master the technique.

11. The manufacturers do not recommend the application of tincture of iodine to the catheter, as this can result in surface erosion. The suggested antiseptic is Betadine or Povidone-Iodine.

12. In the event of extensive skin excoriation or blistering around the catheter site, no dressing should be applied.

Drawing blood from a catheter
Equipment
- One pair of sterile gloves
- One 5-mL syringe
- One syringe suitable for the volume of blood to be collected
- Cannula cap (if no infusion is in progress)
- Two 19-gauge needles
- One dressing pack
- One ampoule of heparinized saline (50 units in 5 mL of saline)
- One Alcowipe, or similar brand
- Appropriate tubes for laboratory tests

Procedure

1. Position the patient. Wash hands and prepare the equipment. Open the ampoule of heparinized saline.
2. Turn off all the intravenous infusions, even with dual-lumen catheters, and clamp all catheters.
3. Repeat hand wash. Put on sterile gloves. Using a 19-gauge needle and 5-mL syringe, aseptically draw up 5 mL of heparinized saline.
4. Drape the patient using a sterile towel. Disconnect the giving set (IVI set) and place it on the sterile towel while blood is being drawn. Using the Alcowipe, swab the connection of the giving set and the catheter thoroughly. Take blood from both lumens when collecting blood cultures, and label the samples separately.
5. Swab the end of the catheter. Connect the 5-mL syringe, and unclamp the catheter. Gently draw off 5 mL of blood. Reclamp the catheter and discard the blood. Do not discard this first 5 mL when taking blood cultures.
6. Connect the remaining syringe, unclamp the catheter, and withdraw the required amount of blood. Clamp the catheter.
7. Swab around the end of the catheter once again to clean away any blood that may remain around the catheter. Connect the syringe that contains heparinized saline. Unclamp the catheter. Flush the catheter with 5 mL of heparinized saline. Clamp the catheter.
8. Swab the end of the catheter once again. Reconnect the giving set if any infusion is in progress. If there is no infusion in progress, connect the cannula cap.
9. Repeat steps 5 to 8 if both lumens require the withdrawal of blood.
10. Fill the appropriate tubes with blood. Ensure that all are labeled with the patient's name, medical record number, ward, and date and time of collection.

Capping and flushing the catheter
Equipment

- One dressing pack
- One or two 19-gauge needles
- One or two Alcowipes, or similar brand
- One pair of sterile gloves
- One or two 5-mL syringes
- One or two ampoules of heparinized saline (50 units in 5 mL of saline)
- One or two cannula caps

Procedure

1. Position the patient. Wash hands and prepare the equipment. If an infusion is in progress, turn it off and clamp the catheter.
2. Repeat hand wash. Put on sterile gloves. Use the 19-gauge needles and the 5-mL syringes to draw up 5 mL of heparinized saline in each syringe.
3. Drape the patient using a sterile dressing towel. Using an Alcowipe, swab the connection of the giving set and the catheter thoroughly. Disconnect the catheter from the giving set, and rest the giving set on the dressing towel.

4. Connect a syringe containing heparinized saline. Unclamp the catheter. Flush the catheter with 5 mL of heparinized saline. Reclamp the catheter.
5. Connect the cannula cap. The catheter should remain clamped when there is no infusion running.
6. Flushing the catheter with heparinized saline is necessary

   (a) if the infusion is discontinued for any length of time, and
   (b) following each blood sampling.

Removing the catheter

Equipment

- One IV cutdown tray and suture material
- One pair of sterile gloves
- One 5-mL syringe
- Local anesthetic
- One sterile gown
- One 19-gauge needle
- One 25-gauge needle
- Nonadherent sterile dressing (Primapore or similar brand)
- Extra swabs, gauze
- Sterile container for catheter tip
- Betadine

Removal of the catheter is usually performed as a sterile procedure under local anesthetic. A premedication may be ordered. Fasting is not usually necessary.

Before removal, check that the platelet count is more than 50×10^9/L. If the platelet count is less than 50×10^9/L, the patient will require a platelet transfusion as close to the time of removal as possible.

Procedure

1. Position the patient in the supine position.
2. After instilling local anesthetic, expose the Dacron cuff, and release any fibrosis; the cuff should be freed using gentle but firm tension. Slowly remove the catheter. After removal, apply pressure to both the exit site and the venous entry site for five minutes. Suturing may be necessary if the exit site has been enlarged during removal.
3. The catheter tip should be sent to the microbiology laboratory for culture.
4. The site must be observed for bleeding or hematoma formation.

Management of a nonfunctioning catheter

Difficulty in sampling blood

If the catheter will accept infusions without a problem, but aspiration from the line is difficult, it is probable that the tip of the catheter is lodged against the wall of the vein or the right atrium. Use of less suction while aspirating may help. Sometimes a change in position, raising the arms, or a deep inhalation will reposition the tip of the catheter.

If these methods are unsuccessful, obtain a cathetergram (venogram), which should help distinguish between malpositioning and the presence of a clot. If malpositioning is the problem, get a vascular surgeon to reposition it. If there is a clot, proceed as given in the following section.

Catheter malfunction due to clotting

Equipment
- One pair of sterile gloves
- One dressing pack
- One 1-mL syringe
- One 2-mL syringe
- One 5-mL syringe
- One 10-mL syringe
- Two Alcowipes, or similar brand
- One 19-gauge needles
- Cannula cap
- Two ampoules of heparinized saline (50 units in 5 mL of saline)

Procedure
1. Position the patient, wash hands, and open the equipment. Clamp the catheter.
2. Wash hands and put on sterile gloves. Aseptically draw up heparinized saline into the 1-mL, 2-mL, and 5-mL syringes.
3. Drape the patient and swab the end of the catheter. Connect the 1-mL syringe and inject the heparinized saline; using the same syringe, attempt to aspirate from the catheter.
4. Repeat the procedure with the 2-mL syringe. If the catheter will allow aspiration, use the 10-mL syringe to aspirate 5 mL of blood.
5. Flush the catheter with 5-mL of heparinized saline and connect to IV infusion or attach the cannula cap.
6. If the catheter is still blocked, the following procedure should be followed:

Equipment
- One pair of sterile gloves
- One dressing pack
- One 1-mL syringe
- One 2-mL syringe
- One 10-mL syringe
- One Alcowipe, or similar brand
- Three 19-gauge needles
- Cannula cap
- One ampoule of heparinized saline (50 units/mL)
- One ampoule of normal saline
- One ampoule of heparin (5000 units/mL)

Procedure

1. Position the patient, wash hands, and prepare the equipment. Break open the ampoules of heparin, normal saline, and heparinized saline. Ensure that the catheter is clamped.
2. Repeat hand wash and put on sterile gloves. Aseptically draw up 5 mL of heparinized saline into the 5-mL syringe, 1 mL of heparin in the 1-mL syringe, and 2 mL of normal saline in the 2-mL syringe.
3. Drape the patient using the sterile dressing towel. Using the Alcowipe, swab the end of the Hickman catheter thoroughly.
4. Connect the 1-mL syringe containing the heparin (5000 units) and inject it into the catheter; clamp the catheter.
5. Connect the cannula cap to the end of the Hickman catheter and leave it for one hour.
6. One hour later, using an aseptic technique, attempt to aspirate from the catheter using the 5-mL or 10-mL syringe. If aspiration is possible, then flush the catheter well and recommence infusion.
7. If the catheter is still blocked, repeat the injection of heparin (5000 units in 1 mL) or try streptokinase injection as given in the following section.

Streptokinase/urokinase/tissue plasminogen activator (t-PA) instillation into a CVC

Do not instill if there is thrombocytopenia or coagulopathy.

1. Dilute a 250 000-unit ampoule in 100 mL of normal saline. Flush each lumen with 2 mL (=5000 units).
2. Leave the streptokinase in the catheter for 10 minutes.
3. Attempt to aspirate blood using the attached syringe. If unable to aspirate blood, leave the streptokinase in the catheter for a further 10 minutes. If still unable to aspirate blood, leave it for a further 10 minutes–a total of 30 minutes–and attempt to aspirate blood again. If unsuccessful, leave for a further 30 minutes before reattempting. If unable to aspirate blood one hour after instillation, withdraw the streptokinase from the catheter. Clamp the catheter.
4. Attach a syringe containing 10 mL of normal saline. Release the clamp and flush.
5. Attach IV fluid or lock off, as per protocol.
6. Clamp and cap the catheter.

If the patient has previously had streptokinase, use urokinase to avoid the risk of anaphylaxis (again, 5000 units/lumen).

An alternative treatment would be to inject 2 mg recombinant t-PA (Alteplase, Cathflo® Activase®) in 2 mL into the occluded catheter. After 30 minutes, try to aspirate. If catheter is not functional, wait for additional 60 minutes. If catheter is still not functional, inject another dose of 2 mg, and wait another 30 minutes. Then aspirate blood and t-PA (total of 5–10 mL). If catheter functions, then gently irrigate with sterile 0.9% saline solution.

Other potential problems

1. Exit site infection
   Signs: erythema, tenderness, induration and/or purulent discharge around the skin exit site of the catheter.

Management: take a swab from the exit site for culture. Start IV vancomycin and continue until the swab result is known.

Prevention: careful insertion technique, meticulous daily dressing of exit site, adherence to aseptic technique.

2. Tunnel infection

Signs: erythema, tenderness, induration along the subcutaneous tunnel of the catheter with or without signs of inflammation and purulent discharge at the exit site.

Management: intravenous antibiotics, including vancomycin. Removal of the catheter is often necessary for satisfactory resolution of the infection.

Prevention: as for exit site infection.

3. Catheter tip infection

Signs: fevers and rigors occur after catheter flushing, even when the WBC count is adequate.

Management: intravenous antibiotics until fever resolves. Removal of the catheter is usually necessary for resolution.

4. Venous occlusion

Signs: distended veins; swelling in supraclavicular fossa or anterior chest wall.

Management: removal of the catheter is often necessary; the patient may be treated with IV heparin.

5. Air embolism

Each intravenous line directly attached to the catheter should have a screw-on Luer lock. If a screw-on Luer lock is unavailable, the connection must be taped to avoid accidental disconnection and possible air embolism. A malfunctioning infusion pump is also a potential source of air embolism.

Symptoms and signs: shortness of breath, tachypnea, chest pain, pallor, hypotension, coma.

Management: in the event that an air embolus is known or suspected, proceed as follows:

- Clamp the catheter
- If IV lines have become disconnected, use cannula caps to cover the lumens while the air embolus is being treated
- Call a cardiac arrest team if necessary
- Place the patient in bed (lying left side down) and elevate the foot of the bed
- Administer oxygen via a mask. Treat the patient as required for maintenance of circulation and oxygenation
- Aspirate the lumens that were disconnected to remove any residual air

6. Trauma or damage to catheter

- Repair kits are available
- Read the labeling carefully, as each repair kit is for a specific catheter (e.g., blue, red, or white lumen)
- Instructions for use are inside the sterile pack. Read them carefully. If you follow instructions, step-by-step repairs are simple
- If possible, always have two people to carry out a repair–one to do the repair and the other to read the instructions and open the equipment

Medications and special considerations regarding conditioning regimens

Conditioning regimens are described on pages 282–285. Special problems involving cytotoxic drugs are discussed on pages 282–285. The most common side effects of conditioning regimens are as follows:

- Nausea, vomiting, diarrhea
- Oropharyngeal mucositis
- Alopecia
- Pancytopenia
- Hemorrhagic cystitis
- Hepatic veno-occlusive disease (sinoidal obstruction syndrome)
- Interstitial pneumonitis
- Secondary malignancy

Fluid regime for conditioning regimens

Intravenous hydration during the conditioning regimen has two purposes. It is intended to

- Minimize the risk of hemorrhagic cystitis by promoting frequent micturition and
- Maintain fluid intake

For regimens that contain cyclophosphamide or ifosfamide, the fluid guidelines are as follows:

1. Give 6 L in 24 hours by IV infusion (IVI).
2. Start four hours before the first dose of cytotoxic drug and continue for 24 hours after the last dose of cytotoxic drug.
3. A typical regimen is
   - Normal saline, 1 L, plus 30 mmol of KCl alternating with
   - 4% dextrose N/5, 1 L, plus 30 mmol of KCl
4. Give furosemide, 40 mg, with each daily dose of cyclophosphamide or ifosfamide.
5. Give MESNA (2-mercaptoethane sulfonate sodium) at 50 mg/kg, divided into three doses for each day when a high dose of cyclophosphamide or ifosfamide is given, starting eight hours before the conditioning; continue MESNA for 24 hours after conditioning is completed (see also page 500).

For other cytotoxic drugs:

1. 4 L in 24 hours by IVI.
2. Watch the patient's daily fluid balance and weight carefully. If the patient's weight increases by 2–3 kg or more, or if the fluid balance becomes 1 L or more positive, give furosemide, 40 mg IV.

Antiemetic regime for conditioning regimens

1. Give lorazepam, 1 mg PO every 12 hours (for anticipatory vomiting), combined with ondansetron, 8 mg IV every 8 hours, or 1 mg/hr by continuous IVI, or 8 mg PO every 8 hours. Ondansetron should be continued until day 13 posttransplant. Lorazepam should

be reviewed on the day of transplant. The dose may need reduction if the patient is excessively sleepy.

2. An alternative 5-HT$_3$ receptor antagonist is tropisetron given as a single daily dose of 5 mg.
3. If the foregoing regimen is ineffective, it can be combined with

- Metoclopramide, 10–60 mg IV every 4 hours or
- Chlorpromazine, 25 mg IV every 8 hours or
- Droperidol, 5 mg IV every 2–4 hours or
- Dexamethasone, 8 mg IV every 8 hours

Antiemetics

Drug	Class	Comment
Metoclopramide	Dopamine and serotonin antagonist	Extrapyramidal effects may occur[a]
Droperidol	Dopamine receptor antagonist	Extrapyramidal effects may occur[a]
Lorazepam	Benzodiazepine	Useful adjunct to ondansetron for anticipatory vomiting
Chlorpromazine	Phenothiazine	Extrapyramidal effects may occur[a]
Ondansetron	Serotonin receptor antagonist	Headache not uncommon
Palonosetron	Serotonin receptor antagonist	Higher potency than ondansetron, similar side effects
Dexamethasone	Corticosteroid	Useful adjunct to ondansetron
Aprepitant	Neurokinin-1 antagonist	For highly emetogenic chemotherapy (in combination with steroid and serotonin receptor antagonist)

[a] use cogentin, 2 mg IV, to treat extrapyramidal side effects.

Total-body irradiation (TBI)

TBI is often used as part of the conditioning regimen for

- Matched unrelated donor transplants
- Mismatched family member transplants
- Some patients with CNS involvement
- Patients with lymphoid malignancies

It can be given in a single session or as multiple fractions. Before each session, remove all heavy metal items (e.g., jewelry, watches).

The most frequent side effects of TBI are as follows:

- Lethargy (immediately following TBI)
- Nausea, vomiting, diarrhea
- Acute parotitis

- Skin erythema
- Oropharyngeal mucositis
- Pancytopenia
- Alopecia
- Hepatic veno-occlusive disease
- Interstitial pneumonitis
- Cataracts
- Growth retardation (in children)

Protocol for the day of transplant

The BM donor

1. The donor must fast from 12 midnight if the BM harvest is to be at 8AM.
2. Consent forms for the operative procedure and tissue donation must be signed.
3. The donor must be seen by the anesthetist, with premedication ordered.
4. Marrow is harvested in an operating theater under general or spinal anesthetic.
5. A unit of autologous blood should be given during the procedure.
6. On return to the ward

    - Routine observations
    - IV fluids until the donor is eating, drinking, and passing urine, then removal of IV cannula
    - Pain relief as required

7. A donor can usually be discharged the same day.
8. Medications on discharge: ferrous sulfate, analgesia.

The response of donors to pain is individual, but some discomfort around the aspiration site may be experienced for 7–10 days, and for up to four weeks in a small minority of donors.

The recipient

The BM cells are infused intravenously via the CVC according to specific guidelines for
    ABO compatibility
    ABO minor incompatibility $\Big\}$ between donor and recipient
    ABO major incompatibility
(See pages 260–262.)

BM harvest

Equipment

- BM harvest kit
- Six 30-mL syringes
- Three 10-mL syringes
- Three 2-mL syringes
- Four large-bore needles
- Three EDTA tubes

- Two bottles of tissue culture medium
- Six ampoules of heparin, 5000 units (5 mL) each

Procedure

1. Collect a specimen of PB for a WBC count (the anesthetist can collect this when cannulating) (specimen 1).
2. Prepare three 10-mL syringes with heparin, 10 000 units (10 mL) each.
3. Add 10 mL (10 000 units) of heparin to one bottle of tissue culture medium.
4. Add 10 mL (10 000 units) of heparin to a jug of saline.
5. Keep 10 mL (10 000 units) of heparin as a spare.
6. Rinse the inside of the syringes with the mixture of tissue culture medium and heparin.
7. Set up a collection stand.
8. Add 30 mL of the mixture of tissue culture medium and heparin to a collection bag.
9. Once the BM volume is 300 mL, take a specimen of BM (specimen 2).
10. Specimens 1 and 2 then go to the hematology laboratory for counts of blood and BM nucleated cells and for calculation of the BM volume that will be required to obtain 3×10^8 nucleated BM cells per kilogram of the recipient's weight.
11. Continue with the collection, adding 10 mL of the medium/heparin mixture per 100 mL of BM until the required volume is obtained.
12. During the collection, use gentle agitation to ensure that the tissue culture medium/heparin solution is being mixed with the BM. Observe the collection for clots.

If clots are detected:
- Add an additional quantity of the tissue culture medium/heparin mixture at once and
- Filter the BM to get rid of clots

If further clotting occurs, give the donor intravenous heparin, 5000 units stat (provided there are no contraindications to anticoagulation).
- Once the collection is complete, filter the BM
- Take another BM sample for a final count of nucleated cells and for microbiological testing
- Label the BM bag appropriately
- Weigh the BM bag

Obese donors

It may be difficult to reach the posterior iliac crest in a donor weighing more than 110 kg. Some trephine needles are longer than BM harvest needles, but not as stout. Giving G-CSF at 5 μg/kg SC daily for four days before BM harvest will reduce the volume of BM needed by increasing the BM nucleated cell count (stimulated BM). Giving heparin, 5000 units IV, at the beginning of the BM harvest will make the BM easier to aspirate, in addition to acting as prophylaxis against deep venous thrombosis. Additional problems and risks with obese donors:
- Increased difficulty in carrying out procedures (e.g., placement of peripheral IV cannula)
- Increased incidence of comorbidities (e.g., diabetes mellitus, arterial disease)
- Increased incidence of anesthetic complications (e.g., deep venous thrombosis)

Bone marrow cell dose

The commonly recommended "dose" of nucleated cells is expressed per kilogram of the recipient's body weight:

1. Autografts: minimum dose, 1.5×10^8 cells per kg
2. HLA-identical sibling allografts for aplastic anemia: minimum dose, 3×10^8 cells per kilogram (Storb et al., 1977)
3. HLA-identical sibling allografts for leukemia, hemoglobinopathies, and IEM dose, 2×10^8 cells per kg
4. Unrelated donor allografts: minimum dose, 3×10^8 nucleated cells per kg

Long-distance transportation of BM:

1. Marrow should be collected in a minimum of two sealed plastic bags.
2. Acid citrate dextrose (ACD) should be the only anticoagulant used, in a ratio of one part ACD to eight parts BM. (Heparin will need to be replenished during a long flight, a task that is difficult to perform aseptically.)
3. Marrow bags should be labeled with the following information:

   - Donor identification number
   - ABO and Rh types
   - Local time and date of collection
   - Name of the intended recipient
   - Name and address of the destination hospital
4. Marrow bags should be wrapped in surgical towels or water-absorbent paper towels.
5. Freezer packs should be wrapped in bubble plastic and then placed in a rigid container with insulating properties. They should line the sides and bottom of the container. Freezer packs should be changed regularly to maintain the desired temperature.

   - NEVER USE DRY ICE.
6. Marrow bags should be stacked vertically or so arranged as to be equally chilled.
7. Marrow bags should be chilled to 4–6°C and monitored by a standardized alcohol thermometer, with the temperature being checked several times during the flight. Thermometers are best placed in between wrapped BM bags (ensures that even a broken thermometer cannot pierce the BM bags).
8. The container should be labeled as follows:

   Human Bone Marrow/Stem Cells for Transplantation
   DO NOT X-RAY
   Do not freeze. Do not delay delivery

9. Samples of PB to be collected:

   - EDTA blood 5 mL
   - Clotted blood 10 mL
   - Heparinized blood 30 mL

The samples should be labeled with the following information:

- Donor identification number
- Local time and date of collection

The tubes should be placed in a plastic specimen bag and then wrapped with bubble plastic. The tubes should not be irradiated. A pair of examination gloves should be included in the transport container so that the airport security guard can examine the BM bags if required.

10. The documents accompanying the BM must contain the following information:

- Donor identification number
- Donor ABO and Rh types
- The most recently available results of the following tests: anti-HIV, HBsAg, anti-HBc, anti-HTLV-I, anti-HCV, anti-CMV, serological test for syphilis, and ALT (alanine transaminase).
- Volume of BM and diluent
- Type and amount of anticoagulant used
- Details of any BM manipulation or treatment

11. Documents required

- A permit to import quarantined material
- A letter of introduction from the director of the BM registry
- A letter of introduction from the director of the hematology department where the harvest was performed
- Signs for the BM container:

**HUMAN BONE MARROW/STEM CELLS FOR TRANSPLANTATION
DO NOT X-RAY**

Guidelines for BM courier:

1. Obtain visa, which requires

- Valid passport
- Visa application
- Photograph

2. Airline ticket/passport and visa
3. Ensure backup airline reservations
4. Foreign cash for immediate use (e.g., taxi, telephone)
5. Have contact phone/fax numbers for

- Harvest center
- Accommodations
- Transplant center

6. Bring only an overnight bag to contain

- BM container and timer
- Two thermometers
- Two surgical towels to wrap BM packs
- Eight freezer packs
- Bubble plastic (to wrap freezer packs and specimens)
- One plastic specimen bag

7. Arrange for transportation from airport to hospital on arrival with BM. Every effort must be made to ensure that the BM arrives at the transplant site within 36 hours of collection.

Although the transport of BM might seem to be a simple, straightforward process, problems can arise. The courier is responsible for ensuring that the following standards are observed:

- BM must be transported in a rigid container at 4°C (unless requested otherwise by the transplant center)
- BM must NEVER be subjected to airport X-ray screening devices. Any security check must be done by hand under direct supervision of the courier
- Alcohol must not be consumed by the courier while transporting the BM
- Immediate alternative flight reservations must be obtained to prevent any delay
- Any change in the original plans must be communicated immediately to the donor and transplant centers involved
- BM must be delivered directly to the person designated, and to no one else

When selecting a courier, the following criteria must be assessed:

1. The courier must understand the importance of the BM transport and must have the maturity to take the task seriously.
2. The courier must be an experienced traveler and in good health.
3. The courier must have a major, internationally recognized credit card.

Transfusion guidelines for BM infusion

The recipient

The BM cells are infused intravenously via a CVC according to the following specific guidelines.

ABO-compatible BM infusion

Irradiation: never

Giving set: a nonfiltered set

Compatibilities: normal saline

Transfusion rate: 150–200 mL per hour

Observations: hourly temperature, pulse, respirations, blood pressure

Storage: it is preferable to infuse the BM immediately after collection. If it is necessary to store the BM, it should be stored in the hospital blood bank

Protocol for ABO-incompatible BM infusion

1. **Major incompatibility** (A, B, or AB donor and O recipient)

Before transplant

- Deplete the marrow inoculum of red cells on a COBE 2991 cell separator or similar machine. The goal is at least 90% depletion
- If a high-titered isoagglutinin or hemolysin is detected in recipient serum against the donor's red cells, carry out plasma exchange on the recipient. Give A or B plasma after the last exchange. Repeat the test for isoagglutinin and hemolysin titers
- The goal is a hemolysin titer of 0, and an agglutinin titer of 1 or ½

Transplant

- Provide intravenous hydration with 1 L of normal saline during BM infusion, with furosemide to maintain diuresis
- Give graduated infusion of BM at 20–80 mL per hour
- Observe for signs of transfusion reaction

Posttransplant

- Transfuse with irradiated blood products of the recipient's group until engraftment occurs
- If the use of donor platelets cannot be avoided, then collect platelets that are red cell poor

2. **Minor incompatibility** (O donor and A, B, or AB recipient, or A_1 donor and A_2 recipient)

Before transplant

- If isoagglutinin is detected in donor serum directed against the recipient's red cells, deplete the BM inoculum of plasma on a COBE 2991 cell separator

Transplant

- Carry out the infusion as for an ABO-matched transplant. Observe for signs of transfusion reaction

Posttransplant

- Transfuse with irradiated group O red cells and platelets of the recipient's blood group. If the use of donor platelets cannot be avoided, then collect platelets that are plasma poor

3. **Mixed incompatibility** (A donor to B recipient, or B donor to A recipient)
    - Treat as for a major and/or minor mismatch, as appropriate
    - Deplete the BM inoculum of red cells on a COBE 2991 cell separator or other instrument
    - Determine isoagglutinin titers in donor plasma against the recipient's red cells (minor mismatch), and in recipient plasma against donor red cells (major mismatch)
    - If high-titers are present in the recipient's plasma, then carry out plasma exchange on the recipient
    - If they are present in the donor's plasma, then deplete the BM inoculum of plasma

Major ABO-incompatible BM infusion

Irradiation: never

Giving set: a nonfiltered set

Compatibilities: normal saline

Administration: commence nonfiltered infusion slowly:

- Give 20 mL/hr for the first 30 minutes
- Then give 40 mL/hr for the next 30 minutes
- Then continue at 40–80 mL/hr until completion of infusion, watching closely for any reaction
- Have epinephrine (adrenaline), hydrocortisone, and antihistamine ready in case of reaction

Observations: hourly temperature, pulse, respirations, blood pressure. Storage: it is preferable to infuse BM immediately after collection. If it is necessary to store BM, it should be stored in the hospital blood bank.

Minor ABO-incompatible BM infusion

Irradiation: never
Giving set: a nonfiltered set
Compatibilities: normal saline
Administration: commence BM infusion slowly:

- Give 60 mL/hr for the first 30 minutes
- Then give 90 mL/hr for the next 30 minutes
- Then continue at 90–100 mL/hr until completion of infusion, watching closely for any reaction
- Have epinephrine (adrenaline), hydrocortisone, and antihistamine ready in case of reaction

Observations: hourly temperature, pulse, respirations, blood pressure.
Storage: it is preferable to infuse BM immediately after collection. If it is necessary to store BM, it should be stored in the hospital blood bank.

Clinical and laboratory features of alloimmune hemolysis in BMT/SCT patients

- Clinical features
- Immediate: fever, back pain, dark urine, dyspnea
- Delayed: unexpected drop in hemoglobin within 24 days, secondary signs of hemolysis rare, but serious complication
- Laboratory features
- Positive direct Coombs test (the finding will be falsely negative if there has been complete consumption of allosensitized cells)
- Isoagglutinin directed against the infused red cells in the patient's serum and/or red cell eluate
- Mixed-field agglutination
- No compensatory reticulocytosis
- Treatment
- May resolve spontaneously, after antibody is identified, transfuse with compatible blood

Autologous BM/PB stem cell infusion

Irradiation: never
Giving set: platelet/leukocyte giving set (i.e., a nonfiltered set).
Compatibilities: normal saline.
Infusion: set up a 37°C water bath at the bedside.

- Remove the cryopreservation bags (125 mL) individually from the liquid nitrogen and place them immediately in the water bath, swirling them gently. Thaw as quickly as possible, such that the bag does not feel obviously cold

- When thawed (~2–3 minutes), remove the cap, swab the connection with methylated spirits, and immediately infuse the platelets via a platelet giving set *with no filter*
- Infuse as quickly as can be tolerated (<5–10 minutes). Slow or stop if the patient reports any adverse reactions. Recommence when the reaction has subsided. Check the bag and line for clumping
- Flush the line with saline, and then remove the next bag from the liquid nitrogen
- Do not give more than 1000 mL of cryopreserved product in a 24-hour period, to avoid dimethyl sulfoxide (DMSO) toxicity

Observations: monitor temperature, pulse, respirations, and blood pressure every 30 minutes during infusion and hourly for four hours postinfusion.

Storage: BM/blood stem cells are stored frozen in liquid nitrogen until administered.

Possible adverse reactions: nausea, coughing, vomiting, flushing, fever, dyspnea, bradycardia, hypertension, coagulopathies, chills.

Side effects: a pungent taste and smell for 24–72 hours, red-stained urine due to dyes in the cryopreservative; hematuria due to hemolysis of red cells during the cryopreservation procedure.

Premedication: acetaminophen, 650 mg PO, and hydrocortisone, 100 mg IV, or antihistamine. Have epinephrine available in case of an anaphylactic reaction to DMSO.

Fluids: give 4 L of saline/dextrose-saline over the 24-hour period following infusion.

Routine tests on BMT/SCT recipients

Test	Frequency
Full blood count; urea, Na^+, K^+, creatinine, glucose	Daily
Liver function tests; Ca^{++}, Mg, phosphate	Monday, Wednesday, Friday
PT, APTT	
Group and hold	Tuesday and Friday
Antibiotic levels	Tuesday and Friday
Levels of immunosuppressants	Monday, Wednesday, Friday (as appropriate)
Diagnosis for CMV disease	Monday, Wednesday, Friday (as appropriate)
Examination of swabs from nose, throat, catheter exit site; midstream urine	Monday, Thursday
	Weekly
For patients on TPN: Ca^{++}, Mg, phosphate	Daily
Chest X-ray	Weekly

TPN, total parenteral nutrition.

Blood bank services

Blood transfusion guidelines for BMT patients

1. All cellular blood products should be checked for the donor's CMV serological status. If the patient is CMV-negative, only CMV-negative blood products should be given. However, some centers consider this as optional, as leukocyte filtration has reduced the likelihood of transmission of CMV to a large extent.
2. All cellular blood products should be irradiated with 25 Gy (2500 rads) to inactivate lymphocytes, in order to prevent transfusion-associated GVHD.
3. All packed red cells and platelet transfusions should be filtered using leukocyte filters to minimize the risk of allosensitization and CMV transfer.
4. *There are different filters for administration of red cells and platelets:* BM and granulocyte infusions must not be put through a leukocyte filter.
5. Acellular blood products such as fresh frozen plasma, albumin, or factor concentrates do not require leukocyte filtration.

Complications of transfusion of fresh blood components

1. Hemolytic transfusion reactions (1 in 12 000 transfusions)
2. Transmission of infectious disease (see the following table)
3. Bacterial contamination of blood components (rare)
4. Alloimmunization of the recipient
5. GVHD (excluded if blood products are irradiated)
6. Febrile reactions (1 in 200 transfusions)
7. Allergic reactions (1 in 100–300 transfusions)
8. Circulatory overload
9. Iron overload (occurs after approximately 30–120 units of blood)
10. Clinically significant depletion of coagulation proteins and platelets can be a complication of massive transfusion
11. Microaggregates consisting of fibrin, white cells, and platelets can develop during storage of blood
12. Metabolic complications can occur when very large amounts of blood are transfused:
    - Hypothermia
    - Citrate toxicity
    - Acidosis
    - Alterations in potassium (hypokalemia or hyperkalemia)

Transmission of infectious disease

Disease	USA
Hepatitis A	Very rare
Hepatitis B	1/200 000
Hepatitis C	1/1 935 000
HIV-1	1/2 100 000

(cont.)

Disease	USA
HTLV-I/II	1/2 900 000
CMV, EBV	Rare
Syphilis	Very rare
Malaria	Very rare
Chagas disease	Very rare
Babesiosis	Very rare (except in endemic regions)

Trypanosomiasis very rare (except in endemic areas)

Risk estimate per unit of blood transfused, if required: testing protocol is followed; risk is different in different parts of the world.

Packed red cell transfusion

Indication: Hb <8 g/dL or <10 g/dL if patient is clinically unstable (e.g., septic)

Irradiation: yes

Giving set: all packed cells should be infused through a leukocyte filter

Transfusion: 3–4 hours per unit (unless patient is hypotensive). Storage: blood bank refrigerator at 4°C; a ward refrigerator is never suitable for storage

CMV status: check the recipient's CMV status; if it is negative or unknown, only CMV-negative blood products should be given

Premedication: some patients with a history of previous blood product reactions may benefit from hydrocortisone, 100 mg IV, with or without promethazine (Phenergan), 12.5 mg IV

Platelet transfusion

Indication	Platelet count
1. Prophylaxis	$<20 \times 10^9$/L (a higher threshold may be appropriate in the presence of sepsis, coagulopathy, asparaginase, or ATG treatment; in some instances also a lower threshold [$<10 \times 10^9$] may be indicated)
2. Invasive procedures (insertion of lines, lumbar puncture, gastroscopy with biopsy, etc.)	$<50 \times 10^9$/L
3. Active bleeding or major surgery	$<100 \times 10^9$/L

Irradiation: yes

Giving set: platelet filter

Transfusion: 20–30 minutes

Storage: store at room temperature on a "rocker" in the blood bank

PLATELETS MUST NEVER BE REFRIGERATED.

CMV status: check the recipient's CMV status; if it is negative or unknown, only CMV-negative blood products should be given.

Premedication: some patients receiving multidonor platelets may require hydrocortisone, 100 mg IV, with or without promethazine (Phenergan), 12.5 mg IV. For patients receiving single-donor platelets, premedicate only if there has been a previous reaction.

Comments

The standard of platelet transfusion is to use platelet concentrates prepared by apheresis. Platelets can be collected by apheresis from a screened volunteer or family member. An apheresis collection of platelets from a single donor will usually give the same yield as six to 10 random blood bank units. Random donor platelets should only be used in emergencies when apheresis concentrates are not available. Whenever possible, give platelets of only one blood group. If sufficient numbers are not available, use cell-compatible rather than serum-compatible platelets (e.g., group O for an A recipient, rather than AB).

Platelet refractory patients

Check for

- Anti-HLA antibodies
- Anti-platelet antibodies

Leukocyte crossmatch-negative platelet donors or HLA-matched donors can sometimes be identified through the blood bank.

To document platelet survival, measure platelet count one hour after platelet transfusion. Intravenous immunoglobulin may be useful in patients with platelet refractoriness and bleeding (Beutler, 1993).

Granulocyte transfusion

Indication: severe infection in a neutropenic patient not responding to an adequate trial of appropriate IV antibiotics. Effective in providing granulocytes to severely neutropenic patients; however, for adult patients clinical efficacy has not been shown in controlled studies (Price, 2006).

Irradiation: yes.

Giving set: a nonfiltered set.

Transfusion: 3–4 hours.

Observations: hourly temperature, pulse, respirations, blood pressure.

Storage: blood bank refrigerator at 4°C.

Premedication: may require hydrocortisone, 100 mg IV, with or without promethazine, 12.5 mg IV, to minimize reaction.

Human serum albumin

Indications: low concentration of serum albumin in an acutely ill patient who has had complications from reduced oncotic pressure; need for plasma expansion

Irradiation: no (acellular product)

Giving set: normal filtered giving set

Compatibility: compatible with normal saline only

Transfusion: 100 mL over 1 hour

Observations: no specific observations

Storage: ward refrigerator

CMV status: not relevant (acellular product)

Premedication: unnecessary

Fresh frozen plasma (FFP)

Indication: coagulopathy

Irradiation: no (acellular product)

Giving set: normal filtered giving set

Administration: FFP should be thawed in a water bath. Once thawed, it cannot be refrozen

Compatibility: compatible with normal saline only

Transfusion: one unit over 30 to 60 minutes

Observations: no specific observations

Storage: blood bank (frozen until needed)

CMV status: not relevant (acellular product)

Premedication: usually unnecessary

Total parenteral nutrition

TPN is used in BMT recipients to avoid severe malnutrition, muscle wasting, and further deterioration of immune competence.

As a direct consequence of the conditioning regimen, most patients will develop oral mucositis and enteritis. Their presence will impede ingestion and absorption of sufficient nutrients to maintain an adequate nutritional status.

TPN should commence when a patient is unable to tolerate an oral intake. It should first be reduced, and then discontinued, when the patient can demonstrate a reasonable oral nutrition intake. Indications for TPN are as follows:

- Severe mucositis with prolonged minimal oral intake (at least 7–10 days)
- Severe malnutrition at admission
- Weight loss of more than 10% during hospitalization

Guidelines

1. 2 L daily of a 25% glucose solution with amino acids. A higher concentration of glucose (e.g., 50%) is often poorly tolerated, especially when the patient is septic. The caloric requirements of TPN are calculated as 30 kcal/kg/day (35 kcal/kg/day in severe infections or other situations with increased caloric demand). The usual amino acid dose is 1.5–2 g/kg/day.

2. If a situation requiring salt restriction arises (pulmonary edema, hepatic VOD, fluid retention), the same TPN preparation, but without electrolytes, can be used.

3. If hyperglycemia occurs (common with prednisone treatment for acute GVHD), add Actrapid insulin, 10 units, to each liter bag of glucose/amino acid TPN solution if the

blood sugar level is 120 mg/dL or higher. Increase the Actrapid dose by 10 units/bag daily, until blood glucose is less than 120 mg/dL.

4. TPN solutions should only be infused through a CVC.

5. TPN supplements:

   - Twice weekly: 20% Intralipid, 500 mL (Tuesday, Saturday)
   - Weekly: vitamin K, 10 mg SC (Friday)
   - Daily: multivitamin preparation; folic acid, 5 mg IV or PO

6. Laboratory monitoring:

   - Daily: biochemistry screen, including blood glucose (in critically ill patients, check electrolytes and glucose several times daily)
   - Weekly: serum zinc; ionized calcium
   - Twice weekly: coagulation screen (PT, APTT)
   - Thrice weekly: liver function tests

7. TPN is associated with infectious and metabolic complications; thus, whenever possible, enteral nutrition should be instituted or re-instituted.

Compatibilities

- TPN can be infused concurrently with saline, glucose, potassium, Intralipid, cyclosporin, or heparin
- Intralipid can be infused with TPN, cyclosporin, or heparin only (cyclosporin and heparin are NOT compatible)

(For a review about nutrition in HSCT recipients, see Martin-Salces et al., 2008.)

Fluid balance

1. A complete daily fluid-balance chart should be kept for each BMT patient because of their propensity to retain fluid (secondary to cyclophosphamide, cyclosporin, high intake of IV fluids).

2. All oral/IV intake should be measured and recorded.

3. All output should be measured and recorded (urine, feces, and vomitus should also be tested for blood, noting whether macroscopic or microscopic).

4. Insensible loss should be recorded as 500 mL when an adult patient is afebrile, and as 800 mL when an adult patient is febrile ($\geq 38.5°C$).

5. Fluid-balance charts should be summarized at 12 midnight.

6. If the fluid-balance chart shows a fluid excess of 1 L or more and/or the patient's weight at 6 am has risen 2 kg or more, the patient should be given furosemide, 40 mg IV.

Oral hygiene

One of the most significant side effects of high-dose chemotherapy and/or radiotherapy is mucositis and/or infection of the oral cavity and/or esophagus.

Mouth care guidelines

On admission, patients should be commenced on

- Sodium bicarbonate mouthwash every 6 hours
- Chlorhexidine (0.02%) mouthwash every 6 hours

Patients should cease using a standard soft toothbrush if neutropenic and should not recommence using a toothbrush until the neutrophil count exceeds $10^9/L$ posttransplant.

Dentures are usually removed by patients, because of discomfort, and are left out for the duration of the mucositis.

Pain relief

Pain relief should be offered promptly and generously and is usually given in the following sequence:

1. Soluble paracetamol, 1–2 tablets every 4 hours, will usually be effective in the early stages when the mouth and/or esophagus become painful, or paracetamol with codeine tablets, 1–2 tablets every 4 hours, or oxycodone, 5–10 mg every 6 hours.
2. Regular doses of oral opioid every 4 hours (e.g., morphine sulfate, 10 mg/mL), absorbed through the buccal mucosa, if swallowing is painful. Alternatively, IV morphine, started at 1 mg/hr will also provide sustained pain relief. This has to be titrated according to side effects (drowsiness, feeling of being out of control) and the dose necessary for appropriate pain control.
3. Escalate oral opioid dose until efficacy is achieved, but remember that efficiency may not exceed 50% and that dose escalation beyond that point may merely increase the side effects.
4. Additional opioid doses can be given as necessary between the doses given every 4 hours.
5. Instruct the patient to avoid swallowing (e.g., expectorate saliva or use a dental suction device).
6. Try to alleviate the patient's anxiety.
7. Control concurrent nausea; ondansetron or other serotonin receptor antagonist is most effective during the conditioning regimen.
8. Additional measures: mouth washes, local anesthetics, prophylactic antifungal agents; clean teeth with sterile cotton buds.
9. Some patients experience some pain relief with the use of oral Xylocaine gel.
10. If excessive saliva secretion is a problem, the use of a dental suction device can offer relief from this annoying symptom. Atropine, 0.4 mg SC, can sometimes be helpful.

Discharge planning

Planning for discharge should begin at the time of a patient's admission. A patient can be discharged from the hospital environment when the following criteria are met:

- A neutrophil count of $10^9/L$
- No obvious signs of infection or bleeding
- Sustained oral nutrition intake of >4000 kJ (1000 kcal) daily
- Reasonable exercise tolerance
- Mastery of the dressing technique for the CVC
- No new evidence of GVHD
- No other clinical problems

Education in the use and care of the CVC for the patient and the principal family member or friend who will be providing assistance should begin as soon as possible after insertion and continued throughout hospitalization. Patients should care for their own catheters, whenever they are well enough, under the supervision of a registered nurse.

Several days before discharge, the patient should be encouraged to read the discharge information (as discussed later) and to ask questions.

On the day of discharge, the patient must be given discharge medications by the nursing staff, who will check the patient's understanding of doses and administration.

The patient should be given a five-day starter pack for care of the CVC.

The physician must go through the discharge instructions with the patient and ascertain that the patient understands how to identify problems that can arise after discharge and whom to contact for help.

Criteria for hospital readmission

1. Shaking chills and/or fever ≥38.5°C
2. Septicemia
3. Gram-negative bacteremia or fungemia
4. Uncontrolled GVHD
5. Graft failure
6. Interstitial pneumonia
7. *Varicella zoster* infection (some cases)
8. Medical emergencies/acute organ failure
9. Failure to thrive:
   - Weight loss (loss of >10% of discharge weight in an adult; loss of >5% of discharge weight in a child)
   - Fluid losses exceeding what can be replaced with maximal support

Vaccinations posttransplant

Recommendations (for recipients of autologous and allogeneic transplants):

1. **Year 1** (only inactivated vaccines, 6–12 months posttransplant, patients with active chronic GVHD may not benefit):
   - Diphtheria, pertussis, tetanus toxoid (DPT), or DT (for adults) (repeat at 14 and 24 months)
   - *H. influenzae* (Hib) conjugate (repeat at 14 and 24 months)
   - Hepatitis B (for adults with risk factors or in countries where universal vaccination is recommended, may be given earlier in special situations) repeat at 14 and 24 months
   - Influenza (annually, lifelong seasonal administration beginning six months Posttransplant)
   - Inactivated poliovirus (repeat at 14 and 24 months) (verify response with serum titers)
   - Pneumococcal vaccine (polysaccharide-based and conjugate vaccines available, in some patients poor responses); begin pneumococcal vaccination 3–6 months posttransplant, give three doses of PPV-13, consider PPV-23 for fourth dose), repeat vaccination at 5 years
2. **Year 2** (only for patients free of chronic GVHD and immune suppressive treatment):
   - Measles, mumps, rubella (MMR)

3. Family members

- No live attenuated poliovirus during year 1 (if the Sabin oral polio vaccine is given to family infants within the first year posttransplant, the marrow graft or stem cell recipient should be isolated from the infant because live virus can be shed for up to 8–12 weeks)

Comment: attenuated varicella vaccine can be given 24 months after transplant if patient is immunocompetent; attenuated zoster vaccine is considered contraindicated (lack of data)

Meningococcal conjugate vaccine may be used 6–12 months posttransplant, as in the general population

(Modified from Antin, 2002; Ljungman et al., 2005, Tomblyn et al., 2009.)

- This should be discussed with an expert
- Current vaccination issues are reviewed by Forlenza & Small (2012)

Useful formulas

Surface area

Most nomograms are based on the Du Bois (1916) formula:

$$SA = H^{0.725} \times W^{0.425} \times 0.2025$$

where SA is surface area in square meters, H is height in meters, and W is weight in kilograms.

Creatinine clearance rate

$$\frac{140 - age\ of\ patient(years)}{814 \times serum\ creatinine(mmol/L)} mL/min/kg$$

Methods for converting units of measure
WBC and platelet counts

$$n \times 10^9 L = \times 1000\ cells/mm^3 (or\ cells/mL)$$

Therefore, to convert counts in cells per cubic millimeter or cells per microliter (μL) to units of 10^9/L, divide by 1000. For example, a WBC count of 4600 cells/mm^3 (or cells/μL) = 4.6 × 10^9/L. Platelets: 240,000 cells/mm^3 (or cells/μL) = 240 × 10^9/L.

Hemoglobin

$$1\ g/dL = 10\ g/L$$

There are 10 deciliters (dL) per liter (L); therefore, values expressed as grams per liter must be divided by 10. For example, a hemoglobin (Hb) concentration of 120 g/L = 12 g/dL.

Creatinine

To convert micromoles per liter (μmol/L) to milligrams per deciliter (mg/dL), multiply by 0.0113. For example,

$$100\ \mu mol/L = 100 \times 0.0113 = 1.1\ mg/dL$$

Bilirubin

To convert micromoles per liter (μmol/L) to milligrams per deciliter (mg/dL), multiply by 0.058. For example:

$$20 \ \mu mol/L = 20 \times 0.058 = 1.16 \ mg/dL$$

Albumin

$$1 \ g/dL = 10 \ g/L$$

Therefore to convert albumin from grams per liter (g/L) to grams per deciliter (g/dL), divide by 10. For example:

$$35 \ g/L = 3.5 \ g/dL$$

Radiation dose

$$1 \ Gy = 100 \ rad$$
$$100 \ cGy = 100 \ rad$$
$$100 \ cGy = 1 \ Gy$$
$$1 \ cGy = 1 \ rad$$

Therefore, to convert rads or centigrays (cGy) to grays (Gy), divide by 100. For example:

$$858 \ rad = 858 \ cGy = 8.58 \ Gy$$

Height and weight

Height

$$1 \ foot \ (ft) = 30.48 \ centimeters \ (cm)$$
$$1 \ inch \ (in.) = 2.54 \ centimeters \ (cm)$$

For example, to convert 5 ft. 10 in. (5' 10") to centimeters:

$$(5\times30.48) + (10\times2.54) = 152.4 + 25.4 = 177.8 \ cm$$

Weight

$$1 \ pound(1b) = 0.4536 \ kilogram(kg)$$

Therefore,

$$160 \ 1b = 160\times0.4536 = 72.6 \ kg$$

Nomograms for calculation of body surface area

A

Nomogram for determining body surface area for adults from height and mass

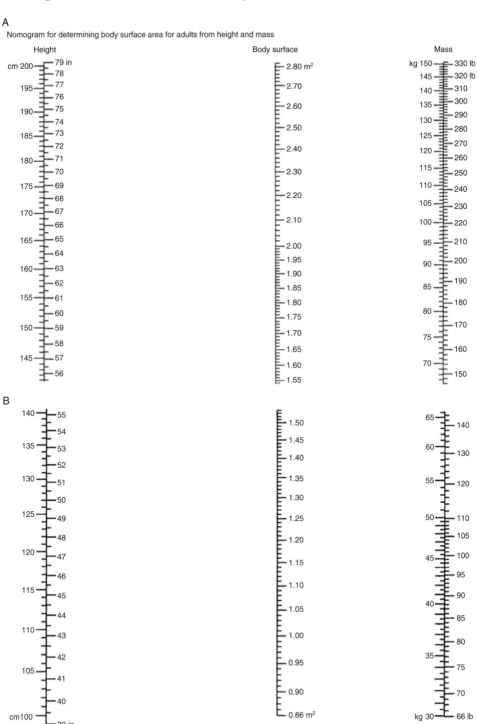

Karnofsky performance score

	%	
Able to carry on normal activity; no special care is needed	100	Normal; no complaints; no evidence of disease
	90	Able to carry on normal activity; minor signs or symptoms of disease
	80	Normal activity with effort; some signs or symptoms of disease
Unable to work; able to live at home and care for most personal needs; varying amounts of assistance are needed	70	Cares for self; unable to carry on normal activity or to do active work
	60	Requires occasional assistance but is able to care for most needs
	50	Requires considerable assistance and frequent medical care
Unable to care for self; requires equivalent of institutional or hospital care; disease may be progressing rapidly	40	Disabled; requires special care and assistance
	30	Severely disabled; hospitalization indicated, although death not imminent
	20	Very sick; hospitalization necessary
	10	Moribund; fatality progresses rapidly
	0	Dead

ECOG/WHO performance status

Summary	Score	Description
Normal activity	0	Fully active; able to carry out all predisease activities without restriction and without the aid of analgesia
Symptoms, but ambulatory	1	Restricted in strenuous activity, but ambulatory and able to carry out light work or pursue a sedentary occupation; patients who are fully active but require analgesia
In bed <50% of time	2	Ambulatory and capable of self-care, but unable to carry out any work; up and about more than 50% of waking hours
In bed >50% of time	3	Capable of only limited self-care; confined to bed or chair more than 50% of waking hours
100% bedridden	4	Completely disabled; unable to carry out any self-care, and confined totally to bed or chair
Dead	5	Dead

Lansky play scale (for children)

The Lansky play performance scale for children is designed to provide a standardized measure of the performance status of the child with cancer and is appropriate for use with children aged 1–16 years.

Parents are asked to select the description that best describes the child's play during the past week, averaging out good days and bad days:

100	–	Fully active, normal
90	–	Minor restrictions in physically strenuous activity
80	–	Active, but tires more quickly
70	–	Both greater restriction of and less time spent in play activity
60	–	Up and around, but minimal active play; keeps busy with quieter activities
50	–	Gets dressed, but lies around much of the day; no active play; able to participate in all quiet play and activities
40	–	Mostly in bed; participates in quiet activities
30	–	In bed; needs assistance even for quiet play
20	–	Often sleeping; play entirely limited to very passive activities
10	–	No play; does not get out of bed
0	–	Unresponsive

Grading organ toxicity after BMT (Seattle criteria, 1988)

Toxicity	Grade I	Grade II	Grade III
Cardiac	Mild ECG abnormality not requiring medical intervention; or noted heart enlargement on chest radiograph, with no clinical symptoms	Moderate ECG abnormalities requiring and responding to medical intervention; requiring continuous monitoring without treatment; or congestive heart failure responsive to digitalis or diuretics	Severe ECG abnormalities with no response or only a partial response to medical intervention; heart failure with no response or only a minor response to intervention; or a decrease in voltage by more than 50%
Bladder	Macroscopic hematuria after two days from last chemotherapy, not caused by infection, with no subjective symptoms of cystitis	Macroscopic hematuria after seven days from last chemotherapy, not caused by infection; or hematuria after two days, with subjective symptoms of cystitis, not caused by infection	Hemorrhagic cystitis with frank blood, necessitating invasive local intervention, with instillation of sclerosing agents, nephrostomy, or other surgical procedure

(cont.)

Toxicity	Grade I	Grade II	Grade III
Renal	Increase in creatinine up to twice the baseline value (usually the last recorded before the start of conditioning)	Increase in creatinine above twice baseline, but not requiring dialysis	Requirement of dialysis
Pulmonary	Dyspnea without chest radiographic changes, not caused by infection or congestive heart failure; or chest radiographic findings of isolated infiltrate or mild interstitial changes without symptoms, not caused by infection or congestive heart failure	Chest radiographic findings of extensive localized infiltrate or moderate interstitial changes combined with dyspnea and not caused by infection or congestive heart failure; decrease in Po_2 ($>10\%$ from baseline) not requiring mechanical ventilation or 50% on mask, and not caused by infection or congestive heart failure	Interstitial changes requiring mechanical ventilatory support or $>50\%$ oxygen on mask, and not caused by infection or congestive heart failure
Hepatic	Mild hepatic dysfunction with bilirubin ≥2.0 mg/dL and <6.0 mg/dL; weight gain $>2.5\%$ and $<5\%$ from baseline, of noncardiac origin; or SGOT increase >2-fold but <5-fold from lowest value preconditioning	Moderate hepatic dysfunction with bilirubin >6 mg/dL and <20 mg/dL; SGOT increase >5-fold from preconditioning; clinical ascites or imaging-documented ascites >100 mL; or weight gain $>5\%$ from baseline, of noncardiac origin	Severe hepatic dysfunction with bilirubin >20 mg/dL; hepatic encephalopathy; or ascites compromising respiratory function
CNS	Somnolence, but patient is easily aroused and is oriented after arousal	Somnolence, with confusion after arousal; or other new objective CNS symptoms, with no loss of consciousness, not more easily explained by other medication, bleeding or CNS infection	Seizures or coma not explained by other medication, CNS infection, or bleeding
Stomatitis	Pain or ulceration not requiring a continuous IV narcotic drug	Pain or ulceration requiring a continuous IV narcotic drug (morphine drip)	Severe ulceration or mucositis requiring preventive intubation or resulting in documented aspiration pneumonia, with or without intubation

(cont.)

Toxicity	Grade I	Grade II	Grade III
Gastrointestinal	Watery stools >500 mL but <2000 mL every day, not related to infection	Watery stools >2000 mL every day, not related to infection; macroscopic hemorrhagic stools with no effect on cardiovascular status, not caused by infection; or subileus not related to infection	Ileus requiring nasogastric suction or surgery and not related to infection; or hemorrhagic enterocolitis affecting cardiovascular status and requiring transfusion

Note: Grade IV regimen-related toxicity is defined as fatal.

Special aspects of haploidentical BMT/SCT

Definition

Haploidentical SCT is by definition a mismatched transplantation. A parent or a child or a partially matched sibling can be considered as a donor for a haploidentical SCT, which results in a 5/10 antigen match. In the absence of special conditioning protocols, a haploidentical SCT usually results in the development of a hyperacute GVH reaction or disease with massive cytokine release, and frequent rejection of the transplant.

Indications

In a consensus meeting, recommendations were made about the eligibility criteria, the graft composition, the timing, and the conditioning for haploidentical SCT (Champlin et al., 2002). Eligible patients should be younger than 55 years old and should lack an HLA-identical related or unrelated donor. The following diagnoses are to be considered:

- AML, refractory, in first relapse, in first remission at high risk of relapse
- ALL, in second or later remission, in first remission with high-risk cytogenetic features

Ineligible are patients with end-stage disease or active bacterial or fungal infections. The decision to proceed with a haploidentical transplant should be made early (within two or three months after diagnosis). A very high dose of CD34-positive PB stem cells should be given ($\geq 10^7$/kg) and the graft should be depleted of T-cells (below 10^5 $CD3^+$ cells/kg). Most experts recommend conditioning to include TBI. Posttransplant prophylaxis against GVHD is not universally recommended as the rates of opportunistic infections are considerably higher than with other allogeneic transplant procedures.

Advantages and disadvantages of haploidentical SCT

The advantages and disadvantages of haploidentical transplants are summarized in the following table:

Advantages	Disadvantages
Donor readily available Availability of donor for subsequent DLI High CD34$^+$ cell doses available Potential for graft engineering (e.g., add back immune cells for CMV or tumor-associated antigens).	High TRM, poor immune recovery and frequent posttransplant opportunistic infections, especially viral reactivation
(Modified from Spitzer, 2005 and Marks et al., 2006.)	

Haploidentical stem cell transplantation should be performed only at centers familiar with high-risk transplantations. Different centers use a variety of conditioning regimens generally including TBI, T-cell depletion, and a high dose of stem cells.

The outline of two different protocols for haploidentical transplantation is reproduced as follows:

Perugia protocol for haploidentical SCT (Aversa et al., 2005)

Day 9: 8 Gy TBI (lungs shielded to receive 4 Gy)
Days 8 and 7: thiotepa (5 mg/kg daily IV)
Days 7, 6, 5, 4, 3: fludarabine (40 mg/m^2 daily IV)
Days 5, 4, 3, 2: ATG or thymoglobuline (IV)
Day 0: CD34-selected CD2-depleted PB progenitor cells are given

Johns Hopkins protocol for reduced-intensity haploidentical BMT (Brunstein et al., 2011)

Days 6 and 5: cyclophosphamide (14.5 mg/kg daily IV)
Days 6, 5, 4, 3, 2: fludarabine (30 mg/m^2 daily IV)
Day 1: 2 Gy TBI
Day 0: BM infusion
Day +3 and +4: cyclophosphamide (50 mg/kg IBW daily IV)

Outcomes in different diseases

The outcomes vary according to disease, disease status, patient age, and other risk factors. In a series of 61 high-risk ALL patients, an OS of 21.5% at a median follow-up of 42 months was reported (Marks et al., 2006). In a large series combining patients with ALL and AML, an OS of 19% at five years was reported (Mehta et al., 2004). In this series about half of the patients had transplants from parents or children, the rest had mismatched sibling transplants. The poor outcomes in this series were mainly caused by patients transplanted with florid, uncontrolled leukemia. In these and other series, patients who survived the acute complications and became tolerant of the haploidentical graft, had a chance of long-term survival and cure not different from other high-risk transplants. In a study from Italy, 104 patients with high-risk leukemia (67 AML and 37 ALL) received a haploidentical transplant (Aversa et al., 2005). The conditioning involved TBI, thiotepa, fludarabine, and ATG. PB progenitor cells were mobilized with recombinant human G-CSF and depleted of T-cells using $CD34^+$ cell selection. No posttransplantation GVHD prophylaxis was administered. A total of 100 among the 101 assessable patients engrafted. Acute GVHD developed in eight of 100 patients, and chronic GVHD in five of 70 assessable patients. Thirty-eight patients died of nonleukemic causes (27 from infections, mainly viral but also fungal or bacterial; 11 from other transplant-associated complications like interstitial pneumonia, GVHD or CNS toxicity). Relapse occurred in nine of 66 patients receiving transplantation in remission and in 17 of 38 receiving transplantation in relapse. Median follow-up of the 40 patients who survived event-free was 22 months (range, 1–65 months). EFS (± standard deviation) rate was 48% ± 8% and 46% ± 10%, respectively, for the 42 AML and 24 ALL patients receiving transplantation in remission. The Kaplan–Meier plot of EFS for these patients is shown in the following figure.

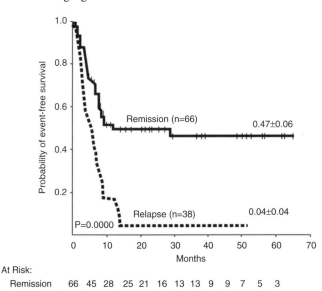

EFS of patients with high-risk leukemia who received a haploidentical SCT. The upper curve shows patients transplanted in remission; the lower curve shows patients transplanted at relapse. (Reproduced with permission from Aversa et al., 2005.)

Recent developments

According to some studies, a mismatch of the KIR and its ligand enhances the immune reactivity of NK cells and this translates into a lower relapse rate in haploidentical transplants. KIRs recognize groups of Class HLA1 alleles. If there is a mismatch in the donor versus recipient direction, the NK cells of the donor (in the situation of maximum immunosuppression) will exert anti-leukemia activity (details are given on page 221). Several newer protocols have been developed which use high-dose immunosuppression but lower-dose chemotherapy (non-myeloablative conditioning). The BMT CTN initiated a study where haploidentical transplants after RIC are compared with double umbilical cord transplants (Brunstein et al., 2011). Some data also show that fetomaternal microchimerism reduced transplant-associated mortality by decreasing the severity of acute GVHD (Spitzer, 2005). Reisner et al. (2011) recently reviewed outcomes and challenges of haploidentical hematopoietic transplantation. The problems of haploidentical transplantation and potential solutions are summarized in the following table.

Problems of haploidentical transplantation and potential solutions

Problems	Current or potential solutions
Graft failure	Megadoses of CD34$^+$ donor cells, immunosuppressive conditioning regimens, selective myeloablative conditioning
Refractory GVHD	Maximal donor cell immune suppression, T-cell depletion of donor graft, co-stimulatory of donor graft, i.e., CTLA-4 blockade
Delayed immune reconstitution	Cytokine manipulation, adoptive cellular immunotherapy, use of non-alloreactive CTLs
Decreased GVT effect	Use of NK-alloreactive donors, expansion of KIR epitope mismatched NK cells

(Modified from Lazarus et al., 2003.)

General points on the administration of cytotoxic drugs

Regarding guidelines for safe handling of antineoplastic agents, see Clinical Oncological Society of Australia (1983) and Connor et al. (2006).

Administration

Check the instructions for individual drugs as to how best they can be given. Vesicant drugs should be injected into the side arm of a fast-running drip, with frequent drawing back of the syringe to check for free return of blood up the tubing. Cannulas used for vesicant drugs should be freshly placed at a secure site. If any pain occurs during administration, discontinue immediately. Where possible, avoid giving vesicant drugs into cannulas placed in the elbow, the wrist, or the back of the hand. Avoid limbs with impaired circulation. Extravasation of those sites poses greater risk for causing extensive damage to nerves and tendons. Whenever possible, central lines are preferred for the administration of vesicant drugs.

Extravasation

The following drugs can cause potentially severe reactions if they extravasate (Ener et al., 2004):

- Daunorubicin/doxorubicin: severe ulceration and soft tissue loss
- Mitomycin C: severe local reactions and soft tissue loss
- Nitrogen mustard: severe local reactions
- Vincristine/vinblastine: local reactions that can be very painful
- Dacarbazine: local reactions

In cases of extravasation, proceed as follows:

1. Aspirate the drug from the vein, and instill antidote:
   - For daunorubicin/doxorubicin, give 5 mL of 8.4% sodium bicarbonate. Apply 100% DMSO topically four times per day for 1 week and then twice per day for 1 week.
   - For mustine, instill 2–4 mL of 10% sodium thiosulfate intravenously (in the area of extravasation); later inject 0.1 mL doses subcutaneously several times over next 3–4 hours.
   - For vinca alkaloids, instill 5 mL of 8.4% sodium bicarbonate or 1 mL of hyaluronidase (150 U/mL), then give 1 mL of hyaluronidase subcutaneously; can be repeated several times over next 3–4 hours.
2. Remove the needle. Use cold compresses for all drugs except vinca alkaloids. Use cold packs for 6–10 hours for anthracyclines. Use hot compresses for vinca alkaloids.
3. Apply hyaluronidase or 1% hydrocortisone cream.
4. Mark the edges of any tissue reaction, and photograph the area.
5. Apply firm dressings/bandage and elevate the affected area.
6. Seek early plastic surgery consultation regarding surgical debridement.

In 2007, the FDA approved the drug dexrazone hydrochloride for the treatment of extravasation resulting from intravenous anthracycline chemotherapy. Dexrazoxane is a cyclic derivative of EDTA. The first dose (1000 mg/m^2) should be given as early as possible (within six hours) by intravenous infusion (over 1–2 hours) through a different venous access. The treatment should be repeated at 24 (1000 mg/m^2) and 48 hours (500 mg/m^2). The maximum daily dose is 2000 mg on days 1 and 2 and 1000 mg on day 3. Dexrazoxan has itself cytotoxic properties; therefore, in patients receiving anthracyclines, additional cytotoxicity (leukopenia, thrombocytopenia) may occur. Dexrazoxan is mainly eliminated by the kidneys. A transient increase in liver enzymes may occur. DMSO (see earlier) should not be used in patients who receive dexrazoxane to treat anthracycline-associated extravasation.

Conditioning regimens
Autologous transplantation
Lymphoma

Regimen	Total (TD) or daily dose (DD) administered
CBV	Cyclophosphamide, 4.8–7.2 g/m^2 (TD) d –5, –4, –3, –2 Carmustine (BCNU), 300–600 mg/m^2 (TD) d –8, –7, –6 Etoposide, 750–2,400 mg/m^2 (TD) d –8, –7, –6
BEAC	Carmustine, 300 mg/m^2 (TD) (over 1 d) Etoposide, 600–800 mg/m^2 (TD) (over 4 d) Cytarabine, 600–800 mg/m^2 (TD) (over 4 d) Cyclophosphamide, 140 mg/kg or 6 g/m^2 (TD) (over 4 d)
BEAM	Carmustine (BCNU), 300 mg/m^2 d –6 (TD) Etoposide, 400–800 mg/m^2 d –5, –4, –3, –2 (TD) Cytarabine, 800–1600 mg/m^2 d –5, –4, –3, –2 (TD) Melphalan, 140 mg/m^2 d –6 (TD)
CY-TBI	Cyclophosphamide, 120–200 mg/kg TBI, 800–1320 cGy
VP-16/CY/TBI (intensified regimen)	Etoposide, 60 mg/kg or 750 mg/m^2 d –4 Cyclophosphamide, 100–120 mg/kg, d –6, –5 TBI, 1200–1375 cGy, d –3, –2, –1
E-M-TBI	Etoposide 60 mg/kg, d –3 Melphalan, 140 mg/m^2, d –2 TBI, 500 cGy, d0

Leukemia

Regimen	Total dose (TD) or daily dose (DD) administered
Bu/CY2	Busulfan, 4 mg/kg/d PO for 4 days Alternatively 3.2 mg/kg/d IV for 4 days Cyclophosphamide, 60 mg/kg/d for 2 days
Bu-MEL	Busulfan, 4 mg/kg/d PO for 4 days Melphalan, 140 mg/m^2
CY-TBI	Cyclophosphamide, 60 mg/kg/d for 2 days TBI, 800–1200 cGy
IV-BU-FLU	Fludarabine 40 mg/m^2 daily for 4 days (d –6, –5, –4, –3) IV busulfan 130 mg/m^2 daily for 4 days (d –6, –5, –4, –3) ± ATG 0.5 mg/kg on day –3, 1.5 mg/kg on day –2 and 2.0 mg/kg on day –1

Myeloma (see also p. 122)

Regimen	Total dose administered
Melphalan	Melphalan, 100 mg/m^2/d for 2 days
Melphalan/Total − body irradiation(TBI)	Melphalan, 140 mg/m^2 for 1 day TBI, 850 cGy
Bu/CY2/E	Busulfan, 4 mg/kg/d PO for 4 days (d −8, −7, −6, −5) (AUC < 1600) Cyclophosphamide, 60 mg/kg/d for 2 days (d −3, −2) Etoposide, 10 mg/kg/d, for 3 days (d −4, −3, −2)

Testicular cancer

Regimen A (Miki et al., 2007)

- ICE
- Etoposide, 250 mg/m^2 IV daily for 5 days (4-hour infusion)
- Ifosfamide, 1500 mg/m^2 IV daily for 5 days (6-hour infusion), plus mesna (bolus IV 300 mg/m^2 every 8 hours, days 1–5)
- Carboplatin, 250 mg/m^2 IV daily for 5 days (6-hour infusion)

Regimen B (tandem) (Einhorn et al., 2007)

- Cycle 1
- Etoposide, 750 mg/m^2/d on days −5, −4, −3
- Carboplatin, 700 mg/m^2 on days −5, −4, −3
- Cycle 2
- Etoposide, 750 mg/m^2/d on days −5, −4, −3
- Carboplatin, 700 mg/m^2 on days −5, −4, −3

Each cycle is supported by infusion of autologous stem cells (harvest enough cells for each transplant before the first transplant); give Cycle 2 after recovery from the toxicity of Cycle 1. Regimen C (Motzer et al., 2007)

- Etoposide, 600 mg/m^2 IV daily for 3 days (1-hour infusion) days 1, 2, 3
- Cyclophosphamide 50 mg/kg IV daily for 4 days (with mesna) days 1, 2, 3
- Carboplatin, 600 mg/m^2 IV daily for 3 days (1-hour infusion) days 1, 2, 3

These agents are followed by infusion of autologous stem cells on day 5.

Allogeneic transplantation (myeloablative)

Definition of myeloablative transplant:

- Myeloablative conditioning regimen: regimens with TBI single doses of ≥500 cGy, or fractionated doses totaling ≥800 cGy, busulfan doses of >9 mg/kg, or melphalan doses of >150 mg/m^2 given either as single agents or in combination with other drugs. (operational definition used by CIBMTR)

HLA-identical sibling transplant.

Hematologic malignancy

1. BU/CY
   - Busulfan, 4 mg/kg/d for 3.5 to 4 days (PO); alternatively 3.2 mg/kg/d IV for 4 days
   - Cyclophosphamide, 60 mg/kg/d for 2 days
2. CY/TBI
   - Cyclophosphamide, 60 mg/kg/d for 2 days d –6, d –5
   - TBI, 12 to 14.4 Gy (one common protocol uses TBI 2 Gy twice daily for 3 days or 2 Gy once daily for 6 days), d –3, –2, –1

A CY/TBI regimen can be used in preference to a chemotherapy-only regimen for patients with

- CNS involvement
- prior exposure to family member blood products
- CLL/NHL

Recently, Gupta et al. (2011) performed a meta-analysis of studies and publications comparing BU/CY with CY/TBI for the conditioning of patients with leukemia. CY/TBI has a modest but not significant advantage in that all cause mortality and relapse of leukemia. In most studies, the TRM was lower with CY/TBI, but due to later complications, no significant survival advantage was observed. Since the randomized studies which Gupta reviewed were performed before the availability of intravenous busulfan, the advantages and disadvantages of similar conditioning regimens may be different in 2012.

Severe aplastic anemia

1. CY-ATG: cyclophosphamide, 50 mg/kg/d (4 doses) (days –5, –4, –3, –2) with or without ATG (horse), 30 mg/kg/d (3 doses, on days –5, –4, –3)

Thalassemia major

The following protocols are currently used for BMT in Class 1, 2, and 3 thalassemia patients (page 184)

Bu/Cy	Busulfan 14–16 mg/kg (total dose over 4 days) given PO every 6 hours (days –9, –8, –7, –6)
	Cyclophosphamide 200 mg/kg (total dose over 4 days) given IV in 1 hour (days –5, –4, –3, and –2)

HLA-partially identical family member transplant or HLA-identical unrelated donor transplant

- CY/TBI: cyclophosphamide, 60 mg/kg/d for 2 days, and TBI, 10–13 Gy

Allogeneic transplantation (reduced-intensity and non-myeloablative)

Definition of a reduced-intensity regimen

- Regimens with lower doses of TBI, fractionated radiation therapy, busulfan, and melphalan than those used to define a myeloablative conditioning regimen (operational definition of CIBMTR)

Regimen	Total or daily dose administered
TBI/fludarabine (Seattle)	TBI, 2 Gy d 0 Fludarabine 30 mg/m^2/d, d −4, d −3, d −2
Fludara/Bu/ATG	Fludarabine 30 mg/m^2/d, d −10, −9, −8, −7, −6, −5 Busulfan 4 mg/kg PO (alternatively 3.2 mg/kg IV)/d, d −5, d −4 ± ATG 10 mg/kg/d, d −4, −3, −2, −1
Fludara/Mel (MDACC, Houston, Popat et al., 2012)	Fludarabine 25–30 mg/m^2/d, for 4–5 days Melphalan 100–140 mg/m^2 ± ATG
Fludara/Mel/alemtuzumab (United Kingdom)	Fludarabine 30 mg/m^2/d, for 5 days Melphalan 140 mg/m^2 Alemtuzumab 20 mg/d, for 5 days
Clofarabine/ Mel (Kirschbaum et al., 2012)	Clofarabine 40 mg/m^2/d, for 5 days Melphalan 100 mg/m^2
FLAMSA-RIC (Munich, Schmid et al., 2008)	Fludarabine 30 mg/m^2/d for 4 days Cytarabine 2 g/m^2/d for 4 days Amsacrine 100 mg/m^2/d for 4 days 3 days rest, then Cyclophosphamide 40–60 mg/kg for 2 days TBI, 4 Gy ATG 10–20 mg/kg for 3 days
FLAMSA-MEL (Saure et al., 2012)	Fludarabine 30 mg/m^2/d for 4 days Cytarabine 2 g/m^2/d for 4 days Amsacrine 100 mg/m^2/d for 4 days 2–3 days rest, then Melphalan 100–200 mg/m^2 ATG 10–20 mg/kg for 3 days

When to choose a myeloablative or reduced-intensity regimen?

Patients who are frail, have significant comorbidities or are older than 55 years are often considered for reduced-intensity protocols. These protocols are also designated as reduced-toxicity protocols. The question has been raised: is RIC the new standard of care for older adults (McClune and Weisdorf, 2010)? The impression from published case series and registry data is that early toxicity and mortality using reduced-intensity protocols is less than with classical myeloablative protocols, but in the long run, these protocols may have less anti-leukemia activity. At present, there is no rigorous comparison between myeloablative and reduced-intensity protocols for patients in good performance status; for example, between the ages 50 and 60 years. The expert opinion is that patients should be enrolled in studies and that conditioning regimens need to be tailored to each patient, his/her disease characteristics and comorbidities. Reduced-toxicity protocols may serve as a platform for posttransplant immunotherapy.

References and further reading

Antin JH. 2002. Long-term care after hematopoietic cell transplantation in adults. *N Engl J Med* **347**: 36–42.

Arfons LM & Lazarus HM. 2005. Total parenteral nutrition and hematopoietic stem cell transplantation: an expensive placebo? *Bone Marrow Transplant* **36**: 281–288.

Aversa F, Terenzi A, Tabilio A, et al. 2005. Full haplotype-mismatched hematopoietic stem-cell transplantation: a phase II study in patients with acute leukemia at high risk of relapse. *J Clin Oncol* **23**: 3447–3454.

Barrett AJ & Savani BN. 2006. Stem cell transplantation with reduced-intensity conditioning regimens: a review of ten years experience with new transplant concepts and new therapeutic agents. *Leukemia* **20**: 1661–1672.

Beutler E. 1993. Red Cross Recommendations. *Blood* **81**: 1411–13.

Brunstein CG, Fuchs EJ, Carter SL, et al. 2011. Alternative donor transplantation after reduced intensity conditioning: results of parallel phase 2 trials using partially HLA-mismatched related bone marrow or unrelated double umbilical cord blood grafts. *Blood* **118**: 282–288.

Cashen AF, Lazarus HM, Devine SM. 2003. Mobilizing stem cells from normal donors: is it possible to improve upon G-CSF? *Bone Marrow Transplant* **39**: 577–588.

Champlin R, Hesdorffer C, Lowenberg B, et al. 2002. Consensus recommendations: haploidentical 'megadose' stem cell transplantation in acute leukemia: recommendations for a protocol agreed upon at the Perugia and Chicago meetings. *Leukemia* **16**: 427–428.

Clinical Oncological Society of Australia. 1983. Guidelines and recommendations for the safe handling of antineoplastic agents. *Med J Aust* **1**: 425.

Connor TH & Mcdiarmid MA. 2006. Preventing occupational exposures to antineoplastic drugs in health care settings. *CA Cancer J Clin* **56**: 354–365.

Einhorn LH, Williams SD, Chamness A, et al. 2007. High-dose chemotherapy and stem cell rescue for metastatic germ-cell tumors. *N Engl J Med* **357**: 340–348.

Ener RA, Meglathery SB, & Styler M. 2004. Extravasation of systemic hematooncologic therapies. *Ann Oncol* **15**: 858–862.

Forlenza CJ & Small TN. 2012. Live (vaccines) from New York. doi: 1038bmt.2012.141.

Gupta T, Kannan S, DantkaleV, et al. 2011. Cyclophosphamide plus total body irradiation compared with busulfan plus cyclophosphamide as a conditioning regimen prior to hematopoietic stem cell transplantation in patients with leukemia: a systematic review and meta-analysis. *Hematol Oncol Stem Cell Ther* **4**: 17–29.

Jantunen E & Lemoli RM. 2012. Preemptive use of plerixafor in difficult-to-mobilize patients: an emerging concept. *Transfusion* **52**: 904–914.

Jones HM, Jones SA, Watts MJ, et al. 1994. Development of a simplified single-apheresis approach for PB progenitor cell transplantation in previously treated patients with lymphoma. *J Clin Oncol* **12**: 1693–1702.

Karanes C, Nelson GO, Chitphakdithai P, et al. 2008. Twenty years of unrelated donor hematopoietic cell transplantation for adult recipients facilitated by the National Marrow Donor Program. *Biol Blood Marrow Transplant* **14**: 8–15.

Kessinger A & Sharp JG. 2003. The whys and hows of hematopoietic progenitor and stem cell mobilization. *Bone Marrow Transplant* **31**: 319–329.

Kirschbaum MH, Stein AS, Popplewell L, et al. 2012. A phase I study in adults of clofarabine combined with high-dose melphalan as reduced-intensity conditioning for allogeneic transplantation. *Biol Blood Marrow Transplant* **18**: 432–440.

Klepin HD & Hurd DD. 2006. Autologous transplantation in elderly patients with multiple myeloma: are we asking the right questions? *Bone Marrow Transplant* **38**: 585–592.

Lazarus HM & Rowe JM. 2003. Haploidentical stem cell transplantation. In Laughlin MJ & Lazarus HM eds. *Allogeneic Stem Cell Transplantation Clinical Research and Practice*. Totowa, NJ: Humana Press, pp. 117–128.

Ljungman P, Engelhard D, de la Cámara R, et al. 2005. Vaccination of stem cell transplant recipients: recommendations of the Infectious Diseases Working Party of The EBMT. *Bone Marrow Transplant* **35**: 737–746.

Marks DI, Aversa F, & Lazarus HM. 2006. Alternative donor transplants for adult acute lymphoblastic leukaemia: a comparison of the three major options. *Bone Marrow Transplant* **38**: 467–475.

Martin-Salces M, de Pat R, Canales MA, et al. 2008. Nutritional recommendations in hematopoietic stem cell transplantation. *Nutrition* **24**: 769–775.

McClune BL & Weisdorf DJ. 2010. Reduced intensity conditioning allogeneic stem cell transplantation for older adults: is it the standard of care? *Curr Opin Hematol* **17**: 133–138.

Mehta J, Mehta J, Singhal S, et al. 2004. Bone marrow transplantation from partially HLA-mismatched donors for acute leukemia: single center experience of 201 patients. *Bone Marrow Transplant* **33**: 389–397.

Miki T, Mizutani Y, Akaza H, et al. 2007. Long-term results of first line sequential high-dose carboplatin, etoposide and ifosfamide chemotherapy with peripheral blood stem cell support for patients with advanced testicular germ cell tumor. *Int J Urol* **14**: 54–59.

Mineishi S. 2011. Overcoming the age barrier in hematopoietic stem cell transplantation. *JAMA* **306**: 1918–1920.

Motzer RJ, Nichols CJ, Margolin KA, et al. 2007. Phase III randomized trial of conventional dose chemotherapy with or without high-dose chemotherapy and autologous hematopoietic stem-cell rescue as first-line treatment for patients with poor prognosis metastatic germ cell tumors. *J Clin Oncol* **25**: 247–256.

Popat U, de Lima MJ, Saliba RM, et al. 2012. Long-term outcome of reduced-intensity allogeneic hematopoietic SCT in patients with AML in CR. *Bone Marrow Transplant* **47**: 212–216.

Price TH. 2006. Granulocyte transfusion therapy. *J Clin Apher* **21**: 65–71.

Reisner Y, Hagin D, & Martelli MF. 2011. Haploidentical hematopoietic transplantation: current status and future perspectives. *Blood* **118**: 6006–6017.

Rowley SD. 1992. Hematopoietic stem cell cryopreservation: a review of current techniques. *J Hematother* **1**: 233–250.

Saure C, Schroeder T, Zohren F, et al. 2012. Upfront allogeneic blood stem cell transplantation for patients with high-risk myelodysplastic syndrome or secondary acute myeloid leukemia using a FLAMSA-based high-dose sequential conditioning regimen. *Biol Blood Marrow Transplant* **18**: 466–472.

Schmid C, Schleuning M, Hentrich M, et al. 2008. High antileukemic efficacy of an intermediate intensity conditioning regimen for allogeneic stem cell transplantation in patients with high-risk acute myeloid leukemia in first complete remission. *Bone Marrow Transplant* **41**: 721–727.

Sorror ML, Maris MB, Storb R, et al. 2005. Hematopoietic cell transplantation (HCT)-specific comorbidity index: a new tool for risk assessment before allogeneic HCT. *Blood* **106**: 2912–2919.

Spitzer TR. 2005. Haploidentical stem cell transplantation: the always present but overlooked donor. *Hematology Am Soc Hematol Educ Program* 390–395.

Storb R, Prentice RL, & Thomas ED. 1977. Marrow transplantation for treatment of aplastic anemia. An analysis of factors associated with graft rejection. *N Engl J Med* **296**: 61–66.

Tomblyn M, Chiller T, Einsele H, et al. 2009. Guidelines for preventing infectious complications among HCT recipients. *Biol Blood Marrow Transplant* **15**: 1195–1238.

22

Umbilical cord blood as an alternative allogeneic graft source: clinical banking and transplant outcomes

Mary J. Laughlin and Reinhold Munker

Introduction and historical background

The clinical applications of UCB comprise growing trends in the fields of transplantation and regenerative medicine. Over 10 000 children and adults worldwide have received UCB transplants, beginning with the first infusion in 1988 (Gluckman et al., 1989). In the ensuing decades, numerous large studies have confirmed the engraftment potential and hematopoietic reconstitution capabilities of UCB grafts, and in addition have revealed multiple unique advantages of UCB as an alternative source of stem cells in patients lacking an available histocompatible sibling allogeneic donor. UCB transplantation has been used effectively to treat hematopoietic malignancies, marrow failures, immunodeficiencies, SCD, β-thalassemia, and inherited metabolic disorders (Eapen et al., 2007; Laughlin et al., 2004; Locatelli et al., 2003; Rubinstein et al., 1998; Staba et al., 2004; Tono et al., 2007). It is estimated that more than 400 000 units of UCB are available worldwide.

The use of UCB addresses several challenges inherent to allo-SCT. Although the availability of HLA-matched adult BM donors through various worldwide registries now approaches 75% for Caucasians, certain ethnic minorities remain difficult to match with available volunteer adult donors (Cicciarelli et al., 2005; Wofford et al., 2007). UCB is readily obtained without risk to mother or infant, and is easily cryopreserved, stored, and transported. Additionally, the use of a patient's autologous stem cells has been considered

The BMT Data Book, Third Edition, ed. Reinhold Munker et al. Published by Cambridge University Press. © Cambridge University Press 2013.

for cellular replacement therapies, but is limited due to the fact that stem cell number and function diminish with advancing age (Chambers & Goodell, 2007; Chambers et al., 2007; Rossi et al., 2007), and an invasive procedure is required to procure these cells from the patient. These advantages are increasingly attractive as UCB banking programs become more widespread, improving both the immediate availability of stored units for clinical use and the representation of the population's genetic background for more robust HLA-matching, impacting transplant outcomes (Ballen et al., 2002; Barker et al., 2002; Krishnamurti et al., 2003).

Immunological features of UCB and hematopoietic engraftment

In addition to the numerous logistic advantages of UCB, clinical reports have highlighted favorable outcomes, particularly in the 4/6 to 6/6 HLA-matched setting. Perhaps the most notable of these findings is the decrease in incidence and severity of acute GVHD despite HLA disparity (Barker et al., 2001; Laughlin et al., 2001, 2004; Rocha et al., 2004; Wagner et al., 2002). The mechanisms by which the neonate maintains a more naive immune system, including reduced mature lymphocyte frequency as well as impaired expression and function of activation coreceptors and signaling molecules associated with inflammation, are believed to contribute to reduced acute GVHD in the unrelated allogeneic setting (Brahmi et al., 2001; Kadereit et al., 1999; Liu et al., 2004; Miller et al., 2002). Despite this observed reduced incidence of acute GVHD, rates of malignancy relapse have remained low and the observed GVL effect has appeared robust in most trials, although the mechanisms underlying the peripheral development of GVL activity following UCB engraftment remain unclear (Parkman et al., 2006). Notably, these reports arose early on from trials involving patients with markedly advanced or nonresponsive malignant disease, suggesting highly acceptable outcomes despite generally poor prognosis. T-cell depletion of UCB units is at best unnecessary and at worst detrimental to engraftment outcomes and GVL (Martin et al., 1988). However, the risk of posttransplant infection at early time points (before day 100) is high (Safdar et al., 2007), potentially related to the naïve immunological phenotype of the graft T-cell population, impacting the kinetics of immune reconstitution (Cohen et al., 2006; Komanduri et al., 2007).

Allogeneic UCB trials have previously shown higher primary failure rates and delayed neutrophil and platelet recovery compared with adult-derived marrow and mobilized PB grafts (Gluckman et al., 2004; Hamza et al., 2004). Rates and kinetics of donor-derived neutrophil recovery in UCB recipients have been shown to correlate with total nucleated and $CD34^+$ cell content (Lemarie et al., 2007). The average total nucleated and $CD34^+$ cell content of UCB grafts is approximately 10 times less than in adult-derived stem cell sources, and it is remarkable that UCB engraftment rates are favorable (Gluckman et al., 2004). This may be attributable in part to the proliferative capacity of UCB-derived hematopoietic progenitors, which has been shown to be significantly higher than those isolated from adult BM or PB (Theunissen & Verfaillie, 2005), and which, with lower acute GVHD rates, results in the incidence of EFS similar to allogeneic adult-derived BM across multiple trials in pediatric and adult patients (Gluckman et al., 2001; Laughlin et al., 2004; Rocha et al., 2001). Attempts to enhance progenitor cell dose ex vivo have been largely unsuccessful to date (Hofmeister et al., 2007), but remain ongoing. However, recent trials have indicated that co-transplantation of two allogeneic UCB units is safe and may overcome graft cell dose limitations, thereby permitting use of lower-intensity non-myeloablative conditioning regimens (Ballen et al., 2002; Barker et al., 2001; Brunstein et al., 2007).

Ultimately, two positions have emerged at North American institutions for UCB indications. Transplant teams at the University of Minnesota advocate 4/6 to 6/6 mismatched UCB as a front-line therapy for acute leukemias in the absence of a fully matched BM donor, particularly in pediatric patients. Transplant physicians at Case Western Reserve University generally defer to 10/10 HLA-matched adult-derived BM or mobilized PB stem cell graft when available, although if a suitably matched UCB unit with a large ($>2.5 \times 10^7$/kg) cell count is available or the transplant is particularly urgent, UCB is prioritized. Both groups have stipulated protocols advocating the use of two UCB units for transplant into patients with malignancies, which has been shown to elicit enhanced GVL activity albeit at the risk of increased acute GVHD. Although in nearly all recipients of multiple units only one unit has shown to contribute to day 100 hematopoietic recovery, attempts to predict the predominating unit have largely failed. Regardless, unit-to-unit HLA matching may be of importance, and both groups require the UCB units to be at least 4/6 matched to each other. In patients receiving single UCB grafts, higher graft nucleated cell dose reduces the risk of adverse events arising from HLA-mismatch, and if a well-matched unit of high enough cell dose ($>2.5 \times 10^7$/kg) exists, this single unit may be preferred.

UCB collection and banking

Cord blood is collected fresh following delivery of a full-term infant. UCB is collected either in utero during the final phase of labor or ex utero, and there are advantages and disadvantages of each approach with respect to the number of cells collected and rates of bacterial contamination (Solves et al., 2003). With the use of either approach, collection of UCB stem cells does not interfere with the normal birthing process and poses no danger to the donating mother or baby. For ex utero collection, the placenta is suspended on a collection frame and the umbilicus is threaded down through an opening, thereby permitting gravity to drain the blood through a venipuncture site relatively low on the clamped cord. The UCB is harvested into a standard blood collection bag containing citrate phosphate dextrose (CPD) anticoagulant. In utero collection involves a similar blood-drawing procedure from the umbilical vein before delivery of the placenta. If the cord is to be used for transplant, the unit is depleted of red blood cells by density gradient separation, and its cell content measured and extensively tested for blood-borne pathogens and inherited disorders, per FDA guidelines. A portion of the collected UCB units is later discarded because the blood tests positive for certain diseases or the amount is too small to be of clinical utility; however, the blood found suitable can be stored for use whenever needed, with no further imposition on the donor or family. UCB viability is maintained potentially indefinitely with liquid nitrogen storage. Testing to date verifies viability after 15 years of liquid nitrogen storage (Broxmeyer et al., 2003).

Clinical and laboratory research with UCB stem cells does not carry the ethical implications of research performed with embryonic stem cells. UCB research and clinical studies are funded currently by all government and private agencies without restriction. Regulatory requirements for the operation of a UCB collection and repository program will continue to be important operational factors. The FDA had planned that all public cord blood banks should become licensed or qualify for an Investigational New Drug (IND) exemption by the end of 2011. CBT is performed under the jurisdiction of the Center for Biologics Evaluation and Research (CBER), FDA. The current regulatory framework has three main goals:

1. Prevent unwitting use of contaminated tissues with the potential for transmitting infectious disease.
2. Prevent improper handling or processing that might contaminate or damage tissues.
3. Ensure that clinical safety and effectiveness is demonstrated for most tissues that are highly processed, used for non-natural purposes, combined with non-tissue components, or that have systemic effects on the body.

To ensure compliance, CBER requires UCB repositories to maintain a comprehensive quality management program, utilize validated methods, supplies, reagents, and equipment, and maintain details of clinical outcomes.

Establishment of a U.S. National Cord Blood Inventory

Each year, more than 20 000 children and adults are diagnosed with a hematologic disorder for which an unrelated blood cell or BM transplant is indicated. Transplant activity during the period 1987 through May 31, 2004 reported by the National Marrow Donor Program included only 18 927 total transplants facilitated, indicating that the adult donor registry has been underutilized both for searching and distributing allogeneic stem cell grafts for a diverse American population. This has set the stage for a federally supported national network of UCB banks in an attempt to build an inventory of the highest quality UCB units for use as unrelated donor grafts for patients who lack HLA-matched sibling donors.

The Health Resources and Services Administration (HRSA), part of the U.S. Department of Health and Human Services, recently awarded funds totaling $12 million to the first group of UCB banks to begin collections for the National Cord Blood Inventory (NCBI). The NCBI will collect and maintain high-quality UCB units and make them available for transplantation through the C.W. Bill Young Cell Transplantation Program. The statutory target for the NCBI, as amended in 2010, was 150 000 new units of high-quality UCB collected from diverse, including minority populations, which historically have been the least able to find a suitable matched adult BM donor.

Recent developments

In a prospective study, the characteristics and outcomes of one versus two cord blood units for adult hematologic malignancies were compared (Kindwall-Keller et al., 2011). The patients were treated with a RIC and had an age median of 50–54 years. Twenty seven patients received one unit and 23 patients received two units. The median time to neutrophil engraftment was comparable (25 and 23 days). However, the survival free of adverse events at three years was improved with two compared with one unit, due to a lower relapse risk (59.3% versus 30.4%). The authors concluded that the transplantation of one cord blood unit is a viable option for adults (if a threshold cell dose of $\geq 2.5 \times 10^7$/kg recipient weight is used), although the infusion of two units confers a lower relapse risk.

Brunstein recently summarized the results of CBT in different hematologic malignancies (Brunstein, 2011). Barker et al. (2011) recently described their experience on how to select units for CBT (see following table).

Total nucleated cell (TNC) dose/ kg	Exact minimum dose unknown, but varies according to HLA match (required dose higher if greater mismatch) Do not use unit <2.5 x 10^7/kg with one or mismatches as single graft
HLA matches for HLA-A, -B, DRB1 alleles	A maximum of two mismatches is acceptable (higher mortality of greater mismatch)
TNC dose and HLA match for double cord bloods	Same principles as for one graft as either unit could engraft, preferably HLA match above TNC of 2.0 x 10^7/kg
Bank of origin	Preferably FACT and/or AABB banks
Confirmatory HLA testing from attached segment	Absolute necessity, unless rapid testing from thawed cells possible
Testing for infectious disease markers and hemoglobinopathies	Complete results should be available before unit is shipped

Summary

While treatment options related to BMT continue to expand, many patients are denied access to this lifesaving therapy because they cannot identify a suitable HLA-matched donor. UCB as an alternate source of donor stem and progenitor cells, which, because of its unique immunological features, can be transplanted across partially mismatched HLA barriers, and thus provides donors for those patients unable to find a full 10/10 antigen/allele HLA match. There is a significant unmet need for graft availability, particularly for Americans of minority ethnic background. UCB is therefore considered part of a continuum, rather than a substitute for cells currently used in transplantation, including BM and PB cells.

Advantages and disadvantages of UCB

UCB as a source of allogeneic hematopoietic stem cells

Benefits

- Abundantly available, easily harvested without risk or pain
- Ethically noncontroversial
- Birthing represents genetic background of given population
- Low CMV/EBV infection, no malignant transformation
- Immune tolerance of neonate, lower GVHD incidence and severity
- Available on demand
- Elimination of age-related graft source concerns
- Lack of isoagglutinin production and immune hemolysis following a minor ABO-incompatible transplantation

Disadvantages

- One-time only donation with low cell dose
- Slower engraftment kinetics
- Difficulty in determining abnormalities that may not yet be apparent in the newborn donor

Comparison of UCB with matched and mismatched BM as a source of stem cells

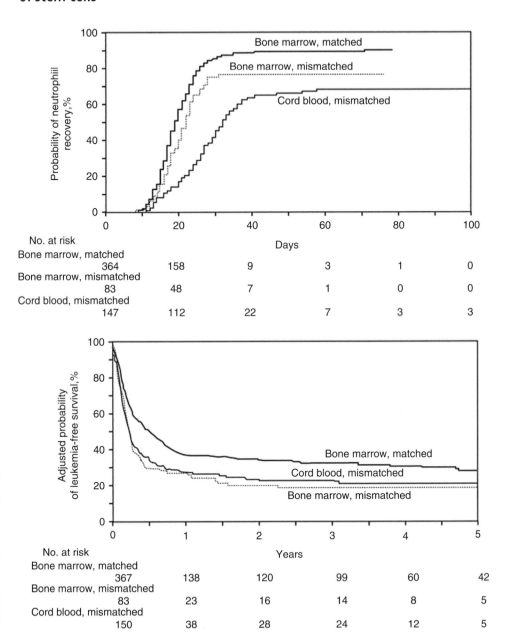

Rate of neutrophil recovery and adjusted probability of LFS compared between matched BM, mismatched BM, and mismatched UCB. The adjusted probability of three-year survival without a recurrence of leukemia was 19% for recipients of mismatched BM, 23% for recipients of UCB, and 33% for recipients of HLA-matched BM. (Reproduced with permission from Laughlin et al., 2004.)

References and further reading

Ballen KK, Hicks J, Dharan B, et al. 2002. Racial and ethnic composition of volunteer cord blood donors: comparison with volunteer unrelated marrow donors. *Transfusion* **42**: 1279–1284.

Barker JN, Byam C, & Scaradavou A. 2011. How I treat: the selection and acquisition of unrelated cord blood grafts. *Blood* **117**: 2332–2339.

Barker JN, Davies SM, DeFor T, et al. 2001. Survival after transplantation of unrelated donor umbilical cord blood is comparable to that of human leukocyte antigen-matched unrelated donor bone marrow: results of a matched-pair analysis. *Blood* **97**: 2957–2961.

Barker JN, Krepski TP, DeFor TE, et al. 2002. Searching for unrelated donor hematopoietic stem cells: availability and speed of umbilical cord blood versus bone marrow. *Biol Blood Marrow Transplant* **8**: 257–260.

Brahmi Z, Hommel-Berrey G, Smith F, et al. 2001. NK cells recover early and mediate cytotoxicity via perforin/granzyme and Fas/FasL pathways in umbilical cord blood recipients. *Hum Immunol* **62**: 782–790.

Broxmeyer HE, Srour EF, Hangoc G, et al. 2003. High-efficiency recovery of functional hematopoietic progenitor and stem cells from human cord blood cryopreserved for 15 years. *Proc Natl Acad Sci USA* **100**: 645–650.

Brunstein CG, Barker JN, Weisdorf DJ, et al. 2007. Umbilical cord blood transplantation after non-myeloablative conditioning: impact on transplantation outcomes in 110 adults with hematologic disease. *Blood* **110**: 3064–3070.

Chambers SM & Goodell MA. 2007. Hematopoietic stem cell aging: wrinkles in stem cell potential. *Stem Cell Rev* **3**: 201–211.

Chambers SM, Shaw CA, Gatza C, et al. 2007. Aging hematopoietic stem cells decline in function and exhibit epigenetic dysregulation. *PLoS Biol* **5**: e201.

Cicciarelli JS, Aswad S, & Mendez R. 2005. Significant HLA matching effect in a large urban transplant center composed primarily of minorities. *Transplant Proc* **37**: 658–660.

Cohen G, Carter SL, Weinberg KI, et al. 2006. Antigen-specific T-lymphocyte function after cord blood transplantation. *Biol Blood Marrow Transplant* **12**: 1335–1342.

Eapen M, Rubinstein P, Zhang MJ, et al. 2007. Outcomes of transplantation of unrelated donor umbilical cord blood and bone marrow in children with acute leukaemia: a comparison study. *Lancet* **369**: 1947–1954.

Gluckman E, Broxmeyer HA, Auerbach, AD, et al. 1989. Hematopoietic reconstitution in a patient with Fanconi's anemia by means of umbilical-cord blood from an HLA-identical sibling. *N Engl J Med* **321**: 1174–1178.

Gluckman E, Rocha V, Arcese W, et al. 2004. Factors associated with outcomes of unrelated cord blood transplant: guidelines for donor choice. *Exp Hematol* **32**: 397–407.

Gluckman E, Rocha V, & Chevret S. 2001. Results of unrelated umbilical cord blood hematopoietic stem cell transplantation. *Rev Clin Exp Hematol* **5**: 87–99.

Hamza NS, Lisgaris M, Yadavalli G, et al. 2004. Kinetics of myeloid and lymphocyte recovery and infectious complications after unrelated umbilical cord blood versus HLA-matched unrelated donor allogeneic transplantation in adults. *Br J Haematol* **124**: 488–498.

Hofmeister CC, Zhang J, Knight KL, et al. 2007. Ex vivo expansion of umbilical cord blood stem cells for transplantation: growing knowledge from the hematopoietic niche. *Bone Marrow Transplant* **39**: 11–23.

Kadereit S, Mohammad SF, Miller RE, et al. 1999. Reduced NFAT1 protein expression in human umbilical cord blood T lymphocytes. *Blood* **94**: 3101–3107.

Kindwall-Keller TL, Hegerfeld Y, Meyerson HJ, et al. 2012. Prospective study of one- vs two-unit umbilical cord blood transplantation following reduced intensity conditioning in adults with hematological malignancies. *Bone Marrow Transplant* **47**: 924–933.

Komanduri KV, St John LS, de Lima M, et al. 2007. Delayed immune reconstitution after cord blood transplantation is characterized by impaired thymopoiesis and late memory T cell skewing. *Blood* **110**: 4543–4551.

Krishnamurti L, Abel S, Maiers M, et al. 2003. Availability of unrelated donors for hematopoietic stem cell transplantation for hemoglobinopathies. *Bone Marrow Transplant* **31**: 547–550.

Laughlin MJ, Barker J, Bambach B, et al. 2001. Hematopoietic engraftment and survival in adult recipients of umbilical-cord blood from unrelated donors. *N Engl J Med* **344**: 1815–1822.

Laughlin MJ, Eapen M, Rubinstein P, et al. 2004. Outcomes after transplantation of cord blood or bone marrow from unrelated donors in adults with leukemia. *N Engl J Med* **351**: 2265–2275.

Lemarie C, Esterni B, Calmels B, et al. 2007. CD34(+) progenitors are reproducibly recovered in thawed umbilical grafts, and positively influence haematopoietic reconstitution after transplantation. *Bone Marrow Transplant* **39**: 453–460.

Liu E, Law HK, & Lau YL. 2004. Tolerance associated with cord blood transplantation may depend on the state of host dendritic cells. *Br J Haematol* **126**: 517–526.

Locatelli F, Rocha V, Reed W, et al. 2003. Related umbilical cord blood transplantation in patients with thalassemia and sickle cell disease. *Blood* **101**: 2137–2143.

Martin PJ, Hansen JA, Torok-Storb B, et al. 1988. Graft failure in patients receiving T cell-depleted HLA-identical allogeneic marrow transplants. *Bone Marrow Transplant* **3**: 445–456.

Miller RE, Fayen JD, Mohammad SF, et al. 2002. Reduced CTLA-4 protein and messenger RNA expression in umbilical cord blood T lymphocytes. *Exp Hematol* **30**: 738–744.

Parkman R, Cohen G, Carter SL, et al. 2006. Successful immune reconstitution decreases leukemic relapse and improves survival in recipients of unrelated cord blood transplantation. *Biol Blood Marrow Transplant* **12**: 919–927.

Rocha V, Cornish J, Sievers EL, et al. 2001. Comparison of outcomes of unrelated bone marrow and umbilical cord blood transplants in children with acute leukemia. *Blood* **97**: 2962–2971.

Rocha V, Labopin M, Sanz G, et al. 2004. Transplants of umbilical-cord blood or bone marrow from unrelated donors in adults with acute leukemia. *N Engl J Med* **351**: 2276–2285.

Rossi DJ, Bryder D, & Weissman IL. 2007. Hematopoietic stem cell aging: mechanism and consequence. *Exp Gerontol* **42**: 385–390.

Rubinstein P, Carrier C, Scaradavou A, et al. 1998. Outcomes among 562 recipients of placental-blood transplants from unrelated donors. *N Engl J Med* **339**: 1565–1577.

Safdar A, Rodriguez GH, De Lima MJ, et al. 2007. Infections in 100 cord blood transplantations: spectrum of early and late posttransplant infections in adult and pediatric patients 1996–2005. *Medicine (Baltimore)* **86**: 324–333.

Solves P, Moraga R, Saucedo E, et al. 2003. Comparison between two strategies for umbilical cord blood collection. *Bone Marrow Transplant* **31**: 269–273.

Staba SL, Escolar ML, Poe M, et al. 2004. Cord-blood transplants from unrelated donors in patients with Hurler's syndrome. *N Engl J Med* **350**: 1960–1969.

Theunissen K & Verfaillie CM. 2005. A multifactorial analysis of umbilical cord blood, adult bone marrow and mobilized peripheral blood progenitors using the improved ML-IC assay. *Exp Hematol* **33**: 165–172.

Tono C, Takahashi Y, Terui K, et al. 2007. Correction of immunodeficiency associated with NEMO mutation by umbilical cord blood transplantation using a reduced-intensity conditioning regimen. *Bone Marrow Transplant* **39**: 801–804.

Wagner JE, Barker JN, DeFor TE, et al. 2002. Transplantation of unrelated donor umbilical cord blood in 102 patients with malignant and nonmalignant diseases: influence of CD34 cell dose and HLA disparity on treatment-related mortality and survival. *Blood* **100**: 1611–1618.

Wofford J, Kemp J, Regan D, et al. 2007. Ethnically mismatched cord blood transplants in African Americans: the Saint Louis Cord Blood Bank experience. *Cytotherapy* **9**: 660–666.

Chapter

23

Pathobiology of graft-versus-host disease

Pavan Reddy

Introduction

The number of allogeneic HCTs has continued to increase, with more than 20 000 allogeneic transplantations performed annually. The GVL/GVT effect during allogeneic HCT effectively eradicates many hematologic malignancies (Appelbaum, 2001). The development of novel strategies that use DLI, non-myeloablative conditioning, and CBT have helped expand the indications for allogeneic HCT over the last several years, especially among older patients (Welniak et al., 2007). Improvements in infectious prophylaxis, immunosuppressive medications, supportive care and DNA-based tissue typing have also contributed to improved outcomes after allogeneic HCT (Appelbaum, 2001). Yet the major complication of allogeneic HCT, GVHD, remains lethal and limits wider application (Ferrara & Reddy, 2006; Welniak et al., 2007). Depending on the time at which it occurs after HCT, GVHD can be either acute or chronic (Deeg, 2007; Lee, 2005; Weiden et al., 1979; Weiden et al., 1981). Acute GVHD is responsible for 15%–40% of mortality and is the major cause of morbidity after allogeneic HCT, while chronic GVHD occurs in up to 50% of patients who survive three months after HCT (Appelbaum, 2001; Lee, 2005).

The GVH reaction was first noted when irradiated mice were infused with allogeneic BM and spleen cells (van Bekkum & De Vries, 1967). Although mice recovered from radiation injury and BM aplasia, they later died with "secondary disease" (van Bekkum & De Vries, 1967), a phenomenon subsequently recognized as acute GVHD. Three requirements for the development of GVHD were formulated by Billingham (Billingham, 1966). First, the graft must contain immunologically competent cells, now recognized as mature

The BMT Data Book, Third Edition, ed. Reinhold Munker et al. Published by Cambridge University Press. © Cambridge University Press 2013.

T-cells. In both experimental and clinical allogeneic BMT, the severity of GVHD correlates with the number of donor T-cells transfused (Kernan et al., 1986; Korngold & Sprent, 1987). The precise nature of these cells and the mechanisms they use are now understood in greater detail (discussed later). Second, the recipient must be incapable of rejecting the transplanted cells, that is, immunocompromised. A patient with a normal immune system will usually reject cells from a foreign donor. In allogeneic BMT, the recipients are usually immunosuppressed with chemotherapy and/or radiation before stem cell infusion (Welniak et al., 2007). Third, the recipient must express tissue antigens that are not present in the transplant donor.

Research efforts over years have provided increasing insight into the biology of this complex disease process. This chapter summarizes the current understanding of the pathobiology of acute GVHD and places it in the context of Billingham's postulates.

Genetic basis of acute GVHD

Billingham's third postulate stipulates that GVH reaction occurs when donor immune cells recognize disparate host antigens (Billingham, 1966). These differences are governed by the genetic polymorphisms of the HLA system and the non-HLA systems (Welniak et al., 2007; Krensky et al., 1990).

HLA matching

Alloreactive T-cell antigen recognition can be classified on the basis of whether the presenting MHC molecule is matched or mismatched (Aosai et al., 1991; Man et al., 1992; Wang et al., 1998). In humans, MHC is governed by the HLA antigens that are encoded by the MHC gene complex on the short arm of chromosome 6 and can be categorized as Class I, II, and III. Class I antigens (HLA-A, -B, and -C) are expressed on almost all cells of the body (Petersdorf & Malkki, 2006). Class II antigens include DR, DQ, and DP antigens and are primarily expressed on hematopoietic cells although their expression can also be induced on other cell types following inflammation (Petersdorf & Malkki, 2006). The incidence of acute GVHD is directly related to the degree of MHC mismatch (Anasetti et al., 1989; Flomenberg et al., 2004; Petersdorf et al., 1995, 1997). The role of HLA mismatching in CBT is more difficult to analyze than in unrelated HSCT, because allele level typing of UCB units for HLA-A, B, C, DRB1, and DQB1 is not performed routinely (Barker & Wagner, 2003). Nonetheless, the total number of HLA disparities between recipient and the UCB unit has been shown to correlate with risk of acute GVHD, and the frequency of severe acute GVHD was lower in patients transplanted with matched (6/6) UCB units (Barker & Wagner, 2003; Barker et al., 2005; Laughlin et al., 2004).

Minor histocompatibility antigens (mHCa)

In MHC-matched BMT context, as is the case with most clinical allo-BMT, donor T-cells recognize MHC-bound peptides derived from the protein products of polymorphic genes (mHCa) that are present in the host but not in the donor (de Bueger and Goulmy, 1993; de Bueger et al., 1992; Den Haan et al., 1995; Goulmy et al., 1996; Malarkannan et al., 1998; Murata et al., 2003). Despite HLA identity between a patient and donor, substantial numbers (40%) of patients receiving HLA-identical grafts and optimal post-grafting immune suppression develop acute GVHD (Bleakley & Riddell, 2004; Goulmy et al., 1996). The mHCas are widely expressed, but can differ in their tissue expression (Bleakley & Riddell, 2004;

de Bueger et al., 1992). This might be one of the reasons for the unique target organ involvement in GVHD. A preponderance of mHCas, such as HA-1 and HA-2, are expressed on hematopoietic cells, which might account for making the host immune system a primary target for the GVH response and help explain the critical role of direct presentation by professional recipient APCs in causing anti-tumor and GVHD responses (Riddell et al., 2006). By contrast, other mHCas, such as H-Y and HA-3, are expressed ubiquitously (Bleakley & Riddell, 2004). The mHCas are not equal in their ability to induce lethal GVHD, and instead show hierarchical immunodominance (Choi et al., 2002a, 2002b). Furthermore, difference in single immunodominant mHCas alone is not insufficient for causing GVHD in murine models, although T-cells targeting single mHCas can induce tissue damage in a skin explant model (Fontaine et al., 2001; Dickinson et al., 2002). However, the role of specific and immunodominant mHCas that are relevant in clinical GVHD has not been systematically evaluated in large groups of patients (de Bueger et al., 1993).

Other non-HLA genes

Genetic polymorphisms in several non-HLA genes such as in KIRs, cytokines, and NOD2 genes have recently been shown to modulate the severity and incidence of GVHD.

KIR receptors on NK cells that bind to the HLA Class I gene products are encoded on chromosome 19. Polymorphisms in the transmembrane and cytoplasmic domains of KIR receptors govern whether the receptor has inhibitory potential (such as KIR2DL1, -2DL2, -2DL3, and -3DL1) or activating potential. Two competing models have been proposed for HLA-KIR allorecognition by donor NK cells following HSCT: the "mismatched ligand" and "missing ligand" models (Hsu et al., 2006; Miller et al., 2005, 2007; Petersdorf, 2006; Velardi et al., 2002). Both models are supported by some clinical observations, albeit in patients receiving very different transplant and immunosuppressive regimens (Davies et al., 2002; Hsu et al., 2005; Miller et al., 2007; Ruggeri et al., 2002).

Proinflammatory cytokines, involved in the classical cytokine storm of GVHD (discussed later), cause pathological damage of target organs such as skin, GI tract, and liver (Antin and Ferrara, 1992). Several cytokine gene polymorphisms, both in hosts and donors, have been implicated. Specifically, TNF polymorphisms (TNFd3/d3 in the recipient, TNF-863 and -857 in donors and/or recipients, and TNFd4, TNF-a-1031C, and TNFRII-196R in the donors) have been associated with an increased risk of acute GVHD and TRM (Cavet et al., 1999, 2001; Dickinson & Charron, 2005). The three common haplotypes of the IL-10 gene promoter region in recipients representing high, intermediate, and low production of IL-10, have been associated with the severity of acute GVHD following allo-BMT after HLA-matched sibling donors (Lin et al., 2003). By contrast, smaller studies have found neither IL-10 nor TNF-α polymorphisms to be associated with GVHD after HLA-mismatched CBTs (Dickinson & Charron, 2005; Mullighan & Bardy, 2007). IFN-γ polymorphisms of the 2/2 genotype (high IFN-γ production) and 3/3 genotype (low IFN-γ) have been associated with decreased or increased acute GVHD, respectively (Dickinson & Charron, 2005; Cavet et al., 2001).

NOD2/CARD15 gene polymorphisms in both the donors and recipients were recently shown to have a striking association with GI GVHD and overall mortality after both related and unrelated allogeneic HSCT (Holler et al., 2006). It is likely that non-HLA gene polymorphisms might play differing roles depending on the donor source (related vs. unrelated), HLA disparity (matched vs. mismatched), source of the graft (UCB vs. PB stem cells vs. BM), and the intensity of the conditioning.

The topic of biomarkers in the development, diagnosis, prognosis, and prognostication of GVHD was recently reviewed by Levine et al. (2012). The value of these biomarkers needs to be confirmed by well-designed clinical trials. Examples of biomarkers for potential clinical use are REG3α (high concentrations at diagnosis of GVHD correlating with shorter survival) and BAFF (high concentrations correlating with chronic GVHD).

Immunobiology of acute GVHD

The development of acute GVHD can be conceptualized in three sequential steps or phases: (1) activation of the APCs; (2) donor T-cell activation, proliferation, differentiation, and migration; and (3) target tissue destruction (see following figure).

Three phases of GVHD immunobiology

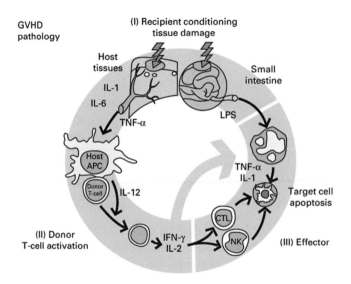

Phase 1: activation of APCs

The first step involves the activation of APCs by the underlying disease and the HCT conditioning regimen (see figure). Damaged host tissues respond by producing "danger signals," including proinflammatory cytokines (e.g., TNF-α), chemokines, increased expression of adhesion, MHC antigens, and co-stimulatory molecules on host APCs (Hill & Ferrara, 2000; Hill et al., 1997; Matzinger, 2002; Paris et al., 2001; Xun et al., 1994). Damage to the GI tract from the conditioning is particularly important because it allows for systemic translocation of additional danger signals, such as microbial products including lipopolysaccharide (LPS) or containing other pathogen-associated molecular patterns that further enhance the activation of host APCs (Hill & Ferrara, 2000). The secondary lymphoid tissue in the GI tract is likely the initial site of interaction between activated APCs and donor T-cells (Murai et al., 2003). These observations have led to an important strategy to reduce acute GVHD by reducing the intensity of the conditioning regimen. Experimental GVHD can be regulated by modulating distinct subsets of dendritic cells, the most powerful APCs (Duffner et al., 2004; Sato et al., 2003). Non-hematopoietic stem cells, such as mesenchymal stem cells or stromal cells, can also reduce allogeneic T-cell responses, although the mechanism for such inhibition remains unclear (Welniak et al., 2007).

The concept of enhanced activation of host APCs unifies a number of seemingly disparate clinical observations that increase the risk of acute GVHD, such as an advanced stage of malignancy, more intense transplant and conditioning regimens, and histories of viral infections. For example, specific viruses such as CMV have been associated with increased risks of GVHD, which may be explained by the ligation of Toll-like receptors that recognize viral DNA or RNA and that activate APCs.

Phase 2: donor T-cell activation

The core of the GVH reaction is Step 2, where donor T-cells proliferate and differentiate in response to host APCs (see figure). In addition to the engagement of the T-cell receptor, TCR, donor T-cells require a second signal generated by ligation of co-stimulatory molecules for activation. The danger signals generated in Phase 1 augment this activation (Dustin, 2001). The second signal is delivered by the co-stimulatory ligands and receptors on APCs and T-cells. As shown in the following table, blockade of co-stimulatory pathways has shown the ability to modulate acute GVHD in animal models; it has, however, not yet been tested in large clinical trials (Welniak et al., 2007).

Co-stimulatory pathways

	T-cell	APC
Adhesion	ICAM-1	LEA-1
	LFA-1	ICAM 1,2,3
	CD2 (LEA-2)	LFA-3
Recognition	TCR/CD4	NIIIC hi
	TCR/CD8	Mi-Icc I
Co-stimulation	CD28	CD80/86
	CD152 (CTLA-4)	CD80/86
	ICOS	B7H/B7RP-1
	PD-1	PD-L1, PD-L2
	Unknown	B7-H3
	CD 154 (CD4OL)	CD4O
	OX40	OX4OL
	4-IBB	4–1IBBL
	HVEM	LIGHT

HVEM HSV glycoprotein D for herpes virus entry mediator; LIGHT, homologous to lymphotoxins, shows inducible expression, and competes with herpes simplex virus glycoprotein D for herpes virus entry mediator (HVEM), a receptor expressed by T-lymphocytes.

T-cell populations consist of several subsets whose responses differ based on antigenic stimulus, activation threshold, and effector function. In mouse models, where genetic differences between donor and recipient strains can be tightly controlled, CD4[+] cells induce acute GVHD to MHC Class II differences, and CD8[+] cells induce acute GVHD to MHC Class I differences (Csencsits & Bishop, 2003; Korngold & Sprent, 1982, 1985). In the majority of HLA-identical HCTs, both CD4[+] and CD8[+] subsets respond to mHCa and can cause GVHD in HLA-identical HCT. Clinical trials that deplete either CD4[+] or CD8[+] subsets have been inconclusive.

In experimental GVHD, naïve (CD62L[+]) T-cells cause acute GVHD but not memory (CD62L[−]) T-cells (Andersonet al., 2003; Chen et al., 2004; Maeda et al., 2007). This subset may contain a population of memory stem cells that are responsible for GVHD (Zhang et al., 2005). Strategies aimed at selective elimination of donor T-cells in vivo after HCT either by targeting a suicide gene to the alloreactive T-cells or by photodynamic cell purging are promising, but are not yet validated in the clinic (Bonini et al., 1997; Chen et al., 2002; Traversari et al., 2007).

Regulatory T-cells can suppress the proliferation of conventional T-cells and prevent GVHD in animal models when added to donor grafts containing conventional T-cells (Cohen & Boyer, 2006). In mice, *Foxp3* functions as a master control gene in the development of regulatory T-cells, which normally constitute 5% of the CD4+ T-cell population (Cohen & Boyer, 2006). They function by secreting inhibiting cytokines IL-10 and TCF-β as well as through contact-dependent inhibition of APCs (Cohen & Boyer, 2006).

NK1.1[+] T-cells of the host form another regulatory T-cell subset that can suppress acute GVHD (Zeng et al., 1999). A recent clinical trial showed that total lymphoid irradiation used as conditioning significantly reduced GVHD and enhanced NK T-cell function (Lowsky et al., 2005). It is likely that the role of regulatory T-cells in clinical acute GVHD will require improved techniques to identify them and expand them in sufficient numbers for clinical trials.

Activation of immune cells results in rapid intracellular biochemical cascades that induce transcription of many genes including those for cytokines and their receptors. The Th1 cytokines (IFN-γ, IL-2, and TNF-α) are preferentially produced in acute GVHD. IL-2 production by donor T-cells remains the principal target of many current clinical therapeutic and prophylactic approaches to GVHD, such as cyclosporin, tacrolimus, and monoclonal antibodies (mAbs) directed against IL-2 and its receptor (Ratanatharathorn et al., 1998). Emerging data indicate an important role for IL-2 in the generation and maintenance of CD4[+]CD25[+] Tregs, suggesting that prolonged interference with IL-2 may have an unintended consequence in the prevention of the development of long-term tolerance after allogeneic HCT (Zeiser et al., 2006).

Similarly, the role of IFN-γ or its inducer can either amplify or reduce GVHD (Fowler et al., 1994; Yang et al., 1998). Th1 polarization of donor T-cells can attenuate acute GVHD, suggesting that some amount of Th1 cytokines is critical for GVHD induction, while ordinate production (extremely low or high) can decrease acute GVHD through negative feedback mechanisms.

IL-10 plays a key role in suppression of immune responses, and clinical data suggest it may regulate acute GVHD (Lin et al., 2003). TGF-β, another suppressive cytokine, can suppress acute GVHD but exacerbate chronic GVHD (Banovic et al., 2005). Taken together, the experimental data demonstrate that the timing and extent of the production of any given cytokine may modulate the outcome of acute GVHD.

Leukocyte migration

Chemokines direct the migration of donor T-cells from lymphoid tissues to the target organs where they cause damage. Macrophage inflammatory protein-1 alpha (MIP-1α) as CCL2–5, CXCL2, CXCL9–11, CCL17, and CCL27 are all overexpressed during experimental GVHD (Wysocki et al., 2005). CXCR3[+] and CCR5[+] cells cause acute GVHD in the liver and intestine (Wysocki et al., 2005). Expression of integrins, such as α4β7 and its ligand MadCAM-1, are also important for the homing of donor T-cells to Peyer's patches during GI GVHD (Murai et al., 2003; Waldman et al., 2006; Welniak et al., 2005).

Phase 3: cellular and inflammatory effector phase

The effector phase of this process is a complex cascade of both cellular mediators such as CTLs and NK cells and soluble inflammatory mediators such as TNF-α, IFN-γ, IL-1, and NO (Welniak et al., 2007; Ferrara & Deeg, 1991) (see figure). These soluble and cellular mediators synergize to amplify local tissue injury and further promote inflammation and target tissue destruction.

Cellular effectors

The cellular effectors of acute GVHD are primarily CTLs and NK cells (Hill & Ferrara, 2000). CTLs that preferentially use the Fas/FasL pathway of target lysis appear to predominate in GVHD liver damage (hepatocytes express large amounts of Fas) whereas GVHD CTLs that use the perforin/granzyme pathways are more important in the GI tract and skin (van den Brink & Burakoff, 2002; Welniak et al., 2006).

Inflammatory effectors

Microbial products such as LPS that leak through a damaged intestinal mucosa or skin may stimulate secretion of inflammatory cytokines through Toll-like receptors (TLRs) (Hill & Ferrara, 2000; Iwasaki & Medzhitov, 2004). In this regard, the GI tract is particularly susceptible to damage from TNF-α, and plays a major role in the amplification and propagation of the "cytokine storm" characteristic of acute GVHD (Hill & Ferrara, 2000). TNF-α can be produced by both donor and host cells, and it acts in three different ways: first, it activates dendritic cells and enhances alloantigen presentation; second, it recruits effector cells to target organs via the induction of inflammatory chemokines; and third, it directly causes tissue necrosis, as its name suggests (Brown et al., 2002; Hill et al., 2000; Piguet et al., 1987; Reddy et al., 2012).

Immunobiology of chronic GVHD

Chronic GVHD generally manifests later (>100 days) and has some features of auto-immune diseases. It may develop either de novo or following resolution or as an extension of acute GVHD. Chronic GVHD is also thought to be induced by donor T-cells, but the nature of relevant antigens, the critical cellular subsets, and the mechanisms of chronic GVHD remain less well understood. It is important to recognize that this traditional definition was based on the temporal rather than the clinical or pathophysiological nature of GVHD. This definition is not satisfactory because acute and chronic GVHD have distinct clinical features that can sometimes present concomitantly and/or independent of the duration after transplant. Recent NIH consensus classification of GVHD includes late-onset (after day 100), acute GVHD, and an overlap syndrome that has features of both acute and chronic GVHD.

Chronic GVHD has myriad manifestations, and unlike acute GVHD, can affect multiple organ systems. Pathologically, depending on the severity, a plethora of features are observed. However, in contrast to acute GVHD, it is most often characterized by fibrosis of the affected organ. On the basis of its clinical features, chronic GVHD has been considered to be an "autoimmune" disease. However, given the lack of impact of acute GVHD rates on chronic GVHD, the time of onset, the organ system involvement, types of tissue damage, and the differences in clinical features and the kinetics suggest that, although both acute and chronic GVHD occur after allogeneic HCT, the underlying immunopathological mechanisms might be distinct.

Advances in the understanding of the biology of chronic GVHD have not been made, in part because of the absence of appropriate experimental models that mimic all the features of chronic GVHD. Some murine models, depending on the strain combinations, conditioning regimen, and type and amount of donor cells, produce certain features of chronic GVHD, such as the fibrosis of skin, lung, or lupus nephritis, or liver damage. But no single model captures all of the features and kinetics of chronic GVHD. This lack of appropriate experimental models might be because of the differences between humans and experimental species. For example, in contrast to murine studies, the kinetics of clinical chronic GVHD is slower and is observed only after prophylaxis and/or treatment for acute GVHD. Even when clinical chronic GVHD raises de novo and in the absence of active immunosuppression, it would not be possible to definitively rule out the impact of either GVH prophylaxis and/or subclinical acute GVHD on the subsequent development of chronic GVHD. It is therefore important to consider these caveats when attempting to understand the biology of chronic GVHD from experimental models.

A recent study demonstrated that acute GVHD in an MHC mismatched model resulted in the emergence of donor-reactive donor T-cells in the host, which caused severe "autoimmune" colitis on adoptive transfer back into donor- but not host-type mice. Some experimental studies have shown that T-cells from animals with chronic GVHD are specific for a common (shared between host and donor) determinant of MHC Class II molecules and are therefore considered to be "autoreactive." These autoreactive cells of chronic GVHD are associated with a damaged thymus and negative selection. Nonetheless, despite the experimental evidence and clinical similarity with autoimmune diseases, there are no clear clinical data on the isolation of donor-derived T-cell clones that recognize nonpolymorphic antigens from both the donor and the recipients. Instead, emerging clinical data show a strong correlation between the presence of immune responses against ubiquitously expressed mHCas and chronic GVHD. Furthermore, because (a) chronic GVHD occurs only after allogeneic HCT, (b) acute GVHD is its main risk factor, and (c) chronic GVHD is distinct from "syngeneic" GVHD caused by improper thymic selection, it is possible that chronic GVHD is caused by T-cells that have undergone chronic antigen stimulation because of the presence of ubiquitous mHCas. The similarity in clinical features with autoimmune diseases therefore might be the result of chronic stimulation-induced target organ damage, which perhaps happens to be mHCas for chronic GVHD and nonpolymorphic "auto-antigens" for autoimmune diseases. This concept is supported by the recent observations demonstrating a strong correlation in female to male HCT and the presence of antibodies to Y chromosome-encoded histocompatibility antigens with chronic GVHD. In any event, even if mHCas are the targets, it remains unknown whether these are the same ones targeted in acute GVHD.

A recent elegant murine study in fact suggested that the type and selection of immuno-dominant mHCas determines the target and character of GVHD damage.

In contrast to the earliest phases of the biology of acute GVHD, little is known about the factors that set into motion the onset of chronic GVHD. Chronic GVHD occurs later, perhaps after complete donor reconstitution, and therefore it stands to reason that indirect antigen presentation by donor APCs might be important in its pathogenesis, a notion supported by (a) clinical correlation between presence of high numbers of donor mono-nuclear cells in PBSCT and greater risk of chronic GVHD; (b) experimental models demonstrating the autoimmune nature of chronic GVHD also suggest a role for donor-derived APCs; and (c) recent experimental data from the MHC-matched mHCa disparate model of CD4$^+$ mediated chronic GVHD demonstrating that either donor or host APCs can initiate chronic GVHD in the skin while only the donor APCs played a dominant role in GI chronic GVHD. Recent clinical data with rituximab indicate that B-cells might be pathogenic in chronic GVHD. These observations, however, do not clarify whether B-cells play a role in priming donor T-cells (as APCs) or function as effectors because of dysregulation of donor T-helper cells.

Th1 cytokines (IFN-γ, IL-2, and TNF-α) have been implicated in the pathophysiology of acute GVHD. By contrast, nonirradiated parent into F1 models of chronic GVHD demon-strated that Th1 polarization reduced while the Th2 phenotype enhanced chronic GVHD. On the other hand, TGF-β suppressed acute GVHD but exacerbated experimental chronic GVHD. Thus the Th1/Th2 paradigm of donor T-cells in the immunopathogenesis of acute and chronic GVHD has evolved over the past years and is complex and incompletely understood. Several studies nonetheless have demonstrated a suppressive role for natural donor CD4$^+$CD25$^+$ Foxp3$^+$ regulatory T (Treg) cells in chronic GVHD, where both host and donor type CD4$^+$CD25$^+$ T-cells reduced the severity of disease. Elegant experimental data have also suggested a role for aberrant thymic education in the development of chronic GVHD. It has been postulated that the thymic damage by conditioning, acute GVHD, and age-related atrophy disrupt thymic education of T-cells and cause chronic GVHD by the emergence of thymic-dependent autoreactive T-cells. Consistent with this notion, thymic-dependent donor BM-derived T-cells that escape from negative selection have the ability to cause lethal chronic GVHD that is similar to human chronic GVHD, which was prevented by thymectomy of the recipients before BMT. By contrast, data from a sublethally irradiated experimental model demonstrated that the host thymus is not required for the development of autoimmune-like chronic GVHD. Taken together, existing experimental data suggest that mature donor T-cells in the allograft are necessary and sufficient for acute GVHD while both mature donor T-cells and host thymic-dependent generation of donor T-cells from the infused hematopoietic stem cells might play a role in the induction of chronic GVHD.

In summary, donor T-cells are critical for the development of both acute and chronic GVHD. However, there might be differences in the prerequisites, target antigens, and cytokine and cellular effectors that cause acute and chronic GVHD.

References and further reading

Anasetti C, Amos D, Beatty PG, et al. 1989. Effect of HLA compatibility on engraftment of bone marrow transplants in patients with leukemia or lymphoma. *N Engl J Med* **320**: 197–204.

Anderson BE, McNiff J, Yan J, et al. 2003. Memory CD4+ T cells do not induce graft-versus-host disease. *J Clin Invest* **112**: 101–108.

Antin JH & Ferrara JL. 1992. Cytokine dysregulation and acute graft-versus-host disease. *Blood* **80**: 2964–2968.

Aosai F, Ohlen C, Ljunggren HG, et al. 1991. Different types of allospecific CTL clones identified by their ability to recognize peptide loading-defective target cells. *Eur J Immunol* **21**: 2767–2774.

Appelbaum FR. Haematopoietic cell transplantation as immunotherapy. 2001. *Nature* **411**: 385–389.

Banovic T, Macdonald KP, Morris ES, et al. 2005. TGF-beta in allogeneic stem cell transplantation: friend or foe? *Blood* **106**: 2206–2214.

Barker JN & Wagner JE. 2003. Umbilical-cord blood transplantation for the treatment of cancer. *Nat Rev Cancer* **3**: 526–532.

Barker JN, Weisdorf DJ, Defor TE, et al. 2005. Transplantation of 2 partially HLA-matched umbilical cord blood units to enhance engraftment in adults with hematologic malignancy. *Blood* **105**: 1343–1347.

Billingham RE. 1966. The biology of graft-versus-host reactions. *Harvey Lect* **62**: 21–78.

Bleakley M & Riddell SR. 2004. Molecules and mechanisms of the graft-versus-leukaemia effect. *Nat Rev Cancer* **4**: 371–380.

Bonini C, Ferrari G, Verzeletti S, et al. 1997. HSV-TK gene transfer into donor lymphocytes for control of allogeneic graft-versus-leukemia. *Science* **276**: 1719–1724.

Brown GR, Lee E, & Thiele DL. 2002. TNF-TNFR2 interactions are critical for the development of intestinal graft-versus-host disease in MHC class II-disparate (C57BL/6J –->C57BL/6J x bm12)F1 mice. *J Immunol* **168**: 3065–3071.

Cavet J, Dickinson AM, Norden J, et al. 2001. Interferon-gamma and interleukin-6 gene polymorphisms associate with graft-versus-host disease in HLA-matched sibling bone marrow transplantation. *Blood* **98**: 1594–1600.

Cavet J, Middleton PG, Segall M, et al. 1999. Recipient tumor necrosis factor-alpha and interleukin-10 gene polymorphisms associate with early mortality and acute graft-versus-host disease severity in HLA-matched sibling bone marrow transplants. *Blood* **94**: 3941–3946.

Chen BJ, Cui X, Liu C, et al. 2002. Prevention of graft-versus-host disease while preserving graft-versus-leukemia effect after selective depletion of host-reactive T cells by photodynamic cell purging process. *Blood* **99**: 3083–3088.

Chen BJ, Cui X, Sempowski GD, et al. 2004. Transfer of allogeneic CD62L-memory T cells without graft-versus-host disease. *Blood* **103**: 1534–1541.

Choi EY, Christianson GJ, Yoshimura Y, et al. 2002a. Real-time T-cell profiling identifies H60 as a major minor histocompatibility antigen in murine graft-versus-host disease. *Blood* **100**: 4259–4265.

Choi EY, Christianson GJ, Yoshimura Y, et al. 2002b. Immunodominance of H60 is caused by an abnormally high precursor T cell pool directed against its unique minor histocompatibility antigen peptide. *Immunity* **17**: 593–603.

Cohen JL & Boyer O. 2006. The role of CD4(+) CD25(hi) regulatory T cells in the physiopathogeny of graft-versus-host disease. *Curr Opin Immunol* **18**: 580–585.

Csencsits KL & Bishop DK. 2003. Contrasting alloreactive CD4+ and CD8+ T cells: there's more to it than MHC restriction. *Am J Transplant* **3**: 107–115.

Davies SM, Ruggieri L, DeFor T, et al. 2002. Evaluation of KIR ligand incompatibility in mismatched unrelated donor hematopoietic transplants. Killer immunoglobulin-like receptor. *Blood* **100**: 3825–3827.

de Bueger M, Bakker A, Bontkes H, et al. 1993. High frequencies of cytotoxic T cell precursors against minor histocompatibility antigens after HLA-identical BMT: absence of correlation with GVHD. *Bone Marrow Transplant* **11**: 363–368.

de Bueger M, Bakker A, Van Rood JJ, et al. 1992. Tissue distribution of human minor histocompatibility antigens. Ubiquitous versus restricted tissue distribution indicates heterogeneity among human cytotoxic T lymphocyte-defined non-MHC antigens. *J Immunol* **149**: 1788–1794.

de Bueger M & Goulmy E. 1993. Human minor histocompatibility antigens. *Transpl Immunol* **1**: 28–38.

Deeg HJ. 2007. How I treat refractory acute GVHD. *Blood* **109**: 4119–4126.

Den Haan JM, Sherman NE, Blokland E, et al. 1995. Identification of a graft versus host disease-associated human minor histocompatibility antigen. *Science* **268**: 1476–1480.

Dickinson AM & Charron D. 2005. Non-HLA immunogenetics in hematopoietic stem cell transplantation. *Curr Opin Immunol* **17**: 517–525.

Dickinson AM, Wang XN, Sviland L, et al. 2002. In situ dissection of the graft-versus-host activities of cytotoxic T cells specific for minor histocompatibility antigens. *Nat Med* **8**: 410–414.

Duffner UA, Maeda Y, Cooke KR, et al. 2004. Host dendritic cells alone are sufficient to initiate acute graft-versus-host disease. *J Immunol* **172**: 7393–7398.

Dustin ML. 2001. Role of adhesion molecules in activation signaling in T lymphocytes. *J Clin Immunol* **21**: 258–263.

Ferrara JLM & Deeg HJ. 1991. Graft versus host disease. *N Engl J Med* **324**: 667–674.

Ferrara JLM, Levine JE, Reddy P, et al. 2009. Graft-versus-host disease. *Lancet* **373**: 1550–1561.

Ferrara JL & Reddy P. 2006. Pathophysiology of graft-versus-host disease. *Semin Hematol* **43**: 3–10.

Flomenberg N, Baxter-Lowe LA, Confer D, et al. 2004. Impact of HLA class I and class II high-resolution matching on outcomes of unrelated donor bone marrow transplantation: HLA-C mismatching is associated with a strong adverse effect on transplantation outcome. *Blood* **104**: 1923–1930.

Fontaine P, Roy-Proulx G, Knafo L, et al. 2001. Adoptive transfer of minor histocompatibility antigen-specific T lymphocytes eradicates leukemia cells without causing graft-versus-host disease. *Nat Med* **7**: 789–794.

Fowler DH, Kurasawa K, Smith R, et al. 1994. Donor CD4-enriched cells of Th2 cytokine phenotype regulate graft-versus-host disease without impairing allogeneic engraftment in sublethally irradiated mice. *Blood* **84**: 3540–3549.

Goulmy E. 2006. Minor histocompatibility antigens: from transplantation problems to therapy of cancer. *Hum Immunol* **67**: 433–438.

Goulmy E, Schipper R, Pool J, et al. 1996. Mismatches of minor histocompatibility antigens between HLA-identical donors and recipients and the development of graft-versus-host disease after bone marrow transplantation. *N Eng J Med* **334**: 281–285.

Hill GR, Crawford JM, Cooke KR, et al. 1997. Total body irradiation and acute graft-versus-host disease: the role of gastrointestinal damage and inflammatory cytokines. *Blood* **90**: 3204–3213.

Hill G & Ferrara J. 2000. The primacy of the gastrointestinal tract as a target organ of acute graft-versus-host disease: rationale for the use of cytokine shields in allogeneic bone marrow transplantation. *Blood* **95**: 2754–2759.

Hill GR, Teshima T, Rebel VI, et al. 2000. The p55 TNF-alpha receptor plays a critical role in T cell alloreactivity. *J Immunol* **164**: 656–663.

Holler E, Rogler G, Brenmoehl J, et al. 2006. Prognostic significance of NOD2/CARD15 variants in HLA-identical sibling hematopoietic stem cell transplantation: effect on long-term outcome is confirmed in 2 independent cohorts and may be modulated by the type of gastrointestinal decontamination. *Blood* **107**: 4189–4193.

Hsu KC, Gooley T, Malkki M, et al. 2006. KIR ligands and prediction of relapse after unrelated donor hematopoietic cell transplantation for hematologic malignancy. *Biol Blood Marrow Transplant* **12**: 828–836.

Hsu KC, Keever-Taylor CA, Wilton A, et al. 2005. Improved outcome in HLA-identical sibling hematopoietic stem-cell transplantation for acute myelogenous leukemia predicted by KIR and HLA genotypes. *Blood* **105**: 4878–4884.

Iwasaki A & Medzhitov R. 2004. Toll-like receptor control of the adaptive immune responses. *Nat Immunol* **5**: 987–995.

Kernan NA, Collins NH, Juliano L, et al. 1986. Clonable T lymphocytes in T cell-depleted bone marrow transplants correlate with development of graft-v-host disease. *Blood* **68**: 770–773.

Korngold R & Sprent J. 1982. Features of T cells causing H-2-restricted lethal graft-vs.-host disease across minor histocompatibility barriers. *J Exp Med* **155**: 872–883.

Korngold R & Sprent J. 1987. Purified T cell subsets and lethal graft-versus-host disease in mice. In Gale RP, Champlin R, eds. *Progress in Bone Marrow Transplantation*. New York, NY: Alan R. Liss, Inc., pp. 213–218.

Korngold R & Sprent J. 1985. Surface markers of T cells causing lethal graft-vs-host disease to class I vs class II H-2 differences. *J Immunol* **135**: 3004–3010.

Krensky AM, Weiss A, Crabtree G, 1987.. 1990. T-lymphocyte–antigen interactions in transplant rejection. *N Engl J Med* **322**: 510–517.

Laughlin MJ, Eapen M, Rubinstein P, et al. 2004. Outcomes after transplantation of cord blood or bone marrow from unrelated donors in adults with leukemia. *N Engl J Med* **351**: 2265–2275.

Lee SJ. 2005. New approaches for preventing and treating chronic graft-versus-host disease. *Blood* **105**: 4200–4206.

Levine JE, Paczesny S, & Sarantopoulos S. 2012. Clinical applications for biomarkers of acute and chronic graft-versus-host disease. *Biol Blood Marrow Transplant* **18**: S116–S124.

Lin MT, Storer B, Martin PJ, et al. 2003. Relation of an interleukin-10 promoter polymorphism to graft-versus-host disease and survival after hematopoietic-cell transplantation. *N Engl J Med* **349**: 2201–2210.

Lowsky R, Takahashi T, Liu YP, et al. 2005. Protective conditioning for acute graft-versus-host disease. *N Engl J Med* **353**: 1321–1331.

Maeda Y, Tawara I, Teshima T, et al. 2007. Lymphopenia-induced proliferation of donor T cells reduces their capacity for causing acute graft-versus-host disease. *Exp Hematol* **35**: 274–286.

Malarkannan S, Shih PP, Eden PA, et al. 1998. The molecular and functional characterization of a dominant minor H antigen, H60. *J Immunol* **161**: 3501–3509.

Man S, Salter RD, & Engelhard VH. 1992. Role of endogenous peptide in human alloreactive cytotoxic T cell responses. *Int Immunol* **4**: 367–375.

Matzinger P. 2002. The danger model: a renewed sense of self. *Science* **296**: 301–305.

Miller JS, Cooley S, Parham P, et al. 2007. Missing KIR-ligands is associated with less relapse and increased graft versus host disease (GVHD) following unrelated donor allogeneic HCT. *Blood* **109**: 5058–5061.

Miller JS, Soignier Y, Panoskaltsis-Mortari A, et al. 2005. Successful adoptive transfer and in vivo expansion of human haploidentical NK cells in patients with cancer. *Blood* **105**: 3051–3057.

Mullighan CG & Bardy PG. 2007. New directions in the genomics of allogeneic hematopoietic stem cell transplantation. *Biol Blood Marrow Transplant* **13**: 127–144.

Murai M, Yoneyama H, Ezaki T, et al. 2003. Peyer's patch is the essential site in initiating murine acute and lethal graft-versus-host reaction. *Nat Immunol* **4**: 154–160.

Murata M, Warren EH, & Riddell SR. 2003. A human minor histocompatibility antigen resulting from differential expression due to a gene deletion. *J Exp Med* **197**: 1279–1289.

Paris F, Fuks Z, Kang A, et al. 2001. Endothelial apoptosis as the primary lesion initiating intestinal radiation damage in mice. *Science* **293**: 293–297.

Petersdorf EW. 2006. Immunogenomics of unrelated hematopoietic cell transplantation. *Curr Opin Immunol* **18**: 559–564.

Petersdorf EW, Longton G, Anasetti C, et al. 1995. Donor-recipient disparities for HLA-C genes is a risk factor for graft failure following marrow transplantation from unrelated donors. *Blood* **86**: S291a.

Petersdorf EW, Longton GM, Anasetti C, et al. 1997. Association of HLA-C disparity with great failure after marrow transplantation from unrelated donors. *Blood* **89**: 1818–1823.

Petersdorf EW & Malkki M. 2006. Genetics of risk factors for graft-versus-host disease. *Semin Hematol* **43**: 11–23.

Piguet PF, Grau GE, Allet B, et al. 1987. Tumor necrosis factor/cachectin is an effector of skin and gut lesions of the acute phase of graft-versus-host disease. *J Exp Med* **166**: 1280–1289.

Ratanatharathorn V, Nash RA, Przepiorka D, et al. 1998. Phase III study comparing methotrexate and tacrolimus (prograf, FK506) with methotrexate and cyclosporine for graft-versus-host disease prophylaxis after HLA-identical sibling bone marrow transplantation. *Blood* **92**: 2303–2314.

Reddy P, Socié G, Cutler C, et al. 2012. GVHD prevention: an ounce is better than a pound. *Biol Blood Marrow Transplant* **18**: S17–S26.

Riddell SR, Bleakley M, Nishida T, et al. 2006. Adoptive transfer of allogeneic antigen-specific T cells. *Biol Blood Marrow Transplant* **12**: S9–S12.

Ruggeri L, Capanni M, Urbani E, et al. 2002. Effectiveness of donor natural killer cell alloreactivity in mismatched hematopoietic transplants. *Science* **295**: 2097–2100.

Sato K, Yamashita N, Baba M, et al. 2003. Regulatory dendritic cells protect mice from murine acute graft-versus-host disease and leukemia relapse. *Immunity* **18**: 367–379.

Traversari C, Marktel S, Magnani Z, et al. 2007. The potential immunogenicity of the TK suicide gene does not prevent full clinical benefit associated with the use of TK-transduced donor lymphocytes in HSCT for hematologic malignancies. *Blood* **109**: 4708–4715.

Van Bekkum DW & De Vries MJ. 1967. *Radiation Chimaeras*. London: Logos Press.

Van Den Brink MR & Burakoff SJ. 2002. Cytolytic pathways in haematopoietic stem-cell transplantation. *Nat Rev Immunol* **2**: 273–281.

Velardi A, Ruggeri L, Moretta A, et al. 2002. NK cells: a lesson from mismatched hematopoietic transplantation. *Trends Immunol* **23**: 438–444.

Waldman E, Lu SX, Hubbard VM, et al. 2006. Absence of beta7 integrin results in less graft-versus-host disease because of decreased homing of alloreactive T cells to intestine. *Blood* **107**: 1703–1711.

Wang W, Man S, Gulden PH, et al. 1998. Class I-restricted alloreactive cytotoxic T lymphocytes recognize a complex array of specific MHC-associated peptides. *J Immunol* **160**: 1091–1097.

Weiden PL, Flournoy N, Thomas ED, et al. 1979. Antileukemic effect of graft-versus-host disease in human recipients of allogeneic-marrow grafts. *N Engl J Med* **300**: 1068–1073.

Weiden PL, Sullivan KM, Flournoy N, et al. 1981. Antileukemic effect of chronic graft-versus-host disease: Contribution to improved survival after allogeneic marrow transplantation. *N Engl J Med* **304**: 1529–1533.

Welniak LA, Blazar BR, & Murphy WJ. 2007. Immunobiology of allogeneic hematopoietic stem cell transplantation. *Annu Rev Immunol* **25**: 139–170.

Welniak LA, Kuprash DV, Tumanov AV, et al. 2005. Peyer's patches are not required for acute graft-versus-host disease after myeloablative conditioning and murine allogeneic bone marrow transplantation. *Blood* **107**: 410–412.

Wysocki CA, Panoskaltsis-Mortari A, Blazar BR, et al. 2005. Leukocyte migration and graft-versus-host disease. *Blood* **105**: 4191–4199.

Xun CQ, Thompson JS, Jennings CD, et al. 1994. Effect of total body irradiation, busulfan-cyclophosphamide, or cyclophosphamide conditioning on inflammatory cytokine release and development of acute and chronic graft-versus-host disease in H-2-incompatible transplanted SCID mice. *Blood* **83**: 2360–2367.

Yang YG, Dey BR, Sergio JJ, et al. 1998. Donor-derived interferon gamma is required for inhibition of acute graft-versus-host disease by interleukin 12. *J Clin Invest* **102**: 2126–2135.

Zeiser R, Nguyen VH, Beilhack A, et al. 2006. Inhibition of CD4+CD25+ regulatory T-cell function by calcineurin-dependent interleukin-2 production. *Blood* **108**: 390–399.

Zeng D, Lewis D, Dejbakhsh-Jones S, et al. 1999. Bone marrow NK1.1(-) and NK1.1 (+) T cells reciprocally regulate acute graft versus host disease. *J Exp Med* **189**: 1073–1081.

Zhang Y, Joe G, Hexner E, et al. 2005. Host-reactive CD8+ memory stem cells in graft-versus-host disease. *Nat Med* **11**: 1299–1305.

Chapter

24

Diagnosis and treatment of graft-versus-host disease

Daniel R. Couriel

Acute graft-versus-host disease (GVHD)

Despite adequate posttransplantation immunosuppressive therapy, acute GVHD remains a major cause of morbidity and mortality in this setting, even when HLA-identical siblings are used as stem cell donors. Up to 30% of the recipients of stem cells or BMT from HLA-identical related donors and most patients receiving cells from other sources (matched unrelated, non-HLA-identical siblings, cord blood) will develop grade ≥2 acute GVHD (Basara et al., 2001; Chao et al., 1993; Goker et al., 2001; Martin et al., 2011; Pidala, 2011).

In this section we will review clinical aspects relevant to the care of patients with this complication.

Definition and staging

Traditionally, the definition of acute and chronic GVHD has followed a chronological approach. Arbitrarily, day 100 posttransplantation has been the dividing line between acute and chronic GVHD. Indeed, the majority of acute and chronic GVHDs occur before and after day 100, respectively. However, because we have gained new insights on these diseases and have become more aware of the existence of acute GVHD after day 100, these two diseases are best differentiated clinically (Couriel et al., 2005; Mielcarek et al., 2003).

The BMT Data Book, Third Edition, ed. Reinhold Munker et al. Published by Cambridge University Press. © Cambridge University Press 2013.

The most common presentation of acute GVHD is a maculopapular, erythematous rash in the extremities, which may spread to other parts of the body (Hymes et al., 2006). The other commonly affected sites are the mucosa of the GI tract, where the disease manifests as profuse diarrhea with or without abdominal cramping and severe nausea and vomiting in case of upper GI involvement. The liver may be involved, leading to elevated levels of total bilirubin and, sometimes, alkaline phosphatase in the blood. Less frequently, acute GVHD can affect the eyes and possibly the lungs as well (Couriel et al., 2003, 2004a). GVHD of the eye more commonly manifests with conjunctival inflammation with sloughing and formation of pseudomembranes in the most severe cases (i.e., pseudomembranous conjunctivitis). The cornea can also be involved with keratitis and occasional loss of corneal epithelium (Jabs et al., 1989).

The management and outcome of acute GVHD are largely determined by the stage of organ involvement and the overall grade based on the stages of various sites involved. The staging and grading of acute GVHD as defined by the consensus conference in 1994 is shown in the following table (Przepiorka et al., 1995). Additionally, there is recent evidence that the timing of acute GVHD may be an important prognostic factor. Thus, early-onset or hyperacute GVHD carries a worse prognosis than acute GVHD manifesting after day 14 posttransplantation (Saliba et al., 2007).

Consensus criteria for staging of acute GVHD*
Organ staging

Stage	Skin	Liver	Gut
0	No rash due to GVHD	Bilirubin, <2 mg/dL	None
1	Maculopapular rash <25% of body surface area without associated symptoms	Bilirubin, 2 to <3 mg/dL	Diarrhea, >500–1000 mL/d, nausea and vomiting
2	Maculopapular rash or erythema with pruritus or other associated symptoms covering ≥25% and <50% of body surface area or localized desquamation	Bilirubin, 3 to <6 mg/dL	Diarrhea, >1,000–1500 mL/d, nausea and vomiting
3	Generalized erythroderma or symptomatic macular, papular, or vesicular eruption, with bullous formation or desquamation covering ≥50% of the body	Bilirubin, 6 to <15 mg/dL	Diarrhea, >1,500 mL/d, nausea and vomiting
4	Generalized exfoliative dermatitis or ulcerative dermatitis or bullous formation	Bilirubin, ≥15 mg/dL	Severe abdominal pain with or without ileus involvement

Overall clinical grading of acute GVHD

Grade	Stage			Functional impairment
	Skin	Liver	Gut	
0 (none)	0	0	0	
I (mild)	1–2	0	0	0
II (moderate)	3	1	1*	1
III (severe)	NA	2–3	2–4	2
IV (life threatening)	4	4	NA	2–4

Adapted from Przepiorka et al. (1995).
*Includes upper GI GVHD.

Prophylaxis of acute GVHD

Posttransplant immunosuppression to prevent GVHD

It is standard of care to administer posttransplant immunosuppressive therapy to suppress alloreactive T-cell activity. Methotrexate was the initial drug used following HLA-identical sibling transplants, and it reduced the development of acute GVHD compared to patients receiving no prophylaxis. The addition of cyclosporin to methotrexate reduced the number of patients developing grade 2–4 acute GVHD to approximately 35%–45% (Chao & Schlegel, 1995; Chao et al., 1993, 2000). Cyclosporin is a calcineurin inhibitor that acts to block the activation and IL-2 production by alloreactive T-cells. Tacrolimus is another calcineurin inhibitor, which acts through a similar mechanism. Tacrolimus is more effective in preventing acute GVHD, but survival has been unchanged in two randomized trials (Nash et al., 2000; Przepiorka et al., 1999; Ratanatharathorn et al., 1998).

Novel agents for prevention of GVHD

Sirolimus (Rapamycin, Rapamune®) is a macrolide structurally related to tacrolimus, which acts through a different mechanism. It does not block the activation of T-cells, but limits their expansion. Sirolimus is extensively used to prevent the rejection of organ allografts and is an effective agent for the treatment of established GVHD (Couriel et al., 2005). Recently, the addition of sirolimus to tacrolimus has been effective in reducing the risk of acute GVHD after unrelated donor SCT (Antin et al., 2003).

Mycophenolate mofetil (MMF, Cellcept®) has been an effective agent for the prevention of GVHD and is commonly combined with cyclosporine for GVHD prophylaxis (Basara et al., 2000; Maloney et al., 2003).

Antithymocyte globulin (ATG) is a rabbit or horse antihuman immune globulin that depletes T-cells. The ATG depletes alloreactive T-cells and is commonly used to prevent GVHD. The addition of rabbit ATG (Thymoglobulin®) has been shown to reduce the incidence of acute GVHD after related and unrelated donor transplants (Bacigalupo et al., 2001).

Treatment of acute GVHD

Initial therapy

The initial management of acute GVHD usually consists of steroids. Steroids in combination with cyclosporin (Jacobsohn & Vogelsang, 2002; Martin et al., 1990) or tacrolimus (Couriel et al., 2004a; Jacobsohn & Vogelsang, 2002) have been considered standard therapy for the initial management of acute GVHD. Their mechanism of action is unclear, but is probably related to the suppression of cytokines and lympholytic activities. Numerous dose schedules have been used in multiple clinical trials, but most centers use methylprednisolone (MP) at doses of 2.0 mg/kg. Higher doses are also effective but at the cost of significant side effects and severe catabolic damage, including hyperglycemia, fluid retention, muscular wasting, avascular bone necrosis, and increased rate of infectious complications (Goker et al., 2001; Lee et al., 2006; Martin et al., 1990). Once a clinical improvement has been noted, there is no consensus regarding the best way of tapering steroids in responding patients, but a faster taper may result in fewer steroid-related complications (Hings et al., 1993). An example of steroid taper used in several clinical trials is shown in the following table.

Suggested steroid taper for patients with acute GVHD

Suggested taper for responders (methylprednisolone IV)	
2 mg/kg/day divided into 2–3 doses, days 0[a]–6	
	0.3 mg/kg/day, days 29–38
1.5–1.0 mg/kg/day once daily, days 7–13	0.2 mg/kg/day, days 39–56
1.0 mg/kg/day, days 14–21	0.1 mg/kg/day, days 57–63
0.5 mg/kg/day, days 22–28	0.1 mg/kg every other day, days 64–69
	Discontinue on day 70
Suggested taper for responders (prednisone orally)	
2.5 mg/kg/day divided into 2–3 doses, days 0–6	
2.0–1.4 mg/kg/day once daily, days 7–13	
1.4 mg/kg/day, days 14–21	0.2 mg/kg/day, days 39–56
0.75 mg/kg/day, days 22–28	0.1 mg/kg/day, days 57–63
0.3 mg/kg/day, days 29–38	0.1 mg/kg every other day, days 64–69
	Discontinue on day 70

[a] day 0 represents the first day of corticosteroid therapy.

Approximately half of the patients treated with steroids in the initial management of acute GVHD will have a partial or complete response to therapy (Martin et al., 1990). The remainder will require additional "salvage" or "secondary" therapy for steroid-refractory acute GVHD, which carries a dismal prognosis. Westin et al. (2011) recently reviewed the predictors and outcomes of steroid-refractory acute GVHD. According to the authors, severity, hyperacute presentation, and gender mismatch predict treatment failure.

Definition of steroid-refractory acute GVHD of the skin: no response to steroids (2 mg/kg of MP) is seen after seven days, or progression (i.e., increase in stage) after 2–3 days.

Role of biopsies in the diagnosis of GVHD

Acute GVHD always requires a biopsy for initial diagnosis. The reason is not only to exclude other differential diagnoses, but also because the treatment of GVHD is generally long and intensive. Once the initial diagnosis of acute GVHD is confirmed by a biopsy, the subsequent involvement of other organs does not necessarily require further biopsies as long as other conditions can be excluded with a reasonable certainty. In many cases, the findings are nonspecific; therefore a close interaction between the clinician and the pathologist is needed. If other diagnoses (e.g., viral infections, allergic reactions) have been excluded and the biopsy or biopsies are inconclusive or nonspecific, then the clinical impression should prevail. In chronic GVHD, a biopsy may be needed in cases that have no diagnostic features according to the NIH classification. However, most cases of chronic GVHD can be diagnosed without a biopsy.

Secondary therapy

Currently there is no consensus regarding the definition of steroid-refractory acute GVHD or its optimal management. The definition of steroid refractoriness varies in different institutions, although there is currently a trend toward earlier intervention in view of the dismal prognosis associated with this condition. We consider acute GVHD to be steroid refractory when there is no response to MP at 2 mg/kg for one week, or when there is progressive disease after 72 hours of MP at this dose. Numerous agents have been and continue to be evaluated; unfortunately, with uniformly poor outcomes.

ATG has been the most common form of immunosuppression used in this setting. Different studies have documented efficacy (Arai et al., 2002; Hsu et al., 2001; Martin et al., 1991), but with significant morbidity and mortality, mainly due to infectious complications. Arai et al. at the Johns Hopkins Oncology Center reported 69 patients with steroid refractory GVHD treated with ATG, with only four survivors in this series (Arai et al., 2002). The largest published ATG study was a retrospective analysis by Khoury et al. (Khoury et al., 2001). Fifty-eight patients with acute GVHD who had failed steroids were treated with ATG in different dose schedules. Overall, 42% had improvement in at least one organ. Ninety percent of the patients died at 40 days, mainly from infections. In many instances, the doses of horse ATG are comparable to doses used for severe aplastic anemia (see page 166; e.g., 40 mg/kg daily over four days).

Pentostatin, a nucleoside analog that inhibits adenosine deaminase, is another immunosuppressant that has been used increasingly for the management of acute GVHD (Jacobsohn & Vogelsang, 2002; Vogelsang, 2000). Objective overall responses in up to 67% have been reported, but the effect on OS remains unknown.

Monoclonal antibodies like daclizumab and infliximab have been evaluated in the prevention and treatment of acute GVHD. Daclizumab is a human monoclonal antibody IgGl that incorporates murine complementary-determining regions, directed against CD25. It is believed that its mechanism of action is the competitive inhibition of the binding of IL-2 to its receptor (Junghans et al., 1990).

Przepiorka et al. (2000) reported 43 patients with advanced, refractory acute GVHD treated with two different schedules of daclizumab at 1 mg/kg. Complete responses were seen in up to 47% of patients with the best schedule, and most of these occurred in GVHD confined to the skin. OS was 53% in this group, and the main causes of death were GVHD and infectious complications (Nash et al., 2000). Lee et al. (2004) completed a multicenter randomized placebo-controlled trial designed to determine whether the addition of dacli-zumab could improve the success of initial steroid therapy for acute GVHD. Unfortunately, a planned interim analysis demonstrated that subjects receiving daclizumab experienced significantly worsened 100-day survival (77% vs. 94%, P=0.02) and one-year OS (29% vs. 60%, P=0.002). These findings appropriately led to premature termination of the trial and the authors' conclusion that daclizumab should not be added to corticosteroids for the initial treatment of acute GVHD. The increased mortality in the experimental arm was due to GVHD-related mortality as well as increased relapse. Importantly, individuals in the daclizumab arm were more likely to develop additional sites of GVHD target organ damage, despite the fact that responses at day +42 were similar in both arms (53% for the arm including daclizumab vs. 51% for steroids alone) and the fact that chronic GVHD occurred similarly in both arms. These results suggest that studies assessing GVHD outcomes should include primary endpoints beyond the likelihood of obtaining a clinical response, and also demonstrate that responses to a given treatment in the setting of primary therapy may not always be concordant with the response in the setting of steroid-refractory disease.

Infliximab is a genetically constructed IgG1 murine–human chimeric monoclonal anti-body that binds both the soluble subunit and the membrane-bound precursor of TNF-α (Scallon et al., 1995), a major mediator of the third phase in the pathogenesis of acute GVHD. Infliximab inhibits a broad range of biological activities of TNF-α by blocking the interaction with its receptors. It may also cause lysis of cells that produce TNF-α (Scallon et al., 1995). The drug has been used with success for the treatment of inflammatory bowel disease and rheumatoid arthritis (Reimold, 2003).

Couriel et al. (2004b) studied the efficacy of infliximab for the treatment of steroid-refractory acute GVHD, with a promising response rate of 65% (especially in GI-GVHD) and an OS of 31%. Infliximab was given at a dose of 10 mg/kg intravenously once weekly, up to eight doses (median, four doses). Infliximab was well tolerated in this study, but others have reported an increased incidence of mold infections associated with its use (Marty et al., 2003).

A toxin fusion, denileukin diftitox, has been evaluated in the treatment of steroid-refractory acute GVHD. Denileukin diftitox is a product of the fusion of IL-2 and diphtheria toxin, with high affinity for the IL-2 receptor, present in activated T-cells. Thus far, it has shown a promising response rate of up to 71%, and 33% of patients are alive at 6–24.6 months (Ho et al., 2004). Further studies are under way, but to date none of all these and other treatment modalities has achieved any improvements in OS in steroid-refractory acute GVHD.

Extracorporeal photopheresis (ECP) has proved to be an effective treatment for GVHD, and most evidence comes from treatment of chronic GVHD (Couriel, 2006b; Greinix, 1998, 2000). Greinix et al. (2006) have shown a high response rate in acute GVHD of the skin, GI tract, and liver with relatively early intervention with ECP after steroid failure. ECP is performed by harvesting blood with a continuous cell separator. Next, a photosensitizer (8-methoxypsoralene) is injected into the bag of leukopheresis. Then, the blood bag is irradiated with a UV-A source. Finally, the treated cell suspension is reinjected into the patient. The mechanism of photopheresis is by inactivating lymphocytes or inducing apoptosis in immunoregulatory lymphocyte subpopulations.

As in the case of primary therapy for acute GVHD, the best treatment for patients with an inadequate response to initial corticosteroids is a clinical trial. Unfortunately, none of the existing options seems promising in the steroid-resistant setting. Therefore, it is difficult to recommend any particular agent over another in this setting. A possible approach in patients who do not qualify for a clinical study can be organ- and evidence-based. Thus, patients with acute GVHD of the skin may benefit from those modalities, such as daclizumab, ATG, or ECP, where current published literature has shown a good or acceptable response rate. In the case of acute GVHD of the GI tract, infliximab and ATG would be acceptable treatment options. Acute GVHD of the liver is more difficult to treat than that of the skin and possibly GI cases as well. ECP has an interesting response rate in cases of liver GVHD. It is important to emphasize that none of these modalities seems to alter survival in a substantial way in the setting of steroid-resistant acute GVHD. Adult mesenchymal stem cells (see pages 220 and 222) showed significant responses in phase II studies and currently are being tested in phase III studies for steroid-refractory acute GVHD. New strategies for the treatment of GVHD were reviewed by Wolf et al. (2012). These strategies include: a modification of the danger signals related to tissue damage; a modification of the host dendritic cells; interfering with the signal transduction of donor T-cells, and also the infusion and expansion of regulatory T-cells (see page 220).

Chronic GVHD
Definitions and staging

Chronic GVHD is the main long-term complication and limitation to successful HSCT. It affects over 50% of all patients undergoing HSCT, and the majority of those with acute GVHD (Couriel et al., 2004a). It has a major impact on both quality of life and survival. Chronic GVHD frequently involves multiple organs and requires prolonged immunosuppressive therapy (Lee et al., 2003; Inamoto & Flowers, 2011). In one report, 15% of cancer-free patients were still on immunosuppressive therapy after seven years (Stewart et al., 2004). The more severe forms of chronic GVHD are clearly associated with a lower DFS. Thus, the potential benefit of a GVL effect is shadowed by significant TRM (Lee et al., 2002).

Chronic GVHD is a disease of deregulated immunity with protean manifestations similar in many ways to autoimmune diseases (Blazar et al., 2012). The relative uncommonness of the disease, the lack of consensus on what represents true manifestations of chronic GVHD, the very limited understanding of its pathophysiology, and the clinical complexity of these patients are all factors that have hindered a systematic approach to the treatment of this problem. It is important to recognize chronic GVHD as a distinct clinical syndrome, different from acute GVHD or the autoimmune disorders it mimics. This has been recognized by the NIH Consensus Development Project on Criteria for Clinical Trials in Chronic GVHD, as shown in the following tables (Filipovich et al., 2005). Thus, as in the case of acute GVHD, the definition of chronic GVHD is eminently clinical. Although the vast majority of cases of chronic GVHD will occur after the classical "100-day" boundary, this should not be part of the definition of chronic GVHD, particularly as it is relatively common to see cases of "late" acute GVHD (Couriel et al., 2005; Mielcarek et al., 2003). The advent of reduced-intensity regimens has often led to a blurring between acute (which may occur later than day 100) and chronic GVHD.

Strategies that have successfully diminished acute GVHD, such as reduced-intensity preparative regimens, seem to have less or no impact on the incidence of chronic GVHD.

Approximately one-third of patients without a history of acute GVHD will have de novo chronic GVHD (Couriel et al., 2004a). On the other hand, not all patients affected by acute GVHD will go on to develop chronic GVHD. Chronic GVHD mimics some aspects of autoimmune conditions like systemic lupus erythematosus or scleroderma. However, the clinical differences here may be just as significant as the similarities. Thus, chronic GVHD is a relatively autonomous entity, and the nature of its association with acute GVHD or similarities with other autoimmune disorders remains unclear.

NIH Consensus Diagnostic Criteria for Chronic GVHD[a]

Organ or site	Diagnostic (sufficient to establish the diagnosis of chronic GVHD)	Distinctive (seen in chronic GVHD, but insufficient alone to establish a diagnosis of chronic GVHD)	Other features (should not be used alone to establish a diagnosis of chronic GVHD*)	Common (seen with both acute and chronic GVHD)
Skin	• Poikilodermia • Lichen-type features • Sclerotic features • Morphea-like features • Lichen sclerosis	• Vitiligo	• Sweat impairment	• Erythema • Maculo-papular rash • Pruritus
Nails		• Dystrophy • Longitudinal ridging, splitting or brittle • Onycholysis • Pterygium • Destruction** (usually symmetric, affects most nails)		
Scalp and body hair		• New alopecia (after recovery from chemoradiotherapy), scarring and nonscarring alopecia; scaling, papulosquamous lesions • Loss of body hair– typically patchy (including eyelashes, eyebrows)	• Thinning scalp hair, coarse or dull (not explained by endocrine or other causes) • Premature gray hair	
Mouth	• Lichen-type features • Hyperkeratotic plaques • Restriction of mouth opening from sclerosis	• Xerostomia • Mucocele • Mucosal atrophy • Pseudomembranes** • Ulcers**		• Gingivitis • Mucositis • Erythema • Pain

(cont.)

Organ or site	Diagnostic (sufficient to establish the diagnosis of chronic GVHD)	Distinctive (seen in chronic GVHD, but insufficient alone to establish a diagnosis of chronic GVHD)	Other features (should not be used alone to establish a diagnosis of chronic GVHD*)	Common (seen with both acute and chronic GVHD)
Eyes		• New onset dry, gritty, or painful eyes[†] • Cicatricial conjunctivitis • Keratoconjunctivitis sicca[†] • Corneal ulceration[**]	• Excessive aqueous tearing • Photophobia • Periorbital hyperpigmentation • Blepharitis (erythema of the eye lids with edema)	
Genitalia	• Lichen-type features • Vaginal stricture or stenosis • Ulcers[**]			

* can be acknowledged as part of the chronic GVHD symptomatology if diagnosis is confirmed;
** In all cases, infection, drug effect, or other causes must be excluded;
[†] diagnosis of chronic GVHD requires biopsy or radiology confirmation (or Schirmer's test for eyes), **and** at least one distinctive manifestation in another organ system;
[a] adapted from Filipovich et al. (2005).

Acute versus chronic GVHD[a]

	Time of symptoms after HSCT or DLI	Presence of acute GVHD features[*]	Presence of chronic GGVHD features[†]
Classic acute GVHD	Usually <6 mo	Yes	No
Persistent, recurrent, or late-onset acute GVHD	No time limit	Yes	No
Acute and chronic overlap	No time limit	Yes	Yes
Chronic GVHD	No time limit	No	Yes

[*] e.g., rash or GI symptoms typical of acute GVHD.
[†] see previous table for diagnostic and distinctive features of chronic GVHD.
[a] adapted from Filipovich et al. (2005).

Organ scoring in chronic GVHD[a]

	Score 0	Score 1	Score 2	Score 3
Performance score: KPS ECOG LPS	• Asymptomatic and fully active (ECOG 0; KPS or LPS 100%)	• Symptomatic, fully ambulatory, restricted only in physically strenuous activity (ECOG 1; KPS or LPS 80%–90%)	• Symptomatic, ambulatory, capable of self-care, >50% of waking hours out of bed (ECOG 2; KPS or LPS 60%–70%)	• Symptomatic, limited self-care, >50% of waking hours in bed (ECOG 3–4; KPS or LPS <60%)
Skin *Clinical features* • Maculopapular rash • Lichen-type features • Papulosquamous or ichtyosis • Hyperpigmentation • Hypopigmentation • Keratosis pilaris • Erythema • Erythroderma • Polikiloderma • Sclerotic features • Pruritus • Hair • Nails • % BSA involved	• No symptoms	• <18% BSA with disease signs but **no** sclerotic features	• 19%–50% BSA **or** substantial involvement with superficial sclerotic features "not hidebound" (able to pinch)	• >50% BSA **or** deep sclerotic features "hidebound" (unable to pinch) **or** interference with ADL due to impaired mobility, ulceration, or severe pruritus
Mouth	• No symptoms	• Mild symptoms with disease signs, but not limiting oral intake significantly	• Moderate symptoms with signs, with partial limitation of oral intake	• Severe symptoms with disease signs on examination, with major limitation of oral intake
Eyes Mean tear test (mm): • 6–10 • <5 • Not done	• No symptoms	• Mild dry eye symptoms not affecting ADL (requiring eye drops <3× per day) **or** asymptomatic signs of sicca keratitis	• Moderate dry eye symptoms partially affecting ADL (requiring drops >3×per day or punctal plugs), **without** vision impairment	• Severe dry eye symptoms significantly affecting ADL (special eyewear to relieve pain) **or** unable to work because of ocular symptoms **or** loss of vision caused by pseudomembranes or corneal ulceration

(cont.)

	Score 0	Score 1	Score 2	Score 3
GI tract	• No symptoms	• Symptoms such as dysphagia, anorexia, nausea, vomiting, abdominal pain, or diarrhea, without significant weight loss (<5%)	• Symptoms associated with mild to moderate weight loss (5%–15%)	• Symptoms associated with significant weight loss (>15%), requires nutritional supplement for most calorie needs **or** esophageal dilation
Liver	• Normal LFT	• Bilirubin, AP*, AST or ALT <2×ULN	• Bilirubin >3 mg/dL or bilirubin, enzymes 2–5×ULN	• Bilirubin or enzymes >5×ULN
Lungs	• No symptoms • FEV1/FVC ratio >0.7 **or** FEV1 >75%, without distinct findings of BO on HRCT	• Mild symptoms (dyspnea with stair climbing) • FEV1/FVC ratio <0.7 **or** FEV1 of 51%–75%, **with** distinct findings of BO on HRCT	• Moderate symptoms (dyspnea with level walking) • FEV1/FVC ratio <0.75 **or** FEV1 of 35%–50%, **with** distinct findings of BO on HRCT	• Severe symptoms (dyspnea at rest; requiring oxygen) • FEV1/FVC ratio <0.75 **or** FEV1 ≤34%, **with** distinct findings of BO on HRCT
Joints and fascia	• No symptoms	• Mild tightness of arms or legs, normal or mild decreased ROM **and** not affecting ADL	• Tightness of arms or legs **or** joint contractures, erythema thought due to fasciitis, moderate decrease ROM **and** mild to moderate limitation of ADL	• Contractures **with** significant decrease of ROM **and** significant limitation of ADL (unable to tie shoes, button shirts, dress self, etc.)

(cont.)

	Score 0	Score 1	Score 2	Score 3
Genital tract	• No symptoms	• Symptomatic with mild distinct signs on examination **and** no effect on coitus and minimal discomfort with GYN examination	• Symptomatic with distinct signs on examination **and** with mild dyspareunia or discomfort with GYN examination	• Symptomatic **with** advanced signs (stricture, labia agglutination, or severe ulceration) **and** severe pain with coitus or inability to insert vaginal speculum

KPS, Karnofsky performance status; LPS, Lanky performance status; BO, bronchiolitis obliterans; HRCT, high-resolution computed tomography; BSA, body surface area; ADL, activities of daily living; ROM, range of motion; GYN, gynecologic.
[a] adapted from Filipovich et al. (2005).

Treatment of chronic GVHD
General aspects and initial therapy

Chronic GVHD is a multisystem disorder that most frequently affects multiple organs as well as psychosocial and sexual aspects of an otherwise cancer-free patient. The involvement of multiple organs dictates the need for a multidisciplinary approach, coordinated by the transplant physician, preferably at a center that has experience in the care of these patients. Larger transplant centers have organized clinics devoted to the follow-up and care of long-term HSCT complications, including GVHD. The participation of subspecialists with an interest, and ideally experience with chronic GVHD patients, is always desirable.

There are two aspects to the management of chronic GVHD, both equally important and interconnected (Shlomchik et al., 2007). The first aspect is systemic treatment with immunosuppressant and immunomodulating agents. Corticosteroids are the single most effective therapy. Although there seems to be no advantage in the combination with cyclosporin, this may reduce long-term complications of corticosteroids (Koc et al., 2002). The alternative use of tacrolimus with corticosteroids does not seem to offer any additional advantage in the initial treatment of chronic GVHD. It is still unclear whether intensifying initial therapy by either higher steroid doses or incorporating new agents to the initial combination of calcineurin inhibitor plus corticosteroid will result in better responses, quality of life, or survival. When mycophenolate mofetil was added to the standard initial corticosteroid therapy for chronic GVHD, no significant benefit could be observed (Martin et al., 2009). Several small studies showed encouraging results with the monoclonal antibody rituximab implicating B-cells in the pathogenesis of chronic GVHD. In a meta-analysis of these studies, an overall response of 66% was reported. Likewise, several small studies reported encouraging results with low doses of the TKI imatinib. These recent data were reviewed by Inamoto and Flowers (2011).

The second component of chronic GVHD therapy, occasionally overlooked, is ancillary and supportive care (Couriel et al., 2006a). This includes education, prevention of flare-ups, infectious disease prophylaxis, physical and occupational therapy, nutrition, alleviation of the chronic manifestations of GVHD and its treatment, and providing the patient with coping mechanisms or resources to deal with the psychosocial, sexual, and financial consequences of the disease. These interventions, when successful, may have the potential to reduce the need for systemic therapy, and the relative impact of these interventions on the outcome of patients with chronic GVHD needs to be explored.

Initial treatment with corticosteroids can control chronic GVHD in about 50% of the patients, and the majority of those without resolution of their chronic GVHD will also suffer the consequences of prolonged immunosuppression (Stewart et al., 2004).

Overview of the most commonly used steroid-sparing therapies

A variety of new drugs and other immunomodulatory treatments have shown activity in the salvage therapy of chronic GVHD. This evidence originates in small pilot and phase II studies, with doses and schedules usually matching those of their FDA-approved use. Thalidomide, sirolimus, extracorporeal photopheresis, rituximab, pentostatin, mycophenolate mofetil, hydroxychloroquine, and clofazimine are just some examples (Couriel et al., 2005, 2006b; Cutler et al., 2006; Lee et al., 2003). The overall response to salvage therapy has ranged between 30% and more than 70%. Unfortunately, with all these different therapies, the vast majority of these responses are partial, and the corticosteroid-sparing effect has not been systematically assessed or reported (Shlomchik et al., 2007). In addition to the difficulties inherent to the assessment of response, it is likely that a substantial proportion of the patients included in chronic GVHD studies that used a chronological definition may have had "late" acute GVHD.

The toxicity of some of these regimens, such as thalidomide (Arora et al., 2001) or the combination of sirolimus and tacrolimus (Couriel et al., 2005), can be substantial. As for initial salvage therapy, the best salvage treatment still remains to be determined.

The evaluation of the role of newer immunomodulating rather than immunosuppressant therapies aimed at facilitating or inducing immune tolerance is under way.

Summary of ancillary and supportive care interventions[a]

Organ system	Organ-specific intervention[*]
Skin and appendages	*Prevention* • Photoprotection. Surveillance for malignancy *Treatment* • For intact skin–topical emollients, corticosteroids, antipruritic agents, and others (e.g., PUVA, calcineurin inhibitors) • For erosions/ulcerations–microbiological cultures, topical antimicrobials, protective films or other dressings, debridement, hyperbaric oxygen, wound care specialist consultation
Mouth and oral cavity	*Prevention* • Maintain good oral/dental hygiene. Consider routine dental cleaning and endocarditis prophylaxis. Surveillance for infection and malignancy *Treatment* • Topical high and ultrahigh potency corticosteroids and analgesics. Therapy for oral dryness
Eyes #	*Prevention* • Photoprotection. Surveillance for infection, cataract formation, and increased intraocular pressure *Treatment* • Artificial tears, ocular ointments, topical corticosteroids or cyclosporin, punctal occlusion, humidified environment, occlusive eye-wear, moisture-chamber eyeglasses, cevimeline, pilocarpine, tarsorraphy, gas-permeable scleral contact lens, autologous serum, microbiological cultures, topical antimicrobials, doxycycline
Vulva and vagina	*Prevention* • Surveillance for estrogen deficiency, infection (herpes simplex virus, human papilloma virus, yeast, bacteria), and malignancy *Treatment* • Water-based lubricants, topical estrogens, topical corticosteroids or calcineurin inhibitors, dilators, surgery for extensive synechiae/obliteration, early gynecology consultation
GI tract and liver	*Prevention* • Surveillance for infection (viral, fungal) *Treatment* • Eliminate other potential etiologies. Dietary modification, enzyme supplementation for malabsorption, gastroesophageal reflux management, esophageal dilatation, ursodeoxycholic acid
Lungs	*Prevention* • Surveillance for infection (*Pneumocystis carinii*, viral, fungal, bacterial) *Treatment* • Eliminate other potential etiologies (e.g., infection, gastroesophageal reflux). Inhaled corticosteroids, bronchodilators, supplementary oxygen, pulmonary rehabilitation. Consideration of lung transplantation in appropriate candidates

(cont.)

Organ system	Organ-specific intervention*
Hematopoietic	*Prevention* • Surveillance for infection (cytomegalovirus, parvovirus) *Treatment* • Eliminate other potential etiologies (e.g., drug toxicity, infection). Hematopoietic growth factors, immunoglobulin for immune cytopenias
Neurologic	*Prevention* • Calcineurin inhibitor drug level monitoring. Seizure prophylaxis including blood pressure control, electrolyte replacement, anticonvulsants *Treatment* • Occupational and physical therapy, treatment of neuropathic syndromes with tricyclic antidepressants, selective serotonin reuptake inhibitors, or anticonvulsants
Immunological and infectious diseases	*Prevention* • Immunizations and prophylaxis against *Pneumocystis jirovecii*, varicella zoster virus, and encapsulated bacteria based on Centers for Disease Control (CDC) guidelines. Consider immunoglobulin replacement based on levels and recurrent infections. No current evidence to support the use of mold-active agents. Surveillance for infection (viral, bacterial, fungal, atypical) *Treatment* • Organism-specific antimicrobial agents. Empiric parenteral broad-spectrum antibacterial coverage for fever
Musculoskeletal	*Prevention* • Surveillance for decreased range of motion, bone densitometry, calcium levels and 25-OH Vitamin D. Physical therapy, calcium, vitamin D, bisphosphonates *Treatment* • Physical therapy, bisphosphonates for osteopenia and osteoporosis

[a] adapted from Arora et al. (2001).
the diagnosis and treatment of chronic GVHD of the eye were recently reviewed in a consensus conference (Dietrich-Ntoukas et al., 2012).

Supportive care and ancillary interventions

Although usually neglected or forgotten as we are struggling with more than one marginally ineffective systemic therapy, this should be an important component in the care of patients with chronic GVHD. Although we know that interventions such as education in photoprotection, physical therapy, and prevention of osteoporosis have a positive impact, we still do not have an accurate idea as to what extent these relatively nontoxic therapies are related to systemic immunosuppression. The relevant supportive and ancillary care measures are summarized in the table on page 324. Therefore, the main questions are whether "intensive" supportive care can contribute to fewer reflares, steroid sparing, fewer adverse effects from systemic immunosuppression, a better quality of life, and ultimately, survival (Couriel et al., 2006a).

Conclusions

Despite our better understanding of histocompatibility and recent advances in transplant immunology, GVHD and its complications continue to be the major limitation to successful allotransplantation. We hope that newer immunomodulatory strategies will make a difference as prophylactic strategies or very early in the course of acute GVHD. Once established, particularly in forms that are not readily responsive to steroids, acute GVHD has a dismal prognosis. Chronic GVHD is a different disease, and prevention of acute GVHD does not naturally lead to a lower incidence of chronic GVHD. Since the clinical redefinition of chronic GVHD by the NIH Consensus Conference, a new baseline has been set for the systematic development of clinical trials that hopefully will provide a better understanding of risk factors, prognosis, and therapy. In the United States, the BMT CTN performs clinical trials for the treatment and prophylaxis of acute and chronic GVHD.

References and further reading

Antin JH, Kim H, Cutler C, et al. 2003. Sirolimus, tacrolimus, and low-dose methotrexate for graft-versus-host disease prophylaxis in mismatched related donor or unrelated donor transplantation. *Blood* **102**: 1601–1605.

Arai S, Margolis J, Zahurak M, et al. 2002. Poor outcome in steroid-refractory graft-versus-host disease with antithymocyte globulin treatment. *Biol Blood Marrow Transplant* **8**: 155–160.

Arora M, Wagner JE, Davies SM, et al. 2001. Randomized clinical trial of thalidomide, cyclosporine, and prednisone versus cyclosporine and prednisone as initial therapy for chronic graft-versus-host disease. *Biol Blood Marrow Transplant* **7**: 265–273.

Bacigalupo A, Lamparelli T, Bruzzi P, et al. 2001. Antithymocyte globulin for graft-versus-host disease prophylaxis in transplants from unrelated donors: 2 randomized studies from Gruppo Italiano Trapianti Midollo Osseo (GITMO). *Blood* **98**: 2942–2947.

Basara N, Blau WI, Kiehl MG, et al., 2000. Mycophenolate mofetil for the prophylaxis of acute GVHD in HLA-mismatched bone marrow transplant patients. *Clin Transplant* **14**: 121–126.

Basara N, Kiehl MG, & Fauser AA. 2001. New therapeutic modalities in the treatment of graft-versus-host disease. *Crit Rev Oncol Hematol* **38**: 129–138.

Blazar B, White ES, & Couriel D. 2012. Understanding chronic GVHD from different angles. *Biol Blood Marrow Transplant* **18**: S184–S188.

Chao NJ & Schlegel PG. 1995. Prevention and treatment of graft-versus-host disease. *Ann N Y Acad Sci* **770**: 130–140.

Chao NJ, Schmidt GM, Niland JC, et al. 1993. Cyclosporine, methotrexate, and prednisone compared with cyclosporine and prednisone for prophylaxis of acute graft-versus-host disease. *N Engl J Med* **329**: 1225–1230.

Chao NJ, Snyder DS, Jain M, et al. 2000. Equivalence of 2 effective graft-versus-host disease prophylaxis regimens: results of a prospective double-blind randomized trial. *Biol Blood Marrow Transplant* **6**: 254–261.

Couriel D, Caldera H, Champlin R, et al. 2004a. Acute graft-versus-host disease: pathophysiology, clinical manifestations, and management. *Cancer* **101**: 1936–1946.

Couriel D, Carpenter PA, Cutler C, et al. 2006a. Ancillary therapy and supportive care of chronic graft-versus-host disease: National Institutes of Health consensus development project on criteria for clinical trials in chronic graft-versus-host disease: V. Ancillary therapy and supportive care working group report. *Biol Blood Marrow Transplant* **12**: 375–396.

Couriel DR, Hosing C, Saliba R, et al. 2006b. Extracorporeal photochemotherapy for the treatment of steroid-resistant chronic GVHD. *Blood* **107**: 3074–3080.

Couriel DR, Saliba R, Escalon MP, et al. 2005. Sirolimus in combination with tacrolimus and corticosteroids for the treatment of resistant chronic graft-versus-host disease. *Br J Haematol* **130**: 409–417.

Couriel DR, Saliba R, Ghosh S, et al. 2003. Graft-versus-host disease of the liver: a clinicopathological analysis. *Blood* **102**: 712a.

Couriel DR, Saliba R, Hicks K, et al. 2004b. Tumor necrosis factor alpha blockade for the treatment of steroid-refractory acute GVHD. *Blood* **104**: 649–654.

Cutler C, Miklos D, Kim HT, et al. 2006. Rituximab for steroid-refractory chronic graft-versus-host disease. *Blood* **108**: 756–762.

Dietrich-Ntoukas T, Cursiefen C, Westekemper H, et al. 2012. Diagnosis and treatment of chronic graft-versus host disease: report from the German-Austrian-Swiss consensus conference on clinical practice in chronic GVHD. *Cornea* **31**: 299–310.

Filipovich AH, Weisdorf D, Pavletic S, et al. 2005. National Institutes of Health consensus development project on criteria for clinical trials in chronic graft-versus-host disease: I. Diagnosis and staging working group report. *Biol Blood Marrow Transplant* **11**: 945–956.

Goker H, Haznedaroglu IC, & Chao NJ. 2001. Acute graft-vs-host disease: pathobiology and management. *Exp Hematol* **29**: 259–277.

Greinix HT, Knobler RM, Worel N, et al. 2006. The effect of intensified extracorporeal photochemotherapy on long-term survival in patients with severe acute graft-versus-host disease. *Haematologica* **91**: 405–408.

Greinix HT, Volc-Platzer B, Kahls P, et al. 2000. Extracorporeal photochemotherapy in the treatment of severe steroid-refractory acute graft-versus-host disease: a pilot study. *Blood* **96**: 2426–2431.

Greinix HT, Valc-Platzer B, Rabitsch W, et al. 1998. Successful use of extracorporeal photochemotherapy in the treatment of severe acute and chronic graft-versus-host disease. *Blood* **92**: 3098–3104.

Hings IM, Filipovich AH, Miller WJ, et al. 1993. Prednisone therapy for acute graft-versus-host disease: short- versus long-term treatment. A prospective randomized trial. *Transplantation* **56**: 577–580.

Ho VT, Zahrieh D, Hochberg E, et al. 2004. Safety and efficacy of denileukin diftitox in patients with steroid refractory acute graft-versus-host disease after allogeneic hematopoietic stem cell transplantation. *Blood* **104**: 1224–1226.

Hsu B, May R, Carrum G, et al. 2001. Use of antithymocyte globulin for treatment of steroid-refractory acute graft-versus-host disease: an international practice survey. *Bone Marrow Transplant* **28**: 945–950.

Hymes SR, Turner ML, Champlin RE, et al. 2006. Cutaneous manifestations of chronic graft-versus-host disease. *Biol Blood Marrow Transplant* **12**: 1101–1113.

Inamoto Y & Flowers ME. 2011. Treatment of chronic graft-versus-host disease in 2011. *Curr Opin Hematol* **18**: 414–420.

Jabs DA, Wingard J, Green WR, et al. 1989. The eye in bone marrow transplantation. III. Conjunctival graft-vs-host disease. *Arch Ophthalmol* **107**: 1343–1348.

Jacobsohn DA & Vogelsang GB. 2002. Novel pharmacotherapeutic approaches to prevention and treatment of GVHD. *Drugs* **62**: 879–889.

Junghans RP, Waldmann TA, Landolfi NF, et al. 1990. Anti-Tac-H, a humanized antibody to the interleukin 2 receptor with new features for immunotherapy in malignant and immune disorders. *Cancer Res* **50**: 1495–1502.

Khoury H, Kashyap A, Adkins DR, et al. 2001. Treatment of steroid-resistant acute graft-versus-host disease with anti-thymocyte globulin. *Bone Marrow Transplant* **27**: 1059–1064.

Koc S, Leisenring W, Flowers ME, et al. 2002. Therapy for chronic graft-versus-host disease: a randomized trial comparing cyclosporine plus prednisone versus prednisone alone. *Blood* **100**: 48–51.

Lee HJ, Oran B, Saliba RM, et al. 2006. Steroid myopathy in patients with acute graft-versus-host disease treated with high-dose steroid therapy. *Bone Marrow Transplant* **38**: 299–303.

Lee SJ, Klein JP, Barrett AJ, et al. 2002. Severity of chronic graft-versus-host disease: association with treatment-related mortality and relapse. *Blood* **100**: 406–414.

Lee SJ, Vogelsang G, & Flowers ME. 2003. Chronic graft-versus-host disease. *Biol Blood Marrow Transplant* **9**: 215–233.

Lee SJ, Zahrieh D, Agura E, et al. 2004. Effect of up-front daclizumab when combined with steroids for the treatment of acute graft-versus-host disease: results of a randomized trial. *Blood* **104**: 1559–1564.

Maloney DG, Molina AJ, Sahebi F, et al. 2003. Allografting with nonmyeloablative conditioning following cytoreductive autografts for the treatment of patients with multiple myeloma. *Blood* **102**: 3447–3454.

Martin PJ, Inamoto Y, Carpenter PA, et al. 2011. Treatment of chronic graft-versus host disease: past, present and future. *Korean J Hematol* **46**: 153–163.

Martin PJ, Schoch G, Fisher L, et al. 1990. A retrospective analysis of therapy for acute graft-versus-host disease: initial treatment. *Blood* **76**: 1464–1472.

Martin PJ, Schoch G, Fisher L, et al. 1991. A retrospective analysis of therapy for acute graft-versus-host disease: secondary treatment. *Blood* **77**: 1821–1828.

Martin PJ, Storer BE, Rowley SD, et al. 2009. Evaluation of mycophenolate mofetil for initial treatment of chronic graft-versus-host disease. *Blood* **113**: 5074–5082.

Marty FM, Lee SJ, Fahey MM, et al. 2003. Infliximab use in patients with severe graft-versus-host disease and other emerging risk factors of non-Candida invasive fungal infections in allogeneic hematopoietic stem cell transplant recipients: a cohort study. *Blood* **102**: 2768–2776.

Mielcarek M, Martin PJ, Leisenring W, et al. 2003. Graft-versus-host disease after nonmyeloablative versus conventional hematopoietic stem cell transplantation. *Blood* **102**: 756–762.

Nash RA, Antin JH, Karanes C, et al. 2000. Phase 3 study comparing methotrexate and tacrolimus with methotrexate and cyclosporine for prophylaxis of acute graft-versus-host disease after marrow transplantation from unrelated donors. *Blood* **96**: 2062–2068.

Pidala J. 2011. Graft-vs-host disease following allogeneic hematopoietic cell transplantation. *Cancer Control* **18**: 268–276.

Przepiorka D, Kernan NA, Ippoliti C, et al. 2000. Daclizumab, a humanized anti-interleukin-2 receptor alpha chain antibody, for treatment of acute graft-versus-host disease. *Blood* **95**: 83–89.

Przepiorka D, Nash RA, Wingard JR, et al. 1999. Relationship of tacrolimus whole blood levels to efficacy and safety outcomes after unrelated donor marrow transplantation. *Biol Blood Marrow Transplant* **5**: 94–97.

Przepiorka D, Weisdorf D, Martin P, et al. 1995. 1994 Consensus Conference on acute GVHD grading. *Bone Marrow Transplant* **15**: 825–828.

Ratanatharathorn V, Nash RA, Przepiorka D, et al. 1998. Phase III study comparing methotrexate and tacrolimus (prograf, FK506) with methotrexate and cyclosporine for graft-versus-host disease prophylaxis after HLA-identical sibling bone marrow transplantation. *Blood* **92**: 2303–2314.

Reimold AM. 2003. New indications for treatment of chronic inflammation by TNF-alpha blockade. *Am J Med Sci* **325**: 75–92.

Saliba RM, de Lima M, Giralt S, et al. 2007. Hyperacute GVHD: risk factors, outcomes, and clinical implications. *Blood* **109**: 2751–2758.

Scallon BJ, Moore MA, Trinh H, et al. 1995. Chimeric anti-TNF-alpha monoclonal antibody cA2 binds recombinant transmembrane TNF-alpha and activates immune effector functions. *Cytokine* **7**: 251–259.

Shlomchik WD, Lee SJ, Couriel D, et al. 2007. Transplantation's greatest challenges: advances in chronic graft-versus-host disease. *Biol Blood Marrow Transplant* **13**: S2–S10.

Stewart BL, Storer B, Storek J, et al. 2004. Duration of immunosuppressive treatment for chronic graft-versus-host disease. *Blood* **104**: 3501–3506.

Vogelsang GB. 2000. Advances in the treatment of graft-versus-host disease. *Leukemia* **14**: 509–510.

Westin JR, Saliba RM, de Lima M, et al. 2011. Steroid-refractory acute GVHD: predictors and outcomes. *Adv Hematol* 2011:601953 [Epub ahead of print].

Wolf D, von Lilienfeld-Toal M, Wolf AM, et al. 2012. Novel treatment concepts for graft-versus host disease. *Blood* **119**: 16–25.

Chapter 25

Management and prophylaxis of infections after BMT/SCT

Nicholas Barber and Alison G. Freifeld

Fever and neutropenia

HSCT preparative regimens are often marked by periods of neutropenia, during which the absolute neutrophil count (ANC) declines and remains at a low level for days or even weeks. Neutropenia as a consequence of cytoreductive chemotherapy is associated with the increased risk of serious infections (Bodey et al., 1966). This risk starts to increase when the ANC decreases to less than 1000 cells/mm^3 and the infection risk increases further dramatically when ANC is less than 500 cells/mm^3. Bloodstream infection develops in approximately 10%–25% of patients with an ANC less than 100 cells/mm^3 (Freifeld et al., 2011; Ramphal, 2004; Wisplinghoff et al., 2003). Less often, pneumonia, cellulitis, CVC-related infections, or herpes virus reactivations will cause fever. The duration of ANC decline is also a critical determinant of infection risk, with longer durations being more likely to incur infection (Bodey et al., 1966). Full intensity HSCT recipients are typically neutropenic for at least 10–14 days or longer, and bacterial

The BMT Data Book, Third Edition, ed. Reinhold Munker et al. Published by Cambridge University Press. © Cambridge University Press 2013.

infections predominate as the infectious etiology of fever. Owing to routine prophylaxis, fungal and viral pathogens are much less common causes.

Reduced-intensity HSCT regimens are generally associated with shorter and less severe neutropenic periods, but these patients remain at high risk for infection in the immediate posttransplant period due to immunosuppression. This chapter focuses on the neutropenic HSCT recipient with fever.

Definitions

Neutropenia is defined as a neutrophil count of <500 cells/mm^3, or an ANC that is anticipated to fall below that level within 48 hours of presentation.

Fever is a single temperature measurement of 38.3°C (101°F) or greater, in the absence of other obvious causes, or a temperature of 38°C or greater for an hour or more.

Evaluation

Fever alone may be the only sign of a severe underlying infection in the neutropenic patient. In the absence of neutrophils, inflammatory signs and symptoms of infection are often attenuated, hence clinical clues may not be apparent (e.g., skin inflammation or pulmonary infiltrates may be minimal or absent despite serious infections at those sites). Signs or symptoms, or blood tests such as C-reactive protein or procalcitonin, will not reliably distinguish those with positive cultures. Therefore, all febrile neutropenic patients must be treated immediately (preferably within one hour) with an empiric regimen of broad-spectrum antibiotics, as there is danger of rapidly progressive sepsis. Neutropenic patients without fever but with the strong suspicion of infection should also be treated accordingly.

All HSCT recipients are considered high risk for a complicated course during fever and neutropenia and should be hospitalized for intravenous antibiotics (Freifeld et al., 2011; NCCN, 2011).

The evaluation of the neutropenic HSCT patient with new fever (or suspected infection) includes:

- History and physical examination: attention to prior infections, recent or ongoing antimicrobials and immunosuppressives, recent procedures or surgeries, and in-dwelling CVC devices
- Blood cultures: 2–3 sets (20–40 mL of blood per set), including a set from each catheter lumen plus a peripheral venipuncture site. If no CVC is present, two sets should be taken from separate venipuncture sites simultaneously
- Complete blood count and differential WBC count (manual differential count)
- Liver and renal function tests
- Chest radiograph is not done routinely: *only* for patients with respiratory signs or symptoms
- Bacterial cultures or viral assays of any suggestive sites of infection: diarrheal stool for *Clostridium difficile* toxin and/or for culture/ova/parasites (only if recent travel to endemic areas); tests and/or cultures of urine, sputum, CSF, skin lesions (for herpesvirus detection by PCR), or nasopharyngeal swab (for respiratory virus detection by PCR)

Treatment algorithms

Empirical antibiotic therapy

For currently available antifungal drugs, see Chapter 27 (pages 448–454).

Monotherapy

Monotherapy with the following broad-spectrum anti-pseudomonal agents is recommended for patients who are hemodynamically stable and have no specific localized symptoms (Freifeld et al., 2011; Paul et al., 2006):

- Cefepime, 2 g IV every 8 hr
- Piperacillin/tazobactam, 4.5 g IV every 8 hr (in some hospitals, extended infusion)
- Imipenem, 500 mg IV every 6 hr or meropenem 1 g IV every 8 hr
- Ceftazidime* 2 g IV every 8 hr

*Note: this agent lacks good streptococcal coverage and is less potent against resistant Gram-negative pathogens.

Penicillin allergy

Penicillin allergy should be assessed by identifying specific reactions to penicillins: patients who claim to be "allergic" because of GI reactions are often misclassified as allergic. Those with a rash (not hives) to penicillins will generally tolerate cephalosporins. True penicillin allergy requires a history of an immediate-type hypersensitivity reaction (hives, bronchospasm, anaphylaxis), and these patients should receive non-β-lactam-containing combinations:

- Aztreonam 2 g IV every 6–8 hr or ciprofloxacin 500 mg IV every 12 hr
  PLUS vancomycin 1 g IV every 12 hr or clindamycin 600 mg IV every 8 hr

Vancomycin (or other agents with enhanced Gram-positive activity) is not a routine part of the empirical regimen and should be added only if the following indications are present:

- Hemodynamic instability or other evidence of severe sepsis
- Pneumonia documented radiographically
- Positive blood culture for gram-positive bacteria, before final identification and susceptibility testing is available
- Clinically suspected serious catheter-related infections (e.g., chills or rigors with infusion through the catheter, cellulitis around the catheter entry/exit site)
- Skin or soft tissue infection at any site
- Colonization with MRSA, VRE, or with penicillin-resistant *Streptococcus pneumoniae*

Antibiotic regimens should be chosen based on local (hospital) antimicrobial susceptibility patterns, the patient's history of prior antibiotic therapy, colonization with resistant bacteria, presumed site of infection, and drug intolerance or allergy.

If there is hypotension, pneumonia diagnosed on a chest X-ray, or a suspected or known antimicrobial resistance are present, then empirical additions of other antimicrobial agents (i.e., aminoglycosides, vancomycin, linezolid, fluoroquinolones, antivirals) may be appropriate.

Adjustments of antibiotic doses must always be made for renal dysfunction.

Management of continued febrile neutropenia in the absence of documented infection (fever of unknown origin [FUO])

Persistent fever in an otherwise stable patient with FUO is *not* an indication for antibiotic changes. Changes or additions to the initial regimen should be based *only* upon emerging microbiological and clinical data. Specifically, there is no clear advantage to the empirical addition of vancomycin or an aminoglycoside if the patient remains febrile after several days of initial empirical antibiotic monotherapy, with negative cultures. A thorough search should be undertaken for the following possibilities:

- Cryptic bacterial infection (e.g., sinusitis)
- In-dwelling catheter infection
- Fungal infection (e.g., invasive mold infection, hepatosplenic candidiasis)
- Oral HSV reactivation
- Drug fever (including antibiotic fever)

Notably, if vancomycin was started empirically during initial therapy and no actual Gram-positive infection is identified after 48 hours of treatment, then the drug should be stopped.

Empirical antibiotics are traditionally continued until the achievement of an ANC greater than 500 cells/mm^3.

Empirical antifungal therapy for persistent fever

Empirical antifungal therapy is indicated for patients who have persistent or recurrent fever after 4–7 days of appropriate empirical antibiotic(s), and are without the prospect for imminent neutrophil recovery (Freifeld et al., 2011; NCCN, 2011; Wingard, 2004). Most HSCT patients typically are already receiving highly effective fluconazole prophylaxis for prevention of *Candida* infections. Rarely, a resistant candidemia due to *C. glabrata* or *C. krusei* may break through fluconazole prophylaxis. However, invasive mold infections (e.g., *Aspergillus* spp.) are of primary concern after a week or more of neutropenia and fever. The lungs and/or sinuses are the most common sites. Empirical IV antifungal therapy directed against *Aspergillus* spp. may be achieved with any of the following:

- Voriconazole – oral or IV
- Caspofungin (other echinocandins are likely as effective)
- Amphotericin-B lipid complex or liposomal amphotericin-B

In patients already receiving a mold-active agent, such as voriconazole, posaconazole, or an echinocandin (see following section on prophylaxis), there are no data to guide therapy; however, many experts suggest a switch to an amphotericin-B product (amphotericin-B lipid complex or liposomal amphotericin-B) for persistent fever. In all cases, symptoms and signs of invasive fungal pneumonia, pneumonia, or sinusitis should be sought, including by CT scans of the chest and/or sinuses, with follow-up nasal endoscopy or bronchoalveolar lavage, as indicated. Lung biopsy with culture and histopathology of any suspected lesions should be pursued aggressively in order to make a definitive mycological diagnosis that will guide therapy.

A preemptive approach is an increasingly acceptable alternative to universal empirical antifungal treatment. High-risk patients on fluconazole (a non-mold agent) prophylaxis but persistently febrile are started on empirical anti-mold agents only on a preemptive basis; that is, only if a CT scan of the chest is abnormal and/or if a serum aspergillus antigen (galactomannan) test is positive, suggesting an invasive mold infection (Cordonnier et al., 2009; Maertens et al., 2011). In the absence of these positive triggers to start empirical antifungal agents, none are given and the patient is simply observed with continued fever. In fact, antifungal therapy may be discontinued in persistently febrile but otherwise clinically stable patients, who are without fungal serum antigen or radiographic evidence of invasive fungal infection.

Management of specific infections

For currently available antibiotic and antifungal drugs see Chapter 27 (pages 422–454).

Bacteremia

Bacteremia occurs in approximately 10%–25% of all patients, with most episodes occurring in the setting of prolonged or profound neutropenia (ANC ≤ 100 neutrophils/mm^3) (Freifeld et al., 2011; Ramphal, 2004; Wisplinghoff et al., 2003). *Pseudomonas aeruginosa* is historically the most lethal bacteremia affecting neutropenic patients. Currently, coagulase-negative *Staphylococci* are the most common blood isolates in most centers; *Enterobacteriaciae* (e.g., *Enterobacter* spp., *Escherichia coli*, and *Klebsiella* sp.) and non-fermenting Gram-negative rods (e.g., *Pseudomonas aeruginosa* and *Stenotrophomonas* sp.) are isolated less often. Drug-resistant Gram-negative bacteria as well as Gram-positive species (MRSA and VRE) are causing an increasing number of infections in febrile neutropenic patients. Penicillin-resistant strains of *S. pneumoniae* and of the viridans group *Streptococci* are less common but may also cause severe infections. It is essential for physicians to be familiar with antibiotic resistance patterns in their institutions in order to anticipate these pathogens.

Management of bacteremia in fever and neutropenia

Blood cultures drawn before antibiotic therapy become positive after empirical antibiotics are started	
Gram-positive*	Add vancomycin pending further identification. Add linezolid or daptomycin if VRE is suspected. If isolate is found susceptible to β-lactam antibiotics, discontinue vancomycin. * a single blood culture for coagulase-negative staphylococcus (CoNS) is considered a contaminant and should not be treated. Two positive sets are required to verify a "true" CoNS bacteremia.
Gram-negative	Maintain regimen if patient is stable and isolate is sensitive. If patient is unstable or if *P. aeruginosa*, *Enterobacter*, *Klebsiella*, or *Citrobacter* is isolated, add an aminoglycoside or ciprofloxacin to cover potentially resistant organisms, until susceptibilities are known. If susceptible to initial β-lactam monotherapy, the second agent may be discontinued.
Organism isolated during empirical antibiotic therapy ("breakthrough" bacteremia or fungemia)	
Gram-positive	Add vancomycin or linezolid (if VRE is suspected), but draw two more blood culture sets prior to addition.
Gram-negative	Change to new combination regimen (e.g., from cefepime to imipenem/meropenem plus aminoglycoside or ciprofloxacin).
Fungi	Switch from azole to echinocandin or amphotericin B product.

If vancomycin or an aminoglycoside are used, serum drug levels should be monitored regularly. Refer to Chapter 27 for specific recommendations.

Antibiotics are continued for standard durations of 10–14 days for bacteremia, even if the ANC returns to >500 cells/mm^3.

Catheter-related bloodstream infections

Most HSCT recipients have surgically implanted catheters including ports, Hickmans or Groshong catheters, while some have peripherally inserted central catheters (PICCs).

Fever and/or rigors occurring after flushing of a catheter indicate an intralumenal infection, although fever alone may be the only symptom.

Staphylococcus epidermidis, S. aureus, Candida, and Gram-negative bacilli are common causes of catheter-related bloodstream infections (CRBSI). Growth of microbes from a blood sample drawn from a catheter at least two hours before microbial growth in a peripheral vein blood sample best defines CRBSI ("differential time to positivity") (Mermel et al., 2010). For suspected or documented CRBSI, IV vancomycin plus broad-spectrum Gram-negative antibiotics are recommended followed by adjustment of drugs when blood culture results are available.

Management of catheter-related bloodstream infections

Fungemia (*Candida* spp.), *S. aureus*, *Bacillus* spp. or myobacteremia (usually rapid growers)	• Remove catheter immediately and start appropriate antimicrobials.
Gram-negative organisms	• If patient is stable and quickly responds to antibiotics–may treat through catheter with appropriate IV antibiotics plus antibiotic lock therapy. • Always repeat blood cultures after 48 hours of appropriate antibiotics and if repeat cultures are positive, catheter must be removed.
Coagulase-negative *Staphylococci*	• Retain catheter and treat with intravenous antibiotics through the catheter; some experts recommend added antibiotic lock therapy.

Exit site infections, with the exception of *Mycobacterium* spp. and *Aspergillus* spp., will usually resolve with oral antibiotics aimed at Gram-positive skin flora such as *S. aureus*. Infections of the catheter tunnel or port pocket are also most often due to *S. aureus* and require early catheter removal, as they rarely resolve with conservative measures.

Antibiotic lock therapy

Antibiotic lock is indicated for patients with CRBSI involving long-term catheters with no signs of exit site or tunnel infection in whom the goal is catheter salvage (Mermel et al., 2010).

Antibiotic lock therapy for CRBSI is used in conjunction with systemic antibiotic therapy and involves installing a high concentration of an antibiotic lock solution to which the causative microbe is susceptible in the catheter lumen, in an amount equal to catheter lumen volume, and leaving it to dwell for hours or even days, usually until the next antibiotic dose. Be sure to aspirate antibiotic lock solution out of the catheter before administering medications. Antibiotic lock solution concentrations:

Vancomycin 2.5 mg/mL

Gentamicin 2 mg/mL

Heparin may be added at 2500 units/mL if needed

Complicated catheter-related infections require catheter removal and prolonged antibiotic therapy (4–6 weeks):

- Deep tissue infection
- Endocarditis
- Septic thrombosis
- Persistent bacteremia/fungemia after 72 hours of appropriate therapy

Infections of the head, eyes, ears, nose, and throat (HEENT)

Management of suspected HEENT infections

Necrotizing or marginal gingivitis	• Add specific anti-anaerobic agent (clindamycin or metronidazole) to empirical therapy.
Vesicular or ulcerative lesions of oral mucosa	• Rapid culture or PCR testing for HSV and begin acyclovir.
Sinus tenderness	• Maxillofacial CT scan to evaluate thickening, sinus opacification, bone erosion. If bacterial infection suspected, broad antimicrobial spectrum. • If fungal infection with *Aspergillus* or *mucormycoses* suspected, initiate amphotericin B product to cover both mold groups until diagnosis is confirmed by ENT biopsy.

Gastrointestinal tract infections

Abdominal pain and diarrhea are common in HSCT patients and may be due to a myriad of problems, including infections. *C. difficile* is the most common infectious cause. Other bacterial pathogens such as *Salmonella*, *Shigella*, *Campylobacter*, and diarrheal *E. coli* are infrequent; it is unnecessary to test for these organisms routinely in HSCT patients with diarrhea unless there is some travel or environmental history of concern.

Management of suspected GI tract infections

Retrosternal burning pain	Suspect esophagitis due to *Candida*, herpes simplex, and/or CMV. Add antifungal therapy and if no response after 48 hours, start acyclovir. Bacterial esophagitis is also a possibility. For patients who do not respond to these interventions, very careful endoscopy should be considered in neutropenic patients.
Acute abdominal pain	Suspect typhlitis if pain in right lower quadrant. Add anti-aerobic coverage (i.e., metronitazole), vancomycin, and aminoglycoside to empiric regimen that covers Gram-negatives, and perform abdominal CT scan to determine diagnosis.
Perianal tenderness	Add specific anti-anaerobic coverage to empiric regimen, and monitor the need for surgical intervention, especially when a patient is recovering from neutropenia.

Respiratory tract infections

Early in the course of transplant, prior to engraftment, bacterial pneumonias predominate. Invasive mold infections, particularly *Aspergillus* infections, become more frequent after prolonged neutropenia of more than about 10 days. In the first 100 days after engraftment, viral infections such as CMV, adenovirus, and respiratory viruses (respiratory syncytial virus [RSV], influenza, parainfluenza) are increasingly problematic, as are pathogens such as *Legionella*, *Pneumocystis jirovecii*, and toxoplasmosis.

Radiographic appearance can help identify the causes of infiltrates:

Infiltrate type	Likely pathogens
Focal	Bacteria, *Aspergillus* spp.
Diffuse interstitial	CMV, respiratory viruses, *Pneumocystis jirovecii* (PjP)
Nodular	*Aspergillus*, mucormycoses, *Nocardia*

Aggressive efforts should be made to diagnose the cause of pulmonary infiltrates. Invasive procedures for diagnosis of pulmonary infiltrates are sometimes critical for determining what antimicrobials will be of greatest benefit to the patient.

Fiber optic bronchoscopy (FOB) with bronchoalveolar lavage (BAL) is a less invasive and more rapid evaluation than lung biopsy, particularly for infectious causes of diffuse pulmonary infiltrates. In HCT patients with new pulmonary symptoms and infiltrates, the diagnostic yield with FOB/BAL for an identifiable infectious pathogen is between 50%–75% (Rabbat et al., 2008; Shannon et al., 2010). Diagnostic yield is highest within 24 hours of presentation. Essential studies on BAL fluid include:

- Culture and stains for bacteria and fungi
- Viral PCR (HSV, CMV, community respiratory viruses)
- Studies for *P. jirovecii* (silver stain)
- Galactomannan antigen (GM sensitivity BAL vs. serum: 88% vs. 42%) (Meersseman et al., 2008)
- Histoplasmosis antigen (BAL sensitivity 93.5%) (Wheat et al., 2007)

For focal infiltrates, percutaneous, transbronchial, or an open lung biopsy (video-assisted thoracoscopic surgery [VATS] or thoracotomy) may identify a pathogen 60%–80% of the time (White et al., 2000). The decision to pursue a transbronchial biopsy or VATS will depend on whether a diagnosis may be obtained otherwise, the severity of illness, platelet transfusion capabilities, location of the lesion, and the skill and comfort of the operator.

Management of suspected respiratory tract infections in neutropenic HSCT recipients

New focal lesion in patient with continuing neutropenia	• Sputum culture if possible. • CT scan to better define lesion. • Bronchoscopy for culture and biopsy (see later) consider needle or open biopsy to make diagnosis. • Consider empirical anti-mold therapy if CT appearance is suggestive. • Lung biopsy may be needed.
New interstitial pneumonitis	• Nasal wash for rapid testing and PCR for respiratory viruses. • FOB with bronchoalveolar lavage BAL. • Consider beginning anti-influenza therapy (during seasonal outbreak) and/or empirical treatment for PjP. • Serum β-glucan test (excellent negative predictive value in PjP). • Consider non-infectious causes and the need for open lung or VATS if condition has not improved after 4 days of empirical therapy.

A number of non-infectious causes can also cause diffuse infiltrates in HSCT recipients:

Septic shock	Pancreatitis
Oxygen toxicity	Hemodialysis/fluid shifts
Renal failure	Lymphocytic bronchitis
Massive blood transfusion	Idiopathic (conditioning regimen, acute GVHD)
Pulmonary embolism	Bronchiolitis obliterans
Cerebral injury	
Disseminated intravascular coagulopathy	

Clostridium difficile infection

In a recent report of over 400 allogeneic HSCT recipients from one center (2004–2007), approximately 13% developed *C. difficile* infection (CDI) (Willems et al., 2012). Most cases occurred in the first month after transplant and were not associated with either severe complications or with an increased mortality risk. CBT, acute GVHD, and TBI were risk factors for CDI. Antecedent or concurrent antimicrobial or antineoplastic therapy is usually present in patients with diarrhea due to *C. difficile* but is not required for the diagnosis (Cohen et al., 2010). The diagnosis of CDI requires:

• Diarrhea (three or more unformed stools in ≤24 hours)

plus

• A stool test positive for toxigenic *C. difficile* (by culture) or its toxins (enzyme immunoassay [EIA] or PCR). Test only diarrheal (unformed stool unless stool is formed due to ileus). EIA that detects both glutamate dehydrogenase (GDH) and toxin A/B is recommended, along with confirmatory PCR for indeterminate EIA tests
• A colonoscopy revealing pseudomembranous colitis is strongly suggestive of CDI

In non-neutropenic patients who are able to mount a WBC count, CDI severity may be assessed by laboratory parameters:

- Mild or moderate–WBC <15 000 cells/μL, serum creatinine <1.5 times ULN
- Severe–WBC >15 000 cells/μL, serum creatinine >1.5 times ULN
- Severe, complicated–severe plus hypotension or shock, ileus, megacolon

Treatment of *C. difficile* infection

Eliminating antibiotics such as cephalosporins and fluoroquines that drive infection is an important first step in treating CDI. In neutropenic patients, empiric therapy with oral metronidazole or vancomycin should be initiated as soon as the diagnosis is suspected.	
Initial episode	
Mild–moderate	Metronidazole 500 mg orally TID for 10–14 days.
Severe	Vancomycin 125 mg orally QID for 10–14 days.
Severe, complicated	Vancomycin 500 mg orally QID, with or without IV metronidazole at 500 mg every 8 hours. Vancomycin retention enemas may be given in patients with ileus or very severe disease, at 500 mg in 100 mL normal saline per rectum every 6 hours. Monitor WBCs and serum lactate. Consider colectomy in severely ill patients with rising leukocytosis and serum lactate. Fecal microbiota transfer may be attempted.
First recurrence	Metronidazole 500 mg orally TID for 10–14 days.
Second recurrence	Vancomycin 125 mg orally QID for 10–14 days.

Fidaxomicin, a new macrocylic antibiotic, appears to be as effective as oral vancomycin for mild to moderate CDI, but may be associated with fewer recurrences (Louie et al., 2011). Data regarding fidaxomicin efficacy in cancer patients is not yet available. Intravenous metronidazole is not recommended generally except in cases where GI intake is not possible. Antimotility agents are contraindicated in CDI.

For prevention of CDI, the use of gowns and gloves by healthcare workers and visitors, thorough handwashing with soap (alcohol-based hand gel is ineffective), and judicious use of antibiotics are essential. Probiotics for primary prevention of CDI are not recommended due to absent definitive evidence.

Fungal infections

Fungal infections occur in about 10%–15% of allogeneic HSCT patients who do not receive anti-mold prophylaxis (Marr et al., 2004). Diagnosis is often difficult. Despite FOB and/or biopsies, mold may not grow (<50% are cultured in the presence of infection) or be seen on histopathology examination due to sampling error. Therefore, the diagnosis is often a "probable" or "possible" fungal infection.

Systemic antifungal treatment

Type of fungal infection	Drug	Daily dose	Treatment duration (days)
Candida fungemia* **Echinocandin initially, until species identified, then Fluconazole for* *Candida albicans* and most other species **except** *C. krusei* and *C. glabrata*	Caspofungin	Caspo: 70 mg IV load on day 1, then 50 mg IV daily (1-hr infusion)	14 days after blood culture becomes negative
	Micafungin	100 mg IV daily	
	Anidulafungin	200 mg IV × 1, then 100 mg IV daily	
	*Fluconazole	400–800 mg IV daily; switch to oral after blood cultures cleared	
Esophageal candidiasis	Fluconazole	400–800 mg	7–14 days following resolution of symptoms
	Amphotericin B or liposomal amphotericin	10–20 mg IV daily, 2–5 mg/kg IV daily (liposomal)	
	Caspofungin	Same as for fungemia	
	Micafungin	150 mg IV daily	
	Anidulafungin	200 mg IV × 1, then 100 mg IV daily	
Invasive candidiasis	Micafungin	150 mg IV daily	Not known
	Lipid Amphotericin B	3–5 mg/kg IV daily	
Invasive aspergillosis	Voriconazole	6 mg/kg IV BID × 2 then 4 mg/kg IV BID or oral load 400 mg BID then 200 mg BID if tolerated	Minimum of 12 weeks
	Posaconazole	200 mg PO QID transition to 400 mg BID once infection stabilized	
	Caspofungin	Same as fungemia dosing	
	Lipid formulation of amphotericin B	3 mg/kg IV daily	Minimum of 12 weeks
Mucormycoses	Lipid formulation of amphotericin B	3–5 mg/kg IV daily	Minimum of 12 weeks
	Posaconazole once patient is clinically improving	200 mg PO QID or 400 mg PO BID	
	Surgical resection/ debridement		

Important antifungal therapy notes

- Azole antifungal drugs will significantly increase cyclosporin and tacrolimus (FK506) serum level. Halving doses of these immunosuppressives and careful monitoring of levels of immunosuppressive drugs is recommended when starting an azole drug
- *C. krusei* and *C. glabrata* strains may be insensitive to fluconazole. Use other agents to treat until susceptibilities are known
- Combinations of antifungals are not clearly more effective than a single agent for aspergillosis or other invasive my cases
- Posaconazole requires high fat food with each dose for proper absorption. Voriconazole is best taken without high fat food
- Continue amphotericin with posaconazole for the first week of therapy, as it takes time to reach a probable therapeutic level (≥ 1 µg/mL) (Thompson, 2009)

P. jirovecii pneumonia

P. jirovecii pneumonia (PjP) onset is usually slow (unlike in HIV/AIDS patients) with fever, cough, and progressive hypoxia over days to weeks, culminating in severe bilateral pneumonia with acute respiratory failure. It typically occurs 6–18 months after autologous or allogeneic HSCT, specifically in patients not taking prophylaxis; prolonged steroid therapy is a significant risk. Trimethoprim-sulfamethoxasole prophylaxis essentially eliminates the risk (Bollee et al., 2007). Mortality rates are 35%–50%.

Treatment of *P. jirovecii* pneumonia (Modified from Limper et al., 2011.)

Drug	Dose	Route
Trimethoprim plus sulfamethoxazole	15–20 mg/kg	Oral of IV
Primaquine plus clindamycin	30 mg daily and 600 mg TID, generally for 3 weeks	Oral
Atovaquone	750 mg twice daily, generally for 3 weeks	Oral
Pentamidine	4 mg/kg/d or 600 mg/d, generally for 3 weeks	IV or aerosol
Corticosteroids–give in addition to antibiotic agent in moderate to severe disease (PaO$_2$ <70 mm Hg on room air)	Prednisone (or IV equivalent) 40 mg bid for 5 days, then 40 mg daily on days 6–11, and then 20 mg daily through day 21	IV or oral

Herpes virus infections

For herpes viruses (HSV, CMV, VZV, EBV), reactivations of latent viruses may occur periodically, particularly during times of immunosuppression. A positive PCR test or culture does not necessarily indicate a clinically significant infection. Clinical signs and symptoms compatible with the diagnosis of an active herpes virus infection must be present to make the diagnosis and direct antiviral use.

Treatment of herpes virus infections.

CMV infections

CMV "syndrome": fever/leucopenia/malaise/myalgia and rising CMV blood viral load is the most common presentation post-allo-HSCT

- Oral valganciclovir 900 mg BID × 2 weeks "induction" course
- Repeat blood CMV viral load (by PCR) after 2 week "induction"
- If negative, then 900 mg QD × another 2–4 weeks
- If positive, continue high doses another 2 weeks and check viral load again

CMV disease – pneumonia, esophagitis, enterocolitis

- Ganciclovir 5 mg/kg IV BID × 2 weeks, then 5 mg/kg IV daily for 2–4 weeks until symptoms resolve (IV immunoglobulin addition may be used for CMV pneumonitis; no advantage to giving CMV-specific IVIG)
- Alternative: foscarnet 60 mg/kg every 8 hours – electrolytes must be closely monitored with foscarnet use

HSV infections

- Severe mucosal disease: acyclovir, 250 mg/m^2 (or 5 mg/kg) IV three times daily for 5–7 days, followed by oral valacyclovir
- Less severe mucosal disease: valacyclovir 500 mg PO BID for 7–14 days
- Acyclovir-resistant HSV is characterized by chronic non-resolving cutaneous or mucosal lesions. Foscarnet is the drug of choice
- HSV encephalitis: acyclovir 10–15 mg/kg IV Q 8 hrs × 14–21 days

Varicella zoster; (VZV) infections

- Disseminated (cutaneous or visceral) zoster: acyclovir, 10 mg/kg IV every 8 hours for 7 days, with hydration to prevent crystallization of drug in kidney
- Localized dermatomal zoster: valacyclovir 1000 mg PO or famciclovir 500 mg TID for 7 days

Viral hepatitis posttransplant

Active hepatitis B or C is a relative contraindication for SCT or a donation. Under certain circumstances, transplant might be considered in individuals previously infected with hepatitis B or C. Hepatitis A generally heals with lasting immunity. The risk of hepatitis B surface antigen seroconversion after allogeneic HSCT is up to 40% or more at five years posttransplant (Viganò, 2011). One study showed evidence that posttransplant vaccination prevents reactivation in recipients with previous HBV infection (Onozawa et al., 2008). A hepatologist should assist in the management of the recipient with hepatitis B or C infection.

Hepatitis B exposed or previously infected recipients

- Perform serological and molecular studies and work with a hepatologist to manage the patient (Liang, 2009)

- Anti-HBc and anti-HBs positive: prophylactic antiviral therapy (lamivudine) may be considered for anti-HBc- and anti-HBs-positive recipients before and for the first six months after HCT
- HBsAg or HBV DNA-positive
  - Perform liver biopsy to rule out cirrhosis
  - Initiate antiviral therapy (lamivudine) for 3–6 months prior to conditioning
- Anti-HBc-positive, HBsAg- and anti-HBs-negative
  - Test for HBV DNA. If negative, vaccinate recipient
  - Monitoring and initiate therapy as anti-HBc/anti-HBs-positive recipients
- Donors with natural immunity (anti-HBs/HBc-positive) are preferred for recipients with evidence of prior exposure (anti-HBc-positive)
- If recipient alanine aminotransferase (ALT) increases posttransplantation, check HBV DNA or HBsAg. If indicative of infection, preemptive antiviral therapy should be given

Hepatitis C infected recipient
- Check serological and molecular markers
- Contact hepatologist (as in hepatitis B)
- Perform a liver biopsy if the patient has evidence of any of the following: iron overload; a history of excess alcohol intake; a history of hepatitis C for >10 years; or clinical evidence of chronic liver disease
- In patients with cirrhosis, fully myeloablative conditioning should not be used and reduced-intensity regimens should be used with extreme caution
- Treat with antiviral drugs if the following requirements have been met:
  - Malignancy has been in remission for ≥2 years posttransplant
  - No significant GVHD
  - Off immunosuppression for six months
  - Normal blood counts and creatinine
- Full dose peginterferon and ribavirin should be used. Daily IFN-α can be used up-front to determine hematologic tolerance prior to peginterferon.

Postsplenectomy infection

Overwhelming sepsis may occur in patients who are asplenic, with high mortality particularly due to encapsulated organisms including *Streptococcus pneumoniae, Haemophilus influenza* and *Neisseria meningities.*

Empirical antiblotics for febrile asplenic adult patients are indicated after a diagnostic evaluation including blood cultures.

Oral antibioltics for non-acute fever:

- Amoxicillin-clavulanate −875 mg twice daily
- Cefuroxime axetil −500 mg twice daily
- Extended-spectrum fluoroquinolones-levofloxacin 750 mg, moxifloxacin 400 mg

Acutely ill patients:

- IV vancomycin plus either ceftriaxone or an extended-spectrum fluoroquinolone

Management of miscellaneous infections

Toxoplasmosis

- Sulfadiazine/pyrimethamine remains the standard first-line treatment for cerebral toxoplasmosis: sulfadiazine, 1–1.5 g PO every six hours and pyrimethamine, 50–75 mg daily
- If allergic to sulfadiazine, substitute clindamycin, 600 mg PO every six hours

Cryptococcosis

- Amphotericin B, 0.7–1 mg/kg IV daily. Amphotericin-B or liposomal amphotericin remains the drug of choice for severe cryptococcal meningitis; may be combined with flucytosine (100 mg/kg) initially. *Cryptococcus* found in the blood, lung, or skin always requires examination of CSF by lumbar puncture to evalutate for cryptococcal meningitis

Legionella pneumonia

- Macrolides (in severe cases, IV azithromycin; alternatively erythromycin, 500 mg IV every six hours). Extended spectrum fluoroquinolones IV (ciprofloxacin, levofloxacin)

Mycobacterium avium complex

- Rifabutin, 300–450 mg PO daily, PLUS
- Ethambutol, 20–25 mg PO daily, PLUS
- Macrolide (clarithromycin, 1 g PO twice daily or azithromycin)

Prophylaxis of infections

Protective environments and reverse isolation

Most infections in neutropenic patients are from endogenous GI or skin organisms; therefore, the role of barrier and other specific precautions is controversial.

- There is no clear evidence that reverse-barrier nursing reduces the incidence of septic episodes in neutropenic patients. Handwashing is most critical
- HEPA filtered environments appear to reduce the incidence of invasive aspergillosis for patients who are likely to have prolonged (>7 days), profound neutropenia ($<0.5 \times 10^9$/L)
- Potted plants and dried or fresh flowers should be avoided in the rooms of transplant recipients as *Aspergillus* spp. and *Fusarium* spp. have been isolated from their surfaces
- It is no longer recommended that a "neutropenic diet" is followed. Patients may eat any foods as long as safe food handling precautions are followed. Well-cleaned, uncooked, raw fruits and vegetables are acceptable as are cooked foods brought from home or restaurants, as long as ingredients are fresh

Pretransplant testing for occult infection

- HCV Ab
- Hep B surface antigen, surface antibody, and core antibody
- Rapid HIV
- HTLV I/II

- RPR (rapid plasma reagin)
- HSV serologies
- CMV IgG/IgM
- VZV IgG/IgM
- PPD (Pirquet test)

Vaccination schedule (see page 270)

Prophylactic antimicrobials

Antibacterial prophylaxis for HSCT

- Levofloxacin 500 mg orally or IV once daily for patients predicted to have prolonged, profound neutropenia (neutrophils $<0.5 \times 10^9$/L) for >7 days
- Stop prophylaxis when ANC recovers

Antifungal prophylaxis for HSCT

- Fluconazole 400 mg oral or IV daily during the first 100 days following allogeneic HSCT. However, fluconazole is not active against *C. krusei* and some isolates of *C. glabrata*
- Micafungin given at 50 mg IV q 24 h IV is also effective prophylaxis for candidiasis during the neutropenic period only
- Voriconazole offers no advantage over fluconazole during the neutropenic period, with no significant difference in freedom from invasive fungal infection or survival (Wingard et al., 2010). Nonetheless, some experts advise that if the risk for invasive *Aspergillus* is high, an anti-mold prophylaxis should be given: very prolonged neutropenia (>14 days), prolonged corticosteroid administration, prolonged antibacterial antibiotic administration, local construction work, or a high local *Aspergillus* prevalence
- Voriconazole, 200 mg twice daily PO or 6 mg/kg q 12 h IV x2, then 3 mg/kg q 12 h IV
- Posaconazole 200 mg PO q 8 hr with a high fat meal has shown a reduction in invasive mold infections and improved OS compared with fluconazole or itraconazole in patients undergoing induction therapy for acute leukemia and MDS (Cornely et al., 2007). In addition, posaconazole may reduce invasive mold infections in patients with GVHD. The role of up-front prophylaxis with posaconazole in HSCT patients is less well defined
- Intermittent liposomal amphotericin IV (3–7 times 3–5 mg/kg per week)
- Continue oral fluconazole through day 100 post-allogeneic transplant (reduced mortality)
- GVHD on high-dose steroids: voriconazole or posaconazole (rather than fluconazole)
- Secondary prophylaxis with voriconazole or posaconazole is required if the patient has had a prior aspergillus infection, before HSCT

Prophylaxis of *P. jirovecii* (PCP)

Prophylaxis against *Pneumocystis* is essential for all patients undergoing HCT. Trimethoprim–sulfamethoxazole (TMP–SMX), 800–160 mg two tablets orally twice per week, should be given starting at engraftment and continuing for at least six months. Prophylaxis should continue in patients who continue to require immunosuppression. In patients with a sulfa allergy, dapsone or inhaled pentamidine may be substituted.

Antiviral prophylaxis

Acyclovir (or valacyclovir) prophylaxis at low doses should be offered to all HSV-seropositive transplant recipients. Prophylaxis should be given until engraftment or recovery of the WBC count or resolution of mucositis, whichever occurs later. The same HSV prophylactic agent can be continued as VZV prophylaxis for up to one year.

- Acyclovir 800–1600 mg PO BID
- Valacyclovir 500 mg PO BID or TID

Preemptive treatment for asymptomatic CMV infection

This is favored over universal prophylaxis for patients at high risk for infection (allotransplant, alemtuzumab) regardless of baseline seropositivity. Once or twice weekly CMV PCR should be done to detect occult infection. Preemptive therapy should be started as soon as CMV DNA is detected.

- Ganciclovir 5 mg/kg IV q 12 hr for 2 weeks; if CMV PCR remains positive, treat for an additional 2 weeks at 6 mg/kg daily 5 days per week
- Valganciclovir 900 mg PO BID for 2 weeks; consider continuing this once daily for an additional 7 days after a negative test

References and further reading

Afessa B & Peters SG. 2006. Major complications following hematopoietic stem cell transplantation. *Semin Respir Crit Care Med* **27**: 297–309.

Bodey GP, Buckley M, Sathe YS, et al. 1966. Quantitative relationships between circulating leukocytes and infection in patients with acute leukemia. *Ann Int Med* **64**: 328–340.

Bollee G, Sarfati C, Thiery G, et al. 2007. Clinical picture of *Pneumocystis jiroveci* pneumonia in cancer patients. *Chest* **132**: 1305–1310.

Cohen SH, Gerding DN, Johnson S, et al. 2010. Clinical practice guidelines for *Clostridium difficile* infection in adults: 2010 update by the Society for Healthcare Epidemiology of America (SHEA) and the Infectious Diseases Society of America (IDSA). *Infect Control Hosp Epidemiol* **31**: 431–455.

Cordonnier C, Pautas C, Maury S, et al. 2009. Empirical versus preemptive antifungal therapy for high-risk, febrile, neutropenic patients: a randomized, controlled trial. *Clin Infect Dis* **48**: 1042–1051.

Cornely OA, Maertens J, Winston DJ, et al. 2007. Posaconazole vs. fluconazole or itraconazole prophylaxis in patients with neutropenia. *N Engl J Med* **356**: 348–359.

Freifeld AG, Bow EJ, Sepkowitz KA, et al., & Infectious Diseases Society of America. 2011. Clinical practice guideline for the use of antimicrobial agents in neutropenic patients with cancer: 2010 update by the Infectious Diseases Society of America. *Clin Infect Dis* **52**: 427–431.

Guidelines for infection control after stem cell transplantation and vaccination schedules can also be found at www.cdc.gov.

Kim YJ, Boeckh M, & Eglund JA. 2007. Community respiratory virus infections in immunocompromised patients: hematopoietic stem cell and solid organ transplant recipients and individuals with human immunodeficiency virus infection. *Semin Respir Crit Care Med* **28**: 222–242.

Liang R. 2009. How I treat and monitor viral hepatitis B infection in patients receiving intensive immunosuppressive therapies or undergoing hematopoietic stem cell transplantation. *Blood* **113**: 3147–3153.

Limper AH, Knox KS, Sarcosi GA, et al. 2011. An official American Thoracic Society statement: treatment of fungal infections in adult pulmonary and critical care patients. *Am J Respir Crit Care Med* **183**: 96–128.

Louie TJ, Miller MA, Mullane KM, et al. 2011. Fidaxomicin versus vancomycin for *Clostridium difficile* infection. *N Engl J Med* **364**: 422–431.

Maertens J, Groll AH, Cordonnier C, et al. 2011. Treatment and timing in invasive mould disease. *J Antimicrob Chemother* **66**: i37–i43.

Marr K, Crippa F, Leisenring W, et al. 2004. Itraconazole versus fluconazole for prevention of fungal infections in patients receiving allogeneic stem cell transplants. *Blood* **103**: 1527–1533.

Meersseman W, Lagrou K, Maertens J, et al. 2008. Galactomannan in bronchoalveolar lavage fluid. *Am J Respir Crit Care Med* **177**: 27–34.

Mermel LA, Allon M, Bouza E, et al. 2010. Clinical practice guidelines for the diagnosis and management of intravascular catheter-related infection: 2009 update by the Infectious Diseases Society of America. *Clin Infect Dis* **49**: 1–45.

NCCN *Practice Guidelines, Prevention and Treatment of Cancer Related Infections*, Ver 2. 2011. Available at www.NCCN.org.

Onozawa M, Hashino S, Darmanin S, et al. 2008. HB vaccination in the prevention of viral reactivation in allogeneic hematopoietic stem cell transplantation recipients with previous HBV infection. *Biol Blood Marrow Transplant* **14**: 1226–1230.

Paul M, Yahav D, Fraser A, et al. 2006. Empirical antibiotic monotherapy for febrile neutropenia: systematic review and meta-analysis of randomized controlled trials. *J Antimicrob Chemother* **57**: 176–189.

Rabbat A, Chaoui D, Lefebvre A, et al. 2008. Is BAL useful in patients with acute myeloid leukemia admitted in ICU for severe respiratory complications? *Leukemia* **22**: 1361–1367.

Ramphal R. 2004. Changes in the etiology of bacteremia in febrile neutropenic patients and the susceptibilities of the currently isolated pathogens. *Clin Infect Dis* **39**: S25–S31.

Sable CA, Strohmaier KM, & Chodakewitz JA. 2008. Advances in antifungal treatment. *Annu Rev Med* **59**: 455–473.

Shannon VR, Andersson BS, Lei X, et al. 2010. Utility of early versus late fiber optic bronchoscopy in the evaluation of new pulmonary infiltrates following hematopoietic stem cell transplantation. *Bone Marrow Transplant* **45**: 647–655.

Shorr AF, Susla GM, & O'Grady NP. 2004. Pulmonary infiltrates in the non-HIV-infected immunocompromised patient: etiologies, diagnostic strategies, and outcomes. *Chest* **125**: 260–271.

Thompson GR. 2009. Posaconazole therapeutic drug monitoring: a reference laboratory experience. *Antimicrob Agents Chemother* **53**: 2223–2224.

Tomblyn M, Chiller T, Einsele H, et al. 2009. Guidelines for preventing infectious complications among hematopoietic cell transplantation recipients: a global perspective. *Biol Blood Marrow Transplant* **15**: 1143–1238.

Viganò M. 2011. Risk of hepatitis B surface antigen seroreversion after allogeneic hematopoietic SCT. *Bone Marrow Transplant* **46**: 125–131.

Wheat LJ, Freifeld AG, Kleiman MB, et al. 2007. Clinical practice guidelines for the management of patients with histoplasmosis: 2007 update by the Infectious Diseases Society of America. *Clin Infect Dis* **45**: 807–825.

White DA, Wong PW, Downey R. 2000. The utility of open lung biopsy in patients with hematologic malignancies. *Am J Respir Crit Care Med* **161**: 723–729.

Willems L, Porcher R, Lafaurie M, et al. 2012. *Clostridium difficile* infection after allogeneic hematopoietic stem cell transplantation: incidence, risk factors, and outcome. *Biol Blood Marrow Trans* **18**: 1295–1301.

Wingard JR. 2004. Empirical antifungal therapy in treating febrile neutropenic patients. *Clin Infect Dis* **39**: S38–S43.

Wingard JR, Carter SL, Walsh TJ, et al. 2010. Randomized, double-blind trial of fluconazole versus voriconazole for prevention of invasive fungal infection after allogeneic hematopoietic cell transplantation. *Blood* **116**: 5111–5118.

Wisplinghoff H, Seifert H, Wenzel RP, et al. 2003. Current trends in the epidemiology of nosocomial bloodstream infections in patients with hematological malignancies and solid neoplasms in hospitals in the United States. *Clin Infect Dis* **36**: 1103–1110.

Chapter 26

Organ-related and miscellaneous complications

Gerhard C. Hildebrandt, Reinhold Munker, Ulrich Duffner, Daniel Wolff, Michael Stadler, Tina Dietrich-Ntoukas, Klemens Angstwurm, Amanda Sun, Binu Nair, Hillard M. Lazarus, and Kerry Atkinson

Transplant-related complications (excluding infections and GVHD)

Definiton of hematopoietic recovery

Neutrophil recovery: absolute neutrophil count (ANC) of $\geq 0.5 \times 10^9$/L for three consecutive laboratory values obtained on different days with the first day defined as date of recovery

Autologous: day +10 to +14

Allogeneic: day +10 to +day 14 (PB SCT); day + 16 to +day 22 (BMT)

Platelet recovery: platelet count $>20 \times 10^9$/L for three consecutive laboratory values obtained on different days and with no platelet transfusions in the previous seven days; the first day defined as date of recovery

Red blood cell recovery: hematocrit $\geq 25\%$ for 20 days without RBC transfusion

Comment: while in auto-HSCT, hematopoietic recovery is consistent with engraftment, in allogeneic HSCT determination of engraftment requires chimerism testing.

Graft failure after allogeneic HSCT (HCT)

- Primary graft failure: lack of initial engraftment of donor cells resulting in insufficient hematopoietic recovery
- Secondary graft failure: loss of donor cells after initial engraftment. The decrease in donor chimerism either can be paralleled by autologous recovery or can result in pancytopenia due to BM aplasia

Incidence

Type of transplant	Failure of sustained engraftment (%)
HLA-identical sibling (myeloablative conditioning)	<1
HLA-identical sibling (RIC)	3–5
Haploidentical family member, negative cross-match	7
Haploidentical family member, positive cross-match*	60
HLA-identical unrelated donor	2–5
HLA-mismatched unrelated donor	5
HLA-identical or partially matched UCB	7–32
* presence of donor-reactive antibodies in recipient	

Causes for graft failure

- Graft rejection mediated by recipient CD8$^+$ T-cells responding to MHC or mHag present on the donor cells; occasionally can be mediated by recipient CD4$^+$ T-cells responding to an MHC Class II difference in the donor
- Allogeneic resistance by recipient NK cells responding to histocompatibility antigen disparity; less likely in patients receiving TBI or Cy prior to and MTX after allogeneic HSCT; well-described in animal models, "hybrid resistance"
- Allosensitization by blood or platelet transfusions or pregnancy; rejection risk in heavily pretransfused recipients 5%–60%; prevention through irradiation and the use of leukocyte depletion filters of transfusion products
- Low stem cell number in PBSC, BM, or UCB inoculums
- Infections (CMV, HHV-6, Parvo-B19, HHV-8)
- Drug toxicity
- Septicemia
- Note: graft failure may also be disease-specific (relapse of severe aplastic anemia)

Risk factors for graft failure

- RIC
- HLA-mismatched donor
- ABO mismatch
- High number of transfusions (RBC, platelets) prior to transplant
- Low progenitor cell number in PBSC, BM, or UCB inoculums
- T-cell depleted graft
- Presence of recipient-anti-donor anti-CD34+/VEGFR-2+ antibodies (Mattson et al., 2008)

Treatment and outcome

- Primary or secondary graft failure is a hematopoietic emergency and will be fatal unless hematopoiesis can be restored
- Temporary bridging of cytopenias through transfusions of blood and platelets, myeloid growth factors, and antibiotics
- In autologous transplantation, a second transplant without conditioning can be performed if additional progenitor cells are stored
- In allogeneic transplantation, a second transplantation can be attempted if the patient experiences severe rejection, same or other donor is available, and the patient is in good general condition and does not have an uncontrolled infection. Consider different conditioning regimen to avoid cumulative toxicity. Most experts recommend that additional immunosuppression be used; consider ATG or alemtuzumab as part of conditioning. Co-transplanted MSCs as facilitators of engraftment are currently being evaluated
- In poor graft function and presence of partial/declining donor chimerism, progenitor cells and/or DLI may be given without further conditioning
- In poor graft function without partial/declining donor chimerism, progenitor cells without additional DLI can be given without additional preparative chemotherapy. If no GVL intended, T-cell depletion can be considered in order to prevent development of GVHD

(See Mattsson et al., 2008.)

Hemorrhagic cystitis
Background

Hemorrhagic cystitis frequently develops in HSCT recipients (incidence: <5%–25%, in earlier studies up to 70%).

Early onset

- 24–72 hours after HSCT
- Secondary to chemotherapy toxicity
- Risk factors:
  - Cyclophosphamide (>1000 mg/m^2), ifosfamide–indirect toxicity through the metabolite acrolein
  - Release of inflammatory mediators (TNF-α, IL-1-β, cyclooxygenase-2, reactive oxygen, and nitric oxide species)
  - Pelvic irradiation or prior busulfan

Late onset

- >72 hours after allogeneic HSCT
- Can occur up to 60 days after HSCT
- Risk factors: allogeneic HSCT, GVHD, conditioning regimen intensity (myeloablative >RIC), donor type (UCB, haploidentical donor), coagulopathy, thrombocytopenia, BK virus (urine PCR positivity prior to HSCT), adenovirus (type 11 >> type 34, 35), CMV, prior early-onset hemorrhagic cystitis
- Cumulative risk profile: urine PCR BK virus positivity + haploidentical or UCB donor source + myeloablative conditioning leads to an eight-fold increase in risk to develop hemorrhagic cystitis (P<0.001) (see de Padua Silva et al., 2010)

BK virus

- Polyomavirus
- Non-encapsulated DNA virus
- 90% of adults have been exposed during life-time
- Dormant persistence in kidneys, urothelium
- Reactivation in the immunocompromised/immunosuppressed host
- Associated with isolated hemorrhagic cystitis in HSCT recipients and nephropathy in HSCT and renal organ transplant recipients
- Significant BK viremia after allogeneic HSCT (>10 000 copies/mL) is associated with increased renal dysfunction and decreased OS

Diagnosis

- Symptom triad
  - Microscopic or macroscopic hematuria
  - Dysuria
  - Urinary frequency

in a patient with a sterile mid-stream specimen of urine (MSU) without evidence of underlying urinary tract infection (UTI) (bacterial, fungal, or parasitic), without bleeding diathesis and in the absence of urinary tract malignancies or mechanical irritation (e.g., catheter)

- Exclusion of bacterial, fungal, and parasitic infection
- PCR of blood and urine for adenovirus/CMV/BK
- Ultrasound of bladder and kidneys to assess for clot formation and hydronephrosis

Grading of hemorrhagic cystitis

0 No symptoms of bladder irritability or hemorrhage
1 Microscopic hematuria with urinary symptoms (e.g., frequency, dysuria)
2 Macroscopic hematuria
3 Macroscopic hematuria with clots
4 Massive macroscopic hematuria with intervention for clot evacuation and/or urinary retention

Prevention of hemorrhagic cystitis

- Hyperhydration (3–6 L /m^2/24 h)
- Diuretics to maintain continuous urine output
- Urine alkalinization
- MESNA
- Ciprofloxacin

Treatment of hemorrhagic cystitis

Systemic

- Hyperhydration (3–6 L/m^2/24 h)
- Diuretics to maintain continuous urine output
- Platelet transfusions
- Factor XIII (50 IU/kg)
- Systemic antifibrinolytic agents (e.g., tranexamic acid)–careful use in concurrent bleeding of the proximal urinary tract (kidney, ureter) due to risk of obstructive clot formation
- Recombinant factor VIIa: effective to stop hemorrhage, no documented benefit on overall outcome, risk of thromboembolic events; while no recommendation can be given at this time, individual use in patients with uncontrollable life-threatening bleeding may be carefully considered
- Antiviral treatment: cidofovir (beneficial and safe both in pediatric and adult patients); less effective: vidarabine, ribavirin
- Leflunomide
- Ciprofloxacin, levofloxacin
- Hyperbaric oxygen (adults; less experience in pediatric patients)
- Palifermine (keratinocyte growth factor) has been used in individual cases parallel to confounding treatments for hemorrhagic cystitis; no recommendation can be given at this time
- Smooth muscle relaxant (e.g., oxybutynin)
- Systemic conjugated estrogens (e.g., a mixture of natural estrogens, as in Premarin)

Local

- Bladder irrigation with
    - Isotonic salt solution–standard to maintain patency of urinary tract
    - Prostaglandin E2 or F2α
    - Alum (toxicity: cardiomyopathy, CNS symptoms, coma)
    - Silver nitrate (0.5%–1.0% conc.)
    - Formalin (toxicity: bladder fibrosis, bladder rupture due to formalin-induced tissue necrosis)
    - Phenol
    - Na hyaluronate
    - Cidofovir
- Cystoscopy, with clot evacuation ± diathermy/laser coagulation
- Fibrin glue administration

- Suprapubic bladder catheter
- Embolization of bladder-directed vasculature; i.e., internal iliac artery
- Cystectomy with urinary diversion (neobladder) only in patients with potentially lethal bleeding and refractory to other treatment option
- Mesenchymal stem cells (under investigation)

(For further references for hemorrhagic cystitis, see Dropulic & Jones, 2008; Haines et al., 2011; Hassan, 2011; Leung et al., 2005; Miller et al., 2011; Tsuboi et al., 2003.)

Hepatic veno-occlusive disease (VOD)/sinusoidal obstruction syndrome (SOD)

Risk factors for VOD

- Pretransplant factors
  - Preexisting liver disease
    - Liver function abnormalities, evidence of liver fibrosis/cirrhosis, chronic hepatitis C infection
    - Iron overload (serum ferritin >1000 ng/dL)
  - Other
    - Female gender, progesterone treatment prior to SCT, prior treatment with gemtuzamab ozogamicin (<3 months prior HSCT), prior radiation to the liver, reduced diffusion capacity for carbon monoxide, older age, CMV positive serological status, malignant infantile osteopetrosis
- Transplant-related factors:
  - Conditioning: single dose TBI, >12 Gy TBI, non-adjusted > targeted busulfan, oral > intravenous busulfan, BCNU, etoposide, cyclophosphamide, cyclosporin A, fever during conditioning, non TCD >TCD graft
  - Risk with myeloablative conditioning > RIC
  - Other: unrelated mismatched donor, allogeneic > autologous
- Incidence:
  - 7%–14%
  - Decrease in incidence due to increased use of RIC over the last years (RIC: incidence 2%)

Pathogenesis

- Endothelial injury through conditioning regimen, cytokines (IL-1, IL-2, TNF, IFN-γ), alloreactive T-cells, neutrophils along with glutathione depletion, nitric oxide depletion, high metalloproteinase activity, high VEGF levels. This leads to endothelial activation, increased permeability, vasoconstriction, endothelial dysfunction with platelet and leukocyte adhesion to the endothelial surface, and endothelial apoptosis. Subsequently, vaso-occlusion of the small venules

Diagnosis of VOD (SOS)

Diagnosis is based on the following clinical/laboratory data

Seattle Criteria

Two of three criteria within 20 days after HSCT

- Serum bilirubin ≥2 mg/dL
- Hepatomegaly or right upper quadrant pain
- >2% weight gain due to fluid retention

Baltimore Criteria

Serum bilirubin ≥2 mg/dL within 21 days after HSCT and at least two of three findings

- Hepatomegaly, usually painful
- >5% weight gain
- Ascites

Differential diagnosis of hepatic VOD (SOS) in BMT/SCT patients

- Infections: cholangitis lenta or sepsis-associated cholestasis, fungal infection, viral hepatitis
- Acute GvHD of the liver
- Drug toxicity: CSA, MTX, azoles, TPN, trimethoprim-sulfamethoxazole and others
- Reduced venous outflow: constrictive pericarditis, congestive heart failure, hepatic vein obstruction
- Increased volume: fluid overload, renal failure
- Others: biliary obstruction, pancreatic disease, peritonitis, infiltration of the liver

Right-sided upper abdominal pain (stretching of hepatic capsule), pleural effusion, oliguria, and sudden and marked thrombocytopenia can also occur.

Other causes of these clinical/laboratory features should be excluded before making the diagnosis of VOD. In addition sometimes VOD can appear several months after HSCT.

Diagnosis

- Doppler ultrasound (reversal of portal vein flow, periportal fluid accumulation)
- CT of abdomen
- Elevated serum levels of plasminogen activator inhibitor type 1 (PAI-1) may be helpful to distinguish VOD from infectious hepatitis or GVHD
- Normal antithrombin plasma levels seem likely to rule out VOD
- In rare situations a liver biopsy may be needed. Because of ongoing thrombocytopenia and coagulopathy a transjugular liver biopsy is the safest way to obtain liver tissue
- Transvenous wedged hepatic vein gradient determination, if >10 mm Hg 90%; specific for VOD (SOS)
- VOD can be of patchy distribution and a normal biopsy does not exclude the diagnosis

Classification

- By clinical course (incidence)
  - Mild (8%–23%): complete resolution on day +100 without treatment

- Moderate (48%–64%): complete resolution on day +100 with treatment
- Severe (23%–28%): no resolution despite treatment or death before or on day +100
- By concurrent clinical status
  - Severe: plus renal and/or pulmonary dysfunction
- By laboratory indicators
  - Severe: total serum bilirubin >10 mg/dL and transfusion-refractory thrombocytopenia

Outcome

- Mortality attributable to VOD (SOS) by day +100
  - 1%–3% of all allogeneic HSCT
  - VOD mortality
    - Mild <5%
    - Moderate: 18%–28%
    - Severe: 75%–95%

Prediction of outcome

An equation taking serum bilirubin and weight gain within 1–2 weeks of HSCT into account can be applied. Probability estimates derived from patient data with this equation are highly specific and moderately sensitive. For example, a patient with a serum bilirubin of more than 6 mg/dL and a weight gain of more than 10% at day +5 to +7 does have a greater than 40% probability of developing a severe VOD. Such estimate may be helpful when considering potential treatments for VOD. (See Bearman et al., 1993.)

Prophylactic treatment

Several prophylactic treatments have shown reduction of frequency and severity of VOD. These treatments need to be initiated before the start of the preparative regimen.

- Ursodeoxycholic acid (10–15 mg/kg × day up to 900 mg/day p.o.); safe, cheap, and efficient. In addition overall decreased TRM was shown in several trials
- Low dose heparin (100 units/kg × day) until 30 days after the transplant or low molecular weight heparin (LMWH) might be considered (however, it should be remembered that VOD is not a coagulation problem, more a fibrotic response to tissue injury)
- Prophylactic defibrotide may be indicated for "high risk" patients
- Iron chelation prior to conditioning may be beneficial (Maradei et al., 2009)
- Parenteral glutamine supplementation has shown to preserve protein C levels. Falling protein C levels have been shown to predict severe VOD (Lakshminarayanan et al., 2010)

Treatment

- Anti-thrombotic treatment

  - Defibrotide is a single-stranded polydeoxyribonucleotide and is currently the most efficient treatment for VOD (SOS). Defibrotide

    - Binds to endothelial cells
    - Enhances fibrinolysis and suppresses coagulation locally
    - Is well tolerated
    - Is expensive
    - Treatment success is more likely with start of treatment within the first 48 hours after diagnosis of VOD
    - Currently in the United States only available in clinical studies
    - Dosing: 6.25 mg/kg IV every 6 hours
    - Keep platelets $\geq$30 000/μL, ht$\geq$30%, INR (international normalized ratio)$\leq$1.5 and serum fibrinogen $\geq$150 mg/dL. (Concomitant treatment with AT III, low molecular weight heparin, or heparin was not permitted for study patients. Resolution of 36%–52% of severe VOD with multiorgan dysfunction and a 47%–60% of survival at day +100 has been reported in adults and children)
    - References for defibrotide: Carreras et al., 2011; Corbacioglu et al., 2012; Richardson et al., 2010

  - Recombinant human TPA, 5–10 mg IV daily for up to 6 days may be effective. Significant risk of hemorrhage

Supportive treatment

1. Maintain intravascular volume and renal perfusion as the primary aim.
   - Packed cell transfusion (keep hematocrit around 40% [>30%])
   - Salt-poor albumin (in patients with albumin <2 g/dL)
   - Monitor central venous pressure and urine output
   - Restrict dietary salt
   - Avoid sodium-containing fluids and drugs
2. Treat secondary hyperaldosteronism: if urine sodium is low, give spironolactone, 200–400 mg per day.
3. Avoid diuretics that deplete intravascular volume (furosemide, thiazides).
4. If ascites causes discomfort or limits breathing, perform midline paracentesis, 1–2 L daily if necessary.
5. Provide chest physical therapy to avoid basal atelectasis.
6. Monitor serum potassium level.
7. Consider renal-dose dopamine infusion.
8. If there is hepatic encephalopathy
   - Avoid psychotropic drugs (if a sedative is needed, use diazepines, e.g., oxazepam, lorazepam)
   - Reduce the gut nitrogen load (lactulose)
   - Maintain the blood glucose concentration
   - Give prophylaxis for stress ulcers (ranitidine)

- Provide coagulation factor and platelet infusions as needed
- Transjugular intrahepatic portosystemic stent shunt and liver transplantation have been reported with possible long-term survival

Transplantation-associated thrombotic microangiopathy (TA-TMA)

TA-TMA happens when endothelial damage in the context of HSCT causes microangiopathic hemolytic anemia and platelet consumption, resulting in thrombosis and fibrin deposition in the microcirculation. The kidney is most frequently affected, but CNS and bowel involvement have been described. In an EBMT survey, the incidence was 7% in allogeneic HSCT, and very rare after auto-HSCT; time of onset has been reported between 2 weeks and 1 year after allogeneic HSCT.

Risk factors

- TBI
- Busulfan
- Fludarabine-based regimens
- Calcineurin inhibitors
- Sirolimus
- Unrelated or mismatched grafts
- GvHD
- CMV/fungal infection
- Older age
- Different pathogenesis from de novo thrombotic–thrombocytopenia purpura; ADAMTS13 levels are generally normal

Diagnostic criteria

- BMT CTN consensus (Ho et al., 2005)
    1. RBC fragmentation and ≥ 2 schistocytes per high-power field (400x magnification) on PB smear
    2. Concurrent increased serum LDH
    3. Concurrent renal (doubling of serum creatinine or 50% decrease in creatinine clearance from baseline) and/or neurological dysfunction without other explanations
    4. Negative direct and indirect Coombs test
- EBMT consensus definition (Ruutu et al., 2007)
    1. $\geq 4\%$ schistocytes in blood
    2. De novo, prolonged or progressive thrombocytopenia (platelet count less than 5×10^9/L or a 50% or greater decrease from previous counts)
    3. Sudden and persistent increase in LDH
    4. Decrease in Hgb concentration or increased RBC transfusion requirement
    5. Decrease in serum haptoglobin concentration

Haptoglobin is an acute-phase reactant. Therefore normal or elevated levels do not exclude TA-TMA.

Creatinine as a marker for renal function is unreliable in patients with decreased muscle mass.

Cystatin C, a non-muscle-based marker of renal function, may prove helpful in assessment of kidney function in HSCT patients.

Other findings potentially associated with TA-TMA

Reticulocytosis, hypertension especially in patients requiring >2 blood pressure medications, proteinuria as diagnosed by elevation of the first-morning spot protein-to-creatinine ratio, fever of non-infectious origin.

Several studies have shown histological evidence for TA-TMA in patients who did not fulfill the clinical/laboratory criteria listed earlier. Therefore, TA-TMA is likely underreported.

Prognosis

A survey by the EBMT found the only factor predictive of resolution of TA-TMA was the absence of nephropathy. The LDH/platelet ratio could also be helpful for outcome prognosis. A retrospective study reported survival of 10/13 patients with a ratio <20 compared to 21/40 patients with a ratio of 20 to 100 and 1/11 patients with a ratio of >100.

Treatment

- Some patients with calcineurin inhibitor-induced nephrotoxicity or neurotoxicity will improve quickly after decreasing the dose or stopping calcineurin inhibitors. Usually this is related to toxic levels. If calcineurin inhibitors need to be stopped, corticosteroids or mycophenolate can be started as replacement
- For patients with TA-TMA not associated with calcineurin inhibitor toxicity, treatment remains a major challenge (see also Batts et al., 2007; Choi et al., 2009; Kojouri & George, 2007; Laskin et al., 2011; Stavrou & Lazarus, 2010)
  - Therapeutic plasma exchange is occasionally used for treatment (to be discouraged). The published results are disappointing with less than 50% response and 70%–90% mortality
  - Small case series reported some success with daclizumab, basiliximab or anti-TNF antibodies (etanercept/infliximab). The rationale for these treatments could be the strong association of TA-TMA with GVHD. Main side effects are serious infections
  - Case reports suggest beneficial effects for thrombomodulin
  - Defibrotide inhibits TNF-mediated endothelial cell apoptosis in vitro and data from a small study with 12 patients reports survival of six patients. In addition, the combination of defibrotide and rituximab was also beneficial
  - Eculizumab is a complement inhibitor FDA approved for the treatment of atypical hemolytic uremic syndrome (HUS). There is a possibility that patients with an underlying genetic defect could develop atypical HUS triggered by the HSCT procedure. At the moment, there are no data to support this hypothesis but eculizumab may have a role in the treatment for a subgroup of patients with TA-TMA

Calcineurin inhibitor-associated hypertension

- Hypertension associated with the use of calcineurin inhibitors (cyclosporin A, tacrolimus) is commonly seen after allogeneic HSCT and in organ transplantation
- Onset usually 2–3 weeks after commencement of calcineurin inhibitor
- Pathophysiology not clear, likely multifactorial, involves stimulation of the sympathetic nervous system (cyclosporin A >tacrolimus) and activation of the renal sodium chloride cotransporter, renal vasoconstriction, and activation of the renin–angiotensin system (see also Bai et al., 2010; Hoorn et al., 2011; Klein et al., 2010)
- Genetic disposition involves genes encoding for angiotensin-converting enzyme, endothelial constitutive nitric oxide synthase, cytochrome P450 3A isoenyzme
- Beware of the combination of diastolic hypertension and thrombocytopenia in the early posttransplant period; both should be treated aggressively to minimize the risk of stroke

Treatment
Acute
- Sublingual nifedipine capsule, 10 mg, punctured (content will be absorbed through the buccal mucosa, thereby avoiding a hepatic first-pass effect)

Continuous
- Calcium channel blocker (e.g., one nifedipine tablet, 10–20 mg twice daily)
- Substitute or add a beta blocker (e.g., atenolol, 25–50 mg at night), if calcium channel blocker is not tolerated or effective, or an ACE inhibitor (e.g., enalapril, 5 mg daily)

Cyclosporin-associated blindness

Cyclosporin-associated blindness is believed to be caused by vasospasm producing ischemia of the occipital cortex. A similar neurotoxicity can also be observed subsequent to other calcineurin inhibitors. Cyclosporin-induced vision loss is a manifestation of posterior reversible encephalopathy syndrome (PRES). Cyclosporin should be held or tapered and the calcium channel blocker nimodipine can be useful in this situation.

Indications for nimodipine
Nimodipine is indicated for prevention and treatment of ischemic neurological deficits caused by cerebral vasospasm. Treatment should commence as soon as possible.

Contraindications
Use nimodipine with caution in patients with cerebral edema or severely elevated intracranial pressure. Do not use in patients who are hypersensitive to it. Monitor renal function closely in patients with renal disease and in those concurrently receiving nephrotoxic drugs, as little is known about the use of nimodipine in patients with renal impairment. Interactions with other drugs such as anticonvulsants need to be observed.

Growth and development

- The amount of growth retardation seen in pediatric patients after conditioning with TBI depends on the age of the child. For example, after fractionated 12 Gy TBI conditioning for children, the final height with a median age of 10.8 years versus 6 years at time of transplant was <-2.0 SD versus <-3.5 SD

- Cranial or craniospinal irradiation in addition to TBI can aggravate the growth retardation
- Accurate measurement of growth through age 17 years for girls and 19 years for boys and bone age if needed can help detecting growth retardation early
- For patients with a height velocity <25th percentile, a dynamic test for growth hormone deficiency should be considered
- Early diagnosis and treatment of growth hormone deficiency result in stronger treatment effect
- Current data do not support the concern that growth hormone treatment may play a role in the development of a relapse or of a secondary malignancy. There might be an increase in benign tumors and bony changes: for children after HSCT, the published rate for benign osteochondromas or exostoses was 12/42 patients with growth hormone treatment compared to 5/48 patients without. In addition, patients treated with growth hormone had a significantly higher incidence of hypothyroidism (14/42 patients). For children that received busulfan/cyclophosphamide conditioning, final height seems to be unaffected
- Prepubertal HSCT recipients are at risk for hypogonadism when entering puberty. With 12 Gy fractionated TBI, Leydig cell function is most often preserved and males are likely to show normal pubertal development. Approximately 50% of prepubertal girls given fractionated TBI will enter and progress through puberty. In most female patients, busulfan/cyclophosphamide conditioning will lead to a need for sex-hormone replacement. Monitoring for development of secondary sex characteristics and measurement of LH and FSH can help to detect gonadal failure. If needed, a physiological regimen of hormone replacement therapy should be initiated at the age of 12–13 years under the guidance of a pediatric endocrinologist
- Pediatric patients who received HSCT are at risk for developing neurocognitive deficiencies, such as the inability to aquire new skills at a rate comparable to their age-matched healthy peers and a decline in long-term memory scores. Patients who received cranial irradiation as part of either their initial therapy or of the HSCT conditioning are at greatest risk. It is important to address these issues during long-term follow-up in an effort to improve the person's overall quality of life

The following measurements to monitor the growth and development of pediatric patients after BMT/SCT should be carried out *at least annually*

- Accurate measurement of height, sitting height, and weight
- Pubertal status assessment
- Palpation of thyroid; thyroid function testing
- Measurements of gonadotropins (LH and FSH) and sex steroids (estradiol or testosterone)
- IGF-1 measurement
- Bone age measurements (every 2–3 years, and at the first sign of puberty)

(For further literature on long-term follow-up, see Consortium, 2012; Majhail et al., 2012; Pulsipher et al., 2012; Sanders et al., 2005.)

Secondary malignancies after HSCT

- Relative risk of developing secondary malignancy in long-term survivors following allogeneic HSCT compared to general population: 4–11-fold increase
- Annual incidence: 3.5% at 10 years–12.8% at 15 years

Risk factors

- TBI
- Younger age at HSCT
- Prolonged and severe chronic GVHD
- Prolonged exposure to immunosuppressive therapy (azathioprine, corticosteroids, cyclosporin)
- T-cell depleted graft
- Use of ATG
- Second or third HSCT
- Chemotherapy (alkylating agents, topoisomerase II inhibitors)

Three major groups

- Therapy-related MDS (t-MDS) also designated as therapy-related myeloid neoplasm (t-MN)/and AML (t-AML)
- Lymphoma/lymphoproliferative disorders
- Solid tumors (Rizzo et al., 2009)

The different types of second malignancies subsequent to allogeneic transplants are described in the following table. (According to Maijhal, 2011; Socié et al., 2012.)

Types of second malignant neoplasms	SIR (standardized incidence ratio)	Cumulative incidence (%)	Comments
Post-transplant lymphoproliferative disorders	29.7–182	1–2	As high as 8%–10% if multiple risk factors. 80% occur in 6–12 months >90% associated with EBV
All solid tumors	2.1	1.2–1.6 at 5 yr 2.2–6.1 at 10 yr 3.8–14.9 at 15 yr	Radiation treatment at young age. Immunosuppression and GVHD increase risk of SCC
Breast cancer	2.2	0.8 at 10 yr 4.6 at 20 yr 11 at 25 yr	Increased risk if received TBI (17% vs. 3% at 25 yr), younger age of transplant, long years posttransplant
Lung cancer	3		Increased risk in smokers, older patients

(cont.)

Types of second malignant neoplasms	SIR (standardized incidence ratio)	Cumulative incidence (%)	Comments
Skin cancer BCC SCC Melanoma	4.1–5	6.5 at 20 y 3.4 at 20 y	TBI, chronic GVHD Acute and chronic GVHD Immunosuppression, TBI Increase with radiation conditioning, immunosuppression
Mouth Lip Tongue	7 26 9–13		Risk increases if chronic GVHD, radiation treatment
Thyroid cancer	3.3–6.6		Female, age <10 yr at time of transplant, radiation to neck, chronic GVHD
Liver cancer	6–7.5		Increase with radiation conditioning, if hepatitis C (16% at 20 yr)
Bone cancer	8–13.4		Increase with radiation conditioning
Soft tissue sarcomas	7–8		Increase with radiation conditioning
CNS malignancies	4–7.6		Increase with radiation conditioning

The cumulative incidence of second solid tumors is shown in the following figure. (Reproduced with permission; Rizzo et al., 2009.)

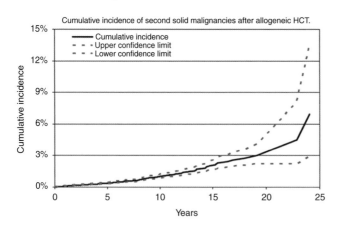

Cumulative incidence of second solid malignancies after allogeneic HCT.

Therapy-related MDS (t-MDS)/AML (t-AML)

- The estimated incidence of t-AML after auto-HSCT for patients with lymphoma or HL ranges between 1% and 14% at 3–15 years
- Therapy-related MDS/AML after auto-HSCT usually appears 4–7 years after exposure to alkylating agent and/or radiation
- Two-thirds of patients present with MDS and one-third with AML with a high incidence of chromosomal abnormalities involving chromosomes 5 [–5/del(5q)] and 7 [–7/del(7q)]
- Topoisomerase II inhibitor-related AML post-auto-HSCT can have a quite short interval between exposure and onset of AML ranging from six months to five years
- Following treatment with epipodophyllotoxins, translocations involving 11q23 are most frequent whereas translocations involving 21q22, inv(16), t (15,17), and t (9,22) are seen posttreatment with anthracyclines
- Specific risk factors for development of t-MDS/t-AML: older age, radiation therapy, topoisomerase II inhibitors, alkylators, >1 HSCT, "poor stem cell mobilizer"
- Poor overall outcome with median survival of six months. Only curative option is allogeneic HSCT with estimated five-year survival of 20% in adults. When four risk factors (age older than 35 years; poor-risk cytogenetics; t-AML not in remission or advanced t-MDS; and donor other than an HLA-identical sibling or a partially or well-matched unrelated donor) are considered, prognosis may be assessed. Five-year survival for subjects with none, 1, 2, 3, or 4 of these risk factors was 50% (95% CI, 38–61), 26% (CI, 20–31), 21% (CI, 16–26), 10% (CI, 5–15), and 4% (CI, 0–16), respectively ($P<0.001$) (Litzow et al., 2010). For children with therapy-related MDS/AML, posttreatment for ALL that was treated with allogeneic HSCT with busulfan/cyclophosphamide/melphalan conditioning, EFS at 5 years was 34%

Posttransplantation lymphoproliferative disorder (PTLD)

- PTLD includes a continuum ranging from EBV-associated polyclonal proliferation to highly aggressive monoclonal monomorphic lymphoma
- Reported incidences for PTLD are in the range of 1% after allogeneic HSCT with full intensity conditioning up to 15% for children receiving allogeneic HSCT with RIC
- Two major risk factors include latent EBV infection or EBV reactivation and T-cell depletion either in vitro by graft manipulation or in vivo with ATG or CD3 antibodies as part of the conditioning regimen
- Other risk factors included unrelated or HLA-mismatched grafts and acute or chronic GVHD with associated immunosuppressive treatment
- Most often the diagnosis is made 1–5 months after HSCT; but for patients with treatment for chronic GVHD a diagnosis much later is possible
- Clinical symptoms include
  - Fever, lymphadenopathy, and enlargement of tonsils, adenoids, liver, spleen, and kidney
  - GI tract symptoms like abdominal pain, vomiting/diarrhea with bloody stools
  - Rare: quite fulminant clinical picture misinterpreted as sepsis syndrome has been described

- PTLD WHO classification 2008

  - Plasmacytic hyperplasia, infectious mononucleosis-like lesion, polyclonal, always EBV+
  - Polymorphic PTLD, monoclonal, always EBV+
  - B-cell lymphoma (DLBCL, Burkitt, plasma cell myeloma, plasmocytoma-like lesions), monoclonal, frequently EBV+
  - Peripheral T-cell lymphoma, hepatosplenic T-cell lymphoma, monoclonal, rarely EBV+
  - Classic HL-like PTLD, monoclonal, frequently EBV

  (Heslop, 2009.)
- Measurement of the EBV-DNA load by quantitative PCR is a helpful screening tool if PTLD is suspected. It can also be used for surveillance in high-risk patients; for example, ATG, Campath, severe GVHD. Interpretation of EBV PCR+ test results depends on the specimen tested and is not specific for disease onset

  - PB mononuclear cell: EBV DNA in normal B-cells and in transformed cells
  - Serum: EBV shedding, EBV DNA from transformed B-cells; EBV shedding from epithelial cells has been reported to occur intermittently in normal EBV seropositive people
  - Whole blood: EBV in normal B-cells, in transformed cells, shedded EBV
- About 50% of HSCT patients with a positive EBV-DNA PCR will develop PTLD. If serial measurements show an increasing EBV-DNA load, further workup and start of treatment even in the absence of clinical symptoms should be considered
- Current recommendation of European Conference in Infections in Leukemia for allogeneic HSCT recipients: weekly screening for EBV DNA for the first three months
- Two-pronged treatment approach

  - Enhance the cellular immune response against EBV

    - If feasible, tapering of the immunosuppressive treatment
    - If the graft donor is EBV positive, infusion of unmanipulated donor T-cells has shown response rates of more than 70%. Careful clinical monitoring due to increased risk of severe GVHD induction
    - Use of EBV-specific T-cells, which have proved to be an effective treatment for more than 80% of patients with overt PTLD. Low risk of GVHD induction. Practical challenges for EBV-specific CTL generation relate to time and site constraints (2–3 months required, specialized laboratory facilities). In the future, the use of partially HLA-matched EBV-specific T-cells stored in a bank may help to have this type of treatment more rapidly available (de Pasquale et al., 2012)

  - Proliferating B-cells as direct target

    - Rituximab, a chimeric murine/human monoclonal anti-CD20 antibody, has been widely used for "preemptive" and therapeutic treatment of PTLD. Response rates between 55% and 100% have been reported
    - Depending on the extent and location of PTLD, radiation therapy, surgery, and chemotherapy (e.g., sequential R-CHOP) can be effective for therapy

- Antiviral treatment (acyclovir, ganciclovir) used for PTLD prophylaxis but has no direct antineoplastic effects in PTLD

(For algorithms for monitoring and treatment of PTLD, see Heslop, 2009.)

Solid tumors
- Incidence of solid tumors as second malignancies after HSCT increases with time (1.2%–1.6% at 5 years, 2.2%–6.1% at 10 years; 3.8%–14.9% at 15 years posttransplant)
- Incidence increases with age
- Occur later than other secondary malignancies after HSCT
- Radiation (TBI or prior local radiation therapy) is single most important risk factor
- Additive risk factors: GVHD, HPV
- The most frequent solid tumors found are
  - Tumors in the oral cavity/buccal mucosa
  - Neoplasms of the skin (squamous cell carcinoma, basal cell carcinoma, melanoma)
  - Uterine cancer
  - Thyroid cancer
  - Breast cancer
  - Brain tumors

The risk for secondary malignancies can be reduced by avoiding additional risk factors regarding smoking, sun exposure, or nutrition. Regarding cancers of the mouth, throat, and cervix, it is possible that the HPV vaccine could help to decrease the risk.

Prognosis
- In many cases, similar to other malignant tumors, especially if early diagnosed. Cancers of the mouth and throat are an exception and generally have a poor prognosis
- Lifelong surveillance is indicated
- Counseling regarding second cancer vigilance and education for self-examination of breast, skin, and testes should be a part of the posttransplantation care. Individualized screening recommendations apply to patients with additional risk factors, such as
  - Chronic GVHD
  - Chronic HCV or HBV infection
  - Radiation exposure of chest (female patients), abdomen or pelvis in addition to TBI
  - Fanconi anemia or dyskeratosis congenita as underlying disease

Long-term follow-up recommendations from the NCI/NHLBI/PBMTC First International Conference on Late Effects after Pediatric Hematopoietic Cell Transplantation 2012 (Majhail et al., 2012):
- Annual risk counseling about risks of secondary malignancy
- Encourage patients to perform self-examination including breast and testis
- Encourage patients to follow general population recommendations for cancer screening
- In patients with chronic GVHD: clinical and dental evaluation to assess for oral and pharyngeal cancer

- Patients with history of TBI or prior thoracic irradiation: mammography starting age 25 years or 8 years after radiation exposure, not later than age 40 years

Organ-related complications
Cardiac and vascular complications
HSCT recipients are at increased risk for cardiac complications and a thorough workup prior to HSCT is required.

Pretransplant workup
Baseline
- Resting ECG /MUGA scan
- Echocardiography (resting) (threshold of ejection fraction: 45%–50%)
- Chest-X ray

Extend (if indicated by medical history/clinical symptoms)
- Exercise ECG
- Exercise echocardiography
- Coronary angiography
- Cardiology consult and clearance

Congestive heart failure (CHF)
- Cumulative incidence after auto-HSCT: 4.8% at 5 years and 9.1%–14.5% at 15 years
- Increased risk with prior diabetes mellitus or essential hypertension
- 4.5 increased overall risk after auto-HSCT to develop CHF
- 50% of all acute cardiac-related mortality
- Chemotherapy-related toxicity from drugs frequently used prior to and during the conditioning regimen; e.g., high-dose cyclophosphamide (cumulative dose independent), anthracyclines (cumulative lifetime dose should be calculated)
- For anthracyclines, 9.9-fold increased risk of developing CHF if cumulative dose exceeded 250 mg/m^2. This threshold is substantially lower than usually considered ([cumulative doxorubicin dose–CHF incidence ratio: 400 mg/m^2–3%, 550 mg/m^2–7%, 700 mg/m^2–18%]), identifying HSCT recipients as specific at-risk population

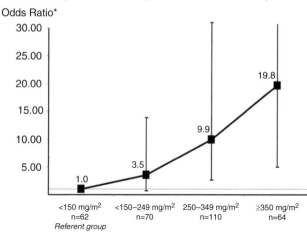

Magnitude of risk of CHF by increments of cumulative anthracycline dose

(Reproduced with permission; Armenian et al., 2011.)

- The following conversion to calculate cumulative anthracycline dose is suggested:
  - 50 mg doxorubicin = 60 mg daunorubicin = 75 mg epirubicin = 10 mg idarubicin = 12.5 mg mitoxantrone
- Risk increased by radiation therapy, chronic hypertension, obesity, diabetes mellitus, smoking, pulmonary hypertension
- Disease-related causes of CHF; e.g., light chain amyloid deposition in AL amyloidosis
- If severe, CHF will preclude subsequent BMT/SCT. If moderate, careful cardiological assessment is required to determine if BMT is feasible, as for example
  - By avoiding hyperhydration regimens for prophylaxis of hemorrhagic cystitis (use MESNA instead)
  - Dose adjustment for cyclophosphamide according to ideal/adjusted body weight
  - By avoiding sodium-containing medications such as ticarcillin (use aminoglycoside/cephalosporin for febrile neutropenia)

Arrhythmia

- Most common: atrial flutter/atrial fibrillation (AF) (Guglin et al., 2009)
- Ventricular tachycardia (VT) less frequent
- Chemotherapy-related toxicity
  - AF: melphalan (especially high-dose melphalan conditioning 6.6%–8.3%), adriamycin, doxorubicin, gemcitabine, ifosfamide, rituximab
  - VT: doxorubicin (rarely), arsenic (hold if QTc>500 ms), gemcitabine, rituximab
  - Bradycardia: thalidomide (27%), rare with cytarabine
- Sinus tachycardia often presents a secondary physiological response to other noncardiac causes; e.g., fever, sepsis, volume depletion, pain

- Pentostatin increases cardiotoxicity of high-dose cyclophosphamide and should be avoided, as fatal arrhythmias and fatal acute cardiomyopathy have been reported
- DMSO toxicity when frozen stem cells are given

(Armenian et al., 2008, 2011.)

Cardiac and cerebrovascular events

- Vascular disease of the arterial system after HSCT leads to increased cardio- and cerebrovascular events
  - Cumulative incidence of arterial vascular events after allogeneic HSCT at 15 years: 7.5%
  - Cumulative incidence of arterial vascular events after auto-HSCT at 15 years: 2.3%

Cumulative incidence of first arterial events after allogeneic HSCT

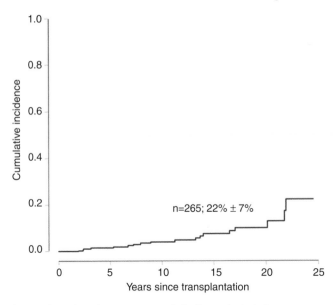

(Reproduced with permission; Tichelli et al., 2007.)

- Increased development of de novo cardiovascular risk factors after treatment with HSCT has been reported. Arterial hypertension, dyslipidemia, and BMI >25 occur more often after allogeneic- than auto-HSCT

- Underlying pathophysiology may involve direct drug toxicity (e.g., calcineurin inhibitors, corticosteroids), secondary drug effects (e.g., calcineurin inhibitor-related hypertension), endothelial activation and injury due to alloreactivity and GVHD synergizing with well-established cardiovascular risk factors
- Education and screening of patients for cardiovascular risk factors should be done rigorously after allogeneic HSCT and management and treatment of hypertension, diabetes, and hyperlipidemia according to current guidelines is strongly recommended

Long-term follow-up recommendations from the NCI/NHLBI/PBMTC First International Conference on Late Effects after Pediatric Hematopoietic Cell Transplantation 2012 (Majhail et al., 2012):

- Routine clinical assessment of cardiovascular risk factors at one year and at least yearly thereafter
- Lifestyle modification (dietary counseling, smoking cessation, weight control/loss, exercise)
- Early treatment of cardiovascular risk factors

Dermatological complications

1. GVHD (see also pages 311–326)
    - Acute (maculopapular rash, pruritus)
    - Chronic (poikiloderma, lichenoid, morphea, scleroderma, dyspigmentation)
2. Treatment-related
    - TBI-induced erythema
    - Chemotherapy-induced; e.g., acral dermatitis
    - Busulfan-induced hyperpigmentation (axillar, submammary, inguinal)
    - Cytarabin-induced erythema
    - Immunosuppression-induced; e.g., cyclosporin-induced hypertrichosis and facial coarsening; corticosteroid acne, skin thinning (parchment paper-like skin), striae
    - Drug allergies and hypersensitivity reactions; e.g., penicillin, cotrimoxazole, allopurinol, etc
    - ATG-induced urticaria
    - Vancomycin erythema (after too rapid IV infusion) transfusion reaction
    - Immediate-type hypersensitivity (e.g., urticaria with ATG)

Alopecia:	complete (secondary to TBI/chemotherapy) focal, with thin and gray hair (secondary to chronic GVHD)
Nail dystrophy:	semilunar ridging (regeneration after chemotherapy), longitudinal ridging (secondary to chronic GVHD)

3. Infections
- Viral: HSV, VZV (localized/generalized), HHV-6, parvovirus B19, CMV (rare)
- Bacterial: cellulitis, boils, IV site infection, septic emboli, paronychia
- Fungal: dermatophytes, *Candida*, *Aspergillus* (subcutaneous nodules–rare)

4. Immune-mediated
- Erythema multiforme
- Eczema
- Transfer of contact sensitivity, psoriasis, etc., from donor to recipient

5. Malignancy
- Extramedullary relapse of underlying malignancy: subcutaneous chloromas
- Secondary malignancy: squamous cell carcinoma, basal cell carcinoma (see page 362)

Long-term follow-up recommendations from the NCI/NHLBI/PBMTC First International Conference on Late Effects after Pediatric Hematopoietic Cell Transplantation 2012 (Majhail et al., 2012):
- Educate patients on routine self-examination of skin
- Avoidance of sunlight exposure/use of sunlight protection (high SPF)

Endocrine complications

Complications of the early posttransplant period

- Disturbances of blood glucose control
  - hyperglycemia
  - hypoglycemia
- Corticosteroid side effects
  - iatrogenic Cushing syndrome
  - hypoadrenalism secondary to rapid corticosteroid reduction
- Abnormal thyroid function tests/sick euthyroid syndrome (low T3 low T4 syndrome)
  - Low T3 or low T3 and low T4 levels in the absence of underlying thyroid disease
  - Commonly seen in hospitalized patients or patients with chronic/critical illness
  - Low T3 syndrome
    - T3 normal, decreased, FT3 decreased
    - T4 normal, TSH normal
    - rT3 increased
  - Low T3/T4 syndrome
    - in severely ill patients, T4 levels decrease following decreased T3 levels
    - both T4 and T3 decreased, FT4 normal/decreased in critical illness
    - TSH normal/decreased/increased
- Syndrome of inappropriate antidiuretic hormone (ADH) secretion (SIADH) (Wei et al., 2010)

- Relatively rare and poorly described for patients undergoing HSCT
- Clinical symptoms often nonspecific: nausea, vomiting, fatigue
- Insidious onset and rapid progression observed
- Early form (<100 days): risk factors include UCB SCT, busulfan-containing conditioning regimen, ifosfamide, vincristine, high-dose cyclophosphamide, MTX, unrelated donor, HLA-mismatch, SSRI, morphine
- Late form (>100 days): varicella zoster infection
- Laboratory findings
  - Hyponatremia <135 mEq/L, P_{Osm} <270 mOsm/kg
  - Urine sodium concentration >20 mEq/L
  - Hypervolemia

- Treatment
  - Fluid restriction
  - Saline infusion (increase in sodium levels should not exceed 12 mEq/liter/day to avoid central pontine myelinolysis)
  - Demecocycline
  - V1/V2 receptor antagonists

Late endocrine complications

- Diabetes mellitus
- Iatrogenic Cushing syndrome
- Gonadal dysfunction (women: >90% primary ovarian failure; men: >90% Sertoli cell/ 10%–50% Leydig cell dysfunction)
  - correlation with infertility, bone loss, ageing (?)
  - → hormonal replacement in young female and hypogonadic male patients
- Gynecomastia (secondary to ciclosporin and/or steroid treatment)
- Growth impairment (risk factors: age at transplantation <10 years, TBI >8 Gy)
  - → growth hormone substitution if height 2 SD lower than expected
- Other abnormalities of hypothalamic-pituitary function
- Thyroid abnormalities
  - hypothyroidism (risk factors: younger age at transplantation, TBI, Bu/Cy)
  - thyroiditis (auto-/alloimmune reaction, associated with chronic GvHD)
  - thyroid carcinoma (secondary cancer, 0.15%–2%, risk: younger transplant age)
- Parathyroid hormone disturbances

(Savani et al., 2011.)

Long-term follow-up recommendations from the NCI/NHLBI/PBMTC First International Conference on Late Effects after Pediatric Hematopoietic Cell Transplantation 2012 (Majhail et al., 2012):

- Thyroid function testing yearly post-HSCT or if patient demonstrates symptoms suggestive of thyroid disease

- Pediatric patients: clinical and endocrinological gonadal assessment within one year of HSCT, further follow-up according to pediatric endocrinologist
- Monitor growth velocity in children annually, growth hormone and thyroid hormone if clinically indicated
- Patients with chronic GVHD: slow tapering of steroids following prolonged exposure due to increased risk of adrenal insufficiency

Eye complications

- Acute GVHD
- Chronic GVHD
- Cataract (due to TBI, steroids, age)
- Hemorrhage (retinal, vitreous, subconjunctival)
- Infection
  - Bacterial: conjunctivitis, keratitis, endophthalmitis, orbital cellulitis
  - Fungal: keratitis, endophthalmitis
  - Viral: HSV keratitis, VZV keratitis, CMV retinitis
- Drug toxicity affecting the eye
- Involvement of the eye by the underlying disease

Eye involvement by GVHD

Tissue	Acute GVHD	Chronic GVHD
Eyelid (skin)	Mild erythema to severe bullae formation and desquamation	Meibomian gland obstruction Anterior and posterior blepharitis, erythema, edema, telangiectasis, trichiasis, madarosis, hyperkeratosis, cicatricial entropion, periorbital hypo- and hyperpigmentation
Conjunctivae	Conjunctivitis, chemosis, ulceration of tarsal conjunctiva	Conjunctival hyperemia, hyperemia with chemosis and/or serosanguineous exudates, (pseudo-)membranous conjunctivitis, cicatricial changes of the palpebral conjunctiva (subtarsal fibrosis), conjunctival necrosis with reduced goblet cell density, epithelial thinning
Cornea	Corneal epithelial thinning, corneal keratinization, mild to severe stippling, filamentary keratitis, sloughing of corneal epithelium	Corneal epithelial thinning, corneal keratinization, mild-to-severe stippling, filamentary keratitis, sloughing of corneal epithelium, keratoconjunctivitis sicca (KCS), superior limbic keratoconjunctivitis, (persistent or recurrent) corneal erosion, corneal

(cont.)

Tissue	Acute GVHD	Chronic GVHD
		thinning, corneal ulceration, corneal scarring, corneal vascularization, corneal perforation, corneal calcification
Lacrimal gland	Dacryoadenitis, cellular infiltration, blocking of acini, lacrimal gland stasis	Fibrosis and obliteration of lumen, fibrosis, atrophy
Lacrimal duct Sclera	Scleritis, episcleritis, posterior scleritis	Occlusion of the lacrimal puncta Scleritis, episcleritis
Uveal tract General	Anterior chamber cells Vitreous cells Choroidal thickening Serous detachment	Pseudoptosis, frequent blinking, constant squinting, photophobia, decrease in visual acuity

Grading system for conjunctival acute GVHD

Stage I	Conjunctival hyperemia
Stage II	Hyperemia with chemosis and/or serosanguineous exudates
Stage III	Pseudomembranous conjunctivitis
Stage IV	Pseudomembranous conjunctivitis with corneal epithelial sloughing

Grading system for ocular GVHD

1. Tissue involvement: (a) the extent of lacrimal gland dysfunction, (b) the involvement of the lids (e.g., blepharitis, meibomian gland dysfunction), (c) the involvement of the conjunctiva (e.g., cicatricial conjunctivitis), (d) the corneal involvement (e.g., keratitis, epithelial defects, corneal ulceration)
2. Inflammatory activity (e.g., hyperemia of the bulbar conjunctiva may be chronically present when ocular chronic GVHD is not well controlled)
3. Presence of complications and functional impairment

Treatment of ocular GVHD

1. Treatment of underlying GVHD
2. Local treatment

   - Tear substitutes, lubricants, ointments
   - Mucolytic agents
   - Punctual occlusion
   - Autologous serum eye drops
   - Warm compresses, lid care with ointments
   - Topical steroids (short term), cyclosporin eye drops (side effects: early itchiness and burning sensation, lock jaw)

- Bandage contact lenses, sclera lenses
- Spectacles with side pieces, goggles
- Prevention of infection
- Tarsorrhaphies (lateral, complete)
- Management of complications (amniotic membrane transplantation or bio-onlay, conjunctival flaps, keratoplasty in case of corneal perforation

3. Lid surgery for ectropion and creams to skin of lid

Long-term follow-up recommendations from the NCI/NHLBI/PBMTC First International Conference on Late Effects after Pediatric Hematopoietic Cell Transplantation 2012 (Majhail et al., 2012):

- Routine clinical evaluation at six months and one year after HSCT and at least yearly thereafter; visual acuity and fundus examination at one year and subsequently according to clinical symptoms and risk factors
- Immediate ophthalmological evaluation in symptomatic patients

Gastrointestinal complications
Major GI complications

Organ	<21 days after BMT/SCT	>21 days after BMT/SCT
Mouth	Conditioning-regimen toxicity/mucositis, *Candida* infection, HSV infection	*Candida* infection, HSV infection, acute GVHD, chronic GVHD, xerostomia due to conditioning regimen
Esophagus	Conditioning-regimen toxicity/mucositis, reflux (peptic), dyspepsia and heartburn (steroids)	HSV and CMV infections, *Candida* infection, reflux (peptic esophagitis), acute GVHD, "pill" ulceration, chronic GVHD
Stomach	Mallory–Weiss tear from persistent vomiting, conditioning regimen gastritis	CMV gastritis, peptic ulceration
Duodenum	Conditioning-regimen duodenitis	CMV duodenitis, peptic ulceration, acute/chronic GVHD
Large intestine	Conditioning-regimen colitis, neutropenic colitis	CMV colitis, acute GVHD, pseudomembranous colitis

Nausea/vomiting
Nausea and vomiting after marrow transplantation can be caused by:

- Direct emetogenic effects from conditioning chemo-/radiotherapy
  - Treatment: antiemetics
- Medications, particularly nystatin or amphotericin oral suspension, itraconazole, voriconazole, co-trimoxazole, oxpentyfilline, trimethoprim-sulfamethoxazole, mycophenolate mofetile, opioids, and occasionally calcineurin inhibitors (cyclosporin, tacrolimus)

- Treatment: replacement of causative drug by alternate medication if possible
- GVHD, particularly upper GI GVHD
  - Diagnosis: endoscopy with biopsy
  - Treatment: immunosuppression (systemic versus GI-restricted steroids; e.g., oral beclomethasone dipropionate)
- Hepatic disease including GVHD and viral hepatitis
  - Diagnosis: viral PCR (see liver disease); transjugular or percutaneous liver biopsy
- Infection involving the esophagus, stomach, or intestine, usually viral (CMV, HSV, VZV) or fungal, occasionally bacterial
  - Diagnosis: endoscopy, biopsy for histology, viral/fungal bacterial cultures, immunohistochemistry
- Adrenal insufficiency, dysmotility, rare: pancreatitis, abdominal abscess
- Impaired upper GI motility
- GI tract infections, such as noro- or rotavirus, parasites
- Be aware of inadequate caloric uptake; identify need for additional oral or parenteral nutrition

Dysphagia/odynophagia

Causes include:

- Oral and esophageal mucositis from conditioning regimen-related toxicity
- Esophageal acute GVHD involvement
- Esophageal chronic GVHD (submucosal fibrosis, strictures, webs, concentric rings, narrowing, decreased peristaltic, xerostomia)
- Esophageal infection (viral, *Candida*)
- Reflux esophagitis (peptic esophagitis)
- Drug-induced esophagitis (doxycycline, tetracycline, potassium, NSAIDS)
- Poor dentition
- Rare: myasthenia gravis as symptom of chronic GVHD
- Workup: endoscopy, barium contrast X-ray
- Treatment: treat underlying cause, mechanical dilation, esophagectomy, interposition surgery, feeding gastrostomy

Diarrhea and abdominal pain

Causes of diarrhea and abdominal pain after BMT include the following:

- Most common within the first 12 months after allogeneic HSCT
- Chemotherapy- and radiation-related toxicity
- Acute/protracted acute GI GVHD
- Intestinal infections: viral (e.g., VZV, CMV, rota-, noro-, adenovirus); parasitic (e.g., *Giardia, Strongyloides, Cryptosporidia*); fungal (*Candida*); *Clostridium difficile*
- Medications (e.g., nonabsorbable antibacterial antibiotics, mycophenolate mofetil ["MMF colitis" versus "GVHD" presents both a clinical and histopathological challenge])
- Liver and gallbladder disease (viral hepatitis, VOD, abscess, gallstones)
- Pancreatitis (e.g., due to hyperlipidemia), pancreatic insufficiency
- Lactose intolerance/disaccharidase deficiency

- Malabsorption
- Inflammatory bowel disease (possibly increased risk in recipients receiving allogeneic HSCT from donors suffering from inflammatory bowel disease; e.g., Crohn's disease, NOD2 variant –related?)
- Workup
    - stool examination, microbiological workup (*C. difficile* toxin, parasites), triglycerides
    - erect and supine abdominal X-rays
    - upper or lower endoscopy (or both) with histology and viral/fungal/bacterial cultures
    - capsule endoscopy
    - abdominal ultrasound/CT/barium contrast
- Treatment
    - treat specific underlying cause
    - symptomatically (analgesics, replacement of pancreatic enzymes, fluids and electrolytes, reduce oral disaccharide intake)

Bleeding
Rarely, bleeding can be voluminous or acute, and the causes can include
- Eosophageal mucosal tears (secondary to nausea and emesis)
- GI tract ulcers
- GVHD
- Viral infections
- Severe esophagitis, gastric erosions, severe hemorrhagic gastritis, colitis
- Workup: endoscopy (upper and/or lower); angiography, nuclear medicine (RBC scan)
- Treatment
    - Cause-specific
    - Platelet transfusions (goal: maintain platelets >50/nL)
    - RBC transfusions (goal: maintain Hb>8 g/dL)
    - Endoscopic (cauterization, ligation)
    - Interventional radiology: embolization
    - If intractable bleeding e-aminocaproic acid, tranexamic acid, desmopressin
    - Use of activated F VII (Novo7) or Factor XIII replacement has been sporadically reported, current value undetermined

Ileus
- Most likely paralytical ileus
    - peritonitis, acute GVHD, sepsis, hypokalemia, morphine derivates, severe infectious colitis, pancreatitis

Hepatobiliary complications
Early (within the first 100 days), following HSCT
- VOD (see page 353)
- GVHD (see page 312)

- Bile duct destruction (secondary to protracted acute hepatic GVHD)
- Infections (bacterial, fungal, viral; e.g., hepatitis A–E, CMV, HSV, HHV-6, parvovirus, enterovirus, adenovirus, rarely VZV, TT-virus, HGV)
- Drug-induced liver disease (e.g., cyclosporin [common], NSAIDs, statins)
- Gallbladder and pancreatic disease
- Hepatic abscess (most likely fungal, septic emboli, mycobacteria)
- Focal nodular hyperplasia (up to 12% in long-term survivors)
- Nodular regenerative hyperplasia (rare)

Late, following HSCT

- GVHD
- Drug-induced liver diseases (e.g., cyclosporin, NSAIDs, statins)
- Focal nodular hyperplasia
- Nodular regenerative hyperplasia
- Viral hepatitis (hepatitis A–E, VZV, HSV)
- Hepatic abscess (most likely fungal, septic embolic)
- Cirrhosis (consider when GOT (glutamic oxaloacetic transaminase) >GPT (glutamic pyruvic transaminase), thrombocytopenia, splenomegaly, irregular liver surface or nodular parenchymal pattern on ultrasound, ascites, INR elevation)
- Recurrence of underlying malignancy
- Cholecystolithiasis, choledocholithiasis
    - Increased risk of gallstone development after allogeneic HSCT
    - Conditioning therapy related (myeloablative >RIC)
    - Biliary sludge in 70% of HSCT patients
    - Calcineurin inhibitor-induced: lithogenic effects
- Degenerative pancreas/pancreatic insufficiency

Overview of liver function abnormalities posttransplant

Disease	Bilirubin	ALT	SAP	Comment
Hepatic VOD	+ to +++	+ to ++	++ to +++	Weight gain, ascites, bilirubin increase and liver pain key indicators
Hepatic GVHD	+ to ++	+ to +++	+ to ++	Rapid ALT elevation to over 500 U/L; often after DLI or associated with tapering off immunosuppressive therapy
Cholestatic GVHD	+ to +++	+ to ++	+ to +++	SAP (serum alkaline phosphatase) increase prior to bilirubin increase
Acute hepatitis	+ to +++	+++	+ (or ++ in cholestatic phase)	
Cyclosporin hepatotoxicity	+	±	±	

(cont.)

Disease	Bilirubin	ALT	SAP	Comment
Hemolysis	+ (indirect and direct)	−	−	
Iron overload	(+)	(+)	(+)	Hepatic dysfunction rare

Hepatotoxic drugs commonly used posttransplant

Drug	Potential liver toxicity
Antilymphocyte globulin/ATG	Hepatitis
Azathioprine	Cholestasis
Cyclosporin	Hyperbilirubinemia; hepatitis (correlated with excessive cyclosporin serum levels)
Ketoconazole; itraconazole; fluconazole; voriconazole	Hepatitis
Methotrexate (long term)	Transient hepatitis, liver fibrosis
Penicillin derivatives	Hepatitis
Phenothiazines	Cholestasis
Total parenteral nutrition	Hepatitis, cholestasis
Trimethoprim/sulfamethoxazole	Hepatitis, cholestasis

Iron overload

- Iron excess occurs in 30%–60% of allo-HSCT recipients
  - High numbers of prior RBC transfusions
  - Dysfunctional iron storage during chronic disease/inflammation
- Serum ferritin levels of ≥1000 ng/mL have been associated with increased risk of blood stream infections, inferior DFS, OS, and increased incidence of acute GVHD
- A potential association between increased serum ferritin levels and the development of VOD has been reported
- Elevated iron stores in the form of unbound pools cause increased organ damage
  - Hepatic iron overload: common in patients after allogeneic HSCT, often clinically without symptoms
  - Cardiac iron overload: incidence in patients after allogeneic HSCT unknown; cardiac iron overload known to be associated with cardiomyopathy and heart failure
  - Iron overload-related endocrine organ damage: pancreas (low insulin), pituitary gland (low growth hormone levels), thyroid (hypothyroidism); incidence in patients after allogeneic HSCT unknown

- Diagnosis
  - Serum ferritin not an accurate marker for organ iron overload, but because of feasibility often used as surrogate marker
  - Serum ferritin is an acute phase protein, can be elevated during infections and inflammatory conditions
  - MRI is a validated method to assess liver and cardiac iron overload
  - Liver biopsy as the classical approach is now being replaced by MRI for noninvasiveness. Correlation between liver biopsy and MRI iron content measurement of the liver has been shown
- Preventive and therapeutic approaches
  - Currently, no standard approach for iron overload pre- or post-HSCT is defined and no recommendation can be given. Based on institutional preferences, it may be considered
    - Determine serum ferritin levels prior to transplant as surrogate marker for iron overload
    - Alternatively, consider pre-HSCT MRI
    - Candidates for allogeneic HSCT as well as survivors after allogeneic HSCT, who have evidence of iron-overload, iron-overload organ damage, or are polytransfused/transfusion-dependent, may benefit from chelation therapy
    - References for iron overload: Kida & McDonald, 2012; Majhail et al., 2008; Pullarkat 2010; Pullarkat et al., 2008

Long-term follow-up recommendations from the NCI/NHLBI/PBMTC First International Conference on Late Effects after Pediatric Hematopoietic Cell Transplantation 2012 (Majhail et al., 2012):
- LFTs every 3–6 months in year 1, then at least yearly
- Hepatitis B and/or C positive patients: quantitative PCR determination of viral load; joint care with infectious disease specialist
- Serum ferritin levels at one year after HSCT (optional MRI, biopsy)

Hormonal changes and related male and female complications after allogeneic HSCT

Andrological problems after BMT
- Fatigue
- Impaired sex drive
- Erectile dysfunction

Gynecological problems after BMT
- Ovarian failure and infertility
- Abnormal uterine bleeding
- Genital tract infections
- GVHD of the vagina
- Vaginal stenosis

Sex hormone monitoring

- Males: testosterone, LH, FSH levels at one year after HSCT or earlier if clinically warranted
- Females: LH/FSH levels at one year after HSCT or earlier if clinically warranted; estrogen levels optional

Adult dosages of testosterone preparations by different routes

Indication: low testosterone levels and no history/increased risk of prostate cancer

Route	Dose
Sublingual	5 mg three times daily
Topical	5–10 mg daily
Transdermal	10–15 mg daily

Adult dosages of estrogen preparations by different routes[a]

Comment: menstrual suppression with various estrogen preparations may be used in protocols/regimens that are expected to induce prolonged thrombocytopenia, which present a risk for menorrhagia. Menstrual suppression does not protect the ovaries and it is not associated with fertility improvement in regards to pregnancy rates later on.

Indication: menopause-related symptoms and/or low LH/FSH levels

Route	Dose
Oral	Piperazine estrone sulfate, 1.25 mg per day, or conjugated equine estrogen, 0.625 mg per day
Percutaneous[b]	Patches equivalent to 0.3, 0.625, or 1.25 mg of oral conjugated estrogens are available; replace every 3–4 days
Intravenous (emergency use only)	Conjugated equine estrogen, 25 mg; repeat in 6–12 hours if necessary; follow up with oral estrogen/progesterone is indicated

[a] accompanied by progesterone treatment for 12 to 14 days per month. In women with intact uterus, do not give estrogen only due to increased risk of carcinoma of the uterus. A typical regimen is Premarin, 0.625 mg PO daily, and Provera, 5–10 mg on days 1–14 or 2.5–5 mg PO daily. An alternative convenient approach is to use a low-dose estrogen contraceptive pill such as Triphasil, one daily, which contains both estrogen (ethinyl estradiol) and progestogen (levonorgestrel).
[b] an estrogen patch can be used short term, in lieu of systemic treatment, for oral estrogen intolerance or LFT abnormalities. Transdermal estrogen may not convey cardiovascular benefits.

Fertility and infertility after HSCT

Because of the increased long-term survival posttransplant, recovery of fertility after autologous and even allogeneic transplantation is assuming increasing importance. Data from CIMBTR indicate that 25% of autologous and more than 60% of allogeneic transplants are performed on recipients younger than age 40 years, and there are more than 12 000 transplants done per year on recipients aged 20 years or younger. A recent study showed that the prevalence of infertility and related concerns is higher among long-term SCT survivors than among age-, gender-, and education-matched controls (Hammond et al., 2007). The survivors have persistent fertility-related needs even 10 years after treatment. Oncologists need to be aware of the fertility consequences and available treatments that can be offered to patients.

Factors that contribute to the development of ovarian or testicular failure

1. Exposure to TBI

TBI is the greatest risk factor of gonadal failure. After TBI, virtually 100% women will develop ovarian failure.

2. Type of chemotherapy agents

Alkylating agents (particularly cyclophosphamide [CY], ifosphamide, nitrosoureas, chlorambucil, melphalan, busulfan [BU], and procarbazine) contribute to the development of ovarian or testicular failure. Several agents are associated with a low or no risk of infertility such as methotrexate, fluorouracil, vincristine, and bleomycin (Lee et al., 2006). The combination of high-dose BU and CY is one of the most potent conditioning regimens to induce gonadal failure (Brennan & Shalet, 2002).

3. Total dosage of chemotherapy received

4. Age at the time of first treatment

High-risk stratification

Definition: high risk

- Males: prolonged/persistent azoospermia posttreatment
- Females: >80% of women develop amenorrhea posttreatment

Regimens associated with impaired fertility

Male and female

- TBI
- Cyclophosphamide >7.5 g/m^2 (all males and females <20 years of age; 5 g/m^2 in females >40 years of age)
- Alkylating chemotherapy for transplant conditioning (cyclophosphamide, busulfan, melphalan)
- Procarbazine-containing regimens (e.g., COPP, MOPP, MOPP/ABVD, COPP/ABVD, BEACOPP)
- Any alkylating agent (e.g., procarbazine, nitrogen mustard, cyclophosphamide) + TBI, pelvic radiation, or testicular radiation
- Cranial/brain radiation ≥40 Gy

Males

- Testicular radiation dose >2.5 Gy in adults (≥6 Gy in boys)

Females

- Whole abdominal or pelvic radiation, doses ≥6 Gy in adult women (≥15 Gy in prepubertal girls, ≥10 Gy in postpubertal girls); CMF, CEF, CAF × 6 cycles in women 40 + years old

Options for preservation of fertility in males

Spermatogonial cryopreservation is an effective method. If no local sperm bank is available, a collection kit can be obtained through www.liveonkit.com. Testicular tissue or spermatogonial cryopreservation and transplantation, which may be promising techniques, have not been tested in humans. Gonadoprotection through hormonal manipulation is largely considered as ineffective.

Summary of fertility preservation options in males

Intervention	Definition	Comment	Considerations
Sperm cryopreservation (S) after masturbation or after alternative methods of sperm collection	Freezing sperm obtained through masturbation or testicular aspiration or extraction, electroejaculation	Masturbation is the most established technique for fertility preservation in men; large cohort studies in men with cancer	• Outpatient procedure • Approximately $1500 for three samples stored for three years; further storage fee for additional years* • Testicular sperm extraction–outpatient surgical procedure
Gonadal shielding during radiation therapy (S)	Use of shielding to reduce the dose of radiation delivered to the testicles	Case series	• Only possible with selected radiation fields and anatomy expertise is required to ensure shielding does not increase dose delivered to the reproductive organs
Testicular tissue cryopreservation Testis xenografting Spermatogonial isolation (I)	Freezing testicular tissue or germ cells and reimplanting after treatment	Has not been tested in humans; successful application in animal models	Outpatient surgical procedure
Testicular suppression with gonadotropin-releasing hormone (GnRH) analogs or antagonists (I)	Use of hormonal therapies to protect testicular tissue during chemotherapy or radiation therapy	Studies do not support the effectiveness of this approach	

S, standard; I, investigational; * costs are estimates based on US providers in 2001.

Options for preservation of fertility in females

Embryo cryopreservation after in vitro fertilization (IVF) is the most established option. To increase efficiency of fertilization, intracytoplasmic sperm injection (ICSI) should be considered. In recent years, the success rate of unfertilized oocyte preservation has improved by adapting a slow freezing or vitrification technique. Vitrification appears to be more effective than regular cryopreservation. However, both techniques require approximately two weeks of ovarian stimulation with FSH. For patients with acute leukemia or a diagnosis for which treatment cannot be delayed, it may not be feasible.

Summary of fertility preservation options in females

Intervention	Definition	Comment	Considerations*
Embryo cryopreservation (S)	Harvesting eggs, in vitro fertilization, and freezing of embryos for later implantation	The most established technique for fertility preservation in women	• Requires 10–14 days of ovarian stimulation from the beginning of menstrual cycle • Outpatient surgical procedure • Requires partner or donor sperm • Approximately $8000 per cycle, $350 per year storage fees
Oocyte vitrification	Harvesting and slow freezing of unfertilized eggs	Rapidly maturing technique. Each thawed egg had an implantation potential of 6–8%	• Outpatient surgical procedure • Approximately $8000* per cycle, $350/yr storage fees
Oocyte cryopreservation (I)	Harvesting and freezing of unfertilized eggs	Small case series and case reports; as of 2005, 120 deliveries reported, approximately 2% live births per thawed oocyte (3–4 times lower than standard IVF)	• Requires 10–14 days of ovarian stimulation from the beginning of menstrual cycle • Outpatient surgical procedure • Approximately $8000* per cycle, $350/yr storage fees
Ovarian cryopreservation and transplantation (I)	Freezing of ovarian tissue and reimplantation after treatment	Case reports; as of 2005, two live births reported	• Not suitable when risk of ovarian involvement is high • Same day outpatient surgical procedure
Gonadal shielding during radiation therapy (S)	Use of shielding to reduce the dose of radiation delivered to the reproductive organs	Case series	• Only possible with selected radiation fields and anatomy • Expertise is required to ensure shielding does not increase dose delivered to the reproductive organs

(cont.)

Intervention	Definition	Comment	Considerations*
Ovarian suppression with GnRH analogs or antagonists (I)	Use of hormonal therapies to protect ovarian tissue during high-dose chemotherapy and SCT	Small randomized studies and case series	• Medication given before and during treatment
Ovarian recovery (I) (Liu et al., 2008)	Use of hormonal replacement therapy after treatment	Small case series	• Medication given after treatment

S, standard; I, investigational.
* modified from Brennan and Shalet, 2002; Lee et al., 2006. Further information can be found at:
http://www.fertilehope.org/toolbar/risk-calculator.cfm

Hematologic complications

Causes of anemia after BMT

1. Inadequate production of RBCs
   - BM suppression by drugs, microbial agents, or coexisting disease
   - Delayed erythroid engraftment associated with ABO incompatibility
   - Pure RBC aplasia associated with ABO incompatibility
   - Sideroblastic anemia associated with pyridoxine deficiency
   - Impaired erythropoietin production
   - BM suppression during GVHD
   - Infection with parvovirus B19
2. Excessive loss of RBCs
   - Bleeding
   - Hemolysis: alloimmune (associated with ABO incompatibility), autoimmune, or microangiopathic (e.g., TTP or HUS)
   - Passenger lymphocyte syndrome (occurs 5–15 days posttransplantation in setting of a minor incompatibility)
   - Hypersplenism

Causes of neutropenia after BMT

1. Inadequate production of neutrophils
   - Delayed engraftment
   - BM suppression by drugs (e.g., ganciclovir, co-trimoxazole, methotrexate), sepsis, or GVHD

2. Excessive loss of neutrophils
   - Autoimmune destruction

Causes of thrombocytopenia after BMT

1. Inadequate production of platelets
   - Delayed megakaryocyte engraftment
   - BM suppression by drugs (e.g., ganciclovir, co-trimoxazole), sepsis, or GVHD
2. Excessive loss of platelets
   - Autoimmune destruction
   - GVHD
   - Hypersplenism
   - Disseminated intravascular coagulation
   - Hepatic VOD (SOS)
   - Thrombotic thrombocytopenic purpura (TTP, respectively transplant-associated microangiopathy, see page 385)

Musculoskeletal complications

Skeletal complications

- Osteoporosis
  - Occurs in up to 50% of allo-BMT patients
  - Risk factors
    - Prolonged corticosteroid/calcineurin-inhibitor therapy/TBI
    - Hypogonadism, hyperparathyroidism
    - Fractures in 10% of patients

- Osteonecrosis
  - Occurs in up to 20% of patients, associated with steroids
  - 5%–10%, mostly hip, often bilateral
- Arthralgia
  - Associated with chronic GVHD, steroid withdrawal, arthrosis
- Septic arthritis
  - Associated with systemic infections or joint replacement
- Osteomyelitis
  - Reactivation or septic metastases
- Spine pain
  - Due to osteoporosis/osteonecrosis and/or vertebral disk prolapse
- Contractures of joints
  - Due to deep sclerosis associated with cGVHD

Patients after allogeneic BMT/SCT have several risk factors for osteoporosis including high-dose chemotherapy, malabsorption syndrome, immobility, and hypogonadism.

GVHD may even increase the risk due to long-term steroid use, and steroid-induced diabetes mellitus.

As a result, the incidence of osteopenia and subsequent osteoporosis in patients with chronic GVHD is between 24% and 40%. There is also an increased rate of osteonecrosis in the axial skeleton, caused by impaired microcirculation.

(Bi-)annual osteodensitometry with dual-energy X-ray absorptiometry (DXA scan) is therefore recommended for all patients, starting one year after alloBMT, and before and during steroid treatment.

The value of osteodensitometry during bisphosphonate treatment is unclear.

All patients receiving steroid treatment should receive calcium (1–1.5 g/day) and vitamin D substitution (1000 IU/day), and physical therapy is recommended.

If osteodensitometry reveals osteoporosis, bisphosphonate treatment should be administered. Additional treatment options are hormone replacement, raloxifene, denosumab, and teriparatide.

If hypogonadism is documented, hormone replacement is recommended.

Avascular osteonecrosis occurs independently of osteoporosis. The best method for diagnosis is MRI of the affected area. There is no specific prophylaxis for osteonecrosis besides avoiding long-term steroid treatment. Treatment is supportive with analgesics, and surgical with bone spur or joint replacement.

Muscle-related complications
- Myopathy (due to steroids, immobilization, catabolism, drug side effects)
- Contractures (due to fasciitis, deep dermal sclerosis associated with GVHD)
- Myalgia (due to steroid withdrawal, GVHD, infectious complications, drug side effects)
- (Poly-)myositis
  - Related to chronic GVHD or septic metastases
  - Proximal muscle weakness, pain
  - Elevated creatine kinase
  - Treatment with steroids ± cyclosporin A

Myopathy and contractures are mainly associated with GVHD; with physical therapy, appropriate nutrition is the most important of the preventive and therapeutic interventions. In the presence of steroid myopathy, a decrease of the steroid dose <0.25 mg/kg prednisone equivalent is crucial.

Others
- Fasciitis
  - Chronic GVHD-associated
  - Diagnosis: MRI, avoid biopsy
  - Treatment: physical therapy, immunosuppression/possibly extracorporeal photopheresis

- Polyserositis
  - Chronic GVHD-associated
  - Pericardial/pleural effusions, ascites, edema
  - Treatment: steroids

- Arthralgia
  - Often related to changes in steroid dosages

- Muscle cramps
  - Often unrelated to electrolyte imbalances

- Preexisting rheumatoid diseases
- Degenerative joint disease
- Mechanical spinal pain
- Intervertebral disk pathologies

Neurological complications

The first step to the neurological diagnosis is to localize signs and symptoms.

Clinical signs of diseases of the CNS

Typical signs of focal brain disease (including transiently, of note: focal signs may disappear in coma):

- Aphasia
- Alexia and other neuropsychological signs
- Hemianopsia
- Hemiparesis
- Hemihypesthesia
- Unilateral ataxia
- Lateralized or exaggerated deep tendon reflexes, spasticity, pyramidal signs
- Focal epileptic seizure (e.g., progression of convulsion with localized beginning, "aura," marked lateralization during seizure)

Typical signs of diffuse brain disease

- Confusion
- Impaired consciousness (somnolence, coma)
- Psychosis
- Epileptic seizures without localizing signs

Typical signs of spinal cord disease

- Sensory or motor deficits affecting both legs and/or arms with exaggerated tendon reflexes, spasticity, or other pyramidal signs (uni- or bilateral)
- Sensory deficits in sacral dermatomes
- Bowel and bladder dysfunction
- Sensory level

Typical signs of radicular disease

- Frequently radicular (e.g., lumboischialgic) pain and sensory deficits
- Decreased or absent deep tendon reflex and palsy in corresponding myotome

Typical signs of polyneuropathy

- Distal symmetric sensory or motor deficits
- Asymmetric sensory or motor deficits with loss of vibration sense and tendon reflexes
- Lesion of several single nerves ("multiplex neuritis")

Typical signs of myasthenic syndromes

- Fatigable pure motor weakness, often pronounced in proximal muscles, often ocular muscle involvement

Typical signs of myopathy

- Pure motor weakness with or without muscle pain, often pronounced in proximal muscles, tendon reflexes normal or weak

Neurological complications occurring in BMT/SCT patients include

Epileptic seizures

Infections

Encephalopathy due to

- Metabolic disturbances
- Treatment-induced leukoencephalopathy; posterior reversible encephalopathy syndrome with visual hallucinations, cortical blindness, seizures

Neurotoxicity due to antineoplastic and immunosuppressive treatment

- Cyclosporin
- Methotrexate
- Cytosine arabinoside

Cerebrovascular lesions

Malignancy and leukemia recurrence in CNS

Disorders of peripheral and cranial nerves

Disorders of muscles

Extrapyramidal disorders

Cognitive impairment and confusion

Hiccup and myoclonic jerks

Benign intracranial hypertension

GVHD

Myositis

Peripheral neuropathy

Myasthenic syndromes

Central nervous system

Benign and iatrogenic disorders

- Headache following lumbar puncture
- Myopathy; e.g., due to corticosteroids
- Migraine

Preexisting neurological disease

Causes of neurological complications in BMT/SCT patients

Disorder	Common causes
Epileptic seizures	Metabolic disorders (e.g., hypoglycemia, hyponatremia), drugs, any other disease involving cerebral cortex
CNS infections	Infections: acute bacterial, viral, or fungal meningitis; focal encephalitis (e.g., toxoplasmosis, progressive multifocal leukoencephalopathy [PML], brain abscess); disseminated encephalitis (e.g., herpes viruses)
Encephalopathy	Metabolic disorders like hyponatremia, hypothyroidism, systemic organ failure, drug toxicity, vitamin deficiency
Leukoencephalopathy	Posterior reversible encephalopathy syndrome (visual hallucinations, cortical blindness, seizures); symmetric: calcineurin inhibitors, prior treatment including whole brain irradiation; asymmetric: infections, malignancy
CNS malignancy	Lymphoma, leukemic recurrence, glioblastoma, metastasis
Cerebrovascular lesions	Intracranial hemorrhage, ischemic stroke, vasculitis
Cognitive impairment	Late complication of brain irradiation and chemotherapy, encephalopathy, cerebrovascular lesions, infections, leukoencephalopathy
Peripheral neuropathy	Herpes zoster infection, toxicity, GVHD-related acute and subacute neuropathy, local nerve compression
Myopathy	Steroid myopathy, myositis

Causes of epileptic seizures in BMT/SCT patients

Metabolic causes	Hypoglycemia (approximately 1/3 with focal signs promptly vanishing at normoglycemia), hyponatremia, hypomagnesemia, hypocalcemia, hypoxia, systemic organ failure (uremia, hepatic failure), vitamin deficiency (especially B vitamins)
Drugs/therapy including immune suppressive agents and therapy	Busulfan, L-asparaginase, high-dose cytosine arabinoside, methotrexate, cyclosporin, corticosteroids, drugs (amphetamines, heroin, cocaine, LSD), rarely theophylline, digitalis, lidocaine (intravenous, intrathecal), antibiotics (penicillins, metronidacol), psychiatric medication (TCAs, neuroleptics) Brain irradiation Discontinuation of preexisting antiepileptic treatment, benzodiazepines or morphine, alcohol withdrawal

(*cont.*)

Cerebrovascular disease (acute/old)	Ischemic stroke, traumatic and non-traumatic intracranial hemorrhage (intracerebral, subdural, epidural, subarachnoidal)
Infections	Meningoencephalitis, rarely meningitis
Malignancy	Recurrence of primary disease including neoplastic meningitis, secondary CNS malignancy
Preexisting epilepsy	

Causes of metabolic encephalopathy in BMT/SCT patients (in order of frequency)

Hypoxia and ischemia
Hepatic failure including hyperammonemia
Electrolyte imbalance, especially sodium, calcium, magnesium, phosphate
Hypo-/hyperglycemia
Renal failure

Antineoplastic and immune suppressive therapy associated with neurotoxicity

Treatment		Neurological side effects
Corticosteroids	CNS	Dysphoria, psychosis, hiccup, headache, lethargy, papilledema, increase of epidural fat
	PNS	Myopathy
Cyclosporin and tacrolimus	CNS	Tremor, seizures, ataxia, leukoencephalopathy, PRES, blindness, headache, psychosis
Methotrexate	CNS	Meningoencephalitis, myelopathy, (transient) encephalopathy, leukoencephalopathy, stroke-like syndromes
Everolimus and other mammalian target of rapamycin inhibitors	CNS	Headache, sleeplessness, dysgeusia, dizziness, sleepiness, depression, intracerebral hemorrhage, infections like progressive multifocal leukoencephalopathy (JC virus), rarely vasculitis
	PNS	Muscle pain
Cytosine arabinoside	CNS	Myelopathy, encephalopathy, cerebellar ataxia, seizures, extrapyramidal signs (dystonia)
	PNS	Neuropathy
Busulfan	CNS	Seizures, Wernicke-like syndrome with ataxia, confusion and diplopia responding to thiamine
Etoposide	CNS	Somnolence, seizures, confusion, motor deficits
Cyclophosphamide	CNS	Synergistic effect with cyclosporin toxicity
Imatinib	CNS	Synergistic effect with cyclosporin toxicity, reduced concentration by inductors of cytochrome CYP3A4

(cont.)

Treatment		Neurological side effects
		(e.g., antiepileptics), headache, sleep disorders, depression, dizziness, tremor, dysgeusia
	PNS	Muscle cramps, muscle pain, restless legs syndrome, rarely polyneuropathy
Procarbazine	CNS	Synergistic effect with cyclosporin toxicity
Monoclonal antibodies (all)	CNS	Headache, aseptic meningitis, infections like progressive multifocal leukoencephalopathy (JC-virus), specific side effects of specific antibodies
Thalidomide	CNS	Sleepiness, tremor, dizziness
	PNS	Axonal polyneuropathy frequently (median after 42 weeks of treatment)
Rituximab	CNS	Sleep disorders, depression, dizziness, dysgeusia
Alemtuzumab	CNS	Sleepiness, tremor, dizziness, dysgeusia, depression
	PNS	Muscle pain
Leukapheresis	CNS	Hemorrhage, ischemic stroke, activation of occult metastasis
Radiation	CNS	Delayed leukoencephalopathy, myelopathy
	PNS	Damage of nerve plexus, nerves in the field of radiation

CNS: central nervous system; PNS: peripheral nervous system including muscles; PRES: Posterior reversible encephalopathy syndrome

Calcineurin-related neurotoxicity: common and reversible syndromes

Syndrome	Frequency	Comment
Tremor	16%–20%	Dose-related, reversible, direct neurotoxicity
Seizures	5%	Dose-related, reversible, direct neurotoxicity Possible contributing risk factors: Hypomagnesemia Hypertension Steroid treatment Capillary leak (??) Hypercholesterolemia (?) Hyperlipidemia (?) Prior chemotherapy
Ataxia	5%	As previously

(*cont.*)

Syndrome	Frequency	Comment
Mental state change or impaired consciousness	5%	Direct neurotoxicity
Mania	Alone rare	Direct neurotoxicity
Subclinical neuropathy	Up to 11%	Mechanism uncertain
Deltoid muscle palsy	Uncommon	Direct peripheral neurotoxicity (?)
Headache	20%	Responds to propranolol

Calcineurin-related neurotoxicity: rare and more serious syndromes

Syndrome	Frequency	Comment
Para- or tetraparesis	Uncommon	Dose-related hypomagnesemia (?), hypocholesterolemia (?), demyelination, prostaglandin-mediated vascular leakage
Leukoencephalopathy cerebellar syndrome	5%	As previously, partially dose related
Akinetic mutism, extrapyramidal syndrome + pseudobulbar palsy	Unusual	Dose-related, potentially reversible
Posterior reversible encephalopathy syndrome	0.5%–2%	Dose-related, reversible changes in brain with typical clinical (visual hallucinations, cortical blindness, seizures) and radiological characteristics

GVHD-related neurological and neuromuscular complications

Peripheral Nervous System

Disorder	Frequency	Specific features	Common differential diagnoses	Time after allo-HSCT	Diagnostics	Therapy
Myositis	2%–3%	Mostly polymyositis, rarely with myocarditis or dermatomyositis; frequently elevated serum creatine kinase (5- to 50-fold, correlates reliably with clinical course), spontaneous activity + myopathic pattern in electromyography	Metabolic, endocrine, drug-induced myopathies (e.g., steroid: serum creatine kinase often normal, in electromyography no spontaneous activity), fasciitis, perimyositis	3–9 months	Serum creatine kinase, electromyography, rarely muscle biopsy	Like GVHD
Immune neuro-pathies acute	1%–2%	*Acute*: like Guillain Barré syndrome: rapidly progressive symmetric ascending motor weakness and numbness, areflexia, in 25% ventilation, autonomic involvement common, cranial nerve palsy possible, peaks in 2–4 weeks, frequently associated with infections (CMV and other) *Chronic inflammatory demyelinating polyneuropathy (CIDP)*: progressive or relapsing, proximal and distal motor weakness, minor sensory deficits, areflexia, occasionally respiratory insufficiency or autonomic involvement CIDP may be triggered by Hodgkin lymphoma and other	Other non-immune-mediated neuropathies (diabetic, toxic/drug-induced, e.g., cyclosporin, tacrolimus, thalidomide, improving or not progressive after cessation of the drug), recurrence of hematologic malignancy in spinal meninges, nerve sheaths, or nerve plexus	≤3 months, rarely later	Nerve conduction, CSF (typically normal cell count, elevated protein content), biopsy of sural nerve only if vasculitis or amyloidosis suspected	Intravenous gammaglobulins, plasma exchange in CIDP, moreover: immunosuppressive therapy (steroids, cyclosporin, mycophenolate mofetil, methotrexate, cyclophosphamide pulse)

(cont.)

Disorder	Frequency	Specific features	Common differential diagnoses	Time after allo-HSCT	Diagnostics	Therapy
		malignancies; may develop 2–10 weeks after initiation of tacrolimus				
Myasthenia gravis	<1%	Fatigable motor weakness: facial weakness (including ptosis, diplopia), dysarthria, dysphagia, dyspnea, limb or axial weakness Antibody mediated autoimmune disease of neuromuscular junction, usually associated with other manifestations of chronic GVHD (associated manifestation) Symptoms start often after reduction or discontinuation of immunosuppressive drugs	Lambert–Eaton myasthenic syndrome, in children congenital myasthenic syndromes	22–60 months	Antibodies against skeletal muscle acetylcholine receptor (up to 40% of HSCT patients positive without symptoms), repetitive (2–5 Hz) nerve stimulation → progresssive decrease of muscle action potential	Oral cholinesterase inhibitor, steroids, immunosuppressives In crisis: intravenous gammaglobulins, plasma exchange

Neurological manifestations of chronic GVHD can affect any part of the PNS or CNS and muscles. They usually occur several months to years after allo-HSCT, affect 23% of allogeneic transplanted patients after one year, and are important prognostic factors for life quality and survival. According to the 2005 NIH consensus criteria for chronic GVHD (Filipovich et al., 2005), the only "distinctive" neurological manifestations of GVHD are myositis and polymyositis; peripheral neuropathies and myasthenic syndromes are considered as "associated features" of chronic GVHD. Muscle cramps, painful contraction of single muscle or muscle groups, seem to be associated with moderate-to-severe chronic GVHD.

CNS manifestation in GVHD-like cerebral vasculitis, demyelinization, and encephalitis-like disease is rare. It has to be distinguished from other CNS diseases like therapy toxicity, infections (especially viral and fungal, other vascular diseases, and other demyelinating diseases like multiple sclerosis (for details, see Grauer et al., 2010; Pulsipher et al., 2008).

Diagnostic workup in patients with suspected chronic GVHD of the nervous system

PNS manifestation
Serum creatine kinase, serum anti-acetylcholine receptor antibodies
Needle electromyography of affected muscles
Neurography of sural, tibial, and other affected nerves (distal motor latency, action potentials, nerve conduction velocity, F-waves)
Repetitive nerve stimulation in myasthenic syndromes
CSF analysis if immune neuropathy or other diseases suspected
Nerve and/or muscle biopsy if indicated
CNS manifestation
Brain MRI with gadolinium
Computed tomography or magnetic resonance angiography
CSF analysis including microbiological and virological testing (PCR more reliable)
Neuropsychological testing if deficits suspected
Evoked potentials and transcranial magnetic stimulation if indicated
Brain biopsy if indicated

Long-term follow-up recommendations from the NCI/NHLBI/PBMTC First International Conference on Late Effects after Pediatric Hematopoietic Cell Transplantation 2012 (Majhail et al., 2012):

- Clinical evaluation for symptoms and signs of neurological dysfunction at one year and yearly thereafter
- Specific functional testing in symptomatic patients should be done together with neurology specialist
- In pediatric patients, annual evaluation for cognitive development

Perianal complications

Prevention of perianal infection

- Avoid rectal examination, suppositories, and enemas, especially when neutropenic
- Avoid constipation, especially when neutropenic
- Keep anal area clean and dry (if there is diarrhea, use soft disposable material, not toilet paper)
- Minimize diarrhea
- Examine stool culture weekly

Conservative treatment for perianal sepsis

- Give appropriate systemic antibiotics, with Gram-negative and anerobe coverage
- Give hemopoietic growth factor (G-CSF, GM-CSF) to accelerate neutrophil recovery
- Employ fastidious local care of lesion (clean, dry)
- Use stool softeners
- Provide analgesia

Psychosocial complications

The eight emotional barriers of BMT/SCT

- Decision to accept treatment (dilemma)
- Preparation for treatment (meditation)
- Chemotherapy/chemoradiotherapy and isolation facilities (physical and emotional discomfort)
- Transplant (anxiety)
- BM rejection/engraftment (increased anxiety)
- GVHD (anxiety, discomfort, and infection)
- Preparation for discharge ("cutting the umbilical cord")
- Adaptation outside hospital (lack of energy, anxiety)

Other factors that can cause stress during BMT/SCT

- Giving up control during hospitalization
- Fatigue
- Anger
- Insomnia
- Death of another patient
- Separation from family and local environment (distant transplant center)

Psychosocial problems after BMT/SCT

- Discomfort from treatment (e.g., oral mucositis, hemorrhagic cystitis)
- Lowered self-esteem and poor body image
- Changes in social habits
- Changes in academic and school performance
- Financial hardship/loss of job
- Difficulties with relationships, low social support

Measures to minimize psychosocial stress posttransplant

- The medical and nursing staff must be alert to the causes of patients' anxieties, and must convey appropriate expressions of understanding and sympathy.
- Conduct detailed information sessions with patient, donor, and family before BMT regarding the transplant procedure, the risks, and the anticipated benefits and outcome.
- Provide early psychological or psychiatric consultation if counseling by the ward staff is insufficient to ameliorate problems.
- Conduct a detailed information session before discharge.
- Clinical assessment during recovery phase, then at 6 months, at 12 months, and then yearly

(For further details, see Parsons et al., 2012.)

Pulmonary complications

Pulmonary complications following allo-HSCT have an incidence of 25%–50% and are associated with significant morbidity and mortality.

Two groups: non-infectious complications and infectious complications (for infectious complications, see page 337).

Non-infectious complications are classically grouped into early- (<day 100) and late-onset complications (>day 100).

Recently, a classification was performed according to site of presumed primary tissue injury (ATS research statement, Panoskaltsis-Mortari et al., 2011, see later).

Categorization of the clinical spectrum of lung injury following HSCT

Clinical spectrum of disease as categorized by presumed site of primary tissue injury

Pulmonary parenchyma	Vascular endothelium	Airway epithelium
Acute interstitial pneumonitis (AIP)*	Peri-engraftment respiratory distress syndrome (PERDS)*	Cryptogenic organizing pneumonia (COP)/ Bronchiolitis obliterans organizing pneumonia (BOOP)*
Acute respiratory distress syndrome (ARDS)*	Noncardiogenic capillary leak syndrome (CLS)*	Bronchiolitis obliterans syndrome (BOS)*
BCNU pneumonitis	Diffuse alveolar hemorrhage (DAH)*	
Radiation pneumonitis	Pulmonary veno-occlusive disease (PVOD)	
Delayed pulmonary toxicity syndrome (DPTS)*	Transfusion-related acute lung injury (TRALI)	
Posttransplant lymphoproliferative disease (PTLD)	Pulmonary cytolytic thrombi (PCT)	

(*cont.*)

Pulmonary parenchyma	Vascular endothelium	Airway epithelium
Eosinophilic pneumonia (EP)	Pulmonary arterial hypertension (PAH)	
Pulmonary alveolar proteinosis (PAP)	Pulmonary thromboembolus (PTE)	

*conditions routinely included under the classification of idiopathic pneumonia syndrome (IPS).

Incidence and mortality of pulmonary complications of the early posttransplant period

	Incidence	Mortality
BM emboli (at day of transplant)	?	0
Pulmonary edema (capillary leakage, fluid overload)	10%–40%	Low
Pneumonia: bacterial/ARDS,	Common	High
fungal (e.g., Aspergilloma),	Rare	High
viral (e.g., HSV, CMV, adenovirus)	Rare	High
Idiopathic pneumonia syndrome, IPS	5%–15%	50%–75%
Diffuse alveolar hemorrhage, DAH	5%–10%	50%–75%
Sinusoidal obstruction syndrome, SOS (VOD), of the lung	Rare	?
Periengraftment respiratory distress syndrome, PERDS	5%–10%	Low
Radiation pneumonitis	Rare	?
Thromboembolism	Rare	?
Pneumothorax (iatrogenic)	Rare	Low

Idiopathic pneumonia syndrome (IPS)

- Definition
  - Evidence of widespread alveolar injury
  - Absence of lower respiratory tract infection
  - Absence of cardiac dysfunction, renal failure, fluid overload

- Clinical symptoms
  - Rapidly evolving dyspnea/respiratory distress
  - +/− Fever
  - +/− Dry cough

- Risk factors:
  - Acute GVHD

- HLA disparity
- Age of recipient
- Conditioning intensity (TBI/myeloablative >>non-myeloablative [2%])

- Diagnosis
  - Chest X-ray/CT: multilobar infiltrates
  - Newly developed restrictive pulmonary function testing pattern or increased alveolar–arterial PO_2 difference
  - Echo for exclusion cardiac dysfunction/fluid overload
  - BAL to exclude infection
  - Rapid clinical deterioration is suggestive

- Pathophysiology
  - Toxic effects of conditioning (TBI, busulfan)
  - Immunologically mediated
  - Danger signals (LPS/LBP)
  - Inflammatory cytokines (TNF, Th17, IL-1b)
  - Cellular effectors (T-cells, neutrophils)
  - Surfactant protein A and/or D deficiency

- Treatment
  - Steroids (starting dose: prednisolone 2 mg/kg BW × 7 days)
  - TNF neutralization (Etanercept 0.4 mg/kg/day, SQ, twice weekly × 8 doses)

    - Yanik et al., 2008:
      - 15 patients, 8/15 requiring mechanical ventilation at therapy onset
      - 0.4 mg/kg (max 25 mg) twice weekly, maximum 8 doses
      - 10/15 CR (defined as ability to discontinue supplement O_2 during study therapy
      - Median time to response 7 days (3–18 days)
      - Day +28 survival 73%
    - Noninvasive/invasive ventilation

Periengraftment–respiratory distress syndrome (PERDS)

(Now included under the classification of IPS; distinct clinical phenotype with very good prognosis)
- Within 5 days of neutrophil engraftment
- Clinical symptoms
  - Progressive dyspnea, cough, hypoxemia, ± fever
  - Weight gain, edema

- Can develop both after auto- and allo-HSCT
- Radiographic: bilateral interstitial infiltrates
- Pathology: endothelial injury >pulmonary edema
- Risk factors: G-CSF, high number of CD34+ cells, rate of neutrophil recovery

- Treatment: high-dose steroids (1–2 mg/kg body weight daily), good response
- Mortality <20%

Diffuse alveolar hemorrhage (DAH)

(Now included under the classification of IPS; distinct clinical phenotype once hemorrhagic)

- Clinical symptoms
    - Progressive dyspnea, cough, hypoxemia, ± fever
    - Frank hemoptysis is rare

- Radiographic: diffuse airspace disease (develops prior to manifest DAH)
- Key finding for Dx: progressively bloodier BAL fluid, >20% hemosiderin-laden macrophages
- Pathology: diffuse alveolar damage, hemorrhagic alveolitis
- Risk factors: GVHD, conditioning intensity, rapidly rising high neutrophil counts, renal insufficiency, TBI, patient age, occult infection
- Treatment: HD steroids (1–2 mg/kg body weight), activated Factor VII (Novo 7), aminocaproic acid
- Mortality
    - Overall: 75%–80%
        - MOF, sepsis 60%–80%
        - Respiratory failure 15%

Incidence and mortality of late pulmonary complications

	Incidence	Mortality
• Pulmonary GVHD:		
(obstructive) bronchiolitis obliterans, BO	5%–15%	50%–70%
(restrictive) cryptogenic organizing pneumonia		
(COP)/BO organizing pneumonia (BOOP)	5%–10%	30%–50%
• Other obstructive lung disease (e.g., COPD, smoking)	Common	Low
• Other restrictive lung disease		
(e.g., pulmonary fibrosis due to TBI, busulfan)	Rare	High
• Late infectious pulmonary complications		
Upper respiratory tract infection, bronchitis	Common	Low
Pneumonia (bacterial, fungal, PcP)	Rare	High

- Late-onset non-infectious pulmonary complications significantly contribute to late mortality after allo-HSCT. In patients surviving longer than two years, a 15.1-fold increased risk of late mortality due to pulmonary dysfunction compared to the general population has been reported.
- Late-onset non-infectious pulmonary complications can present as

  - Restrictive lung function impairment

    - Restrictive pulmonary function (PFT) pattern
    - Late interstitial pneumonitis (IP)
    - Cryptogenic organizing pneumonia (COP), also called bronchiolitis obliterans organizing pneumonia [BOOP])

  - Airway obstruction

    - Obstructive PFT pattern
    - Obliterative bronchiolitis (BO) or bronchiolitis obliterans syndrome (BOS)
    - Combination of both

- BO/BOS is the only pulmonary complication that is currently considered diagnostic of chronic GVHD
- COP/BOOP can be seen both with acute and chronic GVHD

Symptoms of pulmonary chronic GVHD/BO/BOS
- Early

  - Asymptomatic or nonspecific symptoms (mild dyspnea on exertion, dry/nonproductive cough; often delayed recognition)

- On disease progression

  - Significant dyspnea from exertion, exercise intolerance; fever (infection!), dyspnea and productive versus nonproductive cough can be found in any combination or not at all

- End-stage disease

  - O$_2$ dependency, immobility, death due to isolated/combined pulmonary failure and pulmonary infection

Risk factors for pulmonary chronic GVHD/BO/BOS
- Donor type (unrelated versus sibling)
- HLA match/mismatch
- Use of TBI or busulfan
- History of DLI
- Female donor–male recipient
- Patient age
- CMV seropositivity of donor and recipient
- History of smoking (?)

- Allergies (?)
- Lung disease or thoracic irradiation pre-HSCT
- History of acute lung injury following allogeneic HSCT
- History of cGVHD at any other site
- Low serum immunoglobulin levels

Diagnostic workup

- Pulmonary function testing
  - Spirometry, whole-body plethysmography, and single breath CO method
  - Baseline PFT within the last two weeks before starting conditioning therapy
  - Follow-up every three months for the first year, every six months for the second year, and then yearly
  - Restrictive lung function changes
    - Vital capacity (VC) or TLC <80% or FVC less than 80% of predicted value in combination with forced expiratory volume in the first second of expiration (FEV1)/FVC ≥0.7
    - Measured effective resistance (R_{eff}) used in children to identify mild (30%–60% of predicted normal), intermediate (60%–100%), or severe (>100%) restrictive lung impairment
  - Obstructive lung function changes
    - Decrease in FEV1 >5%/year along with FEV1/FVC <0.8 has been reported as indicator for developing air flow obstruction following allo-HSCT
    - FEV1 <75% of predicted normal plus FEV1/FVC <0.7 strongly suggestive for obliterative bronchiolitis

Lung function score (LFS)

FEV1 (%)	Points	TLCO (%)	Points
>80	1	>80	1
70–79	2	70–79	2
60–69	3	60–69	3
50–59	4	50–59	4
40–49	5	40–49	5
<40	6	<40	6
LFS score = summary score FEV1 + TLCO			
LFS I, </=2	LFS II, 3–5	LFS III, 6–9	LFS IV, 10–12

- Imaging studies
  - Chest X-ray

- Inspiratory and expiratory HRCT
- If clinical symptoms of sinus infection and suspected sinubronchial syndrome, a CT of the sinuses

- BAL
  - Exclusion of causative infections, including bacterial cultures, fungal cultures, pneumococci, *Haemophilus influenzae* B, *Chlamydia pneumoniae*, *Mycoplasma pneumoniae*, *Toxoplasma gondii*, *Bordetella pertussis*, *Mycobacterium tuberculosis*, and mycobacteria other than tuberculosis (MOTT), *Pneumocystis jirovecii*, adenovirus, CMV, HHV6, HSV1/2, human metapneumovirus, influenza A/B, parainfluenza 1–3, coronavirus, rhinovirus, respiratory syncytial virus, and *Aspergillus* sp.

- Transbronchial biopsy and open lung biopsy
  - Transbronchial: low sensitivity, poor predictive value of obliterative bronchiolitis; rather helpful in diffuse lung pathology such as interstitial pneumonitis
  - Open lung biopsy: gold standard for the diagnosis of BO or COP/BOOP; overall morbidity of 43% by day +30 post-procedure

NIH consensus project on cGVHD definition of BO/BOS

1. FEV1 <75% of predicted normal and FEV1/FVC <0.7
2. Either signs of air trapping by PFT (RV>120% of predicted normal) or signs of air trapping, small airway thickening, or bronchiectasis by in- and expiratory HRCT or pathological confirmation of constrictive bronchiolitis
3. Absence of active respiratory tract infection
4. In case of lacking histological proof of BO, at least one other distinctive manifestation of cGVHD in a separate organ system in addition to the diagnosis of BOS by pulmonary function and lung imaging studies is required

Treatment

- If possible, treatment should be done within clinical trials
- Suggested treatment algorithm outside of clinical trials (following figure):

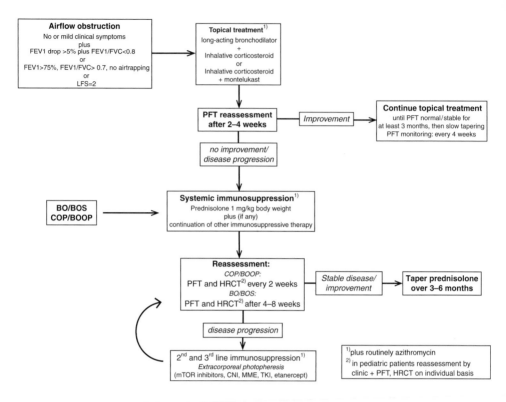

(Reproduced with permission from Hildebrandt et al., 2011.)

For references about pulmonary complications of BMT/SCT see Afessa et al., 2012; Bhatia et al., 2007; Couriel et al., 2006; Filipovitch et al., 2005; Fukuda et al., 2003; Hildebrandt et al., 2011; Pavletic et al., 2006; Sakaguchi et al., 2011; Schlatzer et al., 2012; Tizon et al., 2012.

Renal complications

Renal complications after allo-HSCT

1. Acute kidney injury (AKI)

   - more frequent with myeloablative conditioning than with RIC

     - Renal hypoperfusion due to septic complications
     - Nephrotoxicity
   - Chemotherapy (e.g., cyclophosphamide → nephroprotection by CyP450 2C9 inhibitor fluconazole)
   - Immunosuppression (e.g., methotrexate, calcineurin inhibitors)
   - Antibacterial antibiotics (e.g., aminoglycosides, vancomycin)
   - Antifungals (e.g., amphotericin B)
   - Antivirals (e.g., acyclovir, ganciclovir, foscarnet, cidofovir)

     - Postrenal: urinary tract obstruction
     - Preexisting renal disease, hypertension, or diabetes
     - Hepatic sinusoidal obstruction syndrome, SOS (formerly VOD)

- Transplantation-associated microangiopathy, TAM (CNI; Th.: plasma exchange)
- Tumor lysis syndrome
- Hemoglobinuric kidney failure due to ABO incompatibility (very rare)
- Radiation-induced nephritis (very rare: protective kidney shielding during TBI)

2. Chronic kidney disease (CKD)

- major risk factor: acute kidney injury; incidence 20%, <1% require dialysis
  → life-long surveillance for hypertension, diabetes, renovascular disease

3. Renal GvHD

- contrasting opinions if renal GVHD exists

  - Yes

    - Rare late proteinuria syndromes (membranous glomerulopathies, minimal change, focal segmental glomerulosclerosis, amyloidosis)
    - Association with GvHD or with reduction of immunosuppression
    - Higher incidence after PB SCT compared to BMT
    - Animal models; anti-nuclear antibodies; donor T-cell infiltration (case report)

  - No

    - Proteinuria syndromes also found after autologous transplantation
    - Heterogeneity of posttransplant renal pathologies, due to other causes
    - Nonimmunological conditions: endothelial injury, tubular/interstitial necrosis, relapse-associated paraneoplastic syndromes, podocyte pathology resulting from high-dose chemotherapy
    - Nonspecific improvement of most nephrotic syndromes with steroids or immunosuppressive therapy

Long-term follow-up recommendations from the NCI/NHLBI/PBMTC First International Conference on Late Effects after Pediatric Hematopoietic Cell Transplantation 2012 (Majhail et al., 2012):

- Regular blood pressure monitoring and early therapeutic medical intervention
- Renal function assessment (BUN, creatinine, urine protein) at six months and one year, and at least yearly thereafter

References and further reading

Afessa B, Abdulai RM, Kremers WK, et al. 2012. Risk factors and outcome of pulmonary complications after autologous hematopoietic stem cell transplant. *Chest* **141**: 442–450.

Armenian SH, Sun CL, Francisco L, et al. 2008. Late congestive heart failure after hematopoietic cell transplantation. *J Clin Oncol* **26**: 5537–5543.

Armenian SH, Sun CL, Shannon T, et al. 2011. Incidence and predictors of congestive heart failure after autologous hematopoietic cell transplantation. *Blood* **118**: 6023–6029.

Bai JP, Lesko LJ, & Burckart GJ. 2010. Understanding the genetic basis for adverse drug effects: the calcineurin inhibitors. *Pharmacotherapy* **30**: 195–209.

Batts ED & Lazarus HM. 2007. Diagnosis and treatment of transplantation-associated thrombotic microangiopathy: real progress or are we still waiting? *Bone Marrow Transplant* **40**: 709–719.

Bearman SI, Anderson GL, Mori M, et al. 1993. Venoocclusive disease of the liver: development of a model for predicting fatal outcome after marrow transplantation. *J Clin Oncol* **11**: 1729–1736.

Bhatia S, Francisco L, Carter A, et al. 2007. Late mortality after allogeneic hematopoietic cell transplantation and functional status of long-term survivors: report from the Bone Marrow Transplant Survivor Study. *Blood* **110**: 3784–3792.

Brennan BM & Shalet SM. 2002. Endocrine late effects after bone marrow transplant. *Br J Haematol* **118**: 58–66.

Carreras E, Díaz-Beyá M, Rosiñol L, et al. 2011. The incidence of veno-occlusive disease following allogeneic hematopoietic stem cell transplantation has diminished and the outcome improved over the last decade. *Biol Blood Marrow Transplant* **17**: 1713–1720.

Choi CM, Schmaier AH, Snell MR, et al. 2009. Thrombotic microangiopathy in haematopoietic stem cell transplantation: diagnosis and treatment. *Drugs* **69**: 183–198.

Consortium: National Cancer Institute, National Heart, Lung and Blood Institute/Pediatric Blood and Marrow Transplantation Consortium First International Consensus Conference on late effects after pediatric hematopoietic cell transplantation: the need for pediatric-specific long-term follow-up guidelines. 2012. *Biol Blood Marrow Transplant* **18**: 334–347.

Corbacioglu S, Cesaro S, Faraci M, et al. 2012. Defibrotide for prophylaxis of hepatic veno-occlusive disease in paediatric haemopoietic stem-cell transplantation: an open-label, phase 3, randomised controlled trial. *Lancet* **379**: 1301–1309.

Couriel D, Carpenter PA, Cutler C, et al. 2006. Ancillary therapy and supportive care of chronic graft-versus-host disease: National Institutes of Health consensus development project on criteria for clinical trials in chronic graft-versus-host disease: V. Ancillary therapy and supportive care working group report. *Biol Blood Marrow Transplant* **12**: 375–396.

de Padua Silva L, Patah PA, Saliba RM, et al. 2010. Hemorrhagic cystitis after allogeneic hematopoietic stem cell transplants is the complex result of BK virus infection, preparative regimen intensity and donor type. *Haematologica* **95**: 1183–1190.

De Pasquale MD, Mastronuzzi A, De Vito R, et al. 2012. Unmanipulated donor lymphocytes for EBV-related PTLD after T-cell depleted HLA-haploidentical transplantation. *Pediatrics* **129**: e189–194.

Dropulic LK & Jones RJ. 2008. Polyomavirus BK infection in blood and marrow transplant recipients. *Bone Marrow Transplant* **41**: 11–18.

Filipovich AH, Weisdorf D, Pavletic S, et al. 2005. National Institutes of Health consensus development project on criteria for clinical trials in chronic graft-versus-host disease: I. Diagnosis and staging working group report. *Biol Blood Marrow Transplant* **11**: 945–956.

Fukuda T, Hackman RC, Guthrie KA, et al. 2003. Risks and outcomes of idiopathic pneumonia syndrome after nonmyeloablative and conventional conditioning regimens for allogeneic hematopoietic stem cell transplantation. *Blood* **102**: 2777–2785.

Grauer O, Wolff D, Bertz H, et al. 2010. Neurological manifestations of chronic graft-versus-host disease after allogeneic haematopoietic stem cell transplantation: report from the Consensus Conference on clinical practice in chronic graft-versus-host disease. *Brain* **133**: 2852–2865.

Guglin M, Aljayeh M, Saleemuddin S, et al. 2009. Introducing a new entity: chemotherapy-induced arrhythmia. *Europace* **11**: 1579–1586.

Haines HL, Laskin BL, Goebel J, et al. 2011. Blood, and not urine, BK viral load predicts renal outcome in children with hemorrhagic cystitis following hematopoietic stem cell transplantation. *Biol Blood Marrow Transplant* **17**: 1512–1519.

Hammond C, Abrams JR, & Syrjala KL. 2007. Fertility and risk factors elevated infertility concern in 10-year hematopoietic cell transplant survivors and case-matched controls. *J Clin Oncol* **25**: 3511–3517.

Hassan Z. 2011. Management of refractory hemorrhagic cystitis following hematopoietic stem cell transplantation in children. *Pediatr Transplant* **15**: 348–361.

Heslop HE. 2009. How I treat EBV lymphoproliferation. *Blood* **114**: 4002–4008.

Hildebrandt GC, Fazekas T, Lawitschka A, et al. 2011. Diagnosis and treatment of pulmonary chronic GVHD: report from the consensus conference on clinical practice in chronic GVHD. *Bone Marrow Transplant* **46**: 1283–1295.

Ho VT, Cutler C, Carter S, et al. 2005. Blood and marrow transplant clinical trials network toxicity committee consensus summary. *Biol Blood Marrow Transplant* **11**: 571–575.

Hoorn EJ, Walsh SB, McCormick JA, et al. 2011. The calcineurin inhibitor tacrolimus activates the renal sodium chloride cotransporter to cause hypertension. *Nat Med* **17**: 1304–1309.

Kida A & McDonald GB. 2012. Gastrointestinal, hepatobiliary, pancreatic, and iron-related diseases in long-term survivors of allogeneic hematopoietic stem cell transplantation. *Semin Hematol* **49**: 43–58.

Klein IH, Abrahams AC, van Ede T, et al. 2010. Differential effects of acute and sustained cyclosporine and tacrolimus on sympathetic nerve activity. *J Hypertens* **28**: 1928–1934.

Kojouri K & George JN. 2007. Thrombotic microangiopathy following allogeneic hematopoietic stem cell transplantation. *Curr Opin Oncol* **19**: 148–154.

Lakshminarayanan S, Sahdev I, Goyal M, et al. 2010. Low incidence of hepatic veno-occlusive disease in pediatric patients undergoing hematopoietic stem cell transplantation attributed to a combination of intravenous heparin, oral glutamine, and ursodiol at a single transplant institution. *Pediatr Transplant* **14**: 618–621.

Laskin BL, Goebel J, Davies SM, et al. 2011. Small vessels, big trouble in the kidneys and beyond: hematopoietic stem cell transplantation-associated thrombotic microangiopathy. *Blood* **118**: 1452–1462.

Lee SJ, Schover LR, Partridge AH, et al. 2006. American Society of Clinical Oncology recommendations on fertility preservation in cancer patients. *J Clin Oncol* **24**: 2917–2931.

Leung AY, Yuen KY, & Kwong YL. 2005. Polyoma BK virus and haemorrhagic cystitis in haematopoietic stem cell transplantation: a changing paradigm. *Bone Marrow Transplant* **36**: 929–937.

Litzow MR, Tarima S, Pérez WS, et al. 2010. Allogeneic transplantation for therapy-related myelodysplastic syndrome and acute myeloid leukemia. *Blood* **115**: 1850–1857.

Liu J, Malhotra R, Voltarelli J, et al. 2008. Ovarian recovery after stem cell transplantation. *Bone Marrow Transplant* **41**: 275–278.

Majhail NS. 2011. Secondary cancers following allogeneic haematopoietic cell transplantation in adults. *Br J Haematol* **154**: 301–310.

Majhail NS, Lazarus HM, Burns LJ. 2010. Iron overload in hematopoietic cell transplantation. *Bone Marrow Transplant* **41**: 997–1003.

Majhail NS, Rizzo JD, Lee SJ, et al. 2012. Recommended screening and preventive practices for long term survivors after hematopoietic stem cell transplantation. *Biol Bone Marrow Transplant* **18**: 348–371.

Maradei SC, Maiolino A, de Azevedo AM, et al. 2009. Serum ferritin as risk factor for sinusoidal obstruction syndrome of the liver undergoing hematopoietic stem cell transplantation. *Blood* **114**: 1270–1275.

Mattson J, Ringdén O, & Storb R. 2008. Graft failure after hematopoietic cell transplantation. *Biol Blood Marrow Transplant* **14**: S165–S170.

Miller AN, Glode A, Hogan KR, et al. 2011. Efficacy and safety of ciprofloxacin for prophylaxis of polyomavirus BK virus-associated hemorrhagic cystitis in allogeneic hematopoietic stem cell transplantation recipients. *Biol Blood Marrow Transplant* **17**: 1176–1181.

Panoskaltsis-Mortari A, Griese M, Madtes DK, et al. 2011. An official American Thoracic Society research statement: noninfectious lung injury after hematopoietic stem cell transplantation: idiopathic pneumonia syndrome. *Am J Respir Crit Care Med* **183**: 1262–1279.

Parsons SK, Phipps S, Sung L, et al. 2012. NCI, NHLBI/PBMTC first international conference on late effects after pediatric hematopoietic cell transplantation: health-related quality of life, functional, and neurocognitive outcomes. *Biol Blood Marrow Transplant* **18**: 162–171.

Pavletic SZ, Martin P, Lee SJ, et al. 2006. Measuring therapeutic response in chronic graft-versus-host disease: National Institute of Health Consensus Development Project on criteria for clinical trials in chronic graft-versus-host disease: IV. Response criteria working group report. *Biol Blood Marrow Transpl* **12**: 252–266.

Pullarkat V. 2010. Iron overload in patients undergoing hematopoietic stem cell transplantation. *Adv Hematol* 2010; pii: 345756.

Pullarkat V, Blanchard S, Tegtmeier B, et al. 2008. Iron overload adversely affects outcome of allogeneic hematopoietic cell transplantation. *Bone Marrow Transplant* **42**: 799–805.

Pulsipher MA, Skinner R, McDonald GB, et al. 2008. Progressive declines in neurocognitive function among survivors of hematopoietic stem cell transplantation for pediatric hematologic malignancies. *J Pediatr Hematol Oncol* **30**: 411–418.

Pulsipher MA, Skinner R, McDonald GB, et al. 2012. National Cancer Institute, National Heart, Lung and Blood Institute/Pediatric Blood and Marrow Transplantation Consortium First International Consensus Conference on late effects after pediatric hematopoietic cell transplantation: the need for pediatric-specific long-term follow-up guidelines. *Biol Blood Marrow Transplant* **18**: 334–347.

Richardson PG, Soiffer RJ, Antin JH, et al. 2010. Defibrotide for the treatment of severe hepatic veno-occlusive disease and multiorgan failure after stem cell transplantation: a multicenter, randomized, dose-finding trial. *Biol Blood Marrow Transplant* **16**: 1005–1017.

Rizzo JD, Curtis RE, Socié G, et al. 2009. Solid cancers after allogeneic hematopoietic cell transplantation. *Blood* **113**: 1175–1183.

Ruutu T, Barosi G, Benjamin RJ, et al. 2007. Diagnostic criteria for hematopoietic stem cell transplant associated microangiopathy: results of a consensus process by an international working group. *Haematologica* **92**: 95–100.

Sakaguchi H, Takahashi Y, Watanabe N, et al. 2011. Incidence, clinical features, and risk factors of idiopathic pneumonia syndrome following hematopoietic stem cell transplantation in children. *Pediatr Blood Cancer* **58**: 780–784.

Sanders JE, Guthrie KA, Hoffmeister PA, et al. 2005. Final adult height of patients who received hematopoietic cell transplantation in childhood. *Blood* **105**: 1348–1354.

Savani BN, Griffith ML, Jagasia S, et al. 2011. How I treat late effects in adults after allogeneic stem cell transplantation. *Blood* **117**: 3002–3009.

Schlatzer DM, Dazard JE, Ewing RM, et al. 2012. Human biomarker discovery and predictive models for disease progression for idiopathic pneumonia syndrome following allogeneic stem cell transplantation. *Mol Cell Proteomics* [Epub ahead of print].

Siegal D, Keller A, Xu W, et al. 2007. Central nervous system complications after allogeneic stem cell transplantation: Incidence, manifestations, and clinical significance. *Biol Blood Marrow Transplant* **13**: 1369–1379.

Socié G, Baker KS, Bhatia S, et al. 2012. Subsequent malignant neoplasms after hematopoietic cell transplantation. *Biol Blood Marrow Transplant* **18**: S139–S150.

Stavrou E & Lazarus HM. 2010. Thrombotic microangiopathy in haematopoietic cell transplantation: an update. *Mediterr J Hematol Infect Dis* **2**: e2010033.

Tichelli A, Bucher C, Rovó A, et al. 2007. Premature cardiovascular disease after allogeneic hematopoietic stem-cell transplantation. *Blood* **110**: 3463–3471.

Tizon R, Frey N, Heitjan DF, et al. 2012. High-dose corticosteroids with or without etanercept for the treatment of idiopathic pneumonia syndrome after allo-SCT. *Bone Marrow Transplant* **47**: 1332–1337.

Tsuboi K, Kishi K, Ohmachi K, et al. 2003. Multivariate analysis of risk factors for hemorrhagic cystitis after hematopoietic stem cell transplantation. *Bone Marrow Transplant* **32**: 903–907.

Wei J, Xiao Y, Yu X, et al. 2010. Early onset of syndrome of inappropriate antidiuretic hormone secretion (SIADH) after allogeneic haematopoietic stem cell transplantation: case report and review of the literature. *J Int Med Res* **38**: 705–710.

Yanik GA, Ho VT, White ES, et al. 2008. The impact of soluble tumor necrosis factor receptor etanercept on the treatment of idiopathic pneumonia syndrome after allogeneic hematopoietic stem cell transplantation. *Blood* **112**: 3073–3081.

Chapter

27

The BMT/SCT pharmacopoeia

Jill M. Comeau, Reinhold Munker, and Kerry Atkinson

The BMT Data Book, Third Edition, ed. Reinhold Munker et al. Published by Cambridge University Press. © Cambridge University Press 2013.

The information in this chapter is not all encompassing, but contains the information most significant to the SCT population. Please refer to primary literature or package inserts for more detailed information.

Individual drugs and classes of drugs

Analgesics and adjuvant analgesics

Analgesics
Acetaminophen (APAP)
Indications
Mild-to-moderate pain or fever

Preparations (non-pediatric)

- Capsule, caplet, tablet: 325 mg, 500 mg, 650 mg
- Injection: 10 mg/mL (100 mL vial)
- Liquid: 500 mg/5 mL, 500 mg/15 mL
- Suppositories: 80 mg, 120 mg, 325 mg, 650 mg

Dosing

- 325–650 mg every 4–6 hours, or 1 g every 6–8 hours (maximum 4 g/24 hr)

Contraindications and adverse effects

- Contraindicated with severe hepatic or active liver disease (IV formulation)
- Hepatotoxicity
- Rash

Drug interactions

- Busulfan: APAP may deplete glutathione concentrations, which metabolizes busulfan, avoid APAP starting 72 hours before until after busulfan is cleared from the serum
- Dasatinib and imatinib: may worsen hepatotoxicity, consider alternative therapy
- Ethanol: increase risk of hepatotoxicity, limit to <3 drinks/day
  - One drink is equivalent to 12 ounces of beer, 5 ounces of wine, or 1.5 ounces of liquor

General prescribing information

APAP is an analgesic and antipyretic, but has no anti-inflammatory activity. It is well absorbed orally and rectally. Acetaminophen is metabolized in the liver, and its metabolites are excreted in urine. Its duration of action is about four hours. APAP does not cause gastric irritation and is the analgesic of choice for mild pain. Of note, APAP may mask fevers and lead to serious complications in patients who are neutropenic. Therefore, APAP use should be limited in this patient population.

In patients who are elderly or who have chronic liver disease, intake should be limited to maximum of 2 g/day. APAP is the most common cause of accidental overdose in the United States, as it is combined with other products both over-the-counter and by prescription. Patients should be counseled about this risk and to report all medications they are taking to their physician(s) and pharmacist(s).

Non-steroidal anti-inflammatory drugs (NSAIDS)

Because of the multiple adverse effects of NSAIDs, these medications are rarely used in the hematologic malignancy and SCT population. These include antiplatelet effects, nephrotoxicity, and GI toxicity. Owing to these side effects, they also interact with many drugs used for the treatment of malignancies or GVHD. NSAIDs also have antipyretic effects. Please refer to a drug information resource or package insert for more specific information.

Opioids

Indications

Mild-to-severe pain, also used for cough and medication-induced rigors

Preparations and dosing

- Most opioids have no ceiling dose and should be titrated based upon benefit. Patients who have been on opioids previously will develop tolerance and require much higher doses

Codeine

Preparations

- Tablet: 15 mg, 30 mg, and 60 mg
- Also available in combination products with APAP, guaifenesin (an expectorant), and many others

Dosing

- 15–30 mg every 3–4 hours as needed (maximum dose 1.5 mg/kg due to side effects)

Fentanyl

Preparations

- Buccal film: 200 mcg, 400 mcg, 600 mcg, 800 mcg, and 1200 mcg
- Buccal tablet: 100 mcg, 200 mcg, 400 mcg, 600 mcg, and 800 mcg
- Injection: 0.05 mg/mL solution (2 mL, 5 mL, 10 mL, 20 mL, and 50 mL vials)
- Intranasal solution: 100 mcg/spray and 400 mcg/spray
- Lozenge, oral: 200 mcg, 400 mcg, 600 mcg, 800 mcg, 1200 mcg, and 1600 mcg
- Patch: 12.5 mcg/hr, 25 mcg/hr, 50 mcg/hr, 75 mcg/hr, and 100 mcg/hr
- Tablet, sublingual: 100 mcg, 200 mcg, 300 mcg, 400 mcg, 600 mcg, and 800 mcg

Dosing

- Please refer to package insert for specific dosing recommendations for each formulation
- Severe pain, injection: 50–100 mcg every 1–2 hours as needed
- PCA (patient-controlled analgesia)
  - Demand dose: 20 mcg (range: 10–50 mcg)
  - Lockout interval: 5–8 minutes
  - Basal rate: up to 50 mcg/hr

Hydrocodone

Preparations

Numerous, but only available as a combination product with APAP or ibuprofen
Dosing: 5–10 mg every 3–4 hours as needed (maximum with APAP is 4 g/24 hr)

Hydromorphone

Preparations

- Injection 1 mg/mL (1 mL vial), 2 mg/mL (1 mL and 20 mL vials), 4 mg/mL (1 mL vial), 10 mg/mL (1 mL, 5 mL, and 50 mL vials), and 250 mg powder vial
- Liquid: 1 mg/mL
- Suppository, rectal: 3 mg
- Tablet: 2 mg, 4 mg, and 8 mg
- Tablet, extended release: 8 mg, 12 mg, and 16 mg

Dosing

- IV, opioid-naïve: 0.2–0.6 mg every 2–3 hours as needed
- Oral, opioid-naïve: 2–4 mg every 3–4 hours as needed
- Oral, extended release (Exalgo®): once daily
- Continuous infusion, IV: 0.5–1 mg/hr
- PCA
    - Demand dose: 0.1 mg (range 0.05–0.4 mg)
    - Lockout interval: 5–10 minutes

Meperidine

Preparations

- Injection: 25 mg/mL (1 mL vial), 10 mg/mL (30 mL vial), 50 mg/mL (1 mL vial), 100 mg/mL (1 mL vial)
- Solution, oral: 50 mg/5 mL
- Tablet: 50 mg and 100 mg

Dosing

- 50–150 mg IV, SC, or IM every 3–4 hours as needed
    - Not recommended to be used for more than 24 hours or doses exceeding 600 mg/24 hr
    - Oral route is not recommended for the treatment of pain

Methadone

Preparations

- Injection: 10 mg/mL (20 mL vial)
- Solution, oral: 5 mg/5 mL, 10 mg/5 mL, 10 mg/mL
- Tablet: 5 mg, 10 mg, 40 mg (40 mg tablet only used for opioid addiction)

Dosing: be very cautious due to erratic kinetics and interpatient variability

- IV, opioid-naïve: 2.5 mg every 8–12 hours
- Oral, opioid-naïve: 2.5–10 mg every 8–12 hours

Morphine

Preparations

- Capsule, extended release: 10 mg, 20 mg, 30 mg, 45 mg, 50 mg, 60 mg, 75 mg, 80 mg, 90 mg, 100 mg, 120 mg, 200 mg
- Injection: 1 mg/mL (10 mL vial), 2 mg/mL (1 mL vial), 4 mg/mL (1 mL vial), 5 mg/mL (1 mL vial) 8 mg/mL (1 mL vial), 10 mg/mL (1 mL and 10 mL vials), 10 mg/0.7 mL (0.7 mL vial), 15 mg/mL (1 mL and 20 mL vials), 25 mg/mL (4 mL and 10 mL vials), and 50 mg/mL (20 mL and 50 mL vials)
- Solution: 10 mg/5 mL, 20 mg/5 mL, and 100 mg/5 mL

- Tablet: 15 mg and 30 mg
- Tablet, extended release: 15 mg, 30 mg, 60 mg, 100 mg, and 200 mg

Dosing

- IV, opioid-naïve: 2.5–5 mg every 3–4 hours as needed
- Oral, opioid-naïve: 15 mg every 4 hours as needed
- Long-acting products
    - Capsule, extended release (Avinza®): once daily
    - Capsule, sustained release (Kadian®): once or twice daily
    - Tablet, controlled release (MS Contin®): every 8–12 hours
- Continuous infusion: 0.8–10 mg/hour
- PCA
    - Usual on demand dose: 1 mg (range: 0.5–2.5 mg)
    - Lock-out interval: 5–10 minutes

Oxycodone

Preparations

- Capsule: 5 mg
- Liquid: 20 mg/mL
- Tablet: 5 mg, 10 mg, 15 mg, 20 mg, 30 mg
- Tablet, controlled release: 10 mg, 15 mg, 20 mg, 30 mg, 40 mg, 60 mg, 80 mg

Dosing

- Opioid-naïve: 5–15 mg every 4–6 hours as needed
- Controlled release: every 12 hours

Oxymorphone

Preparations

- Injection: 1 mg/mL (1 mL vial)
- Tablet: 5 mg, 10 mg
- Tablet, extended release: 5 mg, 10 mg, 15 mg, 20 mg, 30 mg, 40 mg

Dosing

- IV, opioid-naïve: 0.5 mg every 4–6 hours as needed
- Oral, opioid-naïve: 10–20 mg every 4–6 hours as needed
- Extended release: every 12 hours

Tramadol

Preparations

- Tablet: 50 mg
- Extended release: 100 mg, 200 mg, 300 mg
- Also available as combination with APAP immediate release and extended release formulations

Dosing

- 50–100 mg every 3–4 hours
- Extended release: 150–600 mg daily

Opioid conversion chart

Agent	IV Dose	PO Dose
Morphine	10 mg	30 mg
Codeine	–	200 mg
Fentanyl	50–100 mcg	NA
Hydrocodone	–	30 mg
Hydromorphone	1.5 mg	7.5 mg
Methadone	Please refer to following reference	
Oxycodone	–	20 mg
Oxymorphone	1 mg	15 mg

When rotating opiates, consider giving 50%–80% of total dose due to incomplete cross-tolerance.

For methadone dosing, see: Indelicato RA, Portenoy RK. 2002. Opioid rotation in the management of refractory cancer pain. *J Clin Oncol* **20**: 348–352.

Contraindications and adverse effects

- Cardiac: bradycardia, hypotension
- CNS: sedation, dependence
- GI tract: constipation, nausea, vomiting
- Pruritus (morphine)
- Respiratory depression
- Urinary or bladder incontinence

Drug interactions

Fentanyl is metabolized extensively by the CYP 3A4 system and therefore has many drug interactions. Please be cautious when coadministering with 3A4 inducers or inhibitors.

- Monitor use of other sedative medications
- Rifamycins: decrease concentrations of morphine, monitor for morphine efficacy
- Serotonergic medications (selective serotonin reuptake inhibitors, tricyclic antidepressants, and monoamine oxidase inhibitors): increase risk for serotonin syndrome with tramadol, consider alternative therapy

General prescribing information

All opioid analgesics have similar side effect profiles and warnings, but to different extents depending on the chemical properties of the particular opioid compound. Even with their extensive side effect profiles, the most important concept in the dosing of opioids is to increase the dose until pain relief is obtained. Just as patients develop tolerance of analgesia, patients also develop tolerance to side effects with the exception of constipation. All patients should receive constipation prophylaxis with a stool softener/laxative combination or osmotic laxative. Constipation is due to activity on the vagus nerve and mesenteric plexus. Opioids do not have antipyretic properties, and therefore are not contraindicated in neutropenic patients.

Codeine, hydrocodone, and tramadol are considered weak opioids. Codeine is not usually tolerated at doses that are needed to obtain adequate pain relief. Hydrocodone is available only as a combination product with APAP or ibuprofen, which limits its use and dose escalation. Tramadol is not a true opioid, but does have some agonistic effects on the mu receptor. Patients are not able to tolerate high doses due to nausea and vomiting from the serotonergic properties. Caution should be taken when administering with other serotonin active agents.

All other opioids listed are considered strong and there is no literature suggesting that one agent is more effective than another. Patient characteristics should be taken into consideration when choosing a pain regimen. Meperidine is no longer recommended for acute or chronic pain management due to the potential for seizure activity, euphoria, and low mu opioid receptor activity. Patients with renal dysfunction and the elderly are at greatest risk. Morphine is also renally cleared and should be used with great caution in the elderly and patients with impaired renal function. Fentanyl transdermal patches are contraindicated in patients who weigh <55 kg because they do not have adequate fat stores to absorb and store the medication.

Methadone prescribing should be limited to physicians and healthcare professionals with adequate experience. Methadone is highly lipid soluble and can accumulate in tissue over time. Additionally, patient pharmacokinetics varies widely. Some benefit has been seen in patients who are poorly controlled on other opioids, who cannot tolerate other opioids, or who have a neuropathic component of their pain.

Variations also exist in the onset and duration of action. This is not only in the difference in chemical structures but also the formulation of the products. Please refer to the following abbreviated table.

Agent and formulation	Onset of action	Duration of action
Fentanyl, IV	"almost immediate"	30–60 minutes
Fentanyl, transdermal patch	6 hours	12 hours after removal of patch
Hydromorphone, IV	5 minutes	4–5 hours
Hydromorphone, PO	15–30 minutes	4–5 hours
Morphine, IV	5–10 minutes	~4 hours
Morphine oral, immediate release	30 minutes	4 hours
Oxycodone, immediate release	10–15 minutes	3–6 hours
Oxycodone, extended release	Peak effect at 4–5 hours	≤12 hours

To reverse opioids, naloxone, an opioid antagonist, should be given at a dose of 2 mg IV, IM, or SC every 2–3 minutes as needed. Response should be seen prior to administration of 10 mg of naloxone. Naloxone has a 30–120-minute duration of action, therefore repeat doses or a continuous infusion may be needed with extended or sustained release opioids.

Adjuvant analgesics

Indications

These are agents with no analgesic properties but may increase the effectiveness of opioids.

Anticonvulsants

Gabapentin

Preparations

- Capsule: 100 mg, 300 mg, 400 mg
- Solution, oral: 250 mg/5 mL
- Tablet: 600 mg, 800 mg

Dosing

- 100–1200 mg orally three times daily

Pregabalin

Preparations

- capsules, 25 mg, 50 mg, 75 mg, 100 mg, 150 mg, 200 mg, 225 mg, 300 mg

Dosing

- 150–300 mg divided into 2–3 doses per day

Contraindications and adverse effects

- CNS: dizziness, somnolence, ataxia
- Edema, weight gain
- Neuromuscular: tremor

Drug interactions

Use caution with other CNS depressants

General prescribing information

Anticonvulsants have been utilized in the treatment of neuropathy for some time. Owing to the adverse effects and drug interactions of other agents, such as carbamazepine, gabapentin has fallen into favor. Pregabalin, a prodrug of gabapentin, is another anticonvulsant used to treat neuropathy. Because these medications are so structurally similar, many of the adverse effects and drug interactions are the same. The most common adverse effect is somnolence, therefore both drugs should start at low doses and be titrated to an effective dose. Both medications are renally cleared and must be adjusted for renal insufficiency.

Serotonin norepinephrine reuptake inhibitors (SNRIs)

Duloxetine

Preparations

- Capsules, 20 mg, 30 mg, and 60 mg

Dosing

- 60 mg orally once or twice daily

Venlafaxine

Preparations

- Capsule, extended release: 37.5 mg, 75 mg, 150 mg
- Tablet: 25 mg, 37.5 mg, 50 mg, 75 mg, 100 mg
- Tablet, extended release: 37.5 mg, 75 mg, 150 mg, 225 mg

Dosing

- 37.5–225 mg given once daily (extended release) or divided into 2–3 doses (immediate release)

Contraindications and adverse effects

- CNS: headache, somnolence, dizziness
- GI: nausea, dry mouth
- Genitourinary: sexual dysfunction
- Sweating
- Tachycardia with high doses
- Weakness

Drug interactions

Both medications are extensively metabolized through the CYP 450 system, so there are multiple drug interactions. The most important are listed as follows:

- Azoles: increase levels of venlafaxine, monitor for toxicity
- Ciprofloxacin: increase levels of SNRIs, consider alternative therapy
- Protease inhibitors: increase levels of SNRIs, consider alternative therapy
- Serotonergic agents: increase risk for serotonin syndrome, consider alternative therapy

General prescribing information

Duloxetine is FDA approved for many neuropathic diseases including diabetic neuropathy, fibromyalgia, and chronic musculoskeletal pain. Both medications are also effective in the treatment of depression. Other medications that have serotonergic properties, such as monoamine oxidase inhibitors, tricyclic antidepressants (TCAs), and selective serotonin reuptake inhibitors (SSRIs), should be avoided due to an increased risk of serotonin syndrome.

Tricyclic antidepressants

Amitriptyline

Preparations

- Tablets, 10 mg, 25 mg, 50 mg, 75 mg, 100 mg, 150 mg

Dosing

- 10–150 mg orally at bedtime

Contraindications and adverse effects

- Contraindications: MAOI used in past 14 days, during recovery from an acute myocardial infarction, or use of cisapride
- Cardiovascular: orthostatic hypotension, tachycardia, arrhythmias
- CNS: restlessness, sedation
- GI: constipation, xerostoma
- Urinary retention

Drug interactions

Amitriptyline has numerous drug interactions, due to adverse effects and extensive metabolism through the CYP 450 system in the liver

- α- or β-agonists: may cause increased tachycardia and vasopressor effects, consider alternative therapy
- Barbiturates: decrease TCA serum concentration, consider alternative therapy
- Metoclopramide: increases risk of extrapyramidal symptoms, neuroleptic malignant syndrome, or serotonin syndrome, consider alternative therapy
- Protease inhibitors: may increase TCA concentration, monitor
- QTc prolonging agents: may potentiate QTc prolongation, contraindicated with nilotinib, thioridazine, and ziprasidone
- Consider alternative therapy with 5HT3 inhibitors or tacrolimus
- Monitor with ciprofloxacin
- Serotonergic medications: avoid coadministration, may cause serotonin syndrome

General prescribing information

TCAs are one of the first classes to be used to treat neuropathic pain. The main concern with this class is the extensive adverse effects. This includes but is not limited to somnolence, orthostatic hypotension, and anticholinergic adverse effects (constipation, dry eyes, and urinary retention). Newer TCAs, such as nortriptyline, have lower incidence of anticholinergic and sedative properties. QTc prolongation and arrhythmias are also widely reported with TCAs. There are rare reports of BM suppression as well. Great caution should be taken when starting this class of medication and all patients should be monitored closely for adverse effects.

Antibiotics
Aminoglycosides
Indications

- Adjunct therapy in the treatment of serious infections with Gram-negative organisms, including *Proteus* sp. and *Pseudomonas* sp. They should never be used as monotherapy in severe, life-threatening infections. Amikacin may retain activity against some resistant strains.
- Steptomycin or gentamicin may be used as synergy for Gram-positive infections along with a penicillin or vancomycin

Preparations

- Amikacin: injection 250 mg/mL solution (2 mL and 4 mL vials)
- Gentamicin

- Infusion, premixed with NS: 60 mg (50 and 100 mL bags), 80 mg (50 mL and 100 mL bags), 120 mg (100 mL bag)
- Injection: 40 mg/mL solution (2 mL and 20 mL vials)
- Tobramycin
  - Infusion, premixed with NS: 80 mg (100 mL bag)
  - Injection: 1.2 g powder
  - Injection: 10 mg/mL solution (2 mL vial), 40 mg/mL solution (2 mL, 30 mL, 50 mL vials)

Dosing

- Weight
  - Ideal body weight (IBW) formulas
    - Male: 50 kg + [2.3 × (height in inches − 60)]
    - Female: 45.5 kg + [2.3 × (height in inches − 60)]
- IBW should be used for aminoglycoside dosing unless the patient's total body weight (TBW) >25% of their IBW, then adjusted body weight (ABW) is recommended
  - ABW = IBW + [0.4 × (TBW − IBW)]
- Gentamicin and tobramycin
  - Traditional dosing
    - Loading dose: pneumonia/life threatening 3 mg/kg, Gram-negative sepsis/serious 2.5 mg/kg
    - Maintenance dose: pneumonia: 2.5 mg/kg, Gram-negative sepsis/serious 2–2.25 mg/kg, UTI/synergy: 1 mg/kg
    - Frequency: varies based upon creatinine clearance (CrCl)
      - CrCl formula: $\frac{[(140-\text{age})\times\text{Weight}]}{72\times\text{serum creatinine}} \times (0.85$ in females only)
    - Use IBW unless obese, then use ABW
    - If patient is >60 years old AND serum creatinine is <1 mg/dL, serum creatinine should be rounded up to 1 mg/dL

CrCl (mL/min)	Frequency
≥60	Every 8 hours
40–60	Every 12 hours
20–40	Every 24 hours
<20	Loading dose, then monitor levels

- Extended interval dosing
- Dose: severe infection: 7 mg/kg, some institutions use 5 mg/kg
- Interval: every 24 hours unless CrCl <60 mL/min

CrCl (mL/min)	Frequency
40–59	Every 36 hours
20–39	Every 48 hours

- Dosing intervals are guided by levels after the initial dosing, please refer to *General prescribing information*
- Amikacin
  - Traditional dosing
  - Loading dose: 10 mg/kg
  - Maintenance dose: 5–7.5 mg/kg
  - Frequency: see previous table, same as gentamicin/tobramycin frequencies
  - Extended interval dosing
- 15 mg/kg once daily
- If CrCl <60 mL/min, refer to gentamicin/tobramycin extended interval frequencies

Contraindications and adverse effects
- Contraindication: myasthenia gravis
- Nephrotoxicity
- Neurotoxicity: gait instability
- Ototoxicity: irreversible auditory and vestibular

Drug interactions
Medications that increase the risk of nephrotoxicity
- Amphotericin B, monitor
- Cyclosporin, monitor
- Loop diuretics, monitor
- Vancomycin, monitor

Medications that increase the risk of ototoxocity
- Loop diuretics, monitor
- Platinum agents, monitor
- Bisphosphonates: aminoglycoside enhances hypocalcemia; monitor therapy
- Extended spectrum penicillins: may decrease aminoglycoside concentrations; consider alternative therapy or separating doses
- NSAIDs: may reduce excretion of aminoglycosides; monitor

General prescribing information
Aminoglycosides have a narrow therapeutic index and must be monitored for both efficacy and toxicity. With traditional dosing, levels should be drawn once a steady state is reached (in 3–5 half-lives). For aminoglycosides, this would be after the third dose unless a bolus dose is given, then peaks and troughs may be drawn within 24 hours of initiating therapy. Peaks should be drawn 30 minutes after a 30-minute infusion or 1 hour after a 1-hour infusion. Troughs should be drawn immediately before the next dose (typically prior to the fourth dose). Goal peaks and troughs are stated as follows.

Monitoring parameter	Indication	Gentamicin/ tobramycin (mg/L)	Amikacin (mg/L)
Peak	Pneumonia or life-threatening	8–12	25–30
Peak	Gram-negative sepsis or serious	6–8	20–25
Peak	UTI Synergy (gent only)	3–5	15–20 (not used for synergy)
Trough	All	<2	<8

Once the aminoglycoside is at its goal levels, peaks and troughs should be repeated at least once weekly. If the patient is not stable, monitoring should occur more frequently. These indications include hemodynamic instability and changes in renal function.

Extended interval dosing is preferred over traditional dosing, while a decrease in adverse effects have been shown, it is easier to administer, and there is an overall cost saving. Because aminoglycosides are concentration-dependent killers, higher doses are more important than the time above the minimum inhibitory concentration (MIC). Extended interval dosing should be used for all patients except those who are pregnant; have cystic fibrosis; are burn victims; have severe liver impairment, ascites, hearing loss, CrCl <20 mL/ min, unstable serum creatinine; are receiving dialysis, aged <18 or >70 years old; have a enterococcal or staphylococcal endocarditis, meningitis, or an uncomplicated UTI. Once the appropriate dose is given, a random level should be drawn between 6–14 hours after the start of the infusion. Once this level is obtained, refer to the appropriate nomogram for the need to adjust the interval. Gentamicin and tobramycin nomograms can be found in the following reference for 7 kg/mg dosing: Nicolau DP, Freeman CD, et al. 1995. Experiences with a once daily aminoglycoside program administered to 2,184 adult patients. *Antimicrob Agents Chem* **39**: 650. The 5 mg/kg dosing nomogram can be found in: Urban AW & Craig WA. 1997. Daily dosage of aminoglycosides. *Current Clinical Topics in Infectious Diseases*, Vol 17. Malden, MA: Blackwell Science. Amikacin levels can be divided by two and then that number applied to the gentamicin/tobramycin nomogram for the Nicolau nomogram.

Aminoglycosides have a small volume of distribution and penetrate extensively into fluids including any edema or ascites. They have poor penetration into the lungs, CNS, and abscesses. Aminoglycosides are excreted unchanged in the urine, and therefore this must be taken into account in patients with preexisting renal dysfunction. In patients receiving dialysis, around 50% of the drug will be dialyzed out of the serum. Therefore, dosing should be after dialysis or a supplemental dose after dialysis may be necessary. Aminoglycosides exert their nephrotoxicity by direct distal tubular damage after 5–7 days of therapy. Patients at risk for aminoglycoside-induced nephrotoxicity include older patients, those with baseline renal dysfunction, reduced renal perfusion, sepsis, receiving other nephrotoxic medications, and elevated troughs. Additionally, electrolyte abnormalities, specifically hypokalemia and hypomagnesia, usually occur due to the distal tubule destruction. Proper dosing, monitoring, and use of extended interval dosing have been shown to decrease the incidence of both nephrotoxicity and ototoxicity.

β-lactams

β-lactam/β-lactamase inhibitors

Amoxicillin/clavulanate

Indications

Amoxicillin/clavulanate is indicated in the treatment of upper and lower respiratory tract infections (RTIs), skin infections, and UTIs. Coverage includes Gram-positive organisms such as methicillin-sensitive *S. aureus* (MSSA), *Streptococcus* sp., and some Gram-negative bacteria including *H. influenza*. Piperacillin/tazobactam is indicated in more severe infections such as pneumonia and bacteremia including those caused by *Pseudomonas*. Piperacillin/tazobactam covers most Gram-positive organisms, except MRSA and VRE, Gram-negative organisms, and anaerobes.

Preparations

- Suspension: 125 mg/5 mL, 200 mg/5 mL, 250 mg/5 mL, 400 mg/5 mL, 600 mg/5 mL
- Tablets: 250 mg, 500 mg, 875 mg
- Tablets, chewable: 200 mg, 400 mg
- Tablets, extended release: 1000 mg

Dosing (by amoxicillin component)

- 875 mg every 12 hours for severe infections
- Alternative for less severe infections: 250–500 mg every 8 hours

Piperacillin/tazobactam

Preparations

- Infusion: 2.25 g (50 mL bag), 3.375 g (50 mL bag), 4.5 g (100 mL bag)
- Injection: 2.25 g, 3.375 g, 4.5 g, 40.5 g powder vials

Dosing

- 3.375–4.5 g every 6–8 hours (maximum 18 g/24 hr)
- Pneumonia, febrile neutropenia, or pseudomonal infection: 4.5 g every 6 hours
- Severe infections: 3.375 g every 6 hours

Contraindications and adverse effects

- Anaphylactic reaction
- CNS: headache, insomnia, fever, seizures (rare)
- Dermatologic: rash, pruritus
- GI: diarrhea, nausea, vomiting
- Hepatic: transaminase increase

Drug interactions

- Aminoglycosides: increase serum concentrations, consider alternative therapy
- Methotrexate: may decrease methotrexate clearance, monitor

- Mycophenolate: may decrease mycophenolic acid concentrations, monitor
- Tetracyclines: may decrease efficacy of penicillins, avoid concomitant use

General prescribing information

Amoxicillin/clavulanate is mostly utilized in the treatment of RTIs and is indicated for the outpatient treatment of febrile neutropenia along with ciprofloxacin. For the hematologic and SCT population, most patients do not meet the criteria to treat their febrile neutropenia on an outpatient basis. Piperacillin/tazobactam has broad-spectrum coverage that includes *Pseudomonas*. Two other medications exist in this category, ampicillin/sulbactam and ticarcillin/clavulanate. These antibiotics are not addressed in this chapter while ampicillin/sulbactam does not cover *Pseudomonas* and ticarcillin/clavulanate use has fallen out of favor due to the high amount of sodium in the product.

Both of these agents are known to cause false positivity in the galactomannan antigen assay. The galactomannan assay is a diagnostic test that detects the galactomannan antigen or part of the cell wall of *Aspergillus* sp. in the blood. This result can continue up to 5 days after discontinuing these antibiotics. Therefore, these products should be avoided if possible in patients who are at high risk for invasive aspergillosis. All β-lactam/β-lactamase inhibitor antibiotics must be renally adjusted.

CrCl (mL/min)	Amoxicillin/clavulanate dosing	Piperacillin/tazobactam dosing
20–40	–	3.375 g every 6 hours
<20	–	2.25 g every 6 hours
10–30	250–500 mg every 12 hours	-
<10	250–500 mg every 24 hours	-

Patients who have a history of anaphylactic reactions or an allergy to penicillins should avoid these antibiotics.

Carbapenems
Indications

Carbapenems have very broad coverage and can overcome β-lactamase-producing bacteria. The carbapenem spectrum includes Gram-positive organisms, anaerobes, and Gram-negative organisms including *Pseudomonas* and extended-spectrum β-lactamases (ESBLs). Carbapenems do not cover *Stenotrophomonas maltophila*, *Enterococcus faecium*, *Klebsiella pneumoniae* carbapenemases (KPCs), and MRSA. Of note, ertapenem, which will not be discussed in this chapter, does not cover *Pseudomonas* but covers ESBLs. Imipenem and meropenem are indicated as monotherapy for febrile neutropenia and in other serious infections resistant to penicillins and cephalosporins.

Imipenem/cilastatin
Preparations

- Injection 250 mg and 500 mg powder vials

Dosing

- 250–1000 mg every 6–8 hours (maximum 4 g/24 hr) infused over 20–60 minutes
- Febrile neutropenia or *Pseudomonas* infections: 500 mg every 6 hours

Meropenem

Preparations

- Injection 500 mg and 1 g powder vials

Dosing

- 500 mg–2 g every 8 hours infused over 15–30 minutes
- Febrile neutropenia: 1 g every 8 hours
- Meningitis: 2 g every 8 hours

Contraindications and adverse effects

- Allergic reactions, anaphylaxis
- CNS: headache, seizures
- GI tract: nausea and vomiting, diarrhea
- Phlebitis
- Rash

Drug interactions

- Cyclosporin: may enhance imipenem neurotoxicity and decrease concentration of cyclosporin, monitor
- Divalproex and valproic acid: may decrease concentration of valproic acid, consider avoiding carbapenem or if necessary give additional anti-seizure prophylaxis
- Ganciclovir and valganciclovir: may lower seizure threshold with imipenem, monitor therapy

General prescribing information

There are currently four carbapenems available in the United States. This includes doripenem, ertapenem, imipenem/cilastatin, and meropenem. Ertapenem does not cover *Pseudomonas* and doripenem has only been studied in the treatment of intra-abdominal infections and UTIs. Both of these carbapenems have not been extensively studied in the febrile neutropenia or SCT population. Carbapenems are considered time-dependent killers, therefore time above the MIC is most important.

All carbapenems are eliminated renally and therefore must be renally adjusted. For febrile neutropenia, imipenem is adjusted as follows: CrCl 41–70 mL/min 500 mg every 8 hours, CrCl 21–40 mL/min 250 mg every 6 hours, CrCl 6–20 mL/min 250 mg every 12 hours. Meropenem renal dose adjustments for febrile neutropenia are as follows: CrCl 26–50 mL/min 1 g every 12 hours, CrCl 10–25 mL/min 500 mg every 12 hours, CrCl <10 mL/min 500 mg every 24 hours.

Carbapenems have been associated with seizures, which is most common with imipenem/cilastatin compared to the other agents. Caution should be used in patients with brain lesions or a history of seizures. Supratherapeutic concentrations, which can occur if patients who have renal insufficiency are overdosed, increase the risk of seizures. The cross reactivity with penicillin is considered to be 0%–11%. Therefore, patients with anaphylactic reactions to penicillins should avoid carbapenems.

Cephalosporins

Indications

First-generation cephalosporins are indicated in Gram-positive infections and limited Gram-negative organisms (*E. coli*, *Klebsiella* spp., and *Proteus*). Third-generation cephalosporins cover Gram-negatives almost exclusively, but may cover some sensitive Gram-positives. Only ceftazadime and cefepime are active against *Pseudomonas*. Ceftaroline, a fifth-generation cephalosporin, was approved by the FDA in 2010 for the treatment of skin and soft tissue infections and community-acquired pneumonia. Although this medication has not been studied in the SCT patients to date, it does have activity against MRSA as well as other Gram-positive organisms and *Enterobacteriaceae*.

Cefazolin

Preparations

- Infusion: 1 g (50 mL bag)
- Injection: 500 mg, 1 g, 10 g, 20 g, 100 g, 300 g powder vials

Dosing

- Endocarditis with *Streptococcus* sp. or MSSA: 2 g every 8 hours
- Severe infection: 1–1.5 g every 6 hours
- Moderate-to-severe: 500–1000 mg every 6–8 hours

Cephalexin

Preparations

- Capsule: 250 mg, 500 mg, 750 mg
- Suspension: 125 mg/5 mL, 250 mg/5 mL
- Tablet: 250 mg, 500 mg

Dosing

- 250–1000 mg every 6 hours (maximum 4 g/24 hr)

Ceftriaxone

Preparations

- Infusion, in D_5W: 1 g (50 mL bag), 2 g (50 mL bag)

Dosing

- 1–2 g every 12–24 hours
- Endocarditis (*Streptococcus* sp.) and other severe infections: 2 g every 24 hours
- Meningitis: 2 g every 12 hours

Ceftazidime

Preparations

- Infusion: 1 g (50 mL bag), 2 g (50 mL bag)
- Injection: 500 mg, 1 g, 2 g, 6 g powder vials

Dosing

- Severe infections including febrile neutropenia, CNS infections, complicated pneumonia: 2 g every 8 hours

Cefepime

Preparations

- Infusion, with dextrose: 1 g (50 mL bag) and 2 g (100 mL bag)
- Injection: 500 mg, 1 g, 2 g powder vials

Dosing

- Febrile neutropenia: 2 g every 8 hours

Contraindications and adverse effects

- Allergic reactions
- Dermatologic: rash and pruritus
- GI: nausea, vomiting, diarrhea
- LFT abnormalities

Drug interactions

- Metformin: cephalexin may increase serum concentrations of metformin, monitor for toxicity
- Phenytoin: cefazolin may decrease the protein binding of phenytoin, therefore causing higher free phenytoin levels, monitor for toxicity

General prescribing information

Cephalosporin antimicrobial coverage varies based upon the generation of the agent and even among the agents themselves within a generation. There are currently five generations of cephalosporins, but only the most commonly used in the hematologic and SCT population are discussed here. The most important factor for cephalosporin efficacy is the time above the MIC. Ceftazidime and cefepime are indicated in the treatment of febrile neutropenia as monotherapy or along with other antimicrobials. Of note, resistant *Pseudomonas* strains have been increasing with ceftazidime so it has fallen out of favor as empiric coverage (Paul et al., 2010). In 2007, a meta-analysis was published that showed there was a statistically significant increase in mortality in patients who received cefepime for the treatment of febrile neutropenia compared to those who received other antibiotics. Following this publication in 2010, the FDA completed and published their own meta-analysis reviewing this data and did not find any mortality difference with cefepime (US FDA Website, 2009).

Patients who are allergic to penicillins have a 0.2%–8.4% reaction to cephalosporins, which varies among medications. Patients who have an anaphylactic reaction to penicillins should not receive a cephalosporin. If a patient reports a mild reaction, cephalosporins can be given with the patients being monitored closely for signs and symptoms of an allergic reaction.

The majority of cephalosporins are cleared renally, except for ceftriaxone. Therefore, these medications must be renally adjusted. Cefepime adjustments for febrile neutropenia are as follows: CrCl 30–60 mL/min 2 g every 12 hours, CrCl 11–29 mL/min 2 g every 24 hours, CrCl <11 mL/min 1 gram every 24 hours, and should be administered after hemodialysis if given on dialysis days.

Aztreonam

Indications

Utilized in the treatment of Gram-negative organisms including *Pseudomonas*, may be used in patients with a penicillin allergy.

Preparations

- Infusion: 1 g (50 mL bag) and 2 g (50 mL bag)
- Injection: 1 g and 2 g powder vials

Dosing

- 2 g every 6–8 hours (maximum 8 g/24 hr)

Contraindications and adverse effects

- GI: nausea, vomiting, diarrhea
- Injection site pain, thrombophlebitis
- Rash

Drug interactions

- None of relevance

General prescribing information

Aztreonam is utilized mostly in patients with severe Gram-negative infections or to replace penicillins in patients who have anaphylactic allergic reactions (Buonomo et al., 2011). Even though there is a low chance, there are reports of anaphylactic reaction in patients who are allergic to penicillins and cephalosporins. Sixty to seventy percent of aztreonam is excreted unchanged in the urine and must be adjusted for patients with renal insufficiency in patients with a CrCl <30 mL/min. The recommended dosing adjustments are as follows: CrCl 10–30 mL/min 1 gram every 6–8 hours, CrCl <10 mL/min 500 mg every 6–8 hours. Aztreonam is dialyzable and should be dosed with a loading dose of 2 g followed by 500 mg every 12 hours.

Penicillins

Indications

Penicillin is indicated in the treatment of *Streptococcal* infections and other Gram-positive infections but rates of resistance are high. Nafcillin and oxacillin treat *Staphylococci* that produce penicillinases and are the drugs of choice for MSSA. Second-generation penicillins (aminopenicillins) have broader coverage that extends to some Gram-negative coverage including *E. coli*, *H. influenza*, *Salmonella*, and *Shigella*. Ampicillin is the drug of choice for the treatment of pan-sensitive *Enterococcus*.

Amoxicillin

Preparations

- Capsule: 250 mg and 500 mg
- Suspension: 125 mg/5 mL, 200 mg/5 mL, 250 mg/5 mL, and 400 mg/5 mL
- Tablet: 500 mg and 875 mg
- Tablet, chewable: 125 mg, 200 mg, 250 mg, and 400 mg
- Tablet, extended release: 775 mg

Dosing

- 250–500 mg every 8 hours OR 500–875 mg twice daily

Ampicillin

Preparations

- Capsule: 250 mg and 500 mg
- Injection: 125 mg, 250 mg, 500 mg, 1 g, 2 g, and 10 g powder vials
- Suspension: 125 mg/5 mL, and 250 mg/5 mL

Dosing

- Oral: 250–500 mg every 6 hours
- Severe infections: 2 g IV every 4 hours

Nafcillin

Preparations

- Infusion, in dextrose: 1 g (50 mL bag) and 2 g (100 mL bag)
- Injection: 1 g, 2 g, and 10 g powder vials

Dosing (severe infections)

- 2 g every 4 hours

Oxacillin

Preparations

- Infusion: 1 g (50 mL bag) and 2 g (50 mL bag)
- Injection: 1 g, 2 g, 10 g powder vials

Dosing (severe infections)

- 2 g every 4 hours

Penicillin

Preparations

- Infusion(Penicillin G), in dextrose: 1 million units (50 mL bag), 2 million units (50 mL bag), and 3 million units (50 mL bag)
- Injection (Penicillin G): 5 million units and 20 million units powder vials
- Oral (Penicillin VK)
  - Suspension: 125 mg/5 mL and 250 mg/5 mL
  - Tablet: 250 mg and 500 mg

Dosing

- Encapsulated bacteria prophylaxis after SCT: 500 mg orally every 12 hours or 250 mg every 6 hours
- Severe infections: 3–4 million units IV every 4 hours
- *Streptococcal* pharyngitis: 500 mg orally every 6–8 hours

Contraindications or adverse effects

- Anaphylactic reactions
- Dermatologic: rash
- GI: diarrhea, vomiting, nausea, pseudomembranous colitis (ampicillin)

Drug interactions

Nafcillin is a strong 3A4 inducer, therefore it causes multiple drug–drug interactions.

- Allopurinol: may increase risk for allergic reaction to amoxicillin, monitor
- Atenolol: ampicillin decreases bioavailability, monitor
- Azoles: nafcillin decreases serum concentration, monitor
- Brentuximab: nafcillin decreases concentration of active metabolite of brentuximab, monitor
- Calcium channel blockers: nafcillin may decrease serum concentrations of calcium channel blockers, consider alternative therapy
- Cyclosporin: nafcillin decreases serum concentration, monitor
- Dasatinib: nafcillin decreases serum concentration, monitor
- Doxorubicin: nafcillin decreases serum concentration, monitor
- Oral contraceptives: decrease serum concentration, use alternative barrier method while receiving penicillins
- Imatinib: nafcillin may decrease imatinib levels; increase imatinib dose by 50% and monitor for toxicity
- Methotrexate: decrease methotrexate excretion, monitor for toxicity
- Mycophenolate: decrease serum concentrations of mycophenolic acid, monitor
- Nilotinib: nafcillin decreases concentrations; avoid
- Tetracyclines: decrease efficacy of penicillins, consider alternative therapy
- Vinca alkaloids: nafcillin decreases serum concentration, monitor

General prescribing information

Penicillins are indicated for the treatment of susceptible Gram-positive organisms. Owing to antibiotic use over the years, resistant patterns for the majority of these agents are extensive. Therefore, these agents should not be used as empiric therapy until susceptibilities are available. Patients with penicillin allergies should obviously avoid this class of antibiotics. All the penicillins, except for nafcillin and oxacillin, must be renally adjusted. High levels of penicillin are associated with an increased risk of seizures. On the other hand, nafcillin is adjusted only in severe hepatorenal failure, but no dosing specifics are given.

CrCl (mL/min)	Amoxicillin dosing	Ampicillin dosing	Penicillin oral dosing	Penicillin IV dosing
31–50	–	Give every 6–12 hours	Give every 8–12 hours	–
10–30	250–500 mg every 12 hours	Give every 6–12 hours	Give every 8–12 hours	–
<10	250–500 mg every 24 hours	Give every 12–24 hours	Give every 12–16 hours	Give full dose once, then half dose every 8–10 hours

Clindamycin

Indications

Susceptible Gram-positive and anaerobic infections

Preparations

- Infusion, in D_5W: 300 mg (50 mL bag), 600 mg (50 mL bag), and 900 mg (50 mL bag)
- Injection: 150 mg/mL solution (2 mL, 4 mL, 6 mL, and 60 mL vials)
- Capsule: 75 mg, 150 mg, and 300 mg
- Granules for oral solution: 75 mg/5 mL
- Topical

Dosing

- Oral: 150–450 mg every 6–8 hours (maximum 1.8 g/24 hr)
- IV: 600–900 mg every 6–8 hours

Contraindications and adverse effects

- GI tract: abdominal pain, diarrhea, nausea, vomiting, pseudomembranous colitis
- Hepatic: LFT abnormalities, jaundice

Drug interactions

- Erythromycin: decrease efficacy of clindamycin: avoid concomitant use
- Neuromuscular-blockers: clindamycin increases efficacy, monitor

General prescribing information

Clindamycin is active against most *Streptococcus* and MSSA. Of note, clindamycin is indicated in the treatment of community-acquired MRSA, but patterns of resistance do exist in the United States. Local resistance patterns and sensitivities should be obtained before using this agent for the treatment of MRSA. Some Gram-positive anaerobes are also covered by clindamycin including, but not limited to, *Peptostreptococcus* and *Fusobacterium*. The most concerning adverse effect is the incidence of CDIs, which can be observed even up to a few months after treatment with clindamycin is complete. Patients should be monitored closely for signs and symptoms of *C. difficile*-induced diarrhea or stools with blood or mucus. If this occurs, clindamycin should be stopped immediately.

Daptomycin

Indications

Daptomycin is indicated in the treatment of aerobic Gram-positive organisms including skin and skin structure infections, bacteremia, and endocarditis. Both MRSA and some VRE are susceptible to daptomycin.

Preparations

- Injection 500 mg powder vial

Dosing

- 6 mg/kg once daily for severe infections per package insert (some inserts recommend 8–10 mg/kg once daily for complicated bacteremia, endocarditis, or VRE-related infections)

Contraindications and adverse effects

- Electrolyte abnormalities
- Eosinophilic pneumonia (rare), should discontinue daptomycin and start corticosteroids
- GI: nausea, vomiting, diarrhea, constipation
- Hematologic: anemia, eosinophilia
- Musculoskeletal: creatinine phosphokinase (CPK) increase, limb or back pain, weakness, peripheral neuropathy

Drug interactions

- Statins: may enhance the muscle toxicity, avoid concomitant use, or if this is not possible, monitor weekly CPK levels

General prescribing information

Daptomycin is most commonly used in Gram-positive infections resistant to vancomycin. Daptomycin has poor penetration into the lungs, bone, and meninges. In the lung, daptomycin is inactivated by the lung surfactant and therefore should not be utilized to treat pneumonia. Approximately 2.8% of patients in clinical trials had asymptomatic elevation of CPK levels, with 0.2% suffering from the signs and symptoms of myopathy (see package inserts). This usually occurs within one week of starting the medication and CPK elevation can continue for a few weeks after daptomycin has been stopped. Baseline and weekly CPK level monitoring is recommended. Seven cases of eosinophilic pneumonia have been reported in the literature (see package inserts), and can progress to respiratory failure if daptomycin is not discontinued and corticosteroids are not initiated. These cases all occurred 2–4 weeks after starting this antibiotic.

The majority of daptomycin is renally excreted as unchanged drug and therefore must be dose adjusted in patients with renal insufficiency. For CrCl <30 mL/min, daptomycin should be dosed every 48 hours for severe infections. In patients receiving dialysis, the dose should be administered after hemodialysis three days per week.

Fluoroquinolones

Indications

This class of medication is indicated in a broad range of infections including UTIs, GI infections, pneumonia, and sensitive bacteremia. The majority of fluoroquinolones cover Gram-negative organisms including *Enterobacteriaceae*. Ciprofloxacin, levofloxacin, and moxifloxacin have the greatest activity against *Pseudomonas*. Fluoroquinolones also have activity against respiratory organisms including *S. pneumonia*, *H. influenza*, and atypical respiratory bacteria. Of note, moxifloxacin and levofloxacin are considered respiratory fluoroquinolones and have the best activity against MSSA, as well as pneumonia caused by *Streptococcus*, *Legionella*, *Mycoplasma*, or *Chlamydia*.

Ciprofloxacin

Preparations

- Infusion, in D_5W: 200 mg (100 mL bag) and 400 mg (200 mL bag)
- Injection: 10 mg/mL solution (20 mL and 40 mL vials)

- Ophthalmic drops
- OTIC drops
- Suspension: 250 mg/5 mL and 500 mg/5 mL
- Tablet: 250 mg and 500 mg
- Tablet, extended release: 500 mg and 1000 mg

Dosing

- Febrile neutropenia, severe infections: 400 mg IV every 8 hours (use with caution due to increased resistance)
- Febrile neutropenia prophylaxis, intra-abdominal infections: 500 mg orally twice daily (400 mg IV dose)

Levofloxacin

Preparations

- Infusion, in D_5W: 250 mg (50 mL bag), 500 mg (100 mL bag), 750 mg (150 mL bag)
- Injection: 25 mg/mL solution (20 mL and 30 mL vials)
- Ophthalmic drops
- Solution, oral: 25 mg/mL
- Tablet: 250 mg, 500 mg, 750 mg

Dosing

- 500 mg orally once daily (IV same as oral dosing)
- Pneumonia, complicated skin infections: 750 mg once daily

Moxifloxacin

Preparations

- Infusion, in sodium chloride: 400 mg (250 mL bag)
- Ophthalmic drops
- Tablet: 400 mg

Dosing

- 400 mg once daily (IV same as oral dosing)

Contraindications and adverse effects

- Allergic reactions: rash, photosensitivity
- Cardiac: QTc prolongation
- Endocrine: hyperglycemia
- CNS: headache, dizziness
- GI: nausea, vomiting, anorexia, abdominal discomfort, diarrhea
- Tendinopathy and arthropathy (rare)

Drug interactions

- Antacids and sucralfate: decrease absorption of fluoroquinolones, give fluoroquinolone 2 hours before or 6 hours after offending agent
- Bendamustine: ciprofloxacin may increase bendamustine concentration, monitor
- Caffeine: fluoroquinolones increase caffeine concentrations, monitor

- Cyclobenzaprine: ciprofloxacin increases serum concentrations of cyclobenzaprine, consider alternative therapy
- Dacarbazine: ciprofloxacin increases serum concentrations of dacarbazine, consider alternative therapy
- Duloxetine: ciprofloxacin increases serum concentrations of duloxetine, consider alternative therapy
- Ferrous sulfate: decreases absorption of fluoroquinolones, give fluoroquinolone 2 hours before or 6 hours after ferrous sulfate
- Methotrexate: ciprofloxacin may increase methotrexate concentration, monitor for toxicity
- Mirtazepine: ciprofloxacin increases serum concentrations of mirtazepine, consider alternative therapy
- Mycophenolate: may decrease mycophenolic acid levels, monitor
- NSAIDs: reports of increase in seizure potential and increased serum concentration of fluoroquinolones, monitor
- Olanzepine: ciprofloxacin increases serum concentrations of olanzepine, consider alternative therapy
- Phenytoin: ciprofloxacin decreases concentrations of phenytoin, monitor levels
- Propranolol: ciprofloxacin increases serum concentrations of propranolol, consider alternative therapy
- QTc prolonging agents: monitor patient and maintain electrolytes (magnesium and potassium), avoid use with nilotinib, thioridazine, and ziprasidone
- Sulfonylureas: enhance hypoglycemia or hyperglycemia with long-term use, monitor

General prescribing information

In the hematologic and SCT population, fluoroquinolones have been utilized as bacterial prophylaxis during times of neutropenia. Therefore, the benefit of fluoroquinolones for severe and breakthrough infections are limited. One should always refer to their institutions antibiogram for local resistance patterns. Oral fluoroquinolones should be given with food to minimize GI side effects but should not be given with antacids or multivitamin products. These products will bind to fluoroquinolones and inactivate them in the GI tract. Therefore, fluoroquinolones should be given 2 hours before or 6 hours after administration of antacids or calcium supplements.

All fluoroquinolones except for moxifloxacin must be renally adjusted. Refer to the following table for exact dosing recommendations.

CrCl(mL/min)	Ciprofloxacin dosing		Levofloxacin dosing (500 mg/day dosing)	
Route	IV	PO	IV	PO
30–50	–	–	500 mg bolus, 250 mg once daily	500 mg bolus, 250 mg once daily
20–29	200–400 mg every 18–24 hours	250–500 mg every 18 hours	500 mg bolus, 250 mg once daily	500 mg bolus, 250 mg once daily
5–19	200–400 mg every 18–24 hours	250–500 mg every 18 hours	500 mg bolus, 250 mg every 48 hours	500 mg bolus, 250 mg every 48 hours

Linezolid

Indication

Linezolid is indicated to treat infections caused by MRSA, resistant *Streptococcus*, and VRE including bacteremia, pneumonia, and skin and soft tissue infections.

Preparations

- Infusion: 200 mg (100 mL bag) and 600 mg (300 mL bag)
- Suspension, oral: 100 mg/5 mL
- Tablet: 600 mg

Dosing

- 600 mg every 12 hours

Contraindications and adverse effects

- Contraindicated for use within 2 weeks of a MAOI and in patients on SSRIs, TCAs, and other serotonergic medications
- CNS: headache, insomnia
- GI: nausea, vomiting
- Hematologic: thrombocytopenia, anemia, leukopenia
- Hepatic enzyme abnormalities
- Neuropathy: optic and peripheral (rare)

Drug interactions

Linezolid is a weak monoamine oxidase inhibitor (MAOI), and therefore has many of the same interactions as that class of medications. The following medications are recommended to be avoided per the package insert unless otherwise stated.

- Antihypertensives: may increase the risk of orthostatic hypotension, monitor for toxicity
- β-2 agonists (albuterol): may increase toxicity, monitor
- Bupropion
- Carbamazepine
- Cyclobenzaprine
- Hydromorphone
- Methadone
- Methylene blue
- Mirtazepine
- SSRIs
- Serotonin-5HT$_{1D}$ agonists (sumatriptan)
- Stimulants
- Tramadol
- Tricyclic antidepressants

General prescribing information

Linezolid is utilized in Gram-positive infections that are resistant to vancomycin. This antibiotic has excellent penetration into perfused tissues including the lungs and meninges. The most concerning adverse effects are the hematologic toxicities including thrombocytopenia and neutropenia. This usually occurs with more than two weeks of treatment but may occur at any time. There is a predisposition to these toxicities in patients who have myelosuppression, are receiving myelosuppressive agents, or have chronic infections. Monitoring with at least a weekly complete blood count is recommended and discontinuing this agent with occurrence or worsening myelosuppression.

Metronidazole

Indications
Treatment of anaerobic and protozoal infections, including *C. difficile* and other GI-related organisms

Preparations
- Capsule: 375 mg
- Infusion, in sodium chloride: 500 mg (100 mL bag)
- Tablet: 250 mg, 500 mg
- Tablet, extended release: 750 mg
- Topical

Dosing
- 500 mg every 6–8 hours
- Antibiotic-associated pseudomembranous colitis: 500 mg every 8 hours, oral route preferred

Contraindications and adverse effects
- Disulfiram-like reactions
- CNS: dizziness, vertigo, aseptic meningitis (rare), seizures (rare)
- Flu-like syndrome
- GI: nausea, vomiting, metallic taste, abdominal cramping, dry mouth
- Genitourinary: dysuria, cystitis, pelvic pressure

Drug interactions
Metronidazole is metabolized through the CYP 450 system and is a moderate 3A4 inhibitor.
- Alcohol: a disulfiram-like reaction may occur, avoid alcohol use
- Busulfan: increases busulfan concentrations, consider alternative therapy
- Calcineurin inhibitors: increase concentrations, monitor therapy
- Fentanyl: increases fentanyl concentrations, monitor patient or reduce dose if necessary
- Mycophenolate: decreases mycophenolic acid levels, monitor for efficacy
- Phenobarbital: decreases metronidazole concentration, monitor for efficacy
- Phenytoin: decreases metronidazole concentration and may increase phenytoin concentration, monitor for efficacy and toxicity

General prescribing information
Metronidazole is the medication of choice for mild-to-moderate CDIs and is used in combination with vancomycin for severe CDIs. Oral metronidazole should be taken with food to minimize GI side effects. Metronidazole does not have any renal adjustment for impairment, but recommendations vary in terms of dosing with dialysis. Metronidazole doses should be reduced with severe liver disease but no specific dosing recommendations are given in the package insert.

Sulfamethoxazole/trimethoprim (SMZ/TMP) and other related agents
Indications
All of these agents are indicated in the prophylaxis and treatment of *P. carinii (jirovecii)* (PCP). SMZ/TMP is also utilized in the treatment of Gram-negative infections as well as other opportunistic infections. SMZ/TMP is also the treatment of choice for *S. maltophilia* and *Nocardia* sp. and is active against community-acquired MRSA. Dapsone, atovaquone, and pentamidine are also used in other rare infections and diseases besides PCP.

Atovaquone
Preparation
- Oral suspension, 750 mg/5 mL

Dosing
- PCP prophylaxis: 1500 mg once daily
- PCP treatment (mild-to-moderate only) 750 mg twice daily

Dapsone
Preparation
- Tablet, 25 mg and 100 mg

Dosing
- PCP prophylaxis: 100 mg once daily or 50 mg twice daily
- PCP treatment: 100 mg once daily combined with trimethoprim

Pentamidine
Preparations
- Inhalation, nebulizer
- Injection: 300 mg powder vial

Dosing
- PCP prophylaxis: 300 mg inhaled every 4 weeks via Respirgard® II nebulizer
- PCP treatment: 4 mg/kg IV once daily

SMZ/TMP
Preparations
- Injection: SMZ 80 mg and TMP 16 mg/mL solution (5 mL, 10 mL, and 30 mL vials)
- Suspension: SMZ 200 mg and TMP 16 mg/5 mL
- Tablet, single strength: SMZ 400 mg and TMP 80 mg
- Tablet, double strength: SMZ 800 mg and TMP 160 mg

Dosing
- PCP prophylaxis: one double-strength tablet once daily or three times weekly
- PCP treatment (PO or IV based upon trimethoprim component): 15–20 mg/kg/day divided into 3–4 doses

Contraindications and adverse effects

Atovaquone
- CNS: headache, insomnia
- Dermatologic: rash, pruritus
- GI: diarrhea, nausea, vomiting
- Hepatic: LFT abnormalities
- Neuromuscular: weakness
- Flu-like syndrome

Dapsone
- CNS: fever, headache, insomnia
- Dermatologic: rash, pruritus
- GI: anorexia, nausea, vomiting
- Hematologic: anemia, reticulocyte increase, shorten red blood cell life span, rare hemolytic anemia or methemoglobinemia with glucose-6-phosphate dehydrogenase deficiency
- Hepatic: hepatitis, cholestatis

Pentamidine (IV)
- Cardiac: arrhythmias, hypotension
- Electrolyte abnormalities: hyperkalemia, hypoglycemia
- LFT elevation
- Nephrotoxicity
- Inhalation: fatigue, fever, dizziness, anorexia, cough, dyspnea, wheezing

SMZ/TMP
- Allergic reactions
- CNS: fever
- Dermatologic: rash, Stevens-Johnson syndrome
- GI: nausea, vomiting, anorexia
- Hematologic: neutropenia
- Hepatotoxicity
- Hyperkalemia
- Nephrotoxicity

Drug interactions

Atovaquone
- Etoposide: increases concentration of etoposide, separate administration of both by 1–2 days
- Hypoglycemic agents: increase risk of hypoglycemia, monitor
- Rifamycin: decreases concentration of atovaquone, consider alternative therapy
- Ritonavir: decreases concentrations of atovaquone, monitor

Dapsone
Dapsone is extensively metabolized by the CYP 450 system in the liver, and therefore has numerous drug interactions.

May decrease dapsone levels
- Rifamycins: consider alternative therapy

May increase dapsone levels
- Azoles: consider alternative therapy
- Dasatinib: monitor
- Protease inhibitors: consider alternative therapy
- SMZ/TMP: monitor

Pentamidine (IV)
- Fluconazole: increases serum concentrations of pentamidine, consider alternative therapy
- Isoniazid: increases serum concentrations of pentamidine, consider alternative therapy
- QTc prolonging agents: avoid use (nilotinib, thioridazine, ziprasidone, etc.)

SMZ/TMP
- ACE inhibitors and angiotensin II receptor blockers: monitor for hyperkalemia
- Carvedilol: increases concentration of carvedilol, monitor
- Cyclosporin: worsens nephrotoxicity, monitor
- Dapsone: increases concentration of dapsone and trimethoprim, monitor
- Fluconazole and ketoconazole: increase concentration of SMZ/TMP, consider alternative therapy
- Leucovorin calcium: diminishes efficacy of SMZ/TMP, monitor
- Methotrexate: enhances toxicity, consider alternative agent
- Phenytoin: increases concentrations of phenytoin, monitor

General prescribing information
SMZ/TMP is considered first line for the prophylaxis and treatment of PCP. In moderate-to-severe PCP, consider the addition of corticosteroids with a partial pressure of oxygen ≤70 mmHg. Treatment should last for 14–21 days. A sulfa allergy is one of the more common drug allergies. Patients with this allergy should avoid use of this agent, as the sulfa moiety is part of the SMZ component. Owing to the prevalence of this allergy, other medications such as atovaquone, dapsone, and pentamidine allow for other prophylaxis and treatment options. Of note, clindamycin and primaquine may also be used in the treatment of PCP in patients with a sulfa allergy. Many of these medications cause blood dyscrasias, even though the overall incidence is rare. Blood dyscrasias include but are not limited to agranulocytosis, aplastic anemia, hemolysis, methemoglobinemia, and pure red cell aplasia. Specifically, these adverse effects have been reported with dapsone and SMZ/TMP and are more common in patients who have a G6PD deficiency. Patients who are planning on receiving dapsone should be tested for this deficiency. SMZ/TMP has been linked to neutropenia and thrombocytopenia. This risk is even more pronounced in the hematologic malignancy and SCT population when they have myelosuppression. A risk–benefit analysis should be undertaken prior to giving this medication to any patient and they should also have their CBCs monitored regularly. Most centers will hold PCP prophylaxis during myelosuppression and restart treatment once counts recover.

SMZ/TMP is not recommended in patients with a CrCl <15 mL/min, and should be reduced to 50% of the recommended dose in patients with a CrCl between 15–30 mL/min.

Intravenous pentamidine should be avoided in patients with renal dysfunction. If the CrCl is <10 mL/min, the recommended dosing for pentamidine is 4 mg/kg every 24–36 hours.

Vancomycin

Indications

Vancomycin is used in the treatment of infections caused by Gram-positive organisms including MRSA. Oral vancomycin is only indicated in the treatment of moderate-to-severe CDIs.

Preparations

- Capsule: 125 mg and 250 mg
- Infusion, in dextrose: 500 mg (100 mL bag), 750 mg (150 mL bag), and 1 g (200 mL bag)
- Injection: 500 mg, 750 mg, 1 g, 5 g, and 10 g powder vials

Dosing

- For IV dosing, use ABW
- Severe infections: 15–20 mg/kg IV every 8–12 hours (may give 25–30 mg/kg loading dose)
- *C. difficile* treatment
  - Severe infection: 125 mg orally every 6 hours for 10–14 days
  - Severe, complicated infection: 500 mg orally every 6 hours with or without metronidazole

Contraindications and adverse effects

- GI (oral formulation only): nausea, vomiting, bitter taste
- Nephrotoxicity (rare)
- Ototoxocity (rare)
- Red man syndrome: erythema on face and neck that occurs when vancomycin is infused too rapidly

Drug interactions

- Aminoglycosides: increase risk of nephrotoxicity, monitor
- NSAIDs: may increase concentration of vancomycin, monitor

General prescribing information

Vancomycin is effective against most Gram-positive organisms and *C. difficile*. Because it is not absorbed from the GI tract, it is given IV, except for the treatment of pseudomembranous colitis. Vancomycin troughs should be monitored for efficacy. Troughs have been found to be related to the AUC:MIC ratio, which is the most important pharmacokinetic measurement that relates to clinical efficacy. In severe infections, troughs should be between 15–20 mcg/mL. Troughs <10 mcg/mL have been associated with resistance and should be avoided. Of note, patients whose organisms have an MIC ≥2 with normal weight and renal function may not reach the optimal AUC:MIC ratio and should be switched to an alternative agent if their clinical status does not improve. The first trough should be taken once a steady state is reached, which is prior to the fourth dose if the patient did not receive a loading dose. Once the patient has a therapeutic trough, levels should be drawn at least once weekly, or more often in those who are hemodynamically unstable or changing renal function (Rybak et al., 2009). The major excretion route is renal, so considerable dosage modification is required in the presence of renal failure. For a CrCl 20–49 mL/min, dose vancomycin every 24 hours and for a CrCl <20 mL/min, vancomycin should be dosed at 15–20 mg/kg and repeated once the levels are at or below the trough goal (pulse dosing). Oral vancomycin is primarily excreted in the feces and does not require renal dosing.

Nephrotoxicity and ototoxicity are rare and usually occur when vancomycin is given with another toxic agent. Red man syndrome is a histamine-induced reaction that occurs when vancomycin is infused too quickly at a rate of 500 mg over <30 minutes. If this syndrome occurs, slow the infusion to ≥2 hours and consider the use of antihistamines or corticosteroids for symptom management.

Antidiarrheals
Indication
Diarrhea not related to infectious causes

Diphenoxylate/atropine
Preparation
- Tablet, 2.5 mg/0.025 mg

Dosing
- Two tablets (5 mg diphenoxylate) four times daily until diarrhea is controlled, then reduce dose as needed (maximum 20 mg diphenoxylate/day)

Loperamide
Preparations
- Caplet or capsule: 2 mg
- Liquid or solution: 1 mg/5 mL

Dosing
- Acute diarrhea: 4 mg with first loose stool, followed by 2 mg with each loose stool thereafter (maximum of 16 mg/day)
- Chronic: 4–8 mg daily in divided doses, titrate as needed for symptom management

Octreotide
Preparations
- Injection: 100 mcg/mL (1 mL vial), 200 mcg/mL (5 mL vial), 1000 mcg/mL (5 mL vial)
- Injection, preservative free: 50 mcg/mL (1 mL vial), 100 mcg/mL (1 mL vial), 200 mcg/mL (5 mL vial), 500 mcg/mL (1 mL vial)

Dosing for severe or refractory diarrhea: 50–100 mcg IV (or SC) every 8 hours, may increase by 100 mcg/dose every 48 hours (maximum, 500 mcg every 8 hours)

Contraindications and adverse effects
Avoid using antidiarrheals when an infection is present, such as *Shigella*, *Salmonella*, *C. difficile*, etc.

- Diphenoxylate/atropine: constipation, abdominal cramps, anticholinergic adverse effects, and CNS adverse effects (confusion, euphoria, lethargy, etc.)
- Loperamide: constipation, abdominal cramps, dizziness
- Octreotide: bradycardia, hyperglycemia (hypoglycemia in diabetes mellitus type I), abdominal pain, nausea, diarrhea, flatulence, cholelithiasis (long-term use), and injection site reactions

Drug interactions

- Anticholinergic medications: may worsen the anticholinergic effects of diphenoxylate/atropine, monitor therapy
- Octreotide: avoid other QTc prolonging agents, including but not limited to dronedarone, nilotinib, thioridazine, and ziprasidone
    - Ciprofloxacin may be used, but QTc monitoring is encouraged

General prescribing information

Stool culture should be obtained and infectious etiologies for diarrhea prior to starting antimotility therapy should be ruled out to prevent worsening infections. According to Benson et al. (2004), loperamide is recommended for mild-to-moderate diarrhea and octreotide is recommended for loperamide refractory or complicated diarrhea related to chemotherapy. Adjunct and nonpharmacologic therapy should be undertaken such as dietary management and fluid and electrolyte replacement. Subcutaneous octreotide has been utilized to treat diarrhea in patients with GVHD. If no benefit is seen after 7 days of treatment, octreotide should be discontinued.

Diphenoxylate/atropine, loperamide, and octreotide should be used cautiously in patients with hepatic impairment due to an increased risk of CNS toxicity. Octreotide has dosing recommendations with both dialysis and hepatic impairment. Diphenoxylate should also be used sparingly in patients with renal dysfunction. Patients receiving octreotide for the duration of >1 year should be monitored for hypothyroidism, pancreatitis, and cholelithiasis.

Antiemetics

Aprepitant and fosaprepitant
Indications

Prophylaxis of acute and delayed chemotherapy-induced nausea and vomiting in patients receiving high or moderate emetogenic chemotherapy along with a serotonin-5HT$_3$ inhibitor and dexamethasone

Aprepitant
Preparation

- Tablet, 40 mg, 80 mg, 125 mg

Dosing

- 125 mg on day 1 given 1 hour prior to chemotherapy, then 80 mg once daily on days 2 and 3

Fosaprepitant

Preparation: injection, 150 mg powder vial

Dosing

- Single dose: 150 mg IV 30 minutes prior to chemotherapy on day 1 only
- 3-day dosing: 115 mg IV 30 minutes prior to chemotherapy on day 1, followed by 80 mg orally once daily on days 2 and 3

Contraindications and adverse effects

- Contraindications: use with cisapride or pimozide
- Constipation
- Fatigue
- Hiccups
- Weakness

Drug interactions

Aprepitant is extensively metabolized through the CYP 450 enzyme system and is also an inhibitor or an inducer of multiple enzymes.

- Azoles: increase aprepitant levels, monitor
- Benzodiazepines: may increase benzodiazepine levels, monitor
- Budesonide: increases serum concentration of budesonide, consider dose reduction with oral budesonide
- Oral contraceptives: may decrease concentration of oral contraceptives, use alternative method
- Corticosteroids: may increase steroid levels, consider alternative therapy or decrease dose
- Dasatinib, imatinib, and nilotinib: may increase levels of these medications, monitor for toxicity
- Docetaxel: may increase docetaxel concentration, monitor for toxicity
- Doxorubicin: may increase doxorubicin serum concentration, monitor
- Etoposide: may increase etoposide serum levels, monitor
- Fentanyl: may increase fentanyl concentration, monitor and make dose reductions as needed
- Ifosfamide: may increase ifosfamide concentration, monitor for toxicity
- Irinotecan: may increase irinotecan serum concentration, monitor
- Paclitaxel: may increase paclitaxel concentration, monitor for toxicity
- Paroxetine: may decrease aprepitant and paroxetine serum levels, monitor
- Rifamycins: may decrease aprepitant serum concentration, monitor for efficacy
- Vinca alkaloids: may increase vinca alkaloid concentration, monitor

General prescribing information

Aprepitant is not indicated in the treatment of breakthrough or chronic nausea and vomiting. It should always be given with a $5HT_3$ inhibitor and dexamethasone. When dosed with dexamethasone, the dose of dexamethasone should be reduced to 12 mg. Case reports of ifosfamide-associated neurotoxicity with aprepitant use exist, but the literature is conflicting.

Serotonin-5HT$_3$ inhibitors

Indications

Prevention of acute chemotherapy-induced nausea and vomiting in high and moderate emenogenic regimens and palonosetron is indicated in delayed nausea and vomiting

Dolasetron

Preparation
- Tablet, 50 mg, 100 mg

Dosing
- 100 mg 1 hour prior to chemotherapy

Granisetron

Preparations
- Injection: 1 mg/mL (1 mL and 4 mL vials)
- Injection, preservative free: 0.1 mg/mL (1 mL vial) and 1 mg/mL (1 mL vial)
- Transdermal patch: 3.1 mg/24 hr
- Solution, oral: 2 mg/10 mL
- Tablet: 1 mg

Dosing
- 2 mg orally or 1 mg IV prior to chemotherapy
- Patch: apply 24–48 hours prior to first dose of chemotherapy

Ondansetron

Preparations
- Film, oral: 4 mg, 8 mg
- Infusion: 32 mg premixed in D_5W 50 mL or NS 50 mL
- Injection: 2 mg/mL (2 mL and 20 mL vial)
- Infection, preservative free: 2 mg/mL (2 mL vial)
- Solution, oral: 4 mg/5 mL
- Tablets: 4 mg, 8 mg (both also available as oral disintegrating tablets)

Dosing
- Highly emetogenic: 24 mg oral or 8 mg IV given 30 minutes prior to start of therapy
- Moderately emetogenic: 16 mg orally or 8 mg IV given 30 minutes prior to chemotherapy

Palonosetron

Preparation
- Injection 0.05 mg/mL (1.5 mL and 5 mL vials)

Dosing
- 0.25 mg injected 30 minutes prior to the start of chemotherapy

Contraindications and adverse effects
- CNS: headache, malaise
- GI: constipation
- QTc prolongation (rare)

Drug interactions

- Avoid use with other QTc prolonging medications (nilotinib, thioridazine, and ziprasidone)

General prescribing information

All $5HT_3$ inhibitors are equally effective for acute nausea and vomiting, but palonosetron is preferred for delayed nausea and vomiting in many of the clinical guidelines (Basch et al., 2011). Palonosetron has a half-life of 40 hours; therefore, it lasts longer than all the other oral and IV agents. No clinical trials have been done to compare multiday dosing of a short-acting $5HT_3$ antagonist compared to palonosetron.

In 2011, IV dolasetron was taken off the market in the United States due to the incidence of arrhythmias and QTc prolongation. This is a class effect and is found to be more prevalent in the IV formulations compared to the oral. All patients who are receiving other QTc prolonging agents should be monitored closely and undergo aggressive electrolyte replacement. The highest incidence is at 1–2 hours after infusion and most arrhythmias reported in the literature are not clinically significant (US FDA website, 2011). $5HT_3$ inhibitors have not been studied in the treatment of breakthrough nausea and vomiting.

Antifungals: systemic use

Azoles

Indications

- Fluconazole is effective against *Candida* sp., *Cryptococcus* sp., and coccidiomycosis. It is ineffective against *Aspergillus* sp. and other mold infections as well as some species of *Candida*.
- Itraconazole is effective against aspergillosis in immunosuppressed patients, histoplasmosis, and in patients in whom resistance to other antifungal agents has developed.
- Ketoconazole is effective against local *Candida* sp. infections in which topical preparations are ineffective.
- Posaconazole is used for the prevention and treatment of invasive *Aspergillus* sp. and *Candida* sp. infections in immunocompromised patients at high risk for invasive fungal infections.
- Voriconazole is effective in the treatment of invasive aspergillosis, fluconazole-resistant *Candida* sp., and has been used as prophylaxis in patients at risk for invasive fungal infections.

Fluconazole

Preparations

- Infusions: 100 mg (50 mL NS), 200 mg (100 mL NS or D_5W), 400 mg (200 mL NS or D_5W)
- Suspension: 10 mg/mL and 40 mg/mL
- Tablet: 50 mg, 100 mg, 150 mg, 200 mg

Dosing

- Candidiasis: 100–200 mg once daily for 14 days, may use up to 400 mg daily in esophageal candidiasis
- Systemic candidiasis: 800 mg on first day then 400 mg once daily for 14 days, use 800 mg daily for patients with *C. glabrata*

- Cryptococcal meningitis: 400–800 mg once daily for 8 weeks for consolidation, then 200 mg once daily for 6–12 months for maintenance
- Neutropenia prophylaxis: 400 mg once daily for duration of neutropenia

Itraconazole
Preparations
- Capsule: 100 mg
- Solution: 10 mg/mL

Dosing
- 200 mg twice daily on an empty stomach or with an acidic beverage (not grapefruit juice)

Ketoconazole
Preparation
- Tablets, 200 mg

Dosing
- 200–400 mg daily with food for a maximum of 14 days

Posaconazole
Preparation
- Oral suspension, 40 mg/mL

Dosing
- Prophylaxis: 200 mg TID with full meal
- Treatment: 400 mg BID

Voriconazole
Preparations
- Injection: 200 mg powder vial
- Suspension: 40 mg/mL
- Tablet: 50 mg, 200 mg

Dosing
- Candidiasis and prophylaxis: 200 mg every 12 hours
- Invasive infection: initial dose of 6 mg/kg IV every 12 hours for 2 doses, then continue at 4 mg every 12 hours for maintenance; oral maintenance dose is 200 mg BID

Contraindications and adverse effects
GI adverse effects are the most common, including nausea, vomiting, abdominal pain, and diarrhea. Ketoconazole has the highest prevalence of GI side effects. Headaches, rash, and hepatotoxicity can also occur with all agents. QTc prolongation has been reported. Azoles should be avoiding during pregnancy, especially in the first trimester, due to reports of craniofacial abnormalities with fluconazole.

- Itraconazole: hypertension, hypokalemia, and peripheral edema
- Ketoconazole: gynecomastia and adrenal suppression can happen at large doses (not commonly used for this indication)
- Posaconazole: fatigue, dizziness, edema, tachycardia, nausea, hyperglycemia, electrolyte disturbances, arthralgias
- Voriconazole: temporary vision changes, electrolyte disturbances, pruritus, peripheral edema, photophobia, skin photosensitivity, periostitis
    - Neurological toxicity including visual hallucinations, confusion, agitation, and myoclonus can be seen at high concentrations

Drug interactions

All azoles have multiple drug interactions, mainly caused by the interaction with the hepatic cytochrome P450 enzyme. The most common enzyme inhibited, CYP3A4, is the strongest with ketoconazole and itraconazole and weakest with fluconazole. Other CYP450 and p-glycoprotein interactions exist and vary among agents.

Decrease azole levels

- Can continue up to 2 weeks after the interacting agent is discontinued
- Rifamycins: rifampin contraindicated with voriconazole
- Rifabutin is the drug of choice if azole coadministration is necessary

    - Anticonvulsants: carbamazepine (contraindicated with voriconazole), phenytoin, and phenobarbital
    - Agents that increase gastric pH: H_2 antagonist, proton-pump inhibitors, and antacids (ketoconazole, itraconazole, and posaconazole)

Increase level of concomitant drug

- Cyclosporin

    - Consider reducing dose to 50% of total dose if administered with voriconazole
    - Consider reducing dose to 75% of total dose if administered with posaconazole
- Sirolimus: consider avoiding

    - Reports suggest decreasing dose to 10% of total dose if administered with voriconazole
- Tacrolimus: consider reducing dose to 1/3 of total daily dose if administered with voriconazole or posaconazole
- Digoxin (itraconazole)
- Increase INR with warfarin (voriconazole and fluconazole)

QTc prolongation

- May occur if administered with any other QTc prolonging agents
- Cisapride, quinidine, haloperidol

General prescribing information

Treatment with systemic antifungal drugs should rarely be given for less than 2–3 weeks, the total duration being dependent on the clinical, mycological, and serological response.

The spectrum of antifungal coverage varies among azole antifungal agents. Fluconazole, considered to have the narrowest coverage, is ineffective in aspergillosis and C. krusei infections. Most C. glabrata isolates have increasing resistance to fluconazole. Of note, there are reports of an increased incidence of mucormycosal infections in high-risk patients who received voriconazole prophylaxis.

Ketoconazole and itraconazole use as first-line agents has fallen out of favor due to low patient tolerability and profound drug interactions as compared to other azoles. Voriconazole is considered the treatment of choice in invasive aspergillosis. In clinical trials, posaconazole prophylaxis has shown to have a survival benefit in patients receiving intensive chemotherapy for AML or MDS compared to fluconazole or itraconazole. In patients receiving immuno-suppression for the treatment of GVHD, posaconazole prophylaxis decreased the rate of invasive fungal infections compared to fluconazole but did not show any OS benefit.

Absorption of posaconazole, itraconazole capsules, and ketoconazole is significantly decreased when administered at a high gastric pH. Therefore, use of the proton pump and H_2 inhibitors should be avoided. Small studies have shown that administering ketoconazole or itraconazole with a carbonated, acidic beverage may overcome this issue (Chin et al., 1995). Posaconazole should be given with food or acidic carbonated beverage to increase absorption. On the other hand, voriconazole should be administered on an empty stomach, while absorption decreases significantly when taken with a high fat meal.

Fluconazole is excreted renally; for patients with renal impairment (CrCl <40 mL/min), the dosage should be reduced. Intravenous voriconazole should be avoided in patients with a CrCl <50 mL/min to prevent accumulation of the vehicle cyclodextrin.

Hepatic dosing adjustment and/or caution is recommended in all azole antifungals except fluconazole.

Echinocandins
Indications
- Anidulafungin: treatment of *Candida* sp. and refractory *Aspergillus* sp.
- Caspofungin: invasive aspergillosis, refractory to intolerance of other antifungal agents, presumed fungal infections, and persistent candemia
- Micafungin: prophylaxis (and treatment) of *Candida* sp. infections in recipients of HSCT, active against *C. albicans*, *C. glabrata*, *C. krusei*, and *C. tropicalis*

Anidulafungin
Preparation
- Injection 50 mg and 100 mg powder vials

Dosing
- Candidemia and non-esophageal candidiasis: 200 mg loading dose on day 1, 100 mg daily for 14 days
- Esophageal candidiasis: 100 mg loading dose on day 1, 50 mg daily for 14 days

Caspofungin
Preparations
- Injection 50 mg and 75 mg powder vials

Dosing
- 70 mg loading dose on day 1, followed by 50 mg daily

Micafungin

Preparation

- Injection 50 mg and 100 mg powder vials

Dosing

- Treatment: 100 to 150 mg daily over 1 hour (latter dose is specifically for esophageal candidiasis)
- Prophylaxis: 50 mg daily

Contraindications and adverse effects

Adverse effects that occur with all echinocandins include liver function abnormalities, headache, electrolyte abnormalities especially hypokalemia, infusion-related reactions, injection site pain, and GI upset. Hepatotoxicity can occur but is less frequent than with azoles. There are also case reports of myelosuppression with the total incidence occuring in <1% of patients.

- Caspofungin: fever and injection site pain (highest incidence of echinocandins)

Drug interactions

- Cyclosporin: caution for use with caspofungin due to increased risk for hepatoxocity
- Micafungin reduces the clearance of cyclosporin, close cyclosporin level monitoring is recommended
- Sirolimus: micafungin reduces the clearance, close monitoring is recommended
- Tacrolimus: caspofungin decreases tacrolimus levels by 20%, close monitoring is recommended
- 3A4 enzyme inducers: include dexamethasone, efavirenz, phenytoin, and rifampin
  - Decrease caspofungin levels, increase dose to 70 mg once daily

General prescribing information

Treatment with systemic antifungal drugs should rarely be given for less than 2–3 weeks, the total duration being dependent on the clinical, mycological, and serological response.

Echinocandins have a very similar spectrum of coverage, which includes most *Candida* and *Aspergillus* species. These antifungals are not commonly used first-line for invasive aspergillosis. Outside of these organisms, echinocandins have very little activity against other yeasts and molds including *Cryptococcus* sp. echinocandins should not be used to treat fungal urinary tract infections.

Echinocandins have minimal renal clearance and therefore have no renal adjustments and are not dialyzable. Hepatic dosing adjustments are recommended for caspofungin. These agents are very well tolerated in terms of adverse effects.

Polyene macrolide

Indications

Amphotericin is effective against systemic *Candida* sp. infections, invasive aspergillosis, blastomycosis, cryptococcosis, coccidioidomycosis, histoplasmosis, mucormycosis, and other mold infections.

Amphotericin deoxycholate
Preparation
- Injection 50 mg powder vial

Dosing
- Must give with a bolus infusion of normal saline both before and after the amphotericin infusion
- Invasive infections: 0.5–1 mg/kg once daily infused over 4–6 hours
- Cryptococcal meningitis: 0.7–1 mg/kg once daily

Amphotericin B cholesteryl sulfate complex
Preparation
- Injection 50 mg and 100 mg powder vials

Dosing
- 3–4 mg/kg/day infused once daily at a rate of 1 mg/kg/hr

Amphotericin B lipid complex
Preparation
- Injection 5 mg/mL suspension (20 mL vial)

Dosing
- 2.5–5 mg/kg once daily

Liposomal amphotericin B
Preparation
- Injection 50 mg powder vial

Dosing
- 3–6 mg/kg once daily

Contraindications and adverse effects
The most common and concerning side effects include infusion-related reactions (fevers, chills, rigors, nausea), phlebitis, electrolyte abnormalities (hypokalemia and hypomagnesemia), and nephrotoxicity. Amphotericin B deoxycholate has the highest incidence of infusion reactions and nephrotoxicity compared to the lipid formulations. Hypotension, edema, and tachycardia have also been reported as well as anaphylactic reactions. With long-term use, there is also a slight risk of developing a reversible, normocytic, normochromic anemia.

Drug interactions
- Avoid administration with other nephrotoxic agents
- Flucytosine: used synergistically with amphotericin to treat cryptococcal meningitis

General prescribing information
Due to toxicity, amphotericin has fallen out of favor as the drug of choice for the majority of invasive fungal infections. It is utilized mostly in invasive fungal infections known to be

resistant to azoles or echinocandins. It is considered the antifungal of choice for systemic mycoses. Lipid-based formulations of amphotericin have reduced some of the toxicities associated with this medication, specifically infusion reaction and nephrotoxicity. These products include amphotericin B cholesteryl sulfate complex (Amphotec®), amphotericin B lipid complex (Abelcet®), and liposomal amphotericin B (Ambisome®). Small clinical trials have found that liposomal amphotericin B has similar efficacy to the amphotericin B deoxycholate, with some studies showing a slightly better clinical outcome for the Ambisome®.

To prevent subsequent infusion-related reactions, premedication with an NSAID with or without diphenhydramine, acetaminophen, and diphenhydramine, or hydrocortisone are all appropriate. Meperidine is recommended to treat rigors due to amphotericin infusions. With renal dysfunction due to amphotericin B deoxycholate nephrotoxicity, it is recommended the dose be decreased by 50% or given every 48 hours. No recommendations are available for the lipid formulations.

Flucytosine
Indications

Flucytosine is used in a synergistic combination with amphotericin against cryptococcosis and also covers some strains of *Candida*.
Preparation: tablets, 250 mg and 500 mg
Dosing: 25 mg/kg every 6 hours for 2 weeks (if converting to fluconazole monotherapy) or for 6–10 weeks with amphotericin B

Contraindications and adverse effects

Flucytosine is known to cause significant myelosuppression due to conversion to 5-FU in vivo. The highest incidence is usually seen during the first two weeks of therapy. If the cause of myelosuppression is due to flucytosine accumulation, an alternate agent should be utilized. Hepatotoxicity including elevated LFT occur in approximately 5% of patients. Flucytosine should be avoided in pregnancy.

Drug interactions

- Cytarabine: reduces efficacy of flucytosine, should be avoided

General prescribing information

Flucytosine should never be used as a single agent to treat fungal infection due to the high incidence of resistance. Its main place in therapy is in the treatment of cryptococcal meningitis or pneumonia along with amphotericin B. It can also be utilized as an adjunct in other cryptococcal or *Candida* infections. Flucytosine is cleared renally and therefore must be adjusted with a CrCl <40 mL/min.

Antifungals: topical oral use
Indications

Topical treatment should only be utilized for the treatment or prevention of mild oropharyngeal candidiasis. Systemic treatment should be used for moderate or severe oropharyngeal candidiasis, esophageal candidiasis, and systemic fungal infections.

Amphotericin suspension

Preparations

- Not available commercially in the United States, must be compounded from powder by compounding pharmacy
- Preparation: suspension, 100 mg/mL

Dosing

- 0.5 to 1 mL of suspension four times daily (rinse around mouth for 2–3 minutes before swallowing).

Clotrimazole

Preparation

- Oral troches, 10 mg

Dosing

- Prophylaxis: 1 troche dissolved orally 3 times daily for duration of chemotherapy
- Treatment: 1 troche dissolved orally 5 times daily for 14 days

Nystatin

Preparation

- Suspension, 100 000 units/mL

Dosing

- 4–6 mL swish and swallow 4 times daily, keep in mouth for several minutes prior to swallowing

Contraindications and adverse effects

- Amphotericin suspension: taste changes, nausea, oral discomfort and burning
- Clotrimazole: elevated LFT
- Nystatin: GI upset such as nausea, vomiting, and diarrhea

Drug interactions

- Clotrimazole has moderate CYP 3A4 enzyme inhibition and will increase the concentration of medications cleared through this pathway. Close monitoring is recommended.
  - Anticonvulsants: carbamazepine, phenytoin, and phenobarbital
  - Azole antifungals
  - Budesonide
  - Cyclosporin
  - Dexamethasone
  - Rifamycins
  - Sirolimus
  - Tacrolimus

General prescribing information

For mild oropharyngeal candidiasis, topical treatment is recommended. If that fails or if the infection is more severe, oral fluconazole is indicated. The majority of studies comparing topical to systemic therapy for oropharyngeal candidiasis are in AIDS patients and may not extrapolate to the SCT population. There have been small clinical trials evaluating the use of amphotericin suspension in the SCT population, but low patient tolerability and compliance confounded results. The suspension is available in Europe, but can be compounded in the United States.

Esophageal candidiasis requires systemic treatment. An addition of topical oral agents in a patient already receiving systemic antifungal treatment has not been studied extensively and does not add any additional antifungal coverage.

If the patient wears dentures, the dentures should be disinfected and the patient should receive preferred topical or oral antifungal therapy.

Antifungals: topical and systemic for dermatological use

Topical preparations

Indications

- Clotrimazole and miconazole are used for fungal skin infections, including tinea (dermatophytes) and *Candida* sp.
- Ketoconazole cream is for use in patients for whom other topical treatments have failed.
- Topical nystatin is used for the treatment of topical *Candida* infections.
- Griseofulvin is used for dermatophyte infections of the skin, scalp, hair, and nails. It is not effective against candidal infections.
- Ketoconazole (oral) is used for dermatophytes, *Candida*, and systemic fungal infections.
- Terbinafine is used for treatment of microbiologically proven onychomycosis due to dermatophyte fungi. Topical terbinafine can be utilized to treat topical dermatophytes.

Clotrimazole

Preparations

- Cream: 1% (15 g, 30 g, 45 g tubes)
- Solution: 1% (10 mL and 30 mL bottles)

Dosing

- Apply twice daily

Ketoconazole

Preparations

- Aerosol foam: 2% (50 g and 100 g containers)
- Cream: 2% (15 g, 30 g, and 60 g tube)
- Gel: 2% (45 g tube)
- Shampoo: 2% (120 mL bottle)

Dosing

- Apply once daily

Miconazole
Preparations
- Aerosol: 2% (90 g or 105 mL containers)
- Cream: 2% (15 g, 30 g, and 45 g tubes)
- Gel: 2% (24 g tube)
- Ointment: 2% (multiple sizes)
- Powder: 2% (30 g, 70 g, and 90 g containers)

Dosing
- Apply twice daily

Nystatin
Preparations
- Cream 100 000 units/g (15 g and 30 g tubes)
- Ointment 100 000 units/g (15 g and 30 g tubes)
- Powder 100 000 units/g (15 g, 30g, and 60 g tubes)

Dosing
- Apply twice to three times daily

Terbinafine
Preparations
- Cream: 1% (15 g and 30 g tubes)
- Gel: 1% (6 g and 12 g tubes)
- Solution: 1% (30 mL bottle)

Dosing
- Apply once daily

Oral preparations

Griseofulvin
Preparations
- Suspension: 125 mg/5 mg
- Tablets: ultramicrosized 125 mg and 250 mg, microsized 500 mg

Dosage
- 500 mg to 1 g microsized daily in divided doses or as a single dose with meals
- 375 mg ultramicrosized daily in divided doses or as a single dose with meals

Ketoconazole: refer to systemic antifungal section

Terbinafine
Preparation
- Tablet: 250 mg

Dosing

- 250 mg daily

Contraindications and adverse effects

- The most common adverse effects for topical antifungals include dermatological reactions such as itching and burning at the site of application.
- Griseofulvin: headaches, nausea, and photosensitivity
  - Contraindicated in pregnancy, porphyria, and liver failure
- Ketoconazole: refer to systemic antifungal section
- Terbinafine: headaches, rare GI upset, and liver enzyme elevation
  - Has exacerbated cutaneous or systemic lupus erythematosus during treatment, should discontinue if this occurs
  - Avoid in patients with renal insufficiency or liver failure

Drug interactions

Griseofulvin

- Alcohol: reports of disulfiram-like reactions, monitor
- Cyclosporin: decreases cyclosporin levels, monitor
- Estrogen contraceptives: decreases estrogen levels, use alternative barrier method of contraception or avoid griseofulvin
- Warfarin: decreases warfarin levels, monitor

Ketoconazole: refer to systemic antifungal section

Terbinafine

- Cyclosporin: decreases cyclosporin levels, monitor
- Rifamycins: decrease terbinafine levels, avoid use or adjust therapy
- SSIs or TCAs: decreases metabolism, avoid use or adjust therapy

General prescribing information

Scalp ringworm is best treated with griseofulvin. Tinea capitis due to *Microsporum* is more sensitive to griseofulvin while tinea due to *Trichophyton* is more sensitive to terbinafine. Topical treatment alone is ineffective and should be used in conjunction with griseofulvin. Treatment of tinea corporis in immunocompromised patients should be given systemically. Fluconazole (2–4 weeks), itraconazole (1–2 weeks), or terbinafine (1–2 weeks) are acceptable options. Tinea cruris can be treated using topical agents with oral agents being utilized for refractory infections. In the treatment of tinea pedis, use of terbinafine has a higher cure rate compared to azoles. If chronic or extensive disease occurs, oral terbinafine or fluconazole may be utilized.

Both oral itraconazole and terbinafine have been found to be more effective in the treatment of onchomycosis than fluconazole or griseofulvin. Terbinafine has a higher rate of long-term cure and has fewer adverse effects and drug interactions compared to itraconazole. Duration of treatment should be at least 6 weeks for fingernails and 12 weeks for toenails. Of note, nystatin is also available in topical form but does not treat any dermatophyte-related infections, only candidal infections. Oral terbinafine is not recommended in patients with impaired renal function (CrCl <50 mL/min) or cirrhosis.

Antineoplastics

Alkylating agents
Busulfan
Indications
Busulfan is currently utilized in allogeneic and autologous transplant conditioning regimens for leukemias and lymphomas.

Preparations
- Injection: 6 mg/mL (10 mL vial)
- Tablet: 2 mg

Dosing
- Varied based upon regimen
- High dose Bu/Cy conditioning oral: 1 mg/kg every 6 hours for 4 days
- IV busulfan
    - 130 mg/kg once daily for 4 days infused over 3 hours
    - 0.8 mg/kg every 6 hours for 4 days
- Dosing should be based upon IBW or ABW, whichever is lower unless the patient is obese. For obese patients, use adjusted IBW

Contraindications and adverse effects
- GI: nausea/vomiting (moderate emetic risk), mucositis, diarrhea
- Myelosuppression
- Pulmonary toxicity
- Seizures
- Sinusoidal obstruction syndrome (dose-limiting toxicity) and liver toxicities

Drug interactions
Busulfan is metabolized mostly through the CYP 450 3A4 enzyme. Therefore, medications that induce or inhibit this enzyme will interact. Pharmacokinetic monitoring may help overcome drug interaction issues. The most common and concerning interactions are listed as follows: Decrease busulfan levels (all recommend monitoring therapy)
- Carbamazepine
- Dexamethasone
- Phenobarbital
- Phenytoin
- Rifamycins

Increase busulfan levels
- Acetaminophen: avoid therapy 72 hours prior to and 48 hours after busulfan administration
- Azoles: consider therapy modification
- Dasatinib: monitor toxicity

- Diltiazem: monitor
- Imatinib: consider therapy modification
- Metronidazole: avoid therapy
- Protease inhibitors: consider therapy modification
- Verapamil: monitor

General prescribing information

For SCT conditioning, intravenous busulfan is more often utilized due to less pharmacokinetic variability. Additionally, vomiting is no longer a concern in terms of the patient receiving their busulfan doses. An area under the curve (AUC) between 900–1500 µmol/min is preferred when busulfan is given every 6 hours; however, goal AUCs may vary depending upon institutional practices. Literature has shown that subtherapeutic dosing may lead to increased rates of relapse in the CML population while supratherapeutic levels increase the risk of hepatic sinusoidal obstruction syndrome (SOS) (Dix et al., 1996; Slattery et al., 1995).

With conditioning doses of busulfan, antiepileptic medication must be given. Both phenytoin, 15–20 mg/kg loading dose followed by 300 mg orally at bedtime, and lorazepam, 0.5–2 mg every 6 hours, have been utilized for this purpose. Of note, phenytoin has been shown to cause an increase in clearance of busulfan and lower measured AUCs. Seizure prophylaxis should start prior to receiving busulfan and continue until at least 24 hours after the infusions are complete. Newer second-generation antiepileptics, such as levetiracetam, may become a favorable option due to decreased adverse effects and minimal drug interactions. Currently, there is minimal literature available supporting the use of second-generation antiepileptic medication for busulfan-induced seizure prophylaxis.

Carboplatin

Indications

Carboplatin is used in the treatment of relapsed lymphomas as well as in autologous conditioning regimens for solid tumor malignancies.

Preparation

- Injection 10 mg/mL (5 mL, 15 mL, 45 mL, 60 mL vials)

Dosing

- Varied based upon regimen
- Dose calculated based upon Calvert formula: Total dose (mg) = AUC $\times$ (GFR + 25)
- Per the FDA, GFR should be capped at 125 mL/min
- Controversy exists about which CrCl and body weight formula to utilize to calculate the dose. Refer to protocol or institutional standards. The Cockcroft-Gault formula can be found in the Antibiotic section under Aminoglycoside *Dosing*.

Contraindications and adverse effects

- Myelosuppression is the dose-limiting toxicity with thrombocytopenia being the common grade 3/4 hematologic toxicity
- Electrolyte abnormalities
- GI: moderate emetic potential
- Transient increase in liver enzymes
- Peripheral neuropathy

- Serum creatinine elevation
- High-dose carboplatin: ototoxicity, nausea, vomiting, renal toxicity (higher incidence compared to standard dose)

Drug interactions

With high-dose carboplatin, avoid use of other ototoxic or nephrotoxic agents (excluding aminoglycosides).

General prescribing information

Carboplatin is usually administered over 15–60 minutes, but can be administered over a longer period of time (24 hours). For high-dose carboplatin in autologous conditioning regimens, aggressive hydration should be utilized to prevent nephrotoxicity. Additional adjustments for renal insufficiency are not necessary, while the Calvert formula accounts for renal function.

Carmustine (BCNU)

Indications

Carmustine is used in autologous conditioning regimens for lymphomas
Preparation: injection 100 mg powder vial
Dosing: varied based upon regimen

Contraindications and adverse effects

- Arrhythmias have been reported at high doses
- GI: high emetic risk, mucositis
- Injection site reactions: pain, burning, erythema
- Liver toxicity including SOS at high doses
- Myelosuppression is the dose-limiting toxicity, which is usually delayed
  - Thrombocytopenia and leukopenia usually occur, with thrombocytopenia being the most severe
  - Anemia is less frequent and severe
- Pulmonary toxicity: cumulative doses >1400 mg/m^2 are at highest risk but have been reported in patients with prolonged treatment of carmustine at lower doses
  - Acute lung injury in transplant occurs around 1–3 months after transplant
    - Signs and symptoms include dyspnea, cough, or fever
  - Patients with underlying history of lung disease or decreased pulmonary function tests are at increased risk
  - Consider baseline and periodic monitoring of pulmonary function tests
- Renal failure can occur at high doses
- Secondary leukemias

Drug interactions

Melphalan: may sensitize patient to pulmonary toxicities, monitor

General prescribing information

Carmustine is infused over at least 2 hours to prevent infusion reactions. Patient's vital signs should be monitored closely for hypotension. Additional fluid support may be needed. Carmustine should be prepared in a non-polyvinyl chloride container (glass or polyolefin). Carmustine should be renally adjusted as follows:

CrCl (mL/min)	Recommendation
46–60	Give 80% of dose
31–45	Give 75% of dose
≤30	Consider using another agent

Hepatic adjustment may be needed but no specifics are addressed in the package insert.

Cyclophosphamide

Indications

Treatment of all hematologic malignancies and is a part of many autologous and allogeneic conditioning regimens. Cyclophosphamide is also used as a mobilization agent to collect stem cells for autologous transplantation.

Preparations

- Injection: 500 mg, 1 g, 2 g powder vials
- Tablet: 25 mg, 50 mg

Dosing

- Varied based upon regimen
- 60 mg/kg IV once daily for 2 days
- 50 mg/kg IV once daily for 4 days
- 4 g/m^2 IV once (mobilization), other doses exist in the literature

Contraindications and adverse effects

- Dose-limiting toxicity: myelosuppression, especially leukopenia
- Alopecia
- Cardiac toxicity and heart failure (high dose)
- Fertility issues (usually reversible)
- GI: moderate emetic risk as well as delayed nausea and vomiting with normal dosing, high emetic risk with high dose, mucositis, metallic taste
- Hemorrhagic cystitis
- Nasal congestion: watery eyes, rhinorrhea, sinus congestion, and sneezing
  - Occurs when IV is infused too quickly
- Secondary leukemias: rare
- Syndrome of inappropriate secretion of antidiuretic hormone (SIADH)

Drug interactions

Cyclophosphamide undergoes extensive hepatic metabolism (especially CYP 450 2B6); therefore has numerous drug interactions. The most important are listed as follows and patients should be monitored.

Decrease cyclophosphamide concentrations

- Carbamazepine
- Phenobarbital
- Phenytoin
- Rifampin

Increase cyclophosphamide concentrations
- Clopidogrel
- Doxorubicin
- Paroxetine
- Sertraline

General prescribing information

To prevent hemorrhagic cystitis, patients should be advised to maintain adequate fluid intake of at least 2 L daily during the infusion and up to 48 hours after. Frequent voiding is also recommended. Aggressive hydration with or without MESNA should be used in patients receiving high-dose cyclophosphamide (>1 gram/m^2). High-dose cyclophosphamide is used mostly in the mobilization and conditioning regimens. Cyclophosphamide infusions occur over 1–24 hours depending upon the regimen and dose.

The package insert does not contain renal or hepatic dosing information, but recommendations exist in the literature. Cyclophosphamide should be administered with a 25% dose reduction if CrCl <10 mL/min. Cyclophosphamide is dialyzable and should be administered at a 50% dose reduction post-dialysis. Hepatic adjustment recommendations are as follows: serum bilirubin 3.1–5 mg/dL or LFTs >3 times ULN, administer 75% of dose; bilirubin >5 mg/dL, avoid use.

Dacarbazine

Indication

Treatment of Hodgkin lymphoma
Preparations: injection 100 mg and 200 mg powder vials
Dosing: 375 mg/m^2 IV once daily on days 1 and 15 every 4 weeks for ABVD regimen

Contraindications and adverse effects

- Dose-limiting toxicity: myelosuppression, especially leukopenia and thrombocytopenia
- Alopecia
- High emetic potential
- Infusion-related pain
- Teratogenicity has been observed in animals

Drug interactions

Dacarbazine is extensively metabolized in the liver, specifically through CYP 450 1A2 and 2E1. Concerning interactions are listed as follows.

Decrease dacarbazine concentrations

- Carbamazepine: consider alternative therapy
- Phenobarbital: consider alternative therapy
- Rifampin: consider alternative therapy

Increase dacarbazine concentrations

- Ciprofloxacin: consider alternative therapy
- Ketoconazole: consider alternative therapy
- Lidocaine: consider alternative therapy

General prescribing information

Dacarbazine is an irritant. If an extravasation occurs, apply cold packs and protect from light. If irritation (not extravasation) occurs, symptoms may be relieved with hot packs. Dacarbazine is usually infused over 30–60 minutes.

Although there are no recommendations in the package insert for renal or hepatic dosage adjustments, caution should be taken with these organ impairments. Suggested renal dosing per Kintzel and Dorr:

CrCl (mL/min)	Recommendation
46–60	Give 80% of dose
31–45	Give 75% of dose
<30	Give 70% of dose

Ifosfamide

Indications

Relapsed lymphomas and germ cell tumors as well as other malignancies

Preparations: injection 1 g and 3 g powder vials and 50 mg/mL solution (20 mL and 60 mL vials)

Dosing

- Varied based upon regimen

Contraindications and adverse effects

- Dose-limiting toxicity: myelosuppression and hemorrhagic cystitis
- Alopecia
- CNS toxicity: somnolence, hallucination, confusion, coma
- Hematuria
- Moderate emetic potential

Drug interactions

Ifosfamide is a major substrate of CYP 450 2A6, 3A4, and 2C19 and is extensively metabolized by the liver.

- Aprepitant: increases serum concentrations of ifosfamide, consider alternative therapy
- Azoles: increases serum concentrations of ifosfamide, consider alternative therapy
- Gemfibrozil: increases serum concentrations of ifosfamide, consider alternative therapy
- Protease inhibitors: increase serum concentrations of ifosfamide, consider alternative therapy
- Rifampin: decreases serum concentrations of ifosfamide, monitor for efficacy

General prescribing information

Hydration of at least 2 L/day with or without MESNA should be utilized to prevent hemorrhagic cystitis, which is caused by the ifosfamide metabolite acrolein. Please refer to MESNA (page 500) for specific recommendations. Encephalopathy is seen in 10%–30% of patients receiving ifosfamide and is more common in patients who have a renal impairment, low albumin, prior cisplatin use, prior history of encephalopathy with ifosfamide, and use with medications that increase ifosfamide levels, including aprepitant and fosaprepitant. In the majority of patients, this encephalopathy, thought to be caused by chloracetaldehyde, is reversible but has also been treated with different agents including methylene blue. The dosing is 50 mg every 4–8 hours until symptoms resolve. Of note, all serotonergic medications should be discontinued immediately with administration of methylene blue to prevent serotonin syndrome.

Ifosfamide is extensively hepatically metabolized and at high doses the majority is renally eliminated as unchanged drug. There are no suggestive dosing adjustments in the package insert for hepatic or renal impairment, but other literature has recommendations. Floyd et al. (2006) recommends giving 25% of the total dose with a serum bilirubin >3 mg/dL and Aronoff et al. (2007) recommends giving 75% of the total dose with a CrCl <10 mL/min. Supplemental dosing is not needed in dialysis patients.

Melphalan

Indications

Lymphoma and multiple myeloma for autologous transplant, oral melphalan is indicated to treat multiple myeloma for patients who are not eligible for transplant

Preparations

- Injection: 50 mg powder vial
- Tablet: 2mg

Dosing

- Varied based upon regimen, examples:
- Multiple myeloma autologous transplant conditioning: 200 mg/m^2 IV once on either day –2 or day –1
- Multiple myeloma palliative treatment: 9 mg/m^2 PO once daily on days 1–4 every 42 days (with VMP)

Contraindications and adverse effects (for IV)

- Dose-limiting toxicities: myelosuppression and oral mucositis
- GI: moderate emetic potential, diarrhea
- Pulmonary toxicity (rare)
- Secondary malignancies

Drug interactions

Carmustine: melphalan can sensitize patient to carmustine-induced pulmonary toxicity, monitor

General prescribing information

Once diluted, melphalan is stable only for 60 minutes and should therefore be infused over 15–30 minutes. When administering melphalan, cryotherapy is recommended to prevent mucositis. Cryotherapy should begin prior to the melphalan infusion, and continue during and after the infusion has ended. There is no consensus in terms of an optimal cryotherapy schedule with melphalan. This medication should be renally adjusted. The package insert recommends decreasing the multiple myeloma conditioning dose to 140 mg/m^2 in the elderly, SCr >2 mg/dL, or in patients receiving hemodialysis. Dialysis patients should receive their melphalan dose(s) after dialysis.

Thiotepa

Indications

Utilized as part of the conditioning regimen for autologous and allogeneic transplantation

Preparation

- Injection 15 mg powder vial

Dosing

- Varies based on regimen

Contraindications and adverse effects

- Dose-limiting toxicity: myelosuppression
- Amenorrhea and spermatogenesis inhibition
- CNS: fever, chills, dizziness, headache, tremors
- Contact dermatitis from thiotepa excretion in sweat (high doses), hyperpigmentation (temporary)
- GI: low emetic risk, diarrhea
- Laryngeal edema
- Secondary leukemias

Drug interactions

Thiotepa is rapidly metabolized by the CYP enzymes and is a strong inhibitor of the CYP2B6 enzyme. Therefore, any medications cleared through the 2B6 system will have higher concentrations when coadministered with thiotepa. Alternative therapies are recommended to avoid this interaction.

- Bupropion
- Efavirenz
- Methadone
- Promethazine

General prescribing information

Because thiotepa causes dermatitis when it comes in contact with skin, strict precautions must be taken. Thiotepa and its active metabolites are excreted through the skin and thus the skin must be bathed multiple times daily (4–6 times) with soap and water starting 3–4 hours after the first dose is administered. If the patient sweats or is very warm, additional baths may be required. Washed areas should then be patted dry to avoid injury to the skin. With each bath all clothes, bed linen, and central line dressing should be changed. Avoid using moisturizers, antiperspirants, deodorants, or other topical agents that would trap in skin moisture. Caregivers should take additional care when performing patient care activities including handling clothes and linen.

Thiotepa is relatively contraindicated in patients who have liver and renal impairment. Dose reduction or avoidance is recommended in this population on a case-by-case basis.

Anthracyclines and anthracenediones (doxorubicin, daunorubicin, idarubicin, and mitoxantrone)

Indications

Anthracyclines are utilized in the induction, consolidation, and/or relapse regimens in hematologic malignancies including ALL, AML, APL, HL and NHL, and multiple myeloma.

Preparations

- Daunorubicin: injection 5 mg/mL (4 ml and 10 mL vials) and 20 mg powder vials
- Doxorubicin: injection 2 mg/mL (5 mL, 10 mL, 25 mL, and 100 mL vials) and 10 mg, 20 mg, and 50 mg powder vials
- Idarubicin: injection 1 mg/mL (5 mL, 10 mL, and 20 mL vials)
- Mitoxantrone: 2 mg/mL (10 mL, 12.5 mL, 15 mL, and 20 mL vials)

Dosing

- Varied based upon regimen

Contraindications and adverse effects

- Myelosuppression is the dose-limiting toxicity
- Cardiac toxicity: ECG abnormalities, chronic heart failure
- Dermatology: alopecia, radiation recall, rash, photosensitivity
- GI: moderate emetic potential, mucositis, diarrhea
- Red urine and other body fluids (tears, saliva, sweat) except mitoxantrone (blue discoloration) which lasts for 24–48 hours after the end of the infusion depending on the particular agent's half-life
- Secondary leukemias: rare

Drug interactions

Doxorubicin is metabolized through multiple hepatic CYP 450 enzymes and is a moderate inhibitor of CYP2B6. Therefore, there are multiple drug interactions with these anthracyclines. The other anthracyclines are mainly cleared through the P-glycoprotein system and have fewer drug interactions.

- Azoles: increase doxorubicin levels, consider therapy modification with itraconazole, ketoconazole, posaconazole, and voriconazole
- Dabigatran: doxorubicin decreases serum concentrations, avoid use
- Dasatinib: may increase doxorubicin levels, monitor therapy
- Digoxin: may decrease effects of digoxin, monitor therapy and cardiac function
- Fluoxetine and paroxetine: increase levels of doxorubicin, consider therapy modification
- Imatinib: may increase levels of doxorubicin, consider therapy modification
- Protease inhibitors: increase levels of doxorubicin, avoid use
- Terbinafine: increases levels of doxorubicin, consider therapy modification
- Warfarin: doxorubicin may enhance warfarin efficacy and bleeding risk, monitor closely

General prescribing information

The principal non-hematologic toxicity is cardiac. Rarely, such cardiac toxicity can be acute, but more commonly it is chronic. ECG changes can be seen in about 10% of patients at all dose levels.

A baseline ECG and gated heart scan are recommended; avoid these drugs if these tests show significant abnormalities. To monitor for chronic or late complications such as heart failure, repeat testing is recommended but there are no standards in terms of which test is preferred or the frequency of testing needed. The risk of cardiac toxicity is directly related to the cumulative lifetime dose of anthracyclines. This risk increases exponentially with increases in lifetime doses. Slower infusions of anthracyclines over 24–72 hours, particularly with doxorubicin, have shown to decrease the risk of cardiac toxicity.

Cumulative cardiotoxic doses of anthracyclines

Agent	5% risk of cardiotoxicity at cumulative dose (mg/m^2)
Daunorubicin	900
Doxorubicin	450
Idarubicin	225
Mitoxantrone	200

All the anthracyclines are vesicants and must be given with extreme care. These drugs should be given into the side arm of a rapidly running infusion. Do not give through another route as severe damage may occur. Avoid giving them concurrently with radiotherapy, as radiation damage may be increased.

Anthracycline dosing must be adjusted for hepatic impairment and varies between products. Daunorubicin and idarubicin have recommended dosing adjustments for renal impairment as well.

Secondary leukemias and MDS have been reported with anthracyclines and usually occur within 1–3 years of treatment. They are also associated with 11q26 and 21q22 chromosomal abnormalities.

Cytarabine

Indications

Pyrimidine analog used for treatment of AML, ALL, relapsed lymphomas, meningeal leukemia prophylaxis and treatment, and as part of autologous transplant conditioning regimens for lymphoma

Preparations

- Injection: 20 mg/mL (25 mL vial), 100 mg/mL (20 mL vial), and 100 mg, 500 mg, 1 g powder vials
- Injection, preservative free: 20 mg/mL (5 mL and 50 mL vials), 100 mg/mL (20 mL vial)
- Injection, liposomal: 10 mg/mL (5 mL) for intrathecal use

Dosing

- Varied based upon regimen

Contraindications and adverse effects

- Dose-limiting toxicity: myelosuppression
- CNS toxicity: cerebellar toxicity (high dose)
- Cytarabine syndrome: bone and chest pain, fever, rash, malaise, myalgias (treat with steroids)
- GI: moderate emetic risk (dose dependent), diarrhea, mucositis
- Liver function abnormalities
- Ocular: conjunctivitis (high dose)

Drug interactions

- No relevant interactions

General prescribing information

High-dose cytarabine, >1 gram/m^2, has a higher incidence of adverse effects compared to lower doses of cytarabine. The most concerning is cerebellar toxicity, which is associated with age >50 years old, impaired renal function, doses >18 grams/m^2 per cycle, and cumulative cytarabine dosing. Patients should be screened for risk factors and be monitored closely for cerebellar toxicity when receiving high-dose cytarabine. In addition, corticosteroid eye drops should be administered four times daily starting prior to cytarabine and continuing up to 24–48 hours after completion of cytarabine to prevent conjunctivitis. Cytarabine syndrome occurs in around 33% of patients and usually 6–12 hours after cytarabine infusion. Signs and symptoms include fever, rigors, sweating, rash, arthralgias and myalgias, and sometimes hypotension. This is not considered a true allergy, and acetaminophen and/or steroids can be used to treat or prevent severe occurrences of this adverse effect.

Cytarabine or liposomal cytarabine can be given intrathecally. The usual dose for cytarabine administered intrathecally is 50–100 mg and 50 mg for cytarabine and liposomal cytarabine, respectively. Patients who are receiving liposomal cytarabine should receive dexamethasone prior to the injection to prevent arachnoiditis either as part of the intrathecal injection or systemically. It is delivered over a 1–5-minute slow push and the patient should stay supine for at least one hour after intrathecal administration.

High-dose cytarabine should be renally adjusted. Kintzel & Dorr (1995) recommend administering 60% of the dose with a CrCl 46–60 mL/min, 50% of dose with a CrCl 31–45 mL/min, and avoiding use in patients with a CrCl <30 mL/min. In patients with hepatic impairment, dose reduction should be considered.

Fludarabine

Indications

Purine analog indicated in the treatment of CLL, relapsed AML, and indolent lymphomas. Fludarabine is also utilized in allogeneic transplant conditioning regimens.

Preparations

- Injection: 50 mg powder vial and 25 mg/mL solution (2 mL vial)
- Tablet: 10 mg

Dosing

- Varied based upon regimen
- Conditioning with busulfan: 40 mg/m^2 IV once daily for 4 days starting 6 days prior to transplant
  - Reduced intensity: 30 mg/m^2 IV once daily for 6 days starting 10 days prior to transplant
- RIC with melphalan: 25–30 mg/m^2 IV once daily for 4–5 days starting 6 days prior to transplant

Contraindications and adverse effects

- Dose-limiting toxicity: myelosuppression, especially lymphopenia and thrombocytopenia
- Autoimmune hemolytic anemia and thrombocytopenia (rare)
- Edema
- Fever, malaise, pain, chills
- Minimal emetic risk
- Neurotoxicity (doses above those recommended in elderly patients)
- Pulmonary: cough, dyspnea

Drug interactions

Imatinib: decreases active metabolite of fludarabine, discontinue imatinib at least 5 days prior to starting fludarabine

General prescribing information

Fludarabine causes severe prolonged lymphopenia which puts patients at risk for opportunistic infections. Anti-infectives should be utilized in patients at risk for complications. Neurotoxicity has been seen in clinical trials with high doses (up to 96 mg/m^2 daily for 5–7 days). Signs and symptoms include delayed blindness, coma, and death. With normal doses agitation, coma, and seizures have been reported. Caution should be used when driving or in patients who have a history of neurological disorders, such as epilepsy.

Fludarabine is renally eliminated and therefore must be adjusted for renal impairment. Adjustment is based upon route of administration, indication for treatment, and CrCl. In the treatment of CLL, the package insert does not recommend the use of fludarabine with a CrCl of <30 mL/min. Recommendations according to Aronoff et al. (2007) are as follows:

CrCl (mL/min)	Recommendation
10–50	Give 75% of dose
<10	Give 50% of dose

Methotrexate

Indications

Folate analog indicated in the treatment of ALL, CNS lymphomas, highly aggressive NHL (such as Burkitt's lymphoma), and acute GVHD prophylaxis after allo-SCT.

Preparations

- Injection: 1 gram powder vial and 25 mg/mL solution (2 mL and 10 mL vials)
- Injection, preservative free: 25 mg/mL solution (2 ml, 4 mL, 8 mL, 10 mL, and 40 mL vials)
- Tablet: 2.5 mg, 5 mg, 7.5 mg, 10 mg, 15 mg

Dosing

- Varied based on regimen
- Acute GVHD prophylaxis: 15 mg/m^2 IV once on day +1, 10 mg/m^2 IV once daily on days +3, +6, and +11
  - Some protocols leave off the day +11 dose
- Acute GVHD prophylaxis, "mini-methotrexate": 5 mg/m^2 IV once daily on days +1, +3, +6, and +11

Contraindications and adverse effects

- Dose-limiting toxicity: myelosuppression
- GI: moderate emetic potential (dose related), mucositis
- Hepatotoxicity
- Rash
- Renal toxicity: not commonly seen with GVHD dosing

Drug interactions

Methotrexate is excreted mainly in the urine but also undergoes some hepatic metabolism.

- Bile acid sequestrants: decrease absorption of oral methotrexate, monitor for efficacy
- Ciprofloxacin: increases methotrexate levels, monitor
- Loop diuretics: may increase levels of methotrexate; methotrexate may decrease efficacy of diuretics, consider alternative therapy or close monitoring
- NSAIDs: decrease excretion, consider alternative therapy
- Penicillins: may decrease excretion of methotrexate, monitor
- Proton pump inhibitors: may increase methotrexate concentrations, monitor therapy
- Salicylates: may increase concentrations, consider alternative therapy
  - Low-dose salicylates for cardioprotective benefit are not likely to cause this interaction
- Sulfonamides/trimethoprim: increase methotrexate toxicity, avoid use if possible

General prescribing information

To prevent prolonged myelosuppression, leucovorin rescue of 10–15 mg/m^2 every 6 hours for 8–10 doses is required in methotrexate doses >500 mg/m^2. Rescue should begin 24–48 hours after the start of the methotrexate infusion unless otherwise specified in the protocol. Leucovorin treatment should continue until serum levels are $\leq$0.1 micromole/L, although some centers require $\leq$0.05 micromole/L. At these levels, methotrexate is considered to be clinically cleared from the body. If the level is >1 micromole/L at 48 hours or >0.2 micromole/L at 72 hours, leucovorin doses should be increased to 100 mg/m^2 IV every 6 hours until methotrexate is cleared. Of note, this dosing schema is just one example of many different dosing strategies utilized. High-dose methotrexate should be avoided in patients with renal dysfunction. Aggressive hydration and urine alkalinization should be utilized to facilitate methotrexate clearance and prevent crystal formation. This is usually accomplished with IV fluids with 100–150 mEq of sodium bicarbonate administered as a continuous infusion. Urinary pH should be $\geq$7 prior to the methotrexate infusion and pH monitoring should continue to maintain this goal until methotrexate is cleared.

Methotrexate distributes into third-space fluids and is released slowly over time similar to that of a depot injection. Therefore, high-dose methotrexate is contraindicated in patients with third spacing, such as those with ascites or pleural effusions. If the patient has already received methotrexate prior to the effusion or ascites being identified, continue supportive-care medications (leucovorin) and urine alkalinization until methotrexate is cleared.

Glucarpidase is an antidote to methotrexate in patients with severe toxicity. Glucarpidase hydrolyzes extracellular methotrexate into its inactive metabolites. It is given for serum toxicity at 50 units/kg IV over 5 minutes and may be repeated 24 hours after the first injection. Intrathecal glucarpidase may also be used to treat intrathecal toxicity at a flat dose of 2000 units. When glucarpidase is given, all supportive measures should continue unless otherwise specified.

Methotrexate must be renally and hepatically adjusted. There are no package insert recommendations or consensus in the literature. Example adjustments are listed as follows.

CrCl (mL/min)	Serum bilirubin (mg/dL)	Recommendation
–	3.1–5 or LFTs >3x ULN	Give 75% of dose
46–60	–	Give 65% of dose
31–45	–	Give 50% of dose
<30	>5	Avoid use

With acute GVHD prophylaxis dosing, methotrexate levels and possible leucovorin rescue should be considered in patients suffering for severe adverse effects. Dosing adjustments for hepatic and renal insufficiency are listed as follows.

Serum creatinine (mg/dL)	Serum bilirubin (mg/dL)	Recommendation
1.5–1.7	–	Give 75% of dose
1.8–2	2.1–3	Give 50% of dose
–	3.1–5	Give 25% of dose
>2	>5	Do not give

Epipodophyllotoxins (topoisomerase II inhibitors)
Etoposide
Indicated in relapsed AML, relapsed lymphomas, and as part of autologous conditioning regimens

Preparations
- Capsule: 50 mg (not commonly used in hematologic malignancies or with SCT)
- Injection: 20 mg/mL (5 mL, 25 mL, and 50 mL vial)

Dosing
- Varied based upon regimen

Contraindications and adverse effects

- Dose-limiting toxicity: myelosuppression, specifically leukopenia and thrombocytopenia
- Alopecia
- Anaphylaxis (rare)
- GI: moderate emetic potential, mucositis, diarrhea
- Hepatic toxicities
- Infusion-related reactions: hypotension (with rapid infusion)
- Secondary leukemias

Drug interactions

Etoposide is extensively metabolized in the liver and therefore has numerous drug–drug interactions.

Decrease etoposide concentrations

- Barbiturates
- Carbamazepine
- Phenytoin
- Rifamycins

Increase etoposide concentrations

- Atazanavir: avoid combination
- Atovaquone: separate by 1–2 days, do not use concomitantly
- Azoles (itraconazole, ketoconazole, posaconazole, and voriconazole): avoid combination
- Clarithromycin: avoid combination
- Cyclosporin: reduce dose of etoposide by 50% or avoid combination
- Darunavir: avoid combination
- Dasatinib: monitor therapy
- Diltiazem and verapamil: consider alternative therapy
- Imatinib: avoid combination
- Ritonavir: avoid combination

General prescribing information

Precipitation of etoposide at high doses, such as those given in transplant, is a pharmaceutical concern. Etoposide is very unstable in a concentration >0.4 mg/mL and usually will precipitate within minutes. If a more dilute solution cannot be compounded, a slow infusion of undiluted drug is recommended or use of etoposide phosphate. Etoposide must be administered over at least 30 minutes to prevent hypotension.

Adjustment for renal and hepatic insufficiency is recommended and examples are listed in the following table. Of note, there are differences in dosing based upon which literature one references.

CrCl (mL/min)	Serum bilirubin (mg/dL)	Recommendation
10–50	–	Give 75% of dose
<10 or hemodialysis	1.5–3 or AST >3 × ULN	Give 50% of dose

Methyltransferase inhibitors (azacitidine and decitabine)

Indications

Treatment of MDS and have been studied in the treatment of AML in older patients or patients unfit for traditional chemotherapy

Azacitidine

Preparation

- Injection 100 mg powder vial

Dosing

- 75 mg/m^2 IV/SC once daily × 7 days every 4 weeks
- Alternate dosing schedules for administration convenience
  - 75 mg/m^2 IV/SC daily for 5 days, 2 days rest (weekend), then 75 mg/m^2 daily for 2 more days
  - 75 mg/m^2 IV/SC daily for 5 days
  - 50 mg/m^2 IV/SC daily for 5 days, 2 days rest (weekend), then 50 mg/m^2 daily for 5 days

Decitabine

Preparation

- Injection 50 mg powder vial

Dosing

- 20 mg/m^2 IV daily for 5 days over 1 hour every 4 weeks (outpatient)
- Inpatient: 15 mg/m^2 IV three times daily for 3 days every 6 weeks

Contraindications and adverse effects

- Dose-limiting toxicities: myelosuppression
- Arthralgias and myalgias
- CNS: fever, chills, headache, malaise
- Edema
- GI: moderate emetic risk (azacitidine), minimal emetic risk (decitabine)
- Hepatotoxicity (rare)

Drug interactions

- No relevant interactions

General prescribing information

Azacitidine is metabolized and excreted both hepatically and renally. Patients who had renal or hepatic insufficiency were excluded from clinical trials, so there are no specific dosing recommendations in this patient population. Avoidance in severe organ impairment is recommended and close monitoring and dose reduction for toxicity should be considered. Decitabine does not have specific dosing recommendations at baseline, but holding doses are recommended if there is a significant elevation in serum creatinine, ALT, or bilirubin.

Vinca alkaloids (vinblastine, vincristine)

Indication

Vinblastine is indicated in the treatment of HL as part of the ABVD regimen. Vincristine is utilized in the treatment of ALL and lymphomas.

Vinblastine

Preparation

- Injection 10 mg powder vial and 1 mg/mL solution (10 mL vial)

Dosing

- 6 mg/m^2 IV on days 1 and 15 every 28 days (ABVD)

Vincristine

Preparation

- Injection 1 mg/mL solution (1 mL and 2 mL vials)

Dosing

- 1.4 mg/m^2 or 2 mg flat dose once (maximum dose: 2 mg)

Contraindications and adverse effects

- Dose-limiting toxicity: myelosuppression mostly leukopenia (vinblastine), neurotoxicity (vincristine)
- Alopecia
- GI: minimal emetic potential, constipation, intestinal perforation (rare), paralytic ileus (rare)
- Hypertension
- Neuromuscular: neuropathy, pain, deep tendon reflex losses, sensorimotor dysfunction

Drug interactions

Vinca alkaloids are extensively metabolized by the cytochrome P450 system, especially the 3A4 pathways. Therefore, there are numerous drug interactions. The most concerning are listed as follows.

Decrease vinca alkaloid concentrations

- Carbamazepine
- Phenobarbital
- Phenytoin
- Rifamycins

Increase vinca alkaloid concentrations

- Aprepitant: monitor for toxicity
- Azoles: consider altering therapy with itraconazole, ketoconazole, posaconazole, and voriconazole
- Clarithyromycin and erythromycin: consider alternative therapy
- Dasatinib: monitor for toxicity
- Imatinib: consider alternative therapy

- Nifedipine: monitor
- Protease inhibitors: consider avoiding therapy or if necessary, monitor for toxicity

General prescribing information

Vinca alkaloids should never be given intrathecally. If this occurs, it is almost always fatal due to demyelination of neurons. All necessary precautions should be taken to prevent an incident from occurring. Vinca alkaloids are extensively metabolized in the liver and therefore must be dose-adjusted for hepatic insufficiency. If serum bilirubin is >3 mg/dL, 50% of the dose should be administered. No renal adjustments are needed. Vinca alkaloids are vesicants and if extravasation occurs, warm packs should be applied to the area with a local injection of hyaluronidase.

Other
Asparaginase
Indication

Treatment of ALL

Preparations

- Injection
  - *E. coli* formulation (Elspar®): 10 000 international units powder vial
  - *Erwinia chrysanthemi* formulation (Erwinaze™): 10 000 international units powder vial
  - Pegaspargase (Oncaspar®): 750 international units/mL (5 mL vial)

Dosing

- Please refer to specific protocols; examples are as follows:
- *E. coli* formulation: 6000–10 000 international units/m^2 IM/IV given three times weekly
- *Erwinia* formulation: 25 000 international units/m^2 IM given three times weekly
- Pegaspargase: 2500 international units/m^2 once (do not administer more often than every 14 days)

Contraindications and adverse effects

- Contraindicated in patients with *E. coli* allergy (except *Erwinia* formulation), history of severe hemorrhage, pancreatitis, or severe thrombosis
- Azotemia
- Coagulopathies: increase PT, PTT, low fibrinogen, reports of cerebrovascular hemorrhages
- GI: minimal emetic risk, anorexia
- Hepatotoxicity: temporary
- Hyperglycemia
- Hypersensitivity reaction: fever, rash, urticaria, hypotension, bronchospasm, anaphylaxis
- Pancreatitis
- Thrombotic events

Drug interactions

- Dexamethasone: asparaginase increases dexamethasone concentrations by decreasing proteins involved in dexamethasone metabolism, monitor for toxicity
- Methotrexate: asparaginase decreases methotrexate activity, give asparaginase 9–10 days prior to or shortly after methotrexate infusion
- Vincristine: increased risk of hepatotoxicity, give vincristine 12 hours prior to asparaginase administration

General prescribing information

Allergic reactions occur in 47%–75% of patients and may induce anaphylaxis. Anaphylactic reactions are shown to be more common in patients who receive asparaginase intravenously, large doses (>6000 international units/m^2), received previous cycles, and have had intervals longer than a few days between doses. Fifty to sixty percent of patients report more minor hypersensitivity reactions such as fever, chills, and/or nausea. To prevent infusion-related reaction, premedication should be given and may include acetaminophen, antihistamines, and corticosteroids. Manufacturers recommend administering a test dose of 2 units (0.1 mL) solution, but false negatives are extremely common at rates up to 80%. Owing to this fact, use of test dosing varies among institutions. All patients should be closely monitored while receiving the injection or infusion and for at least one hour after. Medications necessary for the treatment of asparaginase-induced anaphylaxis including epinephrine, diphenhydramine, and hydrocortisone should be at the bedside. The patient should already have IV access. Patients who do have a hypersensitivity reaction may utilize the *Erwinia* formulation or perform densensitization. The *Erwinia* formulation has recently been approved by the FDA and is now available in the United States. Of note, 33% of patients who react to the *E. coli* formulation will also react to the *Erwinia* formulation. Pegaspargase, the pegylated formulation, has a lower incidence of anaphylactic reactions compared to the native formulation, but should be used with extreme caution if patients have had a previous anaphylactic reaction with Elspar®. Pegaspargase is also derived from *E. coli* and has a long half-life of 5–7 days.

Bleomycin

Indication

Treatment of HL

Preparation

- Injection 15 units and 30 units powder vials

Dosing

- Varied based upon regimen, example as follows:
- 10 units/m^2 once daily on days 1 and 15 every 28 days (ABVD), administer over 10 minutes

Contraindications and adverse effects

- Dose-limiting toxicity: pulmonary
- Dermatologic: erythema, rash, peeling of skin mostly of plantar and palmar surfaces of hands and feet, hyperpigmentation, alopecia
- GI: minimal emetic risk, mucositis

- Idiosyncratic reaction (rare): hypotension, confusion, fever, chills, and wheezing
- Respiratory: shortness of breath, interstitial pneumonitis, pulmonary fibrosis

Drug interactions

- Filgrastim and sargramostim: may increase pulmonary toxicity, monitor
- Gemcitabine: may increase pulmonary toxicity, consider alternative therapy

General prescribing information

Idiosyncratic reactions, although rare, may be fatal to patients. Therefore, the manufacturer recommends a test dose of 1–2 units prior to the first 1–2 doses of bleomycin. Vital signs should be monitored for 15 minutes and the rest of the dose should be administered at least 1 hour after the test dose. The literature has suggested that the test dose is not predictive of the reaction and false negatives may occur.

Pulmonary toxicity is the most concerning adverse effect of bleomycin. Interstitial pneumonitis and pulmonary fibrosis occur in 5%–10% of patients. Increased risk of pulmonary toxicity is more common in patients whose age is >70 years and who received a cumulative dose >400 units. Other associations include smoking, prior radiation, and use of concurrent oxygen. The recommended frequency of pulmonary lung function testing varies in the literature; please refer to institutional practices. Bleomycin should not be given if the carbon monoxide diffusing capacity is <60% of predicted value or drops by >30%–35% from baseline. Adjustment for anemia must be taken into account; the Cotes formula is listed as follows. Glucocorticoids have been used in the treatment of pneumonitis and fibrosis related to bleomycin but large controlled trials are lacking. Consider using glucocorticoids, such as prednisone 1 mg/kg daily, if patients are symptomatic or there is impairment in lung function tests.

Bleomycin needs to be dose reduced if the CrCl is ≤50 mL/min. Refer to the following table.

CrCl (mL/min)	Recommendation
40–50	Give 70% of dose
30–39	Give 60% of dose
20–29	Give 55% of dose
10–19	Give 45% of dose
5–9	Give 40% of dose

Cotes formula:

- Males: [(Hb in g/dL + 10.22)/ (Hb × 1.7)] × measured DLCO
- Females and children <15 years old: [(Hb in g/dL + 9.38)/ (Hb × 1.7)] × measured DLCO

Antivirals

Indications

- Acyclovir, famciclovir, and valacyclovir are used for treatment of HSV infections:
  - Oral or cutaneous
  - Genital
  - Generalized herpes simplex in immune-suppressed patients

- Herpes meningoencephalitis (IV acyclovir)
- Herpetic corneal ulceration (topical acyclovir)
- Herpes zoster
- Ganciclovir and valganciclovir are used for prophylaxis and treatment of CMV
- Foscarnet and cidofovir and used in resistant HSV and CMV infections
- Oseltamivir and zanamivir are used in the prophylaxis and treatment of viral influenza

Acyclovir
Preparations
- Capsule 200 mg
- Cream: 5% (2 g and 5 g tubes)
- Injection: 500 mg and 1000 mg powder vials and 50 mg/mL solution (10 mL and 20 mL vials)
- Ointment: 5% (15 g and 30 g tubes)
- Suspension: 200 mg/5 mL
- Tablet: 400 mg, 800 mg

Dosing
- HSV prophylaxis with transplant: 200 mg orally TID or 250 mg/m^2 IV every 8 hours infused over 1 hour
- HSV treatment: 200 mg orally five times daily for 5–7 days or 5 mg/kg IV every 8 hours infused over 1 hour
    - Encephalitis: 10 mg/kg IV every 8 hours for 10 days infused over 1 hour
    - Mucocutaneous: 5 mg/kg IV every 8 hours for 7 days infused over 1 hour
- Herpes zoster prophylaxis with transplant: 800 mg orally twice daily
- Herpes zoster treatment: 10 mg/kg IV every 8 hours (immunocompromised) infused over 1 hour
    - Immunocompetent: 800 mg orally five times daily for 7–10 days

Cidofovir
Preparations
- Injection 75 mg/mL solution (5 mL vial)

Dosing
- 5 mg/kg weekly for 2 doses, then 5 mg/kg every other week for a total treatment of 4 weeks (induction and maintenance) or until CMV PCR is negative
- Must give with probenicid and prehydration prior to transfusion

Famciclovir
Preparations
- Tablets, 125 mg, 250 mg, and 500 mg

Dosing
- HSV treatment: 250 mg three times daily for 7–10 days
- Herpes zoster treatment: 500 mg every 8 hours for 7 days

Foscarnet

Preparation

- Injection, 24 mg/mL solution (250 mL and 500 mL vials)

Dosing

- CMV prophylaxis for transplant: 60 mg/kg every 8–12 hours for 7 days, then 90–120 mg/kg daily until day +100
- CMV preemptive treatment: 60 mg/kg every 12 hours for 14 days, if CMV still detected continue with 90 mg/kg daily for 5 days/week for 14 more days
- CMV treatment: 90 mg/kg every 12 hours for 2 weeks, then 120 mg/kg daily for ≥2 weeks
- HSV, acyclovir resistant: 40 mg/kg every 8–12 hours for 14–21 days

Ganciclovir

Preparation

- Injection, 500 mg powder vial

Dosing

- CMV prophylaxis with transplant: 5 mg/kg every 12 hours for 5–7 days, then 5 mg/kg once daily 5 days/week from engraftment until day 100
- CMV preemptive treatment (<100 days post-SCT): 5 mg/kg every 12 hours × 7–14 days, then 5 mg/kg once daily 5 days/week for a total treatment course of 4 weeks (induction and maintenance)
  - Start maintenance once CMV PCR is declining but still detectable, can discontinue ganciclovir if CMV PCR is negative
- CMV preemptive treatment (>100 days post-SCT): 5 mg/kg twice daily for 7–14 days, then 5 mg/kg once daily × 7–14 days or until CMV PCR is negative
- CMV treatment: 5 mg/kg every 12 hours for 21 days, followed by 5 mg/kg daily maintenance
  - Pneumonia: IVIG 500 mg/kg QOD × 21 days along with ganciclovir

Oseltamivir

Preparations

- Capsule: 30 mg, 45 mg, and 75 mg
- Suspension: 6 mg/mL

Dosing

- Prophylaxis: 75 mg once daily × 10 days
- Treatment: 75 mg twice daily × 5 days

Valacyclovir

Preparations

- Tablets, 500 mg and 1 g

Dosing

- HSV/VZV prophylaxis: 500 mg 2–3 times daily
- HSV/VZV treatment: 1 g three times daily × 7 days

Valganciclovir

Preparations

- Powder for oral solution: 50 mg/mL
- Tablet: 450 mg

Dosing

- CMV prophylaxis with transplant: 900 mg orally daily within 10 days of transplant until day +100 (studied in solid organ transplants)
- CMV preemptive treatment (>100 days posttransplant): 900 mg orally twice daily for 21 days, then maintenance of 900 mg once daily

Zanamivir

Preparation

- Inhalation, 5 mg

Dosing

- Prophylaxis: 10 mg (2 inhalations) once daily for 10 days
- Treatment: 10 mg (2 inhalations) twice daily for 5 days

Contraindications and adverse effects

- Acyclovir: malaise, nausea, vomiting, phlebitis, and acute renal failure
- Cidofovir: fever, chills, GI upset, anemia, neutropenia, renal dysfunction, metabolic acidosis, Fanconi's syndrome, and an increased risk of infection
  - Sulfa-allergy: contraindicated to cidofovir due to necessary coadministration of probenicid
  - Teratogenic: recommend for women to use contraception during treatment and for one month following treatment, men should use barrier contraception for 3 months following treatment
- Famciclovir and valacyclovir: headache, diarrhea, nausea, abnormal LFTs, and neutropenia
- Foscarnet: electrolyte disturbances (hypocalcemia, hypomagnesemia, hypokalemia, and related seizures), renal dysfunction, nausea, vomiting, diarrhea, thrombophlebitis, and anemia
- Ganciclovir and valganciclovir: reversible BM suppression (thrombocytopenia > leukopenia > anemia), fever, diarrhea, renal dysfunction, nausea, and vomiting
  - Valganciclovir does have an increased incidence of hypertension but a decreased incidence of BM suppression compared to ganciclovir
  - Both agents are teratogenic, contraception should be used in both males (barrier contraception until 90 days after treatment is complete) and females (until 30 days after treatment is complete)

- Oseltamivir: nausea, vomiting, abdominal pain, and rare neuropsychiatric events
- Zanamivir: headache, cough, throat pain, nasal discomfort, viral infections, and rare neuropsychiatric events and anaphylaxis

Drug interactions

- Foscarnet: avoid other QTc prolonging agents, including but not limited to dronedarone, nilotinib, thioridazine, and ziprasidone
    - Ciprofloxacin may be used, but QTc monitoring is encouraged
- Imipenem: avoid giving with ganciclovir and valganciclovir due to increased risk of seizures
- Mycophenolate: may increase levels of acyclovir, valacyclovir, ganciclovir, and valganciclovir, as well as mycophenolate serum concentrations; monitor for toxicity
- Nephrotoxic medications: should be avoided if possible with nephrotoxic antiviral agents (cidofovir, foscarnet, ganciclovir)
- Tenofovir: may increase levels of acyclovir, valacyclovir, ganciclovir, and valganciclovir, as well as tenofovir serum concentrations; monitor for toxicity

General prescribing information

High-dose acyclovir or valacylovir along with CMV reactivation screening have been utilized for the prophylaxis of CMV following SCT. These medications are not the agents of choice for this indication according to the American Society for Blood and Marrow Transplantation Guidelines, but there is literature supporting their use.

Cidofovir must be dosed with probenecid, to decrease the clearance of cidofovir and therefore allow for weekly or twice weekly dosing. The dose of probenecid recommended is 2 grams orally 3 hours prior to the cidofovir infusion, 1 gram at 2 hours, and 1 gram at 8 hours after completion of the 1 hour infusion. Along with probenecid, all patients should receive IV hydration with 1 liter of normal saline over 1–2 hours prior to receiving cidofovir. A second liter may be administered either prior to or after the cidofovir infusion if the patient can tolerate the additional fluid.

Owing to the rates of myelosuppression, ganciclovir should be avoided in patients with an ANC <500 cells/mcL. Of note, there are reports of neutropenia and thrombocytopenia improving where the cause of myelosuppression was due to the virus itself. Ganciclovir has a high pH when reconstituted; therefore, generally use caution in its handling. It should be regarded as a cytotoxic agent and should be handled and disposed of as such. Valganciclovir, the prodrug of ganciclovir, is an oral medication and has not been as extensively studied as ganciclovir in the SCT population. However, there are small studies suggesting valganciclovir has higher areas under the curve compared to ganciclovir and equal efficacy in patients receiving preemptive therapy for CMV status post-allo-SCT (O'Brien et al., 2008).

Both neuraminidase inhibitors (oseltamivir and zanamivir) and adamantanes (amantadine and rimantadine) are FDA approved in the prophylaxis and treatment (except amantadine) of viral influenza. Because of resistance patterns of amantadines, neuramidase inhibitors are the drugs of choice for both prophylaxis and treatment of viral influenza in the United States. Zanamivir is a dry powder delivered through inhalation (Diskhaler®) therefore patient education is paramount to the efficacy of this product. Zanamivir should be avoided in patients with asthma or chronic obstructive pulmonary disease (COPD) due to reports of respiratory distress. If zanamivir is necessary, a rescue inhaler should be available for use. In the event of influenza infection, treatment should begin within 48 hours of the onset of signs and symptoms. If treatment is initiated >48 hours after symptom onset, no benefit is achieved.

All antiviral medications are renally eliminated and therefore must be renally dosed, except for zanamivir. Cidofovir is contraindicated in patients with a SCr >1.5 mg/dL, CrCl <55 mL/min or urine protein ≥100 mg/dL. Dehydration and other nephrotoxic medications should be avoided to reduce the risk of acute renal failure. Foscarnet causes electrolyte disturbances, and aggressive electrolyte repletion through the intravenous route should be performed prior to and while receiving this medication. Patients should be monitored closely for signs and symptoms of hypocalcemia, hypokalemia, and hypomagnesemia.

Immunosuppressants
Antithymocyte globulin (horse)
Indications
ATG is used as part of some pretransplant immune suppression regimens to prevent graft rejection, and most commonly in mismatched unrelated or haploidentical transplants. ATG is used for treatment of acute GVHD unresponsive to corticosteroids. ATG is also used in the treatment of aplastic anemia.

Preparation
- Injection 50 mg/mL solution (5 mL)

Dosing
- Varied based upon regimen
- Severe aplastic anemia or as part of conditioning regimen: 40 mg/kg IV once daily for four days
- Treatment of acute GVHD: 15 mg/kg IV on alternate days for 7–14 days

Contraindications and adverse effects
- Contraindicated with horse protein allergy
- Arthralgias
- Dermatologic: pruritus, rash
- GI: gastritis, GI bleed
- Infusion-related reactions: fevers, chills, hypersensitivity, serum sickness (rare)
- Myelosuppression: leukopenia, thrombocytopenia

Drug interactions
No relevant drug interactions

General prescribing information
ATG is immunoglobulin G (IgG) prepared from the plasma of healthy animals hyperimmunized with human thymic lymphocytes. It principally inhibits cell-mediated immune responses by elimination of T-cells in PB.

All patients should be premedicated with acetaminophen, diphenhydramine, and a corticosteroid to prevent infusion-related reactions. Acetaminophen should be given 2 hours before the infusion starts, diphenhydramine 30 minutes prior, and IV corticosteroids 15 minutes prior to the start of the infusion. Skin testing is recommended prior to the first dose and the IV dose should not be given if tachycardia, hypotension, dyspnea, or anaphylaxis occurs. ATG must be administered through a central line due to this substance causing chemical phlebitis. ATG should be infused over a minimum of 4 hours. Medications needed for anaphylactic reactions, such as epinephrine, should be kept at the patient's bedside while receiving ATG. Antimicrobial prophylaxis is recommended.

Antithymocyte globulin (rabbit)

Indication

Same as horse ATG

Preparation

- Injection 25 mg powder vial

Dosing

- Varies depending upon regimen
- Severe aplastic anemia: 3.5 mg/kg IV once daily for 5 days with cyclosporin
- GVHD: 1–1.5 mg/kg IV every other day for 7–14 days

Contraindications and adverse effects and drug interactions

- Contraindicated with rabbit protein allergy
- See horse ATG information

General prescribing information

The same precautions with horse ATG should be taken with rabbit ATG. The first dose of rabbit ATG should be given over at least 6 hours and if no reactions occur, the subsequent infusions may be given over 4 hours. Of note, there are different products of rabbit ATG with different dosing (Thymoglobulin® in United States, Fresenius® in Europe).

Corticosteroids

Indications

Corticosteroids are utilized for adrenal replacement, part of chemotherapy regimens, prophylaxis of acute and delayed chemotherapy-induced nausea and vomiting, and in the treatment of acute or chronic GVHD.

Cortisone acetate

Preparation

- Tablets, 5 mg and 25 mg.

Dosing

- 25 to 35 mg oral daily; two-thirds of the dose should be taken in the morning before 9 AM, and one-third in the afternoon

Dexamethasone

Preparations

- Injection 4 mg/mL solution (1 mL, 5 mL, and 30 mL vials) and 10 mg/mL solution (1 mL and 10 mL vials)
- Ophthalmic

- Solution, oral: 0.5 mg/5 mL and 1 mg/mL
- Tablets: 0.5 mg, 0.75 mg, 1 mg, 1.5 mg, 2 mg, 4 mg, and 6 mg

Dosing

- Antiemetic prophylaxis acute: 10–20 mg 15–30 minutes prior to chemotherapy
- Antiemetic prophylaxis delayed: 4–10 mg once or twice daily for 2–4 days following chemotherapy
- Addisonian crisis: 4–10 mg IV once, may repeat if needed
- Adrenal replacement: 0.03–0.15 mg/kg/day

Fludrocortisone

Preparation

- Tablet, 0.1 mg

Dosing

- 0.05–0.2 mg/day

Hydrocortisone

Preparations

- Injection: 100 mg, 250 mg, 500 mg, and 1000 mg powder vials
- Tablets: 5 mg, 10 mg, and 20 mg

Dosing

- Adrenal insufficiency: 20–30 mg/day divided into two doses
- Stress dosing: moderate 50–75 mg/day, major 100–150 mg/day
- Acute adrenal insufficiency: 100 mg IV every 8 hours

Prednisone

Preparations

- Solution, oral: 1 mg/mL and 5 mg/mL
- Tablets: 1 mg, 2.5 mg, 5 mg, 10 mg, 20 mg, and 50 mg

Dosing

- Treatment of acute GVHD: 2 mg/kg/day with taper, may use 1 mg/kg if Grade I–II GVHD (see page 314)
- Treatment of chronic GVHD: 1 mg/kg every other day ± cyclosporin

Contraindication and adverse effects

- Contraindications: systemic fungal infections
- Cardiac: hypertension, peripheral edema
- CNS: delirium, euphoria, emotional instability
- Dermatologic: acne, dry scaly skin
- Endocrine: hyperglycemia, increased appetite, adrenal suppression
- GI: nausea, ulcers

- Long-term use: fat maldistribution, osteoporosis, cataracts
- Increased risk of infections: fungal, PCP

Drug interactions

Most steroids are extensively metabolized by the CYP450 system and therefore have numerous drug interactions.

- Azoles: increase corticosteroid levels, monitor
- Aprepitant or fosaprepitant: increase corticosteroid levels, reduce dose of dexamethasone for antiemesis to 12 mg, do not reduce corticosteroid doses used for cancer treatment
- Calcium channel blockers (diltiazem and verapamil): increase corticosteroid levels, monitor
- Cyclosporin: may increase corticosteroid levels and steroids may increase cyclosporin levels, monitor
- Estrogens: may increase corticosteroid levels, monitor
- Loop and thiazide diuretics: worsen hypokalemia, monitor
- Quinolones: increase risk of tendon-related adverse effects, monitor
- Rifamycins: decrease corticosteroid levels, monitor
- Ritonavir: increase corticosteroid levels, consider dose reduction and monitor for adverse effects

General prescribing information

Corticosteroids are utilized for multiple indications in the hematologic malignancy and SCT population. The most difficult issue is the numerous adverse effects which are listed earlier. Of note, patients with adrenal insufficiency should notify all healthcare providers. If the patient is undergoing any invasive procedures or has any illnesses where cortisol would be released, their steroid dose will have to be increased.

Even though corticosteroids are considered the gold standard in the treatment of acute and chronic GVHD, response rates are reported at 40%–50% in the literature (Mielcarek et al., 2009). Other treatments are utilized either due to unresponsiveness or intolerability to steroids.

Cyclosporin

Indications

Prevention and treatment of GVHD following SCT, ophthalmic cyclosporin drops can be used to treatment ocular chronic GVHD

Preparations

- Capsules: 25 mg, 100 mg
- Injection: 50 mg/mL solution (5 mL vial)
- Ophthalmic drops
- Solution, oral: 100 mg/mL

Dosing

- Varied based upon reference or protocol
- Acute GVHD prophylaxis: 3 mg/kg/day IV starting day -2 until day +180 (may convert to oral once patient is clinically stable)
- Chronic GVHD: 6 mg/kg orally twice daily alternating every other day with prednisone
- Conversion of IV cyclosporin to PO cyclosporin is 1:3

Contraindications and adverse effects
- Contraindication to IV formulation: allergy to castor oil
- Electrolyte abnormalities: hypomagnesemia, hyperkalemia, hyperglycemia
- Gingival hyperplasia
- Hirsutism
- Hemolytic uremic syndrome, thrombotic thrombocytopenia purpura, thrombotic microangiopathy
- Hepatotoxicity
- Hypertension
- Infections
- Malignancies: lymphomas, skin cancers
- Nephrotoxicity
- Tremors

Drug interactions
Cyclosporin is extensively metabolized by the liver and is a moderate inhibitor of the CYP 450 3A4 enzyme.
- ACE inhibitors: increase risk of nephrotoxicity, consider alternative therapy
- Aminoglycosides: increase risk of nephrotoxicity, monitor
- Amiodarone: increases cyclosporin serum concentration, consider alternative therapy
- Amphotericin B: increases risk of nephrotoxicity, monitor
- Azole antifungals: increase serum levels of cyclosporin, consider alternative therapy
- Calcium channel blockers (diltiazem and verapamil): increase cyclosporin concentrations, consider alternative therapy
- Calcium channel blockers (amlodipine and nifedipine): cyclosporin may increase serum concentrations, monitor
- Caspofungin: increases risk of hepatotoxicity, consider alternative therapy
- Dasatinib and imatinib: may increase serum concentrations of cyclosporin, monitor
- Dexamethasone: may decrease or increase serum concentrations of cyclosporin, monitor
- Efavirenz: decreases serum levels of cyclosporin, increase cyclosporin level monitoring within first two weeks of adding or removing efavirenz
- Grapefruit juice: may increase concentration of cyclosporin, avoid use
- Imipenem: may worsen neurotoxicity and alter cyclosporin levels, monitor
- Methotrexate: may increase concentrations of both methotrexate and cyclosporin, increase risk for nephrotoxicity, monitor
- Metoclopramide: may increase cyclosporin absorption, monitor
- Metronidazole: increase serum concentrations of cyclosporin, monitor
- Mycophenolate: may decrease serum concentration of mycophenolate and active metabolite, consider alterative therapy
- Omeprazole: may increase cyclosporin levels, monitor
- Phenytoin: may decrease cyclosporin levels, consider alternative therapy
- Protease inhibitors: increase cyclosporin levels, consider alternative therapy
- Sirolimus: may worsen risk of hemolytic uremic syndrome, thrombotic thrombocytopenia purpura, or thrombotic microangiopathy, administer sirolimus 4 hours after cyclosporin

- Statins: may increase statin levels, contraindicated with simvastatin or pitavastatin, consider alternative therapy
- Sulfonamides: may worsen nephrotoxicity and decrease cyclosporin levels, monitor
- Terbinafine: may decrease cyclosporin concentrations, monitor

General prescribing information

Cyclosporin, a calcineurin inhibitor, inhibits cell-mediated immune responses such as allograft rejection and GVHD. It inhibits the proliferation and function of lymphocytes, mainly helper T (inducer)-cells and cytotoxic T-cells. Cyclosporin inhibits the release of IL-2 from activated T-cells. IL-2 causes T-cells to differentiate and proliferate, and therefore inhibition of IL-2 release inhibits the proliferation and differentiation of T-lymphocytes. Cyclosporin is not myelosuppressive. IV cyclosporin should be administered over 2–24 hours.

Cyclosporin is poorly absorbed from the GI tract (average bioavailability is 30%), and there is wide pharmacokinetic interpatient and intrapatient variability. There are different oral preparations of cyclosporin: non-modified (Sandimmune®) and modified (Gengraf® and Neoral®). Modified cyclosporin has better absorption and less interpatient variability as compared to the non-modified formulation. Patients should not change brands or formulations of cyclosporin if possible. If this does occur, close monitoring should be used in the first few weeks of switching products.

Cyclosporin troughs should be monitored for both efficacy and safety. The reference range is 100–400 ng/mL but can vary based upon protocol and/or institution. Troughs should be drawn prior to the time of the next dose, usually 12 hours after the previous dose. Close monitoring should occur with any dose changes or addition or removal of any interacting agents.

Amlodipine or nifedipine are considered the antihypertensive agents of choice for concomitant use with calcineurin inhibitors, while they are not nephrotoxic and have little effect on cyclosporin levels. Excessive exposure to sunlight and appropriate preventative measures should be undertaken to decrease the risk of developing skin cancers. Hemolytic uric syndrome, TTP, and hepatic microangiopathy may occur with cyclosporin; monitoring for these adverse effects includes checking hemoglobin, platelet counts, LDH, and serum bilirubin levels.

Mycophenolate mofetil

Indications

Prophylaxis and treatment of GVHD after allo-SCT

Preparation

- Capsule: 250 mg
- Injection: 500 mg powder vial
- Suspension, oral: 200 mg/mL
- Tablet: 500 mg

Dosing

- Prophylaxis of acute GVHD: 15 mg/kg twice daily (some regimens use 3 times a day dosing)
- Treatment of GVHD: 1–1.5 g twice daily

Contraindications and adverse effects

- Cardiac: hypertension, peripheral edema
- CNS: headaches, tremors
- Endocrine: elevated cholesterol, hyperglycemia
- GI: diarrhea, nausea, vomiting
- Infections
- Myelosuppression
- Teratogenic: use caution with handling

Drug interactions

- Acyclovir, ganciclovir, valacyclovir, valganciclovir: may increase concentration of mycophenolate and antiviral agents, monitor
- Antacids: decrease absorption of mycophenolate, avoid if possible or stagger dosing
- Bile acid sequestrants: decreased mycophenolate concentrations, consider alternative therapy
- Ciprofloxacin: decreases mycophenolic acid concentrations, monitor
- Cyclosporin: decreases mycophenolic acid levels, monitor
- Metronidazole: decreases mycophenolic acid serum concentrations, consider alternative therapy
- Oral contraceptives: decreases oral contraceptive serum concentrations, use alternative barrier method for up to 6 weeks after mycophenolate is stopped
- Proton pump inhibitors: decrease mycophenolic acid levels due to increased gastric pH, consider alternative therapy
- Rifamycins: decrease mycophenolic acid levels, consider alternative therapy

General prescribing information

Mycophenolate mofetil is used in acute GVHD prophylactic regimens, especially those for non-myeloablative and CBT. The most substantial adverse effect is myelosuppression, especially leukopenia. This can be a concern when count recovery is a sign of engraftment. Oral mycophenolate must be taken on an empty stomach. In the BMT CTN 0302 study, methylprednisolone plus either etanercept, mycophenolate mofetil, denileukin diftitox, or pentostatin was used for the treatment of newly diagnosed acute GVHD. Mycophenolate had the highest rate of complete response, 82% at day 56, with minimal toxicity.

Mycophenolate does not usually require pharmacokinetic monitoring, but may be utilized if there are potential concerns about efficacy or toxicity. Trough levels of 2–4 mcg/mL (mycophenolic acid) or AUC monitoring are recommended (recommendations vary).

Sirolimus

Indication

Prophylaxis of acute GVHD or treatment of acute or chronic GVHD

Preparations

- Solution, oral: 1 mg/mL
- Tablet: 0.5 mg, 1 mg, and 2 mg

Dosing

- Prophylaxis of acute GVHD: 12 mg PO on day -3, and then 4 mg once daily until day +180
- Treatment of chronic GVHD: 6 mg loading dose, then 2 mg once daily

Contraindications and adverse effects

- Arthralgias
- Cardiovascular: peripheral edema, hypertension
- CNS: headache, insomnia
- Electrolyte abnormalities: elevated triglycerides, elevated cholesterol
- GI: constipation, abdominal pain
- Myelosuppression: anemia, thrombocytopenia
- Nephrotoxicity

Drug interactions

- ACE inhibitors: increase risk of nephrotoxicity, consider alternative therapy
- Azole antifungals: increase serum levels of sirolimus, avoid use with posaconazole and voriconazole, reduce dose of sirolimus by 50%–90% when used with fluconazole, itraconazole, ketoconazole
- Cyclosporin: increases risk for HUS/TTP/TMA and may increase levels of cyclosporin, consider alternative therapy or monitor for toxicity of use of the combination is necessary, administer sirolimus 4 hours after cyclosporin
- Dasatinib and imatinib: may increase serum concentrations of sirolimus, monitor
- Efavirenz: increases serum levels of sirolimus, monitor closely within first 2 weeks of therapy change
- Grapefruit juice: may increase concentration of sirolimus, avoid use
- Phenytoin: may decrease sirolimus levels, consider alternative therapy
- Protease inhibitors: increase cyclosporin levels, consider alternative therapy
- Tacrolimus: may worsen risk of HUS, TTP or TMA, avoid use unless specifically recommended in protocol

General prescribing information

Sirolimus has been utilized in the prophylaxis and treatment of acute GVHD and the treatment of chronic GVHD. Sirolimus binds to the same intracellular binding protein as calcineurin inhibitors, FKBP-12, but its main mechanism of action is inhibiting the mTOR. The mTOR pathway is necessary for the progression from G_1 to the S phase in the cell cycle. Some retrospective studies have shown an OS benefit or decrease in acute GVHD incidence with sirolimus (Rosenbeck et al., 2011), but this has not been observed in all studies. Higher rates of HUS and TTP have been seen in solid organ transplant recipients who have received both sirolimus and a calcineurin inhibitor. Currently, multiple larger trials are ongoing to compare sirolimus-based regimens to standard prophylactic regimens.

The target level of sirolimus in the allogeneic transplant population is between 3–12 ng/mL. Sirolimus has a long half-life, 62 hours, which means the steady state will take around one week to occur without a loading dose. Therefore, changes in sirolimus dosing will not be seen in the levels for a few days.

Tacrolimus

Indication

Prophylaxis and treatment of acute GVHD as well as the treatment of chronic GVHD

Preparations

- Capsule: 0.5 mg, 1 mg, 5 mg
- Injection: 5 mg/mL solution (1 mL vial)

Dosing

- Dose for
- Prophylaxis of acute GVHD: 0.02–0.03 mg/kg/day as continuous infusion starting day -2 until day +180
- GVHD treatment: 0.06 mg/kg orally twice daily
- Conversion of IV tacrolimus to oral tacrolimus is 1:4

Contraindications and adverse effects

- Similar to cyclosporin, but tacrolimus can be used in patient with a castor oil allergy
- Glucose intolerance and GI adverse effects are more common with tacrolimus
- Hirsuitism and gingival hyperplasia occur only with cyclosporin as well as a higher incidence of hypertension compared to tacrolimus

Drug interactions

- Similar to cyclosporin

General prescribing information

Tacrolimus is a calcineurin inhibitor and therefore has similar adverse effects and drug interactions as cyclosporin. Goal tacrolimus levels are between 5–15 ng/mL but may vary based upon protocol or institutional preferences. Tacrolimus has a long half-life of 23–46 hours; therefore dose adjustment effects may not be seen for a few days after they are made. IV tacrolimus is administered by a 24-hour continuous infusion. Tacrolimus may be given without regards to meals. If the two daily doses of tacrolimus differ in strength, the larger dose should be given in the morning.

Targeted therapies

Alemtuzumab

Indications

Treatment of B-type CLL, also used in conditioning protocols for reduced-intensity allogeneic transplantation and prophylaxis or treatment of GVHD
Preparation: injection 30 mg/mL solution (1 mL vial)

Dosing

- Start at 3 mg, if tolerated give 10 mg on day 2 and 30 mg on day 3. Standard dose 30 mg three times weekly
- May be given IV, over 2 hours, or SC

Adverse effects

- Infusion-related reactions: fever, urticaria, rigors, hypotension, cardiac arrest, anaphylactic reaction
- Myelosuppression including fatal cytopenias
- Opportunitistic infections: CMV, HSV, PCP

Drug interactions

- None of relevance

General prescribing information

Alemtuzumab is a humanized monoclonal antibody reacting with CD52; which is found on normal and malignant B-cells, T-lymphocytes, monocytes, and macrophages. Patients should receive premedication with diphenhydramine and acetaminophen 30 minutes prior to the infusion. Corticosteroids, such as hydrocortisone 200 mg, should be utilized for the treatment of severe reactions. Premedication should be given with both the SC and IV routes of administration, with SC administration having higher rates of infusion reactions. Owing to risk of opportunistic infections, all patients should receive prophylaxis for PCP and HSV starting when treatment begins until two months after last dose or until CD4 count is >200 cells/microL, whichever happens last. CMV monitoring should be conducted during therapy and for two months after the last treatment is given. If CMV infection or viremia occurs, hold treatment and give ganciclovir or valganciclovir. Once CMV is treated, alemtuzumab may be restarted.

Bortezomib

Indications

Multiple myeloma and NHL

Preparation

- Injection 3.5 mg powder vial

Dosing

- 1.3 mg/m^2 by IV injection once daily on days 1, 4, 8, and 11 of a 21-day cycle
- May vary based upon regimen

Contraindications and adverse effects

- Cardiac: hypotension, edema
- Hepatotoxicity (rare)
- Infections, especially VZV or HSV reactivation
- Myelosuppression, especially thrombocytopenia and neutropenia
- Neuropathy

Drug interactions

- Ascorbic acid: may diminish effectiveness of bortezomib, avoid vitamin C containing supplements but probably unnecessary to avoid vitamin C containing food and beverages

- Clopidogrel: bortezomib decreases active metabolite of clopidogrel, avoid concomitant use
- Fluconazole: increases bortezomib levels, consider alternative therapy
- Gemfibrozil: increases bortezomib levels, consider alternative therapy
- Green tea: may decrease effectiveness, avoid concomitant use

General prescribing information

Bortezomib is a proteasome inhibitor, which inhibits chymotrypsin-like activity leading to cell-cycle arrest and cell death. Peripheral neuropathy is one of the most concerning adverse effects to patients. Studies have shown a decreased incidence in weekly dosing or subcutaneous administration (Moreau et al., 2011). Bortezomib dose should be reduced if patients have a serum bilirubin >1.5–3 times ULN. The recommended dose in this patient population is 0.7 mg/m^2 with the first cycle, then adjust as tolerated.

Brentuximab

Indications

Treatment of HL relapsed after auto-SCT or two prior regimens and the treatment of relapsed anaplastic LCL

Preparation

- Injection 50 mg powder vial

Dosing

- 1.8 mg/kg every 3 weeks for up to 16 cycles, disease progression, or intolerable toxicity
- Maximum dose: 180 mg
- Infuse over 30 minutes

Contraindications and adverse effects

- Anaphylaxis (rare)
- Edema
- CNS: fatigue, fever, headache
- Dermatologic: rash, pruritus, alopecia
- GI: nausea, vomiting, diarrhea
- Myelosuppression: neutropenia, anemia, thrombocytopenia
- Peripheral neuropathy, arthralgias, myalgias

Drug interactions

- None of relevance

General prescribing information

Brentuximab was approved in 2011 for the treatment of relapsed/refractory HL and ALCL. Premedication for infusion reactions with acetaminophen, an antihistamine, with or without a corticosteroid is only necessary if the patient has had a previous reaction. Brentuximab is metabolized and excreted both renally and hepatically, but it has not been studied in patients with either renal or hepatic impairment.

Rituximab

Indications

CD20-positive lymphomas or treatment of acute and chronic GVHD

Preparation: injection 10 mg/mL solution (10 mL and 50 mL vials)

Dosing: varied based upon regimen

- 375 mg/m^2 or 500 mg/m^2 are the typical doses with most regimens
- Infusion rate: start at 50 mg/hour, increase by 50 mg/hour every 30 minutes if no reaction, maximum rate of 400 mg/hour
  - Subsequent infusion: start at 100 mg/hour and increase by 100 mg/hour every 30 minutes if no reaction, maximum of 400 mg/hour
  - Reaction: slow or stop infusion; once signs and symptoms disappear, restart at 50% of previous infusion rate

Adverse effects

- Cardiac: edema
- Infusion-related reactions: fever, chills, rigors, bronchospasm
- GI: minimal emetic potential, diarrhea
- Myelosuppression: lymphopenia is most common
- Reactivation of viral infections: hepatitis B, hepatitis C, HSV, CMV, etc.

Drug interactions

- Antihypertensives: may enhance hypotension effects, monitor

General prescribing information

Rituximab infusion-related reactions occur in approximately 75% of patients. This occurs usually during the first or second dose within 30–120 minutes after commencement of the infusion. All patients should receive premedication with acetaminophen and diphenhydramine 30 minutes prior to the infusion. Corticosteroids can be used to treat infusion-related reactions and can be added as prophylaxis with subsequent infusions along with a histamine-2 inhibitor. Meperidine can be used as needed to treat rituximab-induced rigors.

Patients who are at high risk for hepatitis B should be screened prior to treatment and monitored up to 1 month following the last dose. Risk for viral infection reactivation may occur any time during treatment up to 1 year after treatment completion.

Tyrosine kinase inhibitors

(TKIs, dasatinib, imatinib, nilotinib and bosutinib)

Indications

Treatment of CML and Philadelphia-positive (Ph+) ALL

Dasatinib

Preparation

- Tablets, 20 mg, 50 mg, 70 mg, and 100 mg

Dosing

- Chronic phase CML: 100 mg once daily, may increase up to 140 mg daily
- Accelerated or blast phase CML or Ph+ ALL: 140 mg once daily, may increase up to 180 mg daily

Imatinib

Preparation

- Tablets, 100 mg and 400 mg

Dosing

- Chronic phase CML: 400 mg once daily, may increase up to 600 mg daily with a meal or large glass of water
- Accelerated or blast crisis CML or Ph+ ALL: 600 mg once daily, may increase up to 800 mg daily

Nilotinib

Preparations

- Capsules, 150 mg and 200 mg

Dosing

- Chronic phase, newly-diagnosed CML: 300 mg twice daily on an empty stomach 1 hour before or 2 hours after food
- Chronic phase resistant or intolerant to other TKIs or accelerated phase CML: 400 mg twice daily

Bosutinib

Preparations

- Tablets, 100 mg and 500 mg

Dosing

- 500 mg orally once daily with food
- Approved for CHL, all phases, failure of first-line treatment

Contraindications and adverse effects

- Arthralgia and myalgia
- Edema (imatinib), pericardial effusions (dasatinib)
- Fever
- GI: nausea, vomiting, and diarrhea
- Hepatotoxicity: elevated LFTs and bilirubin
- Hyperglycemia (nilotinib)
- Myelosuppression: dose-limiting toxicity mostly leukopenia and thrombocytopenia
- Pulmonary hypertension (rare and reported with dasatinib)
- Rash

Drug interactions

All TKIs are metabolized by the CYP450 enzyme system and imatinib and nilotinib are strong inhibitors of 3A4

- Imatinib doses should be increased by 50% when used with the following agents: carbamazepine, dexamethasone, phenobarbital, phenytoin, and rifampin
- Acetaminophen: may worsen hepatotoxicity, consider alternative therapy
- Antacids: may decrease dasatinib absorption, separate by 2 hours
- Azoles: may increase TKI concentrations, monitor
- Cyclosporin: imatinib and nilotinib may increase concentration of cyclosporin, monitor
- Fentanyl: imatinib and nilotinib may increase concentration of fentanyl, consider patient monitoring and dose reduction if necessary
- Fludarabine: imatinib may decrease the active metabolite of fludarabine, discontinue imatinib 5 days prior to starting fludarabine
- Grapefruit juice: increases TKI concentrations, avoid use
- H-2 antagonists: decrease absorption of dasatinib, consider alternative therapy
- Nafcillin: may decrease serum concentration of imatinib and nilotinib, consider alternative therapy
- Protease inhibitors: may increase protease inhibitor and/or imatinib and nilotinib serum concentrations, consider alternative therapy
- Proton pump inhibitors: decrease serum concentrations of dasatinib, consider alternative therapy
- Statins (atorvastatin, lovastatin, simvastatin): imatinib and nilotinib increase concentration of statins, avoid combination
- QTc prolonging agents: should be avoided with nilotinib use and monitored with dasatinib use

General prescribing information

These tyrosine kinases exert their effects by inhibiting the BCR-ABL tyrosine kinase, which is an essential pathway for cell growth and division. Imatinib only binds to the inactive BCR-ABL tyrosine kinase while dasatinib and nilotinib can bind to other conformation and imatinib-resistant mutations. One mutation, known as T315I, is resistant to all currently available TKIs. New medications are in development and clinical trials, including ponatinib, to overcome this resistant mutation. Clinical trials have shown that both nilotinib and dasatinib have higher rates of molecular responses compared to imatinib in patients with chronic phase CML, but currently have had no effect on OS. Therefore, TKI choice should be tailored to each patient.

There is little literature about the outcomes of patients who have received TKIs pretransplant for CML. However, it is known that patients who are transplanted in chronic phase have better outcomes compared to those with more progressive disease.

The addition of TKIs to patients with Ph+ ALL has significantly improved OS compared to previously treated patients who only received chemotherapy (Thomas et al., 2004). It is still controversial whether TKIs should be continued after allogeneic transplant in both Ph+ ALL and CML patients.

Miscellaneous

Defibrotide

Indication

Prevention or treatment of SOS occurring after allo-SCT

Preparation

- Injection

Dosing

- 5–60 mg/kg/day IV once daily for 14 days
- 25 mg/kg dose has been chosen for an ongoing phase III trial

Contraindications and adverse effects

- Cardiac: hypotension
- GI: nausea, vomiting, stomach upset
- Injection site reactions

Drug interaction

- Anticoagulants: increase risk of bleeding

General prescribing information

Not generally available in the United States, but can be obtained on a compassionate need basis. Defibrotide is a polynucleotide derived from porcine intestinal mucosa that stimulates antithrombic and fibrinolytic properties without causing limited systemic anticoagulation. Thirty to sixty percent response rates are reported in phase II trials (Richardson et al., 2009); phase III studies are pending.

Etanercept

Indications

Treatment of acute or chronic GVHD after allo-SCT along with steroids

Preparations

- Injection 25 mg powder vial or 50 mg/mL solution (0.51 mL and 0.98 mL vials)

Dosing

- 25 mg SC twice weekly

Contraindications and adverse effects

- Contraindicated in patients with sepsis or active infection
- Headache
- Infection including tuberculosis
- Hepatitis B reactivation
- Injection reactions: bleeding, bruising, erythema, pain
- Lymphomas

- Pancytopenia
- Rash

Drug interaction

- Cyclophosphamide: may increase risk of solid tumor development, avoid concomitant use

General prescribing information

Blocks or neutralizes TNF-α and has been reported to have response rates of 28% in patients with steroid-refractory acute GVHD. Etanercept has also been utilized in the treatment of idiopathic pneumonia syndrome. There are numerous relative contraindications including patients with hematologic abnormalities and rare incidences of lymphoma. There are case reports of patients who acquired pancytopenia and aplastic anemia after taking etanercept.

Infliximab

Indication

Steroid-resistant, acute GVHD, especially of the GI tract

Preparation

- Injection 100 mg powder vial

Dosing

- 10 mg/kg weekly for four doses infused over 2 hours for 4–8 doses

Contraindications and adverse effects

- Doses >5 mg/kg are contraindicated in patients with moderate or severe heart failure
- Contraindicated in patients with sepsis or active infection
- Headache
- Increase in LFTs, especially ALT: discontinue if jaundice occurs or LFTs ≥5 times ULN
- Infections: tuberculosis, fungal, bacterial, viral, or other opportunistic infections
- Infusion-related reaction
- Nausea

Drug interactions

- Avoid other immunosuppressive agents

General prescribing information

Infliximab is a recombinant monoclonal antibody which blocks TNF-α. Responses are best with skin (60% response rates) and GI (75% response rates) GVHD (Patriarca et al., 2004). In general, this medication is well tolerated. Infusion reactions occur in 20% of patients and usually happen within the first 2 hours of the infusion. Pretreatment for infusion-related reactions should be utilized in patients who have reacted to infliximab previously. Pre-medications may include acetaminophen, histamine-1 inhibitor, histamine-2 inhibitor, and/or corticosteroids. If a reaction does occur, hold until symptoms subside. If possible, the infusion may be restarted at a slower rate. Infectious disease prophylaxis may also be considered for patients at risk for invasive fungal infections.

Intravenous immunoglobulin (IVIG)

Indication

Adjunct treatment for CMV pneumonia with ganciclovir and may boost humoral immunity after transplant in patients with hypogammaglobulinemia (controversial, see *General prescribing information* section)

Preparation

- Injection (multiple products available)

Dosing

- Vary based upon reference
- Give 100–500 mg/kg commencing on the day of transplant weekly for 90 days, then monthly until day +365.
- CMV pneumonitis: 500 mg/kg IV every other day × 21 days

Contraindications and adverse effects

- Anaphylaxis
- Cardiac: chest tightness, hypotension
- CNS: headache, fever, chills
- Dermatologic: facial flushing, pallor, pruritus
- Dyspnea
- GI: nausea, vomiting, abdominal pain

General prescribing information

IVIG was intended to boost humoral immunity after allogeneic and autologous transplantation. However, a placebo-controlled study (Cordonnier et al., 2003) showed no advantage for IVIG as far as infection, GVHD, hepatic SOS, and interstitial pneumonia and OS at 6 months are concerned. Therefore, the administration of IV immunoglobulin during allogeneic transplantation should be restricted to patients with proven hypogammaglobulinemia.

IVIG can be infused undiluted. The infusion rate for the initial dose is 30 mL/hour for 15 minutes, increasing to 60 mL/hour for 15 minutes, then 90 mL/hour for 15 minutes. Infuse the remaining part of the initial dose over 2–4 hours. Infuse each subsequent dose over 2–4 hours.

Lenalidomide and thalidomide

Indications

Treatment of multiple myeloma, MDS (lenalidomide), CLL (lenalidomide), or chronic GVHD (thalidomide)

Lenalidomide

Preparation

- Capsules, 5 mg, 10 mg, 15 mg, and 25 mg

Dosing

- Varied based upon regimen
- Multiple myeloma (with dexamethasone): 25 mg once daily for 21 days with a 28-day cycle
- MDS with deletion 5q: 10 mg once daily

Thalidomide

Preparation

- Capsules, 50 mg 100 mg 150 mg and 200 mg

Dosing

- Multiple myeloma: 100–400 mg once daily
- Chronic GVHD: doses varied based upon reference

Contraindications and adverse effects

- Contraindications: pregnancy or women not taking adequate precautions to prevent pregnancy
- Cardiovascular: edema, thromboembolism
- CNS: somnolence, peripheral neuropathy (worse with thalidomide)
- GI: constipation (worse with thalidomide)
- Myelosuppression: neutropenia and thrombocytopenia most common (worse with lenalidomide)

Drug interactions

- Dexamethasone: increases risk of thromboembolism, monitor and use prophylaxis appropriately

General prescribing information

The exact mechanism of thalidomide and lenalidomide are unknown, but both have immunomodulatory and antiangiogenic properties. Both are regularly used in numerous multiple myeloma regimens, with lenalidomide becoming favored due to a more beneficial adverse effect profile. Patients who receive thalidomide or lenalidomide with steroids have rates of thromboembolism >20%. Patients should receive thrombotic prophylaxis but there is no agreement about which agent (aspirin, low-dose warfarin, or a low molecular weight heparin) or duration of therapy.

Approximately 67% of lenalidomide is excreted unchanged in the urine. Therefore, it must be dose adjusted for renal impairment.

CrCl (mL/min)	Recommendation for multiple myeloma	Recommendation for MDS
30–59	10 mg once daily	5 mg once daily
< 30	15 mg every other day	5 mg every other day
Dialysis	5 mg every day, administer after dialysis	5 mg after dialysis days three days/week

Both lenalidomide and thalidomide have a REMS (Risk Evaluation and Mitigation Strategies) program that the patient and prescriber must be enrolled in because of teratogenicity. RevAssist® is the lenalidomide program and S.T.E.P.S.® is the thalidomide program. For more information, see the websites www.revlimid.com or www.thalomid.com.

Leucovorin, levoleucovorin, or folinic acid

Indication
Prevention or treatment of hematologic toxicities from methotrexate

Preparations
- Injection: 10 mg/mL solution (50 mL vial) and 50 mg, 100 mg, 200 mg, 350 mg powder vials
- Tablets: 5 mg, 10 mg, 15 mg, and 25 mg

Dosing
- Doses for rescue from methotrexate vary from 10–50 mg/m^2 every 6 hours, starting at $\approx$12–24 hours after methotrexate administration. Please refer to methotrexate drug information for more specifics.
- Levoleucovorin should be dosed at half the normal dose of leucovorin

Contraindications and adverse effects
- Contraindicated in patients with vitamin B$_{12}$ deficient megaloblastic anemia
- Allergic reactions (rare)
- Dermatologic: rash, pruritus
- Wheezing

Drug interactions
- Phenytoin: leucovorin may decrease concentration of phenytoin, monitor
- Trimethoprim: leucovorin may decrease trimethoprim efficacy, monitor

General prescribing information
Absorption of oral leucovorin is variable between patients and decreases significantly at doses above 25 mg. Due to the calcium component of leucovorin, this medication should not be infused at a rate faster than 160 mg/minute. Leucovorin must be administered within 40 hours after the start of methotrexate or hematologic toxicities may be irreversible.

2-mercaptoethane sulfonate sodium (MESNA)

Indication
Prevention of hemorrhagic cystitis caused by ifosfamide or high-dose cyclophosphamide

Preparations
- Injection: 100 mg/mL solution (10 mL vial)
- Tablet: 400 mg

Dosing

- Varied based upon regimen
- Short infusion, ifosfamide dose <2.5 g/m^2/day: 20% of ifosfamide dose given at 0, 4, and 8 hours after the start of ifosfamide infusion
- Continuous infusion, ifosfamide dose <2.5 g/m^2/day: 20% of ifosfamide dose given as bolus, 40% of ifosfamide dose as continuous infusion until 12–24 hours after completion of ifosfamide infusion

Contraindications and adverse effects

- CNS: headache, fatigue
- GI: nausea, diarrhea
- Hypotension

Drug interactions

- No relevant drug interactions

General prescribing information

MESNA binds to the metabolite of ifosfamide or cyclophosphamide, acrolein inactivates it and clears it safely from the body. MESNA should not be used in low or normal dose cyclophosphamide, instead aggressive hydration is recommended (Krass et al., 1997). Even with MESNA, studies have shown microscopic bladder edema and lacerations. The dose of oral MESNA should be double the dose of IV MESNA and should only be utilized after the first dose of IV MESNA is given.

Palifermin

Indication

Used in patients receiving conditioning chemotherapy with HSCT to decrease the length and severity of oral mucositis

Preparation

- Injection 6.25 mg powder

Dosing

- 60 mcg/kg/day IV given for 3 days prior to conditioning therapy, and 3 additional doses started on the same day as SCT to equal a total of 6 doses
  - Third dose must be given 24–48 hours before conditioning begins
  - Fourth dose must be given at least 4 days after third dose of palifermin

Contraindications and adverse effects

- Contraindication: allergy to *E. coli*-derived products
- Cardiovascular: edema, hypertension
- Cough
- Fever
- GI: mouth/tongue discoloration and thickening, taste changes, elevate amylase and lipase

- Proteinurea
- Rash, pruritus, erythema

Drug interaction

- Chemotherapy: see *General prescribing information* section
- Unfractioned and low molecular weight heparin: increases exposure to palifermin, avoid coadministration and rinse intravenous line with normal saline prior to and after palifermin administration

General prescribing information

Palifermin is recombinant keratinocyte growth factor that causes growth, proliferation, and differentiation of epithelial cells in the GI tract. It has been shown in clinical trials to decrease the length and severity of mucositis in patients receiving myeloablative chemotherapy with SCT, but does not have any effect on DFS or OS (Nasilowska-Adamska et al., 2007). Spacing of palifermin from chemotherapy, such as mentioned in the prior *Dosing* section, is essential. If palifermin is dosed within 24 hours of chemotherapy, there is a concern for worsening of mucositis due to chemotherapy's effect on rapidly dividing epithelial cells. Of note, there are in vitro studies showing that palifermin causes growth of epithelial-related tumor cells. Therefore, palifermin should not be used outside of non-hematologic malignancies, although there are studies using palifermin in patients with head and neck cancer (Henke et al., 2011; Le et al., 2011).

Rasburicase

Indication

Prevention of high uric acid levels in patients receiving chemotherapy for treatment of a malignancy in those who are at risk for tumor lysis syndrome

Preparation

- Injection 1.5 mg and 7.5 mg powder vials

Dosing

- Varied based upon reference
- Package insert: 0.1–0.2 mg/kg IV daily × 5 days
- Flat dosing: 0.15 mg/kg, 3 mg, 4.5 mg, 6 mg, or 7.5 mg are some doses that have been studied in small trials

Contraindications and adverse effects

- Contraindication: G6PD deficiency
- CNS: fever, headache
- Edema
- GI: nausea, vomiting, abdominal pain
- Hypersensitivity reaction (rare)

Drug interactions

- No relevant drug interactions

General prescribing information

Rasburicase is a recombinant enzyme which converts uric acid to allantoin. It decreases uric acid levels within 4 hours of initial administration. Owing to cost of the medication, use and dosing of rasburicase varies among institutions. Development of antibodies to rasburicase may develop and this risk increases with repeated exposure.

When measuring serum uric acid levels, samples must be in prechilled heparin tubes, be placed in ice immediately, and processed within 4 hours. If the tube is kept at room temperature, rasburicase will still be active in the vial but cause falsely low uric acid levels.

Ursodiol (ursodeoxycholic acid)

Indication

Prophylaxis for hepatic SOS

Preparations

- Capsule: 300 mg
- Tablets: 250 mg, 500 mg

Dosing

- 300 mg orally twice daily

Contraindications and adverse effects

- Back pain
- CNS: headache, dizziness
- GI: diarrhea, nausea, vomiting
- Upper respiratory tract infections

Drug interactions

- Aluminum hydroxide: decreases concentration of ursodiol, give ursodiol 2 hours before or 6 hours after aluminum product
- Bile acid sequestrants: decrease ursodiol concentrations, administer ursodiol at least 5 hours after bile acid sequestrant
- Estrogen: may decrease efficacy of ursodiol, monitor

General prescribing information

Ursodiol has been shown in clinical trials to reduce the incidence of hepatic SOS and TRM associated with SOS (Tay et al., 2007). There is no OS benefit.

References and further reading

Arns da Cunha C, Weisdorf D, Shu XO, et al. 1998. Early gram-positive bacteremia in BMT recipients: impact of three different approaches to antimicrobial prophylaxis. *Bone Marrow Transplant* **21**: 173–180.

Aronoff GR, Bennett WM, Berns JS, et al. 2007. *Drug Prescribing in Renal Failure: Dosing Guidelines for Adults and Children*, 5th edn. Philadelphia, PA: American College of Physicians.

Basch E, Prestrud AA, Hesketh PJ, et al. 2011. Antiemetics: American Society of Clinical Oncology Clinical Practice guidelines update. *J Clin Oncol* **29**: 4189–4198.

Benson AB, Ajani JA, Catalano RB, et al. 2004. Recommended guidelines for the treatment of cancer treatment-induced diarrhea. *J Clin Oncol* **22**: 2918–2926.

Bruns I, Steidl U, Kronenwett R, et al. 2006. A single dose of 6 or 12 mg of pegfilgrastim for peripheral blood progenitor cell mobilization results in similar yields of CD34+ progenitor in patients with multiple myeloma. *Transfusions* **46**: 180–185.

Brunton LL, Chabner BA, & Knollman BC. 2011. *Goodman and Gilman's The Pharmacological Basis of Therapeutics, 12th edn.* New York, NY: McGraw-Hill.

Buonomo A, Nucera E, & De Pasquale T. 2011. Tolerability of aztreonam in patients with cell-mediated allergy to beta-lactams. *Int Arch Allergy Immunol* **155**: 155–159.

Chin TW, Loeb M, & Fong IW. 1995. Effect of an acidic beverage (coca-cola) on absorption of ketoconazole. *Antimicrob Agents Chemother* **39**: 1671–1675.

Cordonnier C, Chevret S, Legrand M, et al. 2003. Should immunoglobulin therapy be used in allogeneic stem cell transplantation? A randomized double-blind, dose effect, placebo-controlled, multicenter trial. *Ann Int Med* **139**: 8–18.

Cornely OA, Maertens J, Winston DJ, et al. 2007. Posaconazole vs. fluconazole or itraconazole prophylaxis in patients with neutropenia. *N Engl J Med* **356**: 348–359.

Couriel D, Saliba R, Hicks K, et al. 2004. Tumor necrosis factor-α blockade for the treatment of acute GVHD. *Blood* **104**: 649–654.

David KA & Picus J. 2005. Evaluating risk factors for the development of ifosfamide encephalopathy. *Am J Clin Oncol* **28**: 277–280.

Dix SP, Wingard JR, Mullins RE, et al. 1996. Association of busulfan area under the curve with veno-occlusive disease following BMT. *Bone Marrow Transpl* **17**: 225–230.

Eberly AL, Anderson GD, Bubalo JS, et al. 2008. Optimal prevention of seizures induced by high-dose busulfan. *Pharmacotherapy* **28**: 1502–1510.

Einsele H, Reusser P, Bornhauser M, et al. 2006. Oral valganciclovir leads to higher exposure to ganciclovir than intravenous ganciclovir in patients following allogeneic stem cell transplantation. *Blood* **107**: 3002–3008.

Epstein JB, Truelove EL, Hanson-Huggins K, et al. 2004. Topical poleyene antifungals in hematopoietic cell transplant patients: tolerability and efficacy. *Support Care Cancer* **12**: 517–525.

Floyd J, Mirza I, Sachs B, et al. 2006. Hepatoxicity of chemotherapy. *Semin Oncol* **33**: 50–67.

Henke M, Alfonsi M, Foa P, et al. 2011. Palifermin decreases severe oral mucositis of patients undergoing postoperative radiochemotherapy for head and neck cancer: a randomized, placebo-controlled trial. *J Clin Oncol* **29**: 2815-2820.

Kantarjian HM, Hochhaus A, Saglio G, et al. 2011. Nilotinib versus imatinib for the treatment of patients with newly diagnosed chronic phase, Philadelphia chromosome-positive, chronic myeloid leukaemia: 24-month minimum follow-up of the phase 3 randomised ENESTnd trial. *Lancet Oncol* **12**: 841–851.

Kantarjian H, Shah NP, Hochhaus A, et al. 2010. Dasatinib versus imatinib in newly diagnosed chronic-phase chronic myeloid leukemia. *N Engl J Med* **362**: 2260–2270.

Katzung BG. 2007. *Basic and Clinical Pharmacology, 10th edn.* New York, NY: McGraw Hill Lange.

Keefe DL. 2001. Anthracycline-induced cardiomyopathy. *Semin Oncol* **28**: S2–S7.

Keefe DM, Schubert MM, Elting LS, et al. 2007. Updated clinical practice guidelines for the prevention and treatment of mucositis *Cancer* **109**: 820–831.

Kintzel PE & Dorr RT. 1995. Anticancer drug renal toxicity and elimination: dosing guidelines for altered renal function. *Cancer Treat Rev* **21**: 33–64.

Krass I, Bajorek B, Bagia M, et al. 1997. An evaluation of three methods used in the prophylaxis of cyclophosphamide-induced haemorrhagic cystitis in bone marrow transplant patients. *J Oncol Pharm Pract* **3**: 193–199.

Lacy CF, Armstrong LL, Goldman MP, et al. 2011. *Drug Information Handbook, 20th edn.* Hudson, OH: Lexi-Comp.

Le QT, Kim HE, Schneider CJ, *et al.* 2011. Palifermin reduces severe mucositis in definitive chemoradiotherapy of locally advanced head and neck cancer: a randomized, placebo-controlled study. *J Clin Oncol* **29**: 2808–2814.

Lexicomp Up-to-date Website: http://www. uptodate.com/contents/search. [Accessed November and December 2011].

Liu C, Bayer A, Cosgrove SE, et al. 2011. Clinical practice guidelines by the Infectious Diseases Society of America for the treatment of methicillin-resistant *Staphylococcus aureus* infections in adults and children: executive summary. *Clin Infect Dis* **52**: 285–292.

MacIntyre N, Crapo RO, Viegi G, et al. 2005. Standardisation of the single-breath determination of carbon monoxide uptake in the lung. *Eur Respir J* **26**: 720–735.

Marty FM, Lowry CM, Cutler CS, et al. 2006. Voriconazole and sirolimus coadministration after allogeneic hematopoietic stem cell transplantation. *Biol Blood Marrow Transplant* **12**: 552–557.

Micromedex Healthcare Series Website. http:// www.thomsonhc.com/micromedex2/ librarian. Accessed November and December 2011.

Mielcarek M, Storer BE, Boeck H, et al. 2009. Initial therapy of acute graft-versus-host disease with lose-dose prednisone does not compromise patient outcomes. *Blood* **113**: 2888–2894.

Moreau P, Pylypenko H, Grosicki S, et al. 2011. Subcutaneous versus intravenous administration of bortezomib in patients with relapsed multiple myeloma: a randomized, phase 3, non-inferiority study. *Lancet Oncol* **12**: 431–441.

Nasilowska-Adamska B, Rzepecki P, & Manko J. 2007. The influence of palifermin (kepivance) on oral mucositis and acute graft versus host disease in patients with hematological diseases undergoing hematopoetic stem cell transplant. *Bone Marrow Transplant* **40**: 983–988.

O'Brien S, Ravandi F, Riehl T, et al. 2008. Valganciclovir prevents cytomegalovirus reactivation in patients receiving alemtuzumab-based therapy. *Blood* **111**: 1816–1819.

Pappas PG, Kauffman CA, Andes D, et al. 2009. Clinical practice guidelines for the management of candidiasis: 2009 update by the Infectious Disease Society of America. *Clin Infect Dis* **48**: 503–535.

Patriarca F, Sperotto A, Damiani D, et al. 2004. Infliximab treatment for steroid-refractory acute graft-versus-host disease. *Haematologica* **89**: 1352-1359.

Paul M, Yahav D, Bivas A, et al. 2010. Anti-pseudomonal beta-lactams for the initial, empirical treatment of febrile neutropenia: comparison of beta lactams. *Cochrane Database Syst Rev* **10**: CD005197.

Pfaller MA, Diekema FJ, Messer SA, et al. 2004. Activities of fluconazole and voriconazole against 1,586 recent clinical isolates of *Candida* species determined by broth microdilution, disk diffusion and Etest methods: report from the ARTEMIS Global Antifungal Susceptibility Program, 2001. *J Clin Microbiol* **41**: 1440–1146.

Richardson P, Linden E, Revta C, et al. 2009. Use of defibrotide in the treatment and prevention of neo-occlusive disease. *Expert Rev Hematol* **2**: 365–376.

Richardson PG, Soiffer RJ, Antin JH, et al. 2010. Defibrotide for the treatment of severe hepatic veno-occlusive disease and multiorgan failure after stem cell transplantation: a multicenter, randomized, dose-finding trial. *Biol Blood Marrow Transplant* **16**: 1005–1017.

Rosenbeck LL, Kiel PJ, Kalsekar I, et al. 2011 Prophylaxis with sirolimus and tacrolimus ± antithymocyte globulin reduces the risk of acute graft-versus-host disease without an overall survival benefit following allogeneic stem cell transplantation. *Biol Blood Marrow Transplant* **17**: 916–922.

Rybak M, Lomaestro B, Rotschafer JC, et al. 2009. Therapeutic monitoring of vancomycin in adult patients: a consensus review of the American Society of Health-system Pharmacists, the Infectious Diseases Society of America, and the Society of Infectious Diseases Pharmacists. *Am J Health System Pharm* **66**: 82–98.

Scheinberg P, Nunez O, Weinstein B, et al. 2011. Horse versus rabbit antithymocyte globulin in acquired aplastic anemia. *N Engl J Med* **365**: 430–438.

Slattery JT, Sanders JE, Buckner CD, et al. 1995. Graft-rejection and toxicity following bone marrow transplantation in relation to busulfan pharmacokinetics. *Bone Marrow Transpl* **16**: 31–42.

Sokos DR, Berger M, Lazarus HM. 2002. Intravenous immunoglobulin: appropriate indications and uses in hematopoietic stem cell transplantation. *Biol Blood Marrow Transplant* **8**: 117–130.

Tay J, Tinmouth A, Fergusson D, et al. 2007. Systematic review of controlled clinical trials on the use of ursodeoxycholic acid for the prevention of hepatic veno-occlusive disease in hematopoietic stem cell transplantation. *Biol Blood Marrow Transplant* **13**: 206–217.

Thomas DA, Faderl S, Cortes J, et al. 2004. Treatment of Philadelphia chromosome-positive acute lymphocytic leukemia with hyper-CVAD and imatinib mesylate. *Blood* **130**: 4396–4407.

Tomblyn M, Chiller T, Einsele H, et al. 2009. Guidelines for preventing infectious complications among hematopoietic cell transplantation recipients: a global perspective. *Biol Blood Marrow Transplant* **15**: 1143–1238.

Trifilio SM, Bennett CL, Yarnold PR, et al. 2007. Breakthrough zygomycosis after voriconazole administration among patients with hematologic malignancies who received hematopoietic stem-cell transplants or intensive chemotherapy. *Bone Marrow Transplant* **39**: 425–429.

Ullmann AJ, Lipton JH, Vesole DH, et al. 2007. Posaconazole or fluconazole for prophylaxis in severe graft-versus-host disease. *N Engl J Med* **356**: 335–347.

Urban AW & Craig WA. 1997. *Daily Dosage of Aminoglycosides. Current Clinical Topics in Infectious Diseases*, Vol **17**. Malden, MA: Blackwell Science.

US Food and Drug Administration Website: http://www.fda.gov/Drugs/DrugSafety/PostmarketDrugSafetyInformationfor PatientsandProviders/ucm198675.htm. 2009. [Accessed November 2011].

US Food and Drug Administration Website: http://www.fda.gov/Safety/MedWatch/Safety-Information/SafetyAlertsforHumanMedical Products/ucm272041.htm. 2011. [Accessed November 2011].

Xhaard A, Rocha V, Bueno B, et al. 2011. Steroid-refractory acute GVHD: lack of long-term improved survival using new generation anticytokine treatment. *Biol Blood Marrow Transplant* **18**: 406–413.

Chapter

28

HLA-testing and laboratory medicine

Nicholas R. DiPaola, Reinhold Munker, and Kerry Atkinson

Histocompatibility typing

HLA-matching or compatibility is the major condition for standard allogeneic transplant-ation. HLA-testing is generally done on PB leukocytes or lymphocytes. By definition, HLA-matching implies identity at class I and II loci. Recently, most transplant centers switched from serological testing to molecular testing, which offers a higher degree of definition for unrelated transplants.

There are four possible scenarios for allogeneic transplantation.

Donor–recipient combination	Serologic match	Molecular match	Comment
Identical twin	Yes	Yes	Low-risk transplant, no GVHD, no graft-versus-malignancy reactions
Sibling match	Yes	Yes	Standard-risk transplant
Unrelated match	Yes	Yes or no	Higher-risk transplant, especially if one or several mismatches are found by molecular typing
Haploidentical transplant	No (only 5/10 antigens match)	No	High-risk transplant, special protocols have to be used

The BMT Data Book, Third Edition, ed. Reinhold Munker et al. Published by Cambridge University Press. © Cambridge University Press 2013.

Overview of HLA typing

Typing involves identifying given polymorphic proteins (known as human leukocyte antigens) expressed on most or all nucleated cells and are intimately involved in the functioning of the immune system. The proteins are separated into two classes based on their structure and function in the immune system; however, their function is beyond the scope of this review (see also Chapter 1).

Class I molecules consist of a single 45-kDa polypeptide and are encoded by three loci (A, B, C) found on chromosome six in a region known as the MHC. Class II molecules are composed of a dimer of an alpha chain and beta chain, also encoded in the MHC region. The alpha and beta chains are encoded separately, and historically it is the beta chain that is polymorphic and can therefore be viewed by the immune system as "non-self" (although newer research suggests that this may not be the case entirely). The beta chains are encoded on six separate genes, three main genes, DPβ1, DQβ1, DRβ1; and three accessory genes, DRβ3, DRβ4, DRβ5, which will be expressed only with specific DRβ1 genes. Expression of the HLA genes is codominant, thus one has two alleles expressed at each locus. A given typing would have two A alleles, two B alleles, two C alleles for class I and two DPβ1 alleles, two DQβ1 alleles, two DRβ1 alleles, and possibly two DRβ3, 4, and 5 alleles.

Typing is broken down into two levels of resolution, serological and molecular. Serological typing is based on the protein structure of the molecule as it is exposed on the cell surface. Allelic type is determined by exposing lymphocytes from a given individual to a panel of antisera having antibodies against the various HLA alleles. By determining which specific antisera react, a typing is deduced. Originally there was a limited set of serologies, but as more individuals were tested and the antisera became more specific, subgroups of serological types were discovered. The table on page 510 lists the current serological groups and where appropriate, the subgroups or "serological split groups."

As gene sequencing became widely utilized, the serological typing was replaced by molecular typing. In molecular typing, the gene sequence of the given HLA molecule is examined, including introns and silent mutations. This is high-resolution typing and the nomenclature has changed to accommodate it. In molecular typing, the serological desig-nation, A1, is replaced by a letter, signifying the locus, and a four-digit number with the first two digits signifying the parent serological group and the second two digits signifying the order in which the allele was discovered. For example, A*0101 would be A1 serological group and the first allele discovered. If only the serological level of typing is needed then the molecular typing is listed as A*01xx, implying that this is a molecular typing but only at a serological level. In some cases, the letter "N" will follow the molecular typing (example A*0104N). This letter designates that the allele has a coding mutation that prevents it from ever being expressed. Thus, an individual with a typing of A*0201; A*0104N serologically would only type serologically as A2 as there is no A1 molecule on the surface of the cell to react with antisera for A1. The tables between pages 510 and 517 list the serological and corresponding molecular typing for the common or well-documented HLA alleles as suggested by the American Society of Histocompatibility and Immunogenetics (2007). Many of the molecular typing results do not associate directly with a given serology; for example, B60 alligusto molecular B*4001. This is due to the fact that the B40 serological group was discovered to have subgroups associated with them. Using the DNA sequences, these subgroups still aligned best with one another compared to other groups and the parent designation of B40 remained in the molecular typing of the B*40xx alleles.

Finally, concerning class II genes, the DRβ1 genes often have associated with them specific DRβ3, β4, or β5 genes. These beta chains also associate with alpha chains on class II expressing cells and thus one can have multiple DR serologies. The β3, β4, and β5 genes are associated with serologies DR52, DR53, and DR51, respectively, and are in strong linkage disequilibrium with the β1 genes. The associations are listed in column three of the table on page 517. Thus, if using the table, an individual having a DR17 should also express a DR52. An individual with DR15 or DR16 should express DR51. A few DR serologies DR1, DR8, and DR10 have no DR51/52/53 associated with it.

Three methods are commonly used for molecular typing:

1. PCR using sequence-specific oligonucleotides (PCR-SSO)
2. PCR using sequence-specific primers (PCR-SSP)
3. PCR sequencing

The mHCa play a major role in the successful outcome of allogeneic transplantation (Rezvani et al., 2008). The mHCa are inherited separately from the major class I and class II antigens. In fully identical sibling allografts, mHCa differences are the basis for the clinical GVHD and the GVT effects of allotransplantation. Currently close to 30 mHCs are described. They are not tested routinely. Research is ongoing to exploit reactivity to mHCa to augment GVT effects without worsening GVHD.

Suggestions for typing for BMT/SCT

Current work suggests that typing for BMT/SCT should include high-resolution typing at A, B, Cw, DRβ1, and DRβ3, 4, and 5, as appropriate. The DPβ1 typing is beginning to be appreciated but its utility varies among institutions. Some centers suggest that low-resolution typing is sufficient for related siblings, but some cases were found where the low-resolution typing (i.e., A*01xx; B*07xx, etc.) matches; yet allelic differences exist, especially when the parents share more common alleles (A1, A2, B7, etc.).

HLA-Class I and Class II serology (broad and split categories)

Broad	Split	Broad	Split	Broad	Split	Broad	Split
A1		B15	B62	B70	B70	DR3	DR3
A2			B63		B71		DR17
A3			B75		B72		DR18
A9	A23		B76	B73		DR4	
	A24		B77	B78		DR5	DR11
A10	A10	B16	B38	B80			DR12
	A25		B39	Cw2		DR6	DR6
	A26	B17	B57	Cw3	Cw3		DR13
	A34		B58		Cw9		DR14
	A66	B18			Cw10	DR7	
A11		B21	B49	Cw4		DR8	

(cont.)

Broad	Split	Broad	Split	Broad	Split	Broad	Split
A19	A29		B50	Cw5		DR9	
	A30	B62	B54	Cw6	Cw6	DR10	
	A31	B63	B55		Cw18	DR51	
	A32	B75	B56	Cw7	Cw7	DR52	
	A33	B27			Cw17	DR53	
	A74	B35		Cw8			
A28	A68	B37		Cw12			
	A69	B40	B60	Cw14			
A35			B61	Cw15			
A43		B41		Cw16			
A80		B42		DQ1	DQ5		
B5	B51	B46			DQ6		
	B52	B47		DQ2			
B7		B48		DQ3	DQ7		
B8		B53			DQ8		
B12	B44	B54			DQ9		
	B45	B55		DQ4			
B13		B56		DR1			
B14	B64	B59		DR2	DR15		
	B65	B67			DR16		

HLA-A serology with corresponding common alleles

Serology	Allele	Serology	Allele	Serology	Allele	Serology	Allele
A1	A*0101	A2	A*0264	A25	A*2501	A34	A*3401
	A*0102	A3	A*0301		A*2502		A*3402
	A*0103		A*0302	A26	A*2601		A*3405
	A*0104N		A*0305		A*2602	A35	A*3601
A2	A*0201	A10	A*2615		A*2603		A*3603
	A*0202	A11	A*1101		A*2605	A43	A*4301
	A*0203		A*1102		A*2607	A66	A*6601
	A*0204		A*1103		A*2608		A*6602
	A*0205		A*1104		A*2609		A*6603
	A*0206		A*1105		A*2612	A68	A*6801
	A*0207	A23	A*2301	A29	A*2901		A*6802
	A*0208		A*2302		A*2902		A*6803
	A*0209	A24	A*2402		A*2903		A*6804
	A*0210		A*2402L	A30	A*3001		A*6805
	A*0211		A*2403		A*3002		A*6806
	A*0212		A*2405		A*3003		A*6807

(cont.)

Serology	Allele	Serology	Allele	Serology	Allele	Serology	Allele
	A*0213		A*2406		A*3004		A*6811N
	A*0214		A*2407		A*3007		A*6812
	A*0216		A*2408		A*3009		A*6815
	A*0217		A*2409N		A*3010		A*6817
	A*0219	A31	A*2410		A*3101		A*6820
	A*0220		A*2413	A69	A*3102		A*6901
	A*0222		A*2414	A74	A*3104		A*7401
	A*0224		A*2417		A*3106		A*7402
	A*0225		A*2420		A*3106		A*7403
	A*0227	A32	A*2421	A80	A*3201		A*8001
	A*0230		A*2422		A*3202		
	A*0235		A*2423		A*3204		
	A*0238		A*2425		A*3206		
	A*0245	A33	A*2428		A*3301		
	A*0253N		A*2433		A*3303		
	A*0260		A*2435		A*3305		

HLA-B serology with corresponding common alleles

Serology	Allele	Serology	Allele	Serology	Allele	Serology	Allele
B5	B*5123	B27	B*2706	B35	B*3543	B44	B*4406
B7	B*0702		B*2707		B*3531		B*4407
	B*0703		B*2709	B37	B*3701		B*4408
	B*0704		B*2714		B*3702		B*4410
	B*0705		B*2708	B38	B*3801		B*4420
	B*0706	B35	B*3501		B*3802		B*4427
	B*0707		B*3502	B39	B*3903		B*4429
	B*0709		B*3503		B*3904		B*4409
	B*0710		B*3504		B*3905	B45	B*4501
	B*0712		B*3505		B*3906		B*5002
	B*0714		B*3506		B*3908	B46	B*4601
	B*0720		B*3508		B*3909	B47	B*4701
B8	B*0801		B*3509		B*3910		B*4702
	B*0802		B*3510		B*3911		B*4703
	B*0809		B*3511		B*3912	B48	B*4801
	B*0812		B*3512		B*3913		B*4803
	B*0804		B*3513		B*3914		B*4804
B12	B*4415		B*3514		B*3915		B*4805
B13	B*1301		B*3516		B*3924		B*4807
	B*1302		B*3517		B*3901		B*4802
B14	B*1403		B*3518		B*3902	B49	B*4901
	B*1405		B*3519	B40	B*4005		B*1303
B16	B*3920		B*3520	B41	B*4101		B*1304

(cont.)

Serology	Allele	Serology	Allele	Serology	Allele	Serology	Allele
B18	B*1801		B*3521		B*4102	B50	B*5001
	B*1802		B*3522		B*4103	B51	B*5101
	B*1803		B*3523		B*4106		B*5104
	B*1804		B*3524	B42	B*4201		B*5105
B27	B*2701		B*3527		B*4202		B*5106
	B*2702		B*3528	B44	B*4402		B*5107
	B*2703		B*3530		B*4403		B*5108
	B*2704		B*3531		B*4404		B*5109
	B*2705		B*3541		B*4405		B*5113
B51	B*5114	B61	B*4004	B70	B*1509		
	B*5119		B*4006		B*1529		
	B*5121		B*4009		B*1537		
	B*5122		B*4011		B*1552		
	B*5102		B*4016		B*1523		
	B*5103		B*4020		B*1547		
B52	B*5201		B*4027	B71	B*1510		
B53	B*5301		B*4040		B*1518		
	B*5302		B*4008	B72	B*1503		
B54	B*5401	B62	B*1501		B*1546		
B55	B*5501		B*1507		B*1554		
	B*5502		B*1520	B73	B*7301		
	B*5504		B*1524	B75	B*1502		
B56	B*5601		B*1525		B*1511		
	B*5602		B*1527		B*1515		
	B*5603		B*1528		B*1531		
	B*5604		B*1530		B*1508		
B57	B*5701		B*1532	B76	B*1512		
	B*5702		B*1533		B*1514		
	B*5703		B*1534	B77	B*1513		
	B*5704		B*1535	B78	B*7801		
	B*5705		B*1538		B*7802		
B58	B*5801		B*1539	B81	B*8101		
	B*5802		B*1548		B*8102		
B59	B*5901		B*1558				
B60	B*4001		B*1540				
	B*4007	B63	B*1516				
	B*4010		B*1517				
	B*4030	B64	B*1401				
	B*4012	B65	B*1402				
B61	B*4002	B67	B*6701				
	B*4003		B*6702				

HLA-Cw serology with corresponding common alleles

Serology	Allele	Serology	Allele	Serology	Allele
Cw2	Cw*0202	Cw7	Cw*0712	Cw16	Cw*1601
	Cw*0203		Cw*0718		Cw*1602
	Cw*0205		Cw*0719		Cw*1604
	Cw*0207		Cw*0722	Cw17/Cw7	Cw*1701
	Cw*0210		Cw*0726		Cw*1703
Cw3	Cw*0305	Cw8	Cw*0801	Cw18/Cw6	Cw*1801
	Cw*0307		Cw*0802		Cw*1802
	Cw*0308		Cw*0803		
	Cw*0310		Cw*0804		
	Cw*0314		Cw*0806		
	Cw*0316	Cw9	Cw*0303		
	Cw*0319	Cw10	Cw*0302		
Cw4	Cw*0401		Cw*0304		
	Cw*0404		Cw*0306		
	Cw*0407		Cw*0309		
	Cw*0409N	Cw12	Cw*1202		
	Cw*0413		Cw*1203		
	Cw*0403		Cw*1204		
	Cw*0406		Cw*1205		
Cw5	Cw*0501		Cw*1209		
	Cw*0502		Cw*1213		
	Cw*0505	Cw14	Cw*1404		
	Cw*0509		Cw*1402		
	Cw*0510		Cw*1403		
Cw6	Cw*0602	Cw15	Cw*1502		
	Cw*0604		Cw*1503		
Cw7	Cw*0701		Cw*1504		
	Cw*0702		Cw*1505		
	Cw*0704		Cw*1506		
	Cw*0705		Cw*1507		
	Cw*0706		Cw*1509		
	Cw*0710		Cw*1511		

HLA-DPB1 common alleles

Allele	Allele
DPB1*0101	DPB1*3401
DPB1*0101	DPB1*3501
DPB1*0201	DPB1*3601
DPB1*0202	DPB1*3801
DPB1*0301	DPB1*3901
DPB1*0302	DPB1*4001
DPB1*0401	DPB1*4501
DPB1*0402	DPB1*4601
DPB1*0501	DPB1*4701
DPB1*0601	DPB1*5001
DPB1*0602	DPB1*5101
DPB1*0901	DPB1*5501
DPB1*1001	DPB1*5901
DPB1*1101	DPB1*6301
DPB1*1301	DPB1*6901
DPB1*1401	DPB1*7201
DPB1*1501	DPB1*7801
DPB1*1601	DPB1*8101
DPB1*1701	DPB1*8501
DPB1*1801	
DPB1*1901	
DPB1*2001	
DPB1*2101	
DPB1*2201	
DPB1*2301	
DPB1*2601	
DPB1*2701	
DPB1*2801	
DPB1*2901	
DPB1*3001	
DPB1*3101	
DPB1*3301	

HLA-DQB1 serology with corresponding common alleles

Serology	Allele
DQ1	DQB1*0610
	DQB1*0611
DQ2	DQB1*0201
	DQB1*0202
	DQB1*0203
DQ3	DQB1*0309
	DQB1*0319
DQ4	DQB1*0401
	DQB1*0402
DQ5	DQB1*0501
	DQB1*0502
	DQB1*0503
	DQB1*0504
DQ6	DQB1*0601
	DQB1*0602
	DQB1*0603
	DQB1*0604
	DQB1*0608
	DQB1*0609
	DQB1*0619
DQ7	DQB1*0301
	DQB1*0304
DQ8	DQB1*0302
	DQB1*0305
DQ9	DQB1*0303

HLA-DRB1 serology with corresponding common alleles

Serology	Allele	Serology	Allele	Serology	Allele	Serology	Allele
DR1	DRB1*0101	DR8	DRB1*0802	DR11	DRB1*1134	DR14	DRB1*1409
	DRB1*0102		DRB1*0803		DRB1*1139		DRB1*1410
	DRB1*0107		DRB1*0804		DRB1*1145		DRB1*1411
	DRB1*0103		DRB1*0806	DR12	DRB1*1201		DRB1*1412
DR3	DRB1*0307		DRB1*0807		DRB1*1202		DRB1*1413
	DRB1*0322		DRB1*0809	DR13	DRB1*1301		DRB1*1414
DR4	DRB1*0401		DRB1*0810		DRB1*1302		DRB1*1418
	DRB1*0402		DRB1*0811		DRB1*1303		DRB1*1420
	DRB1*0403		DRB1*0813		DRB1*1304		DRB1*1421
	DRB1*0404		DRB1*0814		DRB1*1305		DRB1*1448
	DRB1*0405		DRB1*0818		DRB1*1306		DRB1*1454
	DRB1*0406		DRB1*1415		DRB1*1307	DR15	DRB1*1501
	DRB1*0407	DR9	DRB1*0901		DRB1*1310		DRB1*1502
	DRB1*0408	DR10	DRB1*1001		DRB1*1311		DRB1*1503
	DRB1*0409	DR11	DRB1*1101		DRB1*1312		DRB1*1504
	DRB1*0410		DRB1*1102		DRB1*1313		DRB1*1505
	DRB1*0411		DRB1*1103		DRB1*1314		DRB1*1510
	DRB1*0412		DRB1*1104		DRB1*1315	DR16	DRB1*1601
	DRB1*0415		DRB1*1105		DRB1*1316		DRB1*1602
	DRB1*0416		DRB1*1106		DRB1*1318		DRB1*1604
	DRB1*0417		DRB1*1107		DRB1*1320		DRB1*1605
	DRB1*0418		DRB1*1109		DRB1*1329		DRB1*1607
	DRB1*0426		DRB1*1110		DRB1*1331	DR17	DRB1*0301
	DRB1*0438		DRB1*1111		DRB1*1336		DRB1*0304
	DRB1*0440		DRB1*1112	DR14	DRB1*1401	DR18	DRB1*0302
DR6	DRB1*1356		DRB1*1113		DRB1*1402		DRB1*0303
	DRB1*1416		DRB1*1114		DRB1*1403		
	DRB1*1417		DRB1*1115		DRB1*1404		
	DRB1*1424		DRB1*1117		DRB1*1405		
	DRB1*1425		DRB1*1118		DRB1*1406		
DR7	DRB1*0703		DRB1*1119		DRB1*1407		
DR8	DRB1*0801		DRB1*1127		DRB1*1408		

HLA-DRB3, B4, and B5 serology with corresponding common alleles

Serology	Allele	Associates with
DR51	DRB5*0101	
	DRB5*0102	DR15
	DRB5*0103	DR16
	DRB5*0108N	
	DRB5*0110N	
	DRB5*0202	
	DRB5*0203	
DR52	DRB3*0101	
	DRB3*0201	
	DRB3*0202	
	DRB3*0203	DR11
	DRB3*0206	DR12
	DRB3*0207	DR13
	DRB3 0209	DR14
	DRB3*0210	DR17
	DRB3*0211	DR18
	DRB3*0216	
	DRB3*0217	
	DRB3*0301	
	DRB*0303	
DR53	DRB4*0101	
	DRB4*0102	
	DRB3*0103	DR4
	DRB4*0103N	DR7
	DRB4*0201N	DR9
	DRB4*0301N	

Note: All tables were produced from data obtained from a variety of sources including but not limited to:
The Anthony Nolan Trust: www.anthonynolan.org.uk;
Allele Frequencies in Woldwide Population Database: www.allelefrequencies.net;
IMGT/HLA Database: www.ebi.ac.uk/imgt/hla/;
American Society of Histocompatibility and Immunogenetics: www.ashi-hla.org;
HLA Beyond Tears Introduction to Human Histocompatibility, 2nd Edition, 2000;
The HLA Dictionary 2004: a summary of HLA-A, -B, -C, -DRB1/3/4/5 and -DQB1 alleles and their association with serologically defined HLA-A, -B, -C, -DR and -DQ antigens. *Tissue Antigens* **65**: 1–55, 2005.
(Modified from Baron and Sandmaier, 2006.)

Studies for chimerism

The principle of allo-SCT is the replacement of hematopoietic cells by cells of a different individual. This generally involves HLA-matching and leads, in a successful allogeneic transplant, to full chimerism (>95% of hematopoietic cells are of donor type). In the situation of "mixed chimerism," only 5% to 95% of hematopoietic cells are of donor type. If <5% of hematopoietic cells are of donor type, the engraftment is not successful (failure of engraftment).

Tissue used for chimerism testing

Generally, PB mononuclear cells or buffy coat white cells are used, but other tissues like bone marrow or sorted cell fractions (T-cells, NK cells, B-lymphocytes, dendritic cells) can also be used. It is important that the method used for testing is determined before transplant and an adequate specimen (e.g., DNA) is stored before transplant.

Testing for chimerism is important to detect failure of engraftment after a myeloablative transplant and to monitor the degree of engraftment (partial versus full chimerism after an RIC transplant). In some situations, a reduction of chimerism can also be a sign of relapse. In a workshop (Antin et al., 2001), recommendations were given on when chimerism should be monitored.

Especially when T-cell count is depleted, non-myeloablative or reduced-intensity regimens are used for conditioning or new prophylactic treatments are used for GVHD; then chimerism should be monitored at 1, 3, 6, and 12 months after transplantation because interventions (especially DLI) depend on the chimerism status. In non-myeloablative transplantation, the early pattern of chimerism is useful to predict either GVHD or loss of engraftment. Therefore, more frequent measurements (every 2–4 weeks) may be warranted. In nonmalignant disorders, chimerism generally should by analyzed 1, 2, and 3 months after transplantation.

Categories of chimerism

Full chimerism	<<1% *	All hematopoietic cells are of donor origin (usual situation after myeloablative conditioning)
Transient mixed chimerism	1%–5%	Commonly happens after non-myeloablative conditioning, patient later acquires full chimerism
Stable mixed chimerism	1%–20%	No change over time, often observed in transplants for nonmalignant disorders
Progressive mixed chimerism	>10%	Continuous increase of recipient cells (predicts relapse or graft rejection)

* Percentage of cells of recipient origin

Methods used for determining chimerism

Method	Sensitivity	Comments
Red blood cell antigens	0.1%–1%	Limited to erythroid lineage
Cytogenetics	10%–20%	Low sensitivity and accuracy, limited to cells in metaphase and male versus female or normal versus leukemic karyotype
HLA antigens	Variable	Limited to mismatched transplants, reagents for all antigens are not available (flow cytometry)
FISH for X or Y chromosomes	0.1%–3%	Widely used, only applicable to sex-mismatched transplantation, loss of Y chromosome in some situations
RFLP	5%–20%	Moderate sensitivity and accuracy
VNTR/STR	1%–5%	Moderate sensitivity and accuracy
Fluorescence-based STR-PCR (with multiplex PCR)	1%–5%	Moderate sensitivity, high accuracy
Real-time PCR	0.001%–1%	High sensitivity, moderate quantitative accuracy

RFLP, restriction-fragment polymorphism; VNTR, variable number of tandem repeats; STR, short tandem repeats. (Modified from Baron & Sandmaier, 2006.)

Cytogenetic terminology
Terms commonly used in cytogenetics

Structural abnormality	Change to chromosomal material	Abbreviation	Example
Translocation	Transfer of material from one chromosome to another	t	t(9;22) in CML
Duplication	Repetition of a segment of a chromosome	dup	Dup(1) (q12 → q31), seen in some cases of ALL
Deletion	Loss of a segment of a chromosome	del	del(5)(q13q33), seen in myelodysplasia
Inversion	Reversal of chromosome segments between two breakpoints	inv	Inv(16)(p13q22), seen in AML M4 with bone marrow eosinophilia (M4 Eo)
Insertion	Breakage of a chromosome, followed by transfer of the same or another chromosome into that chromosome at the breakpoint	ins	ins(3;7)(q21; q21qter), insertion of segment 7 into chromosome 3

(cont.)

Structural abnormality	Change to chromosomal material	Abbreviation	Example
Isochromosome	A chromosome in which both arms are identical, resulting from transverse rather than longitudinal separation during mitosis	i	i(17q) commonly seen in accelerated phase of CML
Ring	A circular chromosome formed by breakage at two points within the chromosome, followed by rejoining of the broken ends	r	r(22)(p11q13)
Aneuploidy	Numerical deviation from the normal cell chromosome content (the latter known as diploidy; in man 46 chromosomes (i.e., 44 plus two sex chromosomes)		48,XY,+8,+21
Hyperdiploidy	Cells (in man) with more than 46 chromosomes		55,XX,+4,+6,+7,+1,+14, +18,+20,+21, reported in ALL
Hypodiploidy	Cells (in man) with less than 46 chromosomes		44,X,−Y,−21
Pseudodiploidy	Cells (in man) with 46 chromosomes, but abnormalities present		46,XY,(t4;11)(q21; q23), reported in ALL
Monosomy	Loss of a single individual chromosome	−	45,XY,−7, seen in AML
Trisomy	Gain of a single individual chromosome	+	47,XY,+8, seen in AML

Detection of MRD

Potential uses of MRD assays in BMT/SCT

1. Selection of patients in remission but at high risk for relapse after conventional therapy
2. Assessing the efficacy of marrow or stem cell purging protocols
3. Predicting relapse after BMT

Assays for the detection of MRD

Method	Marker	Sensitivity
Routine	Cellular morphology	10^{-1} to 10^{-2}
Cytogenetics	Chromosome number and structure	10^{-1} to 10^{-2}
FISH	Chromosome number and structure	10^{-2}
Gene rearrangement	DNA hybridization	10^{-2} to 10^{-3}
Flow cytometry	Antigen profile	10^{-3} to 10^{-4}
Clonogenic culture	In vitro growth	10^{-2} to 10^{-4}
PCR	DNA/ RNA structure	10^{-4} to 10^{-6}

Molecular markers amenable to detection by PCR for MRD studies

Cytogenetic abnormality	Molecular marker	Disease
None	CDRIII	B-lineage ALL, NHL
None	TCR rearrangement	T-lineage ALL, NHL
t(14;18)	BCL-2 IGH	85% FSCCL, 25% DLCL
Deletion	SIL-TAL	25% T-lineage ALL
t(9;22)	BCR-ABL fusion	95%–100% CML
t(1;19)	E2A-PBX1 fusion	25% pre-B ALL
t(15;17)	PML-RARα-fusion	100% APL
t(6;9)	DEK-CAN fusion	AML-M2, M4
t(17;19)	E2A-HLF fusion	Rare ALL
AML with normal cytogenetics	Mutation of NPM1	30% of AML

References and further reading

Antin JH, Childs R, Filipovich AH, et al. 2001. Establishment of complete and mixed donor chimerism after allogeneic lymphohematopoietic transplantation: recommendations from a workshop at the 2001 Tandem Meetings of the International Bone Marrow Transplant Registry and the American Society of Blood and Marrow Transplantation. *Biol Blood Marrow Transplant* 7: 473–485.

Bacher U, Haferlach T, Fehse B, et al. 2011. Minimal residual disease and chimerism in the post-transplant period in acute myeloid leukemia. *Scientific World Journal* 11: 310–319.

Baron F & Sandmaier BM. 2006. Chimerism and outcomes after allogeneic hematopoietic cell transplantation following nonmyeloablative conditioning. *Leukemia* 20: 1690–1700.

Cano P, Klitz W, Mack SJ, et al. 2007. Common and well-documented HLA alleles; report of the ad-hoc committee of the American Society of Histocompatibility and Immunogenetics. *Hum Immunol* 68: 392–417.

Little AM. 2007. An overview of HLA typing for hematopoietic stem cell transplantation. In Beksac M, ed. *Methods In Molecular Medicine, vol 134: Bone Marrow and Stem Cell Transplantation.* Totowa NJ: Humana Press.

Rezvani AR & Storb RF. 2008. Separation of graft-vs.-tumor effects from graft-vs.-host disease in allogeneic hematopoietic cell transplantation. *J Autoimmun* **30**: 172–179.

Appendix: Guide to the internet and literature databases relevant for BMT/SCT

Websites and organizations specialized in BMT/SCT

Center for International Blood and Marrow Transplantation Research (formerly known as International Bone Marrow Transplant Registry)

Website: www.cibmtr.org

International database on autologous and allogeneic BMT/SCT performs outcomes research and publishes a newsletter with outcomes data and posttransplant guidelines.

Partnership of National Marrow Donor Program and International Bone Marrow and Autologous Blood and Marrow Transplant Registry of Medical College of Wisconsin. Promotes studies to increase safety and success of transplant and improve access to healthcare services.

National Marrow Donor Program

Website: www.marrow.org

Information about the activities of the National Marrow Donor Program (NMDP) facilitating matched unrelated transplantation. This information is directed to potential donors, patients, and physicians. The NMDP maintains the world's largest volunteer donor database and performs accreditation of transplant centers and outcomes research.

American Society for Blood and Marrow Transplantation

Website: www.asbmt.org

Association of North American transplant physicians and scientists.

Promotes research and issues guidelines for blood and marrow transplantation.

Website has links to other transplant-related organizations.

American Society of Hematology

Website: www.hematology.org

The American Society of Hematology (ASH) is the world's largest professional society concerned with causes and treatments of blood disorders. ASH has both physicians and pure scientists as members and merges the clinical and scientific aspects of hematology. Membership is very broad and includes hematologists in the United States and virtually every country of the world. The website has a host of information both for members, nonmembers, and patients. There are educational materials, grant opportunities, news releases, and information about past and future annual meetings.

European Group for Blood and Marrow Transplantation

Website: www.ebmt.org

European association for research and clinical practice in BMT/SCT.

Issues guidelines for transplantation.

Has members in many countries and promotes clinical research in 11 working parties.

Publishes the ESH-EBMT Handbook on Haematopoietic Stem Cell Transplantation (2008 rev. edn. Apperley J, Carreras E, Gluckman E, et al., eds. Can be ordered online).

The BMT Data Book, Third Edition, ed. Reinhold Munker et al. Published by Cambridge University Press. © Cambridge University Press 2013.

Blood and Marrow Transplant Clinical Trials Network

Website: www.web.emmes.com/study/bmt2

Organizes multicenter clinical trials in the area of blood and marrow transplantation.

Currently (1/2012), 16 core clinical centers and 11 open protocols.

Also edits a technical and organizational manual of procedures.

Foundation for the Accreditation of Cellular Therapy (FACT)

Website: www.factwebsite.org

Voluntary organization for the accreditation of transplant units and transplant activities including stem cell collection and processing, thereby promoting excellence in cellular therapy.

Maintains a list of certified facilities (adult, pediatric, autologous, allogeneic, collection of marrow and peripheral stem cells, processing).

Also accredits cord blood banks.

Bone Marrow Donors Worldwide

Collects data from 66 donor registries in 48 countries and 44 cord blood banks in 29 countries.

Website: www.bmdp.org

Facilitates donor searches and stem cell donation. Currently, 19 million volunteer donors registered.

World Marrow Donors Association

The World Marrow Donor Association (WMDA) fosters international collaboration to facilitate the exchange of high quality hematopoietic stem cells for clinical transplantation worldwide and to promote the interests of donors.

Network of 69 donor registries, 140 cord blood banks, 350 donor centers, and 1259 transplant hospitals from 48 different countries.

Website:www.worldmarrow.org

The Cord Blood Forum

Website: www.cordbloodforum.org

Maintains a database about CBT.

Textbooks specifically devoted to BMT/SCT

Allogeneic Stem Cell Transplantation, 2nd edn, 900 p.

Lazarus HM & Laughlin MJ, eds.

Humana Press, 2010.

Comment: overview of basic sciences and clinical advances.

Blood and Marrow Transplant Handbook, Comprehensive Guide for Patient Care, 1st edn., 324 p.

Maziarz RT & Slater S, eds.

Springer Science, 2011.

Comment: multi-authored guide for patient care issues.

Blood and Marrow Transplantation Supportive Care Manual. 1st edn, 206 p.

Champlin R & Ippoliti C, eds.

Summit Communications, 2007.

Comment: pocket book dealing with drugs used and complications commonly seen in a transplant unit.

Bone Marrow Transplantation Across Major Genetic Barriers, 1st edn, 477 p.

Reisner Y & Martelli MF, eds.

World Scientific, 2010.

Comment: text specializing in haploidentical transplantation, complications, procedures.

Clinical Bone Marrow and Blood Stem Cell Transplantation, 3rd edn, 1968 p.

Atkinson K, Champlin R, Ritz J, et al., eds.

Cambridge University Press, 2004.

Comment: standard textbook of clinical BMT/SCT.

Haematopoietic Stem Cell Transplantation in Clinical Practice, 1st edn, 512 p.

Treleaven JG & Barrett AJ, eds.

Churchill Livingstone Elsevier, 2009.

Comment: multiauthored review of clinical studies and management.

Hematopoietic Stem Cell Transplantation, 1st edn, 589 p.

Bishop MR, ed.

Springer Science, 2009.

Comment: multiauthored textbook; gives overview of current literature and practice.

Hematopoietic Stem Cell Transplantation: A Handbook for Clinicians, 1st edn, 729 p.

Wingard JR, Gastineau DA, Leather HL, et al., eds.

American Association of Blood Banks, 2009.

Comment: spiral bound, multiauthored, broadly covers indications, cell processing, donor evaluation, and other topics.

Manual of Stem Cell and Bone Marrow Transplantation, 1st edn, 177 p.

Antin JH & Yolin Raley D, eds.

Cambridge Medicine, 2009.

Comment: practical pocket manual for all members of the BMT/SCT team.

Pediatric Stem Cell Transplantation, 1st edn, 458 p.

Mehta P, ed.

Jones and Bartlett Publishers, 2004.

Comment: textbook focused on pediatric aspects of SCT.

Practical Hematopoietic Stem Cell Transplantation, 1st edn, 216 p.

Cant AJ, Galloway A, & Jackson G, eds.

Blackwell Publishers Ltd., 2007.

Comment: concise textbook focusing on practical aspects and complications.

Stem Cell Transplantation Biology, Processing, and Therapy, 1st edn, 268 p.

Ho AD, Hoffman R, & Zanjani ED, eds.

Wiley-VCH, 2006.

Comment: manual of basic biology, cell processing, and selected clinical applications.

Thomas' Hematopoietic Cell Transplantation, 4th edn, 1600 p.

Appelbaum FR, Forman SJ, Negriv R, et al., eds.

Blackwell, 2009.

Comment: standard textbook of BMT/SCT.

Periodicals specializing in BMT/SCT or putting major emphasis on these topics

Current Impact Factor (2010)

Biology of Blood and Marrow Transplantation 3.27

Blood 10.56

Bone Marrow Transplantation 3.66

British Journal of Haematology 4.94

Blood and Marrow Transplantation Reviews NA

Available in print form and online at www.bloodline.net/bmt-reviews

Patient-oriented databases and sources of information

BMT InfoNet

2310 Skokie Road, Suite 104, Highland Park, IL 60035.

www.bmtinfonet.org

Offers help for patients and family members undergoing BMT/SCT. Publishes a newsletter, several publications including a calendar, maintains a database of transplant centers, mediates contacts between patients, and offers help for insurance issues.

National Bone Marrow Transplant Link

20411 W, 12 Mile Road, Suite 108, Southfield, MI 48076.

www.nbmtlink.org

Non-profit organization giving information for patients, caregivers, families, and healthcare professionals about BMT/SCT. Organizes patient support groups and publishes brochures and a video documentary.

National Library of Medicine

Provides basic information and links to relevant sites.

www.nlm.nih.gov/medlineplus/bone-marrowtransplantation.html

Index